T0210773

Outpatient Nutrition Care

As the number of patients receiving home care nutrition support increases, proper assessment and management of this therapy is crucial, and clinicians need to practice at an advanced level. This second edition provides practical nutrition care information for professionals working with individuals outside the hospital including registered dietitians, nurses, pharmacists, and physicians. It covers screening, assessing, and treating malnutrition; outpatient nutrition care in diabetes, cardiovascular disease, gastrointestinal disease, and home enteral and parenteral nutrition. Each chapter describes the disease process as well as the management of the disease or therapy.

Key Features

- Presents practical information on proper nutrition care of individuals in the outpatient setting and those receiving home nutrition support
- New information on GI tests and procedures; gastroparesis/pancreatitis, parenteral lipids, and bariatric surgery
- Expanded chapter on short bowel syndrome and malabsorptive disorders
- Additional information on feeding options including an overview of oral, oral supplements, and enteral and parenteral nutrition
- Teaches the user additional information on disease processes as well as the management of the disease or therapy

Outpatient Nutrition Care GI, Metabolic, and Home Nutrition Support

Practical Guidelines for Assessment and Management

Second Edition

Edited by

Carol Ireton-Jones, PhD, RD, LD, CNSC, FACN, FASPEN

Associate Editor

Berkeley Limketkai, MD, PhD

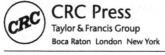

CRC Press
Taylor & Francis Group
Boca Raton London New York

CRC Press is an imprint of the
Taylor & Francis Group, an **informa** business

Second edition published 2024
by CRC Press
2385 NW Executive Center Drive, Suite 320, Boca Raton, FL 33431

and by CRC Press
4 Park Square, Milton Park, Abingdon, Oxon, OX14 4RN

CRC Press is an imprint of Taylor & Francis Group, LLC

© 2024 Taylor & Francis Group, LLC

First edition published by CRC Press 2017

Library of Congress Cataloging-in-Publication Data
Names: Ireton-Jones, Carol S., editor.
Title: Outpatient Nutrition Care : GI, Metabolic, and Home Nutrition Support / edited
    by Carol Ireton-Jones, PhD, RD, LD, CNSC, FACN, FASPEN.
Description: Second edition. | Boca Raton, FL : CRC Press, 2023. | Includes
    bibliographical references and index. | Summary: "As the number of patients
    receiving home care nutrition support increases, proper assessment and management
    of this therapy is crucial, and clinicians need to practice at an advanced level. This
    new edition provides practical nutrition care information for professionals working
    with individuals outside of the hospital including registered dietitians, nurses,
    pharmacists, and physicians. It covers screening, assessing, and treating malnutrition;
    out-patient nutrition care in diabetes, cardiovascular disease, gastrointestinal disease,
    and home enteral and parenteral nutrition. Each chapter describes the disease process
    as well as the management of the disease or therapy"— Provided by publisher.
Identifiers: LCCN 2023010591 (print) | LCCN 2023010592 (ebook) | ISBN
    9780367338800 (hbk) | ISBN 9780367338732 (pbk) | ISBN 9780429322570 (ebk)
Subjects: MESH: Nutrition Therapy—methods | Nutrition Assessment | Home Care
    Services | Ambulatory Care | Outpatients
Classification: LCC RM217 .O88 2023 (print) | LCC RM217 (ebook) |
    DDC 615.8/54—dc23/eng/20230724
LC record available at https://lccn.loc.gov/2023010591
LC ebook record available at https://lccn.loc.gov/2023010592

ISBN: 978-0-367-33880-0 (hbk)
ISBN: 978-0-367-33873-2 (pbk)
ISBN: 978-0-429-32257-0 (ebk)

DOI: 10.1201/9780429322570

Typeset in Times
by Apex CoVantage, LLC

To my colleagues across many disciplines, it is a pleasure to know and collaborate with you,

and to my patients who inspire me,

To my amazing family, Jim, my supportive husband, and all-around best guy,

To my first daughter Lauren and her husband Cody And to my daughter Krissy and her husband Marshall, You all make my work fun and fabulous!

Nutrition is vital and meaningful, from food shared with family and friends to specialized diets for people who need them. There is nothing more rewarding than being part of helping someone reach their goals for good nutrition for good living.

Carol Ireton-Jones

I am deeply indebted and grateful to my family village who supported me as I worked on the book chapters. To my parents, your unconditional love, sacrifice, and discipline molded me during critical formative years and have allowed me to pursue dreams.

To my sons Aidan and Ethan, I truly appreciate your patience during the many moments I could not play with you or attend your competitions. To my wife Dandan, I feel immensely blessed to spend my life with you. Throughout my impossible balancing act as a husband, father, son, physician, and scientific explorer, you helped pick up the pieces and regularly encouraged me to persevere. Thank you!

Berkeley Limketkai

Contents

Preface

After the publication of the first edition of *Outpatient Nutrition Care: GI, Metabolic, and Home Nutrition Support*, there was so much more nutrition to include – a second edition was a must! Besides being updated, the second edition has 14 new chapters courtesy of my Associate Editor Berkeley Limketkai, MD. Special thanks to my colleague Steve McClave, MD, as well.

Nutrition has always been important to me. As a Registered Dietitian Nutritionist (RDN), nutrition is my lifelong career. It is a vital part of life – in fact, without nutrition, there is no life. Food can be satisfying, and it can also be healing. Food can be fresh from the farm, purchased at a store, or prepared in a pharmacy to be administered intravenously.

RDNs have a thorough knowledge of food and the effects of food and nutrition on the human body. RDNs have expertise in disease management and translation of nutrition requirements to foods to consume. However, nutrition care often does not receive the attention in the outpatient setting, which is needed to achieve nutrition goals.

There are many considerations in assuring that intake provides nutrition. The purpose of *Outpatient Nutrition Care: GI, Metabolic, and Home Nutrition Support* is to provide practical guidelines and pertinent and concise information for assessment and nutrition management. This book includes a chapter on digestion and absorption, food intolerances, food allergies, weight management, and alternative methods of receiving nutrition – enteral and parenteral nutrition support. Gastrointestinal conditions such as irritable bowel syndrome, inflammatory bowel disease, celiac disease, and short bowel syndrome, affect nutrition and intake. Small intestinal bacterial overgrowth, diabetes, and oncology may challenge a person's ability to consume adequate nutrition. This second edition is comprehensive although certainly not complete given new questions and new discoveries occurring daily.

Food (nutrition) can provide vital nutrients and energy and can be comforting, life enhancing, fun, and healing. Sometimes "food" is provided in a different way – via a tube or intravenously with the same goals. While food is important and life sustaining, it is not medicine. Applying sound, evidence-based principles to nutrition care is of utmost importance.

Carol Ireton-Jones, PhD, RDN, CNSC, FAND, FASPEN
Good Nutrition for Good Living©

Editors

Editor

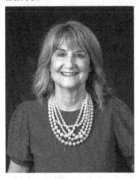

Carol Ireton-Jones, PhD, RDN, LD, CNSC, FAND, FASPEN, earned her PhD and master's degrees in nutrition from Texas Woman's University. Her undergraduate degree in nutrition and dietetics came from Texas Tech University where she also received her clinical training. She developed the Ireton-Jones equations for estimating energy requirements in hospitalized patients and these are widely used nationally and internationally.

Dr. Ireton-Jones is a nutrition therapy specialist, a consultant, speaker, and in private practice. Dr. Ireton-Jones provides outpatient nutrition care for people with GI disorders, including irritable bowel syndrome, gastroparesis, and inflammatory bowel disease (IBD), as well as for those who require home parenteral and enteral nutrition. She teaches graduate nutrition courses at Texas Tech University and is a preceptor for doctoral students from Rutgers University.

She has lectured extensively, nationally, and internationally on a variety of nutrition topics and authored five previous books, numerous book chapters, and peer-reviewed papers. Dr. Ireton-Jones is an active member of several local and national nutrition-related organizations. She has received many honors and awards, including the 2022 Award for Excellence in Entrepreneurial Practice from the Academy of Nutrition and Dietetics and the 2023 Chancellor's Alumni Excellence Award from Texas Woman's University.

Balancing both evidence-based nutrition with sensible and *practical* applications is her strong point!

Associate Editor

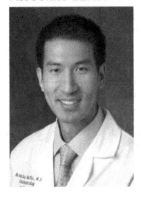

Berkeley Limketkai, MD, PhD, is an Associate Clinical Professor at the David Geffen School of Medicine at UCLA. He received his medical degree from the University of Cincinnati and subsequently completed his internal medicine residency, gastroenterology fellowship, advanced training in IBDs, and PhD education at Johns Hopkins University. Dr. Limketkai specializes in the care of patients with complex IBD. He has a primary research interest in the role of nutrition, nutrient sensing, and the gut microbiome in IBD. His doctoral dissertation explored the role of vitamin D in IBD pathogenesis and severity, and he has several ongoing studies investigating interactions across nutrition, the gut microbiome, and IBD. Dr. Limketkai also focuses on identifying novel treatment approaches for IBD, establishing evidence-based frameworks in the management of gastrointestinal conditions, building artificial intelligence-based tools for nutrition and gastroenterology, and developing clinical practice guidelines. An overarching motivation for all these efforts is to help shape and improve the future care of our patients.

Contributors

Sherifatu Abu, MD, MPH
Assistant Professor of Medicine
Johns Hopkins University School of
    Medicine
Baltimore, MD

Therezia AlChoufete, MS, RD, LDN
Division of Gastroenterology,
    Hepatology and Nutrition
University of Pittsburgh
Pittsburgh, PA

**Elizabeth Bobo, MS, RDN, LDN,
    CNSC, FAND**
Clinical Dietitian Lead
Nemours Children's Health
Jacksonville, FL

Po-Hung (Victor) Chen, MD
Assistant Professor
Division of Gastroenterology
Johns Hopkins University School of
    Medicine
Baltimore, MD

**Julia Fechtner, RD, LDN, CSO,
    CNSC**
Clinical Oncology Dietitian
City of Hope
Chicago, IL

**Trisha Fuhrman, MS, RDN, LDN,
    FAND, FSPEN**
Clinical Liaison Lead
Pentec Health, Inc.
Chicago, IL

Khushboo Gala, MD
Fellow
Gastroenterology and Hepatology
Mayo Clinic
Rochester, MN

Michael Garcia, MD
Assistant Professor of Medicine
Division of Clinical Nutrition
UCLA School of Medicine
Los Angeles, CA

**Christina Terese Gentile, PsyD,
    MA, ABPP**
Clinical Health Psychologist
Division of Digestive Diseases at UCLA
    Health
Los Angeles, CA

Michael Herman, DO
Borland Grover Clinic
Jacksonville, FL

**Carol Ireton-Jones, PhD, RDN, LD,
    CNSC, FAND, FASPEN**
Nutrition Therapy Specialist
Good Nutrition for Good Living
Digestive Nutrition Group
Carrollton, TX

Nancee Jaffe, MS, RD
UCLA Vatche and Tamar
    Manoukian
Division of Digestive
    Diseases
Los Angeles, CA

Matthew Kappus, MD
Assistant Professor
Division of Gastroenterology
Department of Medicine
Duke University School
    of Medicine
Raleigh/Durham, NC

Matthew Kaspar, MD
Bellin Health System
De Pere, WI

Arunkumar Krishnan, MBBS
Clinical Research Fellow
Division of Gastroenterology and
  Hepatology
Johns Hopkins University School of Medicine
Baltimore, MD
and
Senior Research Scientist
Department of Supportive Oncology
Levine Cancer Institute, Atrium Health
Charlotte, NC

Anne Roland Lee, EdD, RDN, LD
Assistant Professor of Nutritional Medicine
Celiac Disease Center
Columbia University
New York, NY

Lauren Lemieux, MD, FACP, Dipl. ABOM
Internist and Obesity Medicine Specialist
Sacramento, CA

Zhaoping Li, MD, PhD
Professor of Medicine and Chief
Division of Clinical Nutrition
UCLA School of Medicine
Los Angeles, CA

Berkeley Limketkai, MD, PhD
Associate Clinical Professor
Division of Digestive Diseases
UCLA School of Medicine
Los Angeles, California

Lisa Lin, MD
Beverly Hills Digestive Disease
Beverly Hills, CA

Beth Lyman, MSN, RN, FASPEN, FAAN
Clinical Nurse Consultant
Kansas City, MO

**Angela Matthewson, MPH, RDN,
  LD/N, CSO**
Florida Cancer Specialists & Research
  Institute
Fort Myers, FL

**Stephen A. McClave, MD, FACN,
  FASGE, FASPEN, AGAF**
Professor of Medicine
Director of Clinical
  Nutrition
University of Louisville School of
  Medicine
Louisville, KY

Martha McHenry, RDN, CDE
Smart Plate Nutrition
Dallas, TX

**Reid Nishikawa, Pharm D, BCNSP,
  FASPEN**
Nutrition Support
  Specialist
Granite Bay, CA

**Endashaw Omer, MD, MPH, AGAF,
  FACG, PNS**
Associate Professor of
  Medicine
Director of Endoscopy
University of Louisville
Louisville, KY

Marianne Opilla, RN
In Memoriam

Lucian Panait, MD
Bhatti GI Clinic
Chaska, MN

**Kristen M. Roberts, PhD, RDN, LD,
  CNSC, FASPEN, FAND**
Associate Professor
College of Medicine
Ohio State University
Columbus, OH

**Michelle Romano, MS, RDN, LD/N,
  CNSC, FASPEN**
Fresenius Kabi USA
Chicago, IL

**Senthilkumar Sankararaman, MD
FAAP, D-ABOM**
Pediatric Gastroenterologist and
    Physician Nutrition Specialist
Division of Pediatric Gastroenterology,
    Hepatology and Nutrition
UH Rainbow Babies and Children's
    Hospital, Cleveland
Associate Professor, Case Western
    Reserve University School of Medicine
Cleveland, OH

**Neha D. Shah, MPH, RD, CNSC,
CHES**
Colitis and Crohn's Disease Center
University of California, San Francisco
San Francisco, CA

Thomas J. Sferra, MD, AGAF, FAAP
Division Chief, Pediatric
    Gastroenterology
UH Rainbow Babies and Children's
    Hospital
Program Director, Pediatric
    Gastroenterology Fellowship, UH
    Cleveland Medical Center
Professor, Case Western Reserve
    University School of Medicine
Cleveland, OH

Taylor Stauble, MS, RD
Louisville KY

Allyson Stout, RD, LD, CNSC
Shelbyville, KY

Aravind Thavamani, MD
Assistant Professor of Pediatrics
Division of Pediatric Gastroenterology,
    Hepatology and Nutrition
UH Rainbow Babies and Children's
    Hospital
Case Western Reserve University
    School of Medicine
Cleveland, OH

Peng-sheng (Brian) Ting, MD
Assistant Professor of Medicine
Division of Gastroenterology and
    Hepatology
Tulane University School of Medicine
New Orleans, LA

Kristen Trukova, PA-C, RD
Gastroenterology/Otolaryngology
City of Hope
Chicago, IL

Pankaj Vashi, MD, AGAF, FSPEN
Department Head of Gastroenterology/
    Nutrition
Vice Chief of Staff
City of Hope
Chicago, IL

Sujithra Velayuthan, MD
Pediatric Gastroenterologist
Division of Pediatric Gastroenterology,
    Hepatology and Nutrition
UH Rainbow Babies and Children's
    Hospital
Cleveland, OH

Carla Venegas, MD
Critical Care Medicine
Mayo Clinic
Jacksonville, FL

Gillian White, MS, RDN, CNSC
Digestive Nutrition Group
Dallas, TX

Tinsay Woreta, MD, MPH
Program Director
Gastroenterology and Transplant
    Hepatology Fellowships
Assistant Professor of Medicine
Division of Gastroenterology and Hepatology
Johns Hopkins University School of
    Medicine
Baltimore, MD

1 Nutrition Screening, Assessment, and Monitoring

Trisha Fuhrman

1.1 INTRODUCTION

Patients are referred to home care and outpatient care from hospitals, healthcare facilities, primary care providers and patient self-referral. No matter what brings the patient to the out-patient or home care setting, the patient's current nutritional status should be evaluated. Sometimes the clinician receiving the referral is given an extensive amount of information about the patient and sometimes there is little or no information provided. Regardless of the quantity and quality of the information provided with the referral, the clinician should perform their own nutrition screening and assessment.

1.2 NUTRITION SCREENING

A nutrition screen should be a simple and quick means of determining which patients will require an in-depth nutrition assessment. It can also be used to collect information on what the patient hopes to accomplish, or goals of therapy, through interactions with the nutrition-focused clinician. For the dietitian working in an outpatient clinic or private practice, the initial form(s) completed by the patient prior to a consult may include nutrition screening questions.

There are several validated tools available for nutrition screening.[1] A systematic review of screening tools for identification of malnutrition in adults found that there were no tools with high validity, high reliability, and strong supportive evidence.[2] Most tools were moderate in their validity and reliability and were found to have a wide variation in results. Also, keep in mind that if the clinician changes the screening tool, it is no longer validated and the clinician should validate the changed tool to determine if it still enables the clinician to identify the patients who require a nutrition intervention versus those who do not. Information generally collected in a nutrition screen includes non-quantified changes in weight and appetite, chewing and/or swallowing problems, and diagnosis or reason for requiring or requesting nutrition care. In the outpatient setting, it is reasonable to have the patient and/or caregiver complete the nutrition screen. Each home care provider and clinic needs to identify who will perform the screen and how the referral to the registered dietitian nutritionist (RDN) or to the nutrition-trained qualified individual will be done. Identification of a patient who requires a nutrition assessment leads to initiation of

DOI: 10.1201/9780429322570-1

the Nutrition Care Process, a standardized process that includes assessment, nutrition diagnosis, nutrition intervention, and monitoring and evaluation.[3] Standards of practice indicators for RDNs working in nutrition support performing the NCP are delineated by level of practice (competent, proficient, and expert) and apply to all practice settings.[4] There are also standards of practice for clinicians working in home care and alternate sites.[5]

1.3   NUTRITION ASSESSMENT

The nutrition assessment incorporates medical and surgical history, laboratory data, medications, anthropometrics, functional status, nutrient intake, nutrition-focused physical exam, and clinical judgment.[4–6] The goal is not only to determine the individualized nutritional and educational needs of the patient, but to also identify whether or not the patient is malnourished. Although malnutrition is typically associated with patients in either a hospital or long-term care facility, shorter hospital stays and preference for keeping patients at home increases the risk for malnutrition in the outpatient setting, emphasizing the importance of evaluating all patients for the presence of malnutrition. Additionally, chronic disease such as inflammatory bowel disease, diabetes, or renal disease may detrimentally affect nutritional status.

The nutrition assessment components that are used to diagnosis malnutrition include anthropometrics, functional status, nutrient intake, and nutrition-focused physical exam (Table 1.1). If the patient is malnourished, the degree of malnutrition and the planned nutrition intervention must be delineated in the care plan and communicated with the entire healthcare team. The clinician should evaluate the patient's and caregiver's nutrition counseling needs and readiness to make nutrition and lifestyle changes.

1.3.1   MALNUTRITION

The Academy of Nutrition and Dietetics and the American Society of Parenteral and Enteral Nutrition created a Malnutrition Workgroup that published the definitions and the characteristics of adult malnutrition.[7] The definitions of malnutrition are etiology-based and are divided into three categories: (1) Chronic starvation due to societal and environmental conditions, (2) chronic disease with mild to moderate inflammation, and (3) acute disease, illness, or injury with severe inflammation. Malnourished patients in the outpatient and home care setting are more likely to suffer from chronic malnutrition without inflammation or chronic disease-related malnutrition with mild to moderate inflammation. The six characteristics used to determine the degree of malnutrition (severe versus non-severe) include amount/ degree of weight loss, insufficient nutrient intake, loss of body fat, loss of subcutaneous fat, fluid accumulation, and diminished functional capacity (Table 1.1). Two characteristics are needed to assign the diagnosis of malnutrition. Assessment of weight loss over time and percent of intake compared to estimated needs are skills regularly used by RDNs. It is not surprising that these characteristics were the most often used to diagnose malnutrition.[8] The challenge is to increase competency in nutrition-focused physical assessment in order to assess the patient's lean body mass,

TABLE 1.1
Characteristics Associated with Chronic Disease and Mild to Moderate Inflammation

Characteristic	Severe Malnutrition		Non-Severe Malnutrition	
	Starvation-related	Chronic disease-related	Starvation-related	Chronic disease-related
Energy Needs (Compare estimated energy needs to patient's past and current intake to estimate adequacy of intake over time.)	≥1 month consuming < 50% energy needs	≥1 month consuming < 75% energy needs	>3 months consuming ≤75% energy needs	>1 month consuming ≤75% energy needs
Actual Body Weight (Consider hydration status when interpreting weight changes from baseline. Fluid accumulations can mask weight changes and loss of fat and lean body mass.)	>5 %, >7.5%, >10%, and >20% weight loss over 1, 3, 6, and 12 months respectively	>5 %, >7.5%, >10%, and >20% weight loss over 1, 3, 6, and 12 months respectively	5%, 7.5%, 10%, and 20% weight loss over 1, 3, 6, and 12 months respectively	>5%, >7.5%, >10%, and >20% weight loss over 1, 3, 6, and 12 months respectively
Muscle Mass (Examine temples, clavicles, shoulders, interosseous muscle, scapula, thigh, and calf muscle for visible signs of losses.)	Severe loss of lean body mass		Mild loss of lean body mass	
Body Fat (Examine orbital, triceps [roll skin between thumb and forefinger to separate fat from muscle in upper arm with arm bent], and ribs for loss of subcutaneous fat.)	Severe loss of subcutaneous body fat		Mild loss of subcutaneous body fat	
Fluid Accumulation (Examine for signs of fluid retention in extremities, vulvar/scrotal edema, or ascites. Physician and nursing notes may provide information on fluid status.)	Severe localized or generalized fluid accumulation		Mild localized or generalized fluid accumulation	
Functional Capacity (Compare measurement to normative standards as provided by manufacturer of measurement device. Occupation therapy evaluation may provide information on functional status and capacity.)	Measurably reduced functional measures, such as hand grip strength		Non-applicable	

Source: Adapted with permission from White J.W., Guenter P., Jensen G., et al. Consensus statement: Academy of Nutrition and Dietetics and American Society for Parenteral and Enteral Nutrition: Characteristics recommended for the identification and documentation of adult malnutrition (undernutrition). *JPEN J Parenter Enteral Nutr.* 2012;36(3):275–283.

subcutaneous fat mass, and fluid status. In general, the clinician can examine the upper body to obtain indicators of lean body mass and subcutaneous fat losses. This is often more feasible in the outpatient setting where patients are wearing their usual clothing versus wearing a hospital gown. It is important for clinicians to be cognizant of the potential for the presence of malnutrition in patients who are obese. For example, an obese patient's temporal muscle may not be visibly sunken, but may depress quickly and feel watery above the bone.

1.3.2 MEDICAL AND SURGICAL HISTORY

The patient's medical and surgical histories are often obtained from the medical chart or through discussion with the referring physician. However, there may be times when the clinician must obtain data from the patient and the patient's family. The more the clinician knows about the patient's medical and surgical history, the more comprehensive the nutrition care plan for the present and future can be developed. The patient's primary reason for referral as well as existing comorbidities impact the plan of care. Past gastrointestinal surgical procedures as well as chronic conditions can affect consumption, digestion, absorption, and excretion of nutrients.

1.3.3 LABORATORY DATA

Laboratory data may have been collected during a hospitalization or the most recent physician office visit. It can provide a historic perspective of the patient's overall health and trends in improvement or deterioration, such as can be seen with sequential lipid panels or HbA1c levels for example. Historically, malnutrition was determined by hepatic protein levels. Unfortunately, this quick and easy way to categorize malnutrition responds more dramatically to inflammation with a slower response to energy and protein intake.[9] The recognition and acceptance of the new definitions and characteristics of malnutrition behoove clinicians to evaluate hepatic proteins within the context of inflammation and nutrient intake.

1.3.4 MEDICATIONS

Each medication the patient is taking should be considered for its potential nutritional impact. Medications can alter nutrient metabolism and availability and nutrients can affect drug effectiveness. The clinician should be aware of prescribed and over-the-counter medication that the patient is taking. Herbal and nutrition supplements should also be investigated since these can impact nutritional status or counter the effects of prescription medications. The pharmacokinetics of medication should be evaluated when the route of providing a medication is being changed from oral to enteral or parenteral.

The following components of nutrition assessment are integral to the diagnosis of malnutrition.

1.3.5 ANTHROPOMETRICS

Ideally weight and height are measured and there is the opportunity to compare current measurements to past measurements to identify the patient's usual weight and changes in body weight. However, usual body weight is often obtained from the patient. As a rule, individuals tend to report being taller with a lower weight compared to actual. Height and weight are used to calculate Body Mass Index or BMI, estimate energy and protein needs, and determine degree of weight change over time. Therefore, a measured height and weight improves the accuracy of the equations. Arm span, summation of body parts, and knee height can be used to indirectly determine height in a patient unable to stand.[10] Evaluation of percent ideal body weight (IBW) and BMI are both used to determine under- and over-nutrition (Table 1.2).[11–13]

Weights can be reported as actual body weight (ABW), usual body weight (UBW), IBW, and estimated dry weight (EDW). Actual body weight is the measured weight at the time of assessment. Usual body weight is either reported by the patient or gleaned from the chart as the weight recorded during previous office visits or hospitalizations. Ideal body weight can be obtained using actuarial tables[14] or epidemiological data[15] or calculated using the Hamwi method.[16] The Hamwi method is a quick and easy way to estimate IBW in the outpatient and home care setting.

- *Men*: 106 pounds for the first 5 feet of height and 6 pounds for each additional inch.
- *Women*: 100 pounds for first 5 feet of height and 5 pounds for each additional inch.

When calculating IBW, subtract for any loss of body parts: 0.7% (hand); 5% (entire arm); 1.5% (foot); 5.9% (foot and lower leg); 16% (entire leg).[17] Spinal cord injury also requires a reduction in IBW calculation with 5–10% subtracted with paraplegia and 10–15% subtracted with quadriplegia.[18]

Estimated dry weight is used in the dialysis population to determine the desired weight of the patient following the removal of fluid with dialysis.[19] The EDW is used in energy and protein calculations in the dialysis population or in any patient population with a propensity to retain fluid, such as liver failure with ascites and congestive heart failure.

TABLE 1.2

Interpretation of Body Mass Index (BMI) and Percent Ideal Body Weight (%IBW)[11–13]

BMI (kg/m²)	%IBW	Interpretation
14–15	< 80%	Associated with mortality
< 18.5	80–90%	Underweight, health risks low
18.5–25	90–110%	Healthy weight
> 25	110–120%	Overweight, health risk increased
> 30	120–140%	Obese, health risk moderate
> 35	141–200%	Severe obesity, health risk severe
> 40	> 200%	Morbid obesity, health risk very severe

Adjusted body weight (AdjBW) is sometimes used to take into account a higher percentage of body fat in a patient who is obese in an attempt to avoid assigning the patient excessive energy requirements. Rather than create an artificial weight for the patient, it may be better for the clinician to decrease estimated needs by 10–20% based on ABW.

1.3.6 FUNCTIONAL STATUS

Functional status indicates the patient's ability to perform activities of daily living and interact with family and friends. It is often an indicator of quality of life. A patient debilitated from a prolonged hospitalization may not be able to transfer from bed to chair or use bathroom facilities independently. Functional capacity will also be used when determining characteristics of malnutrition. Functional capacity can be measured using a hand dynamometer, which has been shown to correlate to muscle mass and nutritional status.[7] Results are compared to standards provided by the manufacturer. Functional parameters can also include wound healing, walking endurance, and Karnofsky's scale[20] which uses activities of daily living to determine functionality (form available at www.npcrc.org/files/news/karnofsky-performance-scale.pdf). The short physical performance battery (SPPB)[21] (instructions available at www.nia.nih.gov/research/labs/leps/short-physical-performance-battery-sppb). The SPPB has three components that determine the score: standing upright for 10 seconds, a 3- or 4-meter walk, and time required to rise from chair 5 times. A higher score indicates higher functional status. Lower scores are associated with increased risk of falling, more dependence for activities of daily living, disability, immobility, hospitalization, and death.[22] In the outpatient and home care setting, the clinician can monitor measurements over time to assess improvement or deterioration in status.

1.3.7 NUTRIENT INTAKE AND NUTRIENT NEEDS

Nutrient intake should be compared to estimated energy and protein needs to determine if the patient needs to increase or decrease the intake of caloric and nutrient dense foods. The amount of food consumed compared to estimated needs over a period of time is part of the diagnosis of malnutrition. Review GI tract integrity when determining if nutrition intake is sufficient. Losses from diarrhea, drains, fistulae, and wounds may contribute to nutrient imbalance. The Mifflin-St. Jeor equation has been reported to be the most accurate predictive equation for energy expenditure at rest (RMR) in healthy individuals [w = weight in kg; h = height in cm; and a = age in years].[23]

- *Male*: RMR = 10 (w) + 6.3 (h) – 4.9 (a) + 5
- *Female*: RMR = 10 (w) + 6.3 (h) – 4.9 (a) – 161

Total daily energy needs are determined by estimating the effect of disease or injury and activity on predicted RMR. Protein needs are estimated based on metabolic demand, ongoing losses, and disease process. Requirements range from 0.8 to 1.5 gm/kg per day.[23] Requirements may be elevated with wounds, excess losses, and metabolic stress. Requirements may be reduced with renal failure without dialysis and hepatic encephalopathy responsive to protein intake. Doses > 1 gm/kg can contribute to hypercalciuria and risk of metabolic bone disease in patients on long-term parenteral nutrition.

Fluid requirements are easily determined by using 35 mL/kg for adults and 30 mL/kg for elderly adults.[24] Fluid needs for patients on tube feeding is often estimated using 1 mL/kcal of tube feeding. Regardless of how fluid needs are estimated, it is important to monitor the physical signs and symptoms of fluid status to avoid over- or under-hydration – particularly in patients who cannot express thirst. Fluid requirements may be reduced with cardiac, renal, and hepatic failure. Requirements may be increased with ongoing fluid losses through drains, fistulae, wounds, and the GI tract. Assessing signs and symptoms of fluid status is part of the nutrition-focused physical assessment and diagnosis characteristics for malnutrition (Table 1.1). Fluid accumulation can mask loss of weight, fat mass, and lean body mass.

Whether a patient is receiving nutrients by mouth, tube feeding, or parenteral nutrition, it is important to ensure that 100% of micronutrient needs are being provided. This can be challenging with periodic injectable micronutrient shortages for patients reliant on parenteral nutrition. Monitoring for signs and symptoms of micronutrient deficiencies are incorporated into the nutrition-focused physical assessment (Table 1.3).[25–27]

In the outpatient setting, surgical procedures such as bariatric surgery, GI surgery/resection, chronic disease including diabetes, renal disease, and inflammatory bowel disease, as well as conditions such as heart disease, diabetes, and anorexia nervosa may cause micronutrient deficiencies and malnutrition which should be identified during a nutrition assessment.

1.3.8 NUTRITION-FOCUSED PHYSICAL EXAM

This is a head-to-toe approach for inspecting the patient. During this process the clinician looks for signs and symptoms of micronutrient deficiencies as well as characteristics of malnutrition: muscle wasting, loss of subcutaneous fat, and fluid accumulation. There is currently a focus to increase the competency and confidence of RDNs in performing nutrition-focused physical assessment in order to diagnosis malnutrition. However, RDNs should not lose sight of using inspection and light palpation to monitor for micronutrient deficiencies and to assess the patient's overall condition. A head-to-toe approach ensures that the RDN methodically examines the skin, nails, hair, head and eyes, oral cavity, neck and chest, and musculoskeletal system.[25–27] Table 1.3 provides a list of micronutrients and signs and symptoms associated with deficiency and toxicity. Individuals at risk for malnutrition and nutrient deficiencies include patients with chronic conditions and illnesses that interfere with ingestion, absorption, assimilation, or excretion of nutrients (Table 1.4).

TABLE 1.3

Micronutrient Assessment Guide[20-22]

Nutrient	Signs and Symptoms of Deficiency	Potential Etiology (in addition to deficient diet)	Signs and Symptoms of Toxicity	Potential Etiology of Toxicity	Assessment of Status	DRI (Adults)	IV Standard Dose (adults)
Vitamin A	• Night blindness • Bitot's spots • Conjunctival xerosis • Scaling of skin • Nasolabial seborrhea • Follicular hyperkeratosis • Blindness • Impaired mucus secretion • Depressed T-helper cell activity	• Liver disease • Critical illness • Steatorrhea	• Alopecia • Ataxia • Muscle and bone pain • Cheilitis • Headache • Conjunctivitis • Skin and vision disorders • Hepatotoxicity • Pruritis • Hyperlipidemia • Membrane dryness • Renal osteodystrophy	• Liver disease • Malnutrition • ETOH abuse • Chronic kidney disease	Serum retinol	RDA: Male/Female 900/700 mcg RE	3300 IU/d
Ascorbic Acid, Vitamin C (Scurvy)	• Petechiae (perifollicular) • Swollen/bleeding gums • Purpura • Follicular hyperkeratosis • Poor wound healing • Pressure ulcers • Retracted gums • Corkscrew hair • Anorexia • Fatigue • Muscle pain	• Surgical and burn patients • Wounds/pressure ulcers • Acute inflammation/ metabolic stress hinders vitamin C transport	• Nausea • Vomiting	• Renal failure • Kidney stones • Iron overload disease • Individuals on warfarin or heparin therapy should avoid high doses	Plasma ascorbic acid analysis via high-pressure liquid chromatography	RDA: Male/Female 90/75 mg	200 mg

Nutrient	Deficiency Signs/Symptoms	Risk Factors	Toxicity		Assessment	RDA/AI	
Biotin	• Alopecia • Pallor • Glossitis • Nausea/vomiting • Depression/lethargy • Muscle pain • Erythematous seborrheic dermatitis • Increased chol and bile pigments	• Deficiency rarely reported • Long-term PN • Alcoholism • S/p partial gastrectomy	No known toxic effects	N/A	Serum and 24-hr urine collections	AI (adequate intake): 30 mcg	60 mcg
Cyanocobalamin, B$_{12}$	• Atrophic lingual papillae • Dementia • Peripheral neuropathy with weakness and paresthesias • Ataxia • Poor memory • Confusion/depression • Delusions • Megaloblastic anemia with macrocytosis • Hypersegmentation of neutrophil nuclei • Bone marrow changes • Leucopenia • Thrombocytopenia • Glossitis • Constipation/diarrhea	• Malabsorption syndromes (s/p gastrectomy, gastric bypass, ileal resection) • Vegetarianism • Impaired HCl production • Overgrowth of *H. pylori*	No known toxic effects	N/A	Serum B$_{12}$ Increased methylmalonic acid and homocysteine with deficiency (homocysteine also increased with folic acid deficiency)	RDA: 2.4 mg	5 mcg

(Continued)

TABLE 1.3 (Continued)
Micronutrient Assessment Guide[20-22]

Nutrient	Signs and Symptoms of Deficiency	Potential Etiology (in addition to deficient diet)	Signs and Symptoms of Toxicity	Potential Etiology of Toxicity	Assessment of Status	DRI (Adults)	IV Standard Dose (adults)
Vitamin D	• Tetany • Rickets or osteomalacia	• Limited sun exposure • Steatorrhea • Long-term PN • Hepatic/renal disease • Gastric resection • Antiepileptic medications (phenytoin, Phenobarbital)	• Hypercalcemia • Hypercalciuria • Soft tissue calcification	Excessive supplementation	Serum 25-hydroxyvitamin D	AI: 19–50 years 5 mcg 51–70 years 10 mcg >70 years Male/Female 15/10 mcg	200 IU
Vitamin E	• Increased platelet aggregation • Decreased red blood cell survival • Hemolytic anemia • Neuronal degeneration • Creatinuria	• Steatorrhea • Fat malabsorption • Requirement for high oxygen concentration via mechanical ventilation	• Impaired neutrophil function • Impaired coagulation • Prolonged toxicity: skeletal muscle lesions	Excessive supplementation	Plasma or serum alpha-tocopherol Vitamin E, plasma	RDA: 15 mg α-TE	10 IU
Folic Acid	• Atrophic lingual papillae • Megaloblastic or macrocytic anemia • Diarrhea • Weight loss • Decreased cell-mediated immunity • Dementia • Neural tube defects in infants born to mothers who are deficient	• Chronic alcoholism • Medications (phenytoin, cholestyramine, sulfasalazine, amphotericin B) • Increased risk with pregnancy due to increased demand for DNA synthesis for embryonic development	No known toxic effects	N/A	Stage I (early): serum folate levels Stage II (tissue depletion): RBC folate levels Stage III (erythropoiesis): neutrophil hypersegmentation and abnormal deoxyuridine suppression test Stage IV (clinical deficiency): megaloblastic anemia or macrocytic anemia	RDA: 400 mcg	600 mcg

Nutrient	Deficiency Signs & Symptoms	Risk Factors/Causes	Toxicity	Excessive	Laboratory Assessment	RDA/AI	Upper Limit
Vitamin K	• Purpura • Bleeding	• Fat malabsorption • Antibiotic therapy • Oral anticoagulants • Infant hemorrhagic disease	Prolonged bleeding	Excessive supplementation	Prothrombin time International normalized ratio	AI: Male/Female 120/90 mcg	150 mcg
Niacin, B₃ (Pellagra)	• 3 Ds: dermatitis, diarrhea, dementia • Pigmentation of skin • Desquamation of sun exposed areas • Atrophic lingual papillae • Angular stomatitis • Cheilosis	• Deficiency rare in US due to food fortification • Synthesized from tryptophan [60 gm = 1 mg niacin equivalent (NE) or 1 mg niacin] • Alcoholism • Severe malabsorption	• Flushing of skin • Pharmacological doses (3 g/d) cause vasodilation, itching, sensation of heat, headaches, GI irritation, glucose intolerance	Pharmacological dosing	Urinary measurement of N-methylnicotinamide (NMN) and 2-pyridone	RDA: Male/Female 16/14 mcg	40 mcg
Pantothenic Acid	• Listlessness • Fatigue • Irritability • Restlessness • Malaise • Sleep disturbances • Nausea/vomiting • Diarrhea/abdominal cramps • Neuromuscular imbalance – numbness, staggering gait, paresthesias, muscle cramps • Hypoglycemia • Increased insulin sensitivity	• Occurs in conjunction with other nutrient deficiencies • Increased risk with diabetes, inflammatory bowel disease, alcoholism	Rare – can cause mild GI distress	N/A	Whole blood 24-hr urinary pantothenic acid concentration	AI: 5 mg	15 mg

(Continued)

TABLE 1.3 (Continued)

Micronutrient Assessment Guide[20-22]

Nutrient	Signs and Symptoms of Deficiency	Potential Etiology (in addition to deficient diet)	Signs and Symptoms of Toxicity	Potential Etiology of Toxicity	Assessment of Status	DRI (Adults)	IV Standard Dose (adults)
Pyridoxine, B$_6$	• Seborrheic dermatitis • Redness/fissuring in corners of eyes • Scaling of skin • Nasolabial seborrhea • Cheilosis • Angular stomatitis • Peripheral neuropathy with weakness and paresthesias • Ataxia • Microcytic anemia • Epileptiform convulsions • Confusion/depression	• Alcoholism • Dialysis • Elderly • Medications (isoniazid, penicillamine, corticosteroids, anticonvulsants)	• Sensory neuropathy • Sensory ataxia • Areflexia • Impaired cutaneous and deep sensations • Dermatologic lesions	Excessive oral supplement doses	Pyridoxal 5-phosphate, Combination of 3 tests: 1. Direct plasma PLP level 2. 24-hr urinary excretion of 4-pyridoxic acid 3. Activation of erythrocyte aspartate aminotransferase (EAST) and alanine aminotransferase (EALT)	RDA: 19–50 years 1.3 mg 51–70 years Male/Female 1.7/1.5 mg	6 mg
Riboflavin, B$_2$	• Redness/fissuring in corners of eyes • Magenta tongue • Photophobia • Scaling of skin • Nasolabial seborrhea • Cheilosis • Angular stomatitis • Atrophic lingual papillae • Sore throat • Hyperemia and edema of pharyngeal and oral mucosa	• Deficiency rarely occurs in isolation – generally is in conjunction with other B vitamins • Diet low in dairy products and animal protein • At-risk populations: thyroid deficiency, alcoholism, chronic malabsorption	Rare	N/A	Erythrocyte glutathione reductase activity (not valid in patients with glucose 6-phosphate deficiency)	RDA: Male/Female 1.3/1.1 mg	3.6 mg

Nutrient	Deficiency Signs/Symptoms	Risk Factors for Deficiency	Toxicity	Toxicity Risk Factors	Assessment	RDA/AI	PN Dose
Thiamin, B$_1$ (Beriberi)	• Seborrheic dermatitis of face and scrotum • Corneal vascularization *Wet beriberi* • Cardiac failure • Hepatomegaly • Tachycardia • Oliguria *Dry beriberi* • Peripheral neuropathy with weakness and paresthesias • Ataxia • Foot/wrist drop *Wernicke's encephalopathy* *Korsakoff's psychosis*	• Alcohol abuse • Refeeding syndrome • Malabsorption • Dialysis • Hyperemesis gravidarum • PN MVI shortages	Rare	N/A	Erythrocyte transketolase activity	RDA: Male/Female 1.2/1.1 mg	6 mg
Chromium	• Hyperglycemia refractory to insulin • Glucosuria • Impaired amino acid utilization • Increased LDL–cholesterol • Peripheral neuropathy • Weight loss	• Trace elements omitted from PN	• Occurs with Cr^{3+} (muscle rhabdomyolysis, liver dysfunction, renal failure	Intake of chromium picolinate (Cr^{3+}) supplements	Deficiency difficult to determine due to very low concentration in blood	AI: Male/Female 19–50 years 35/25 mcg > 50 years 30/20 mcg	10–15 mcg
Copper	• Pancytopenia (hypochromic and microcytic anemia, leucopenia, neutropenia) • Hypercholesterolemia • Decreased ceruloplasmin and erythrocyte Cu/Zn SOD • Increased erythrocyte turnover • Abnormal electrocardiogram	• Omitted from PN due to hyperbilirubinemia • Decreased absorption (intestinal surgery) • Increased GI losses (chronic diarrhea) • Hemodialysis • Excessive zinc supplementation	Rare – liver damage	• Impaired liver function • Chronic ingestion of excessive copper • Genetic predisposition to store copper in liver (Wilson's disease)	Serum copper and/or ceruloplasmin can be used but may not reflect liver stores and can be impacted by inflammation.	RDA: 900 mcg	0.3–0.5 mg

(Continued)

TABLE 1.3 (Continued)
Micronutrient Assessment Guide[20-22]

Nutrient	Signs and Symptoms of Deficiency	Potential Etiology (in addition to deficient diet)	Signs and Symptoms of Toxicity	Potential Etiology of Toxicity	Assessment of Status	DRI (Adults)	IV Standard Dose (adults)
Manganese	• Poor reproductive performance • Congenital abnormalities • Abnormal bone/cartilage formation • Ataxia • Growth retardation • Defects in CHO and lipid metabolism	• Deficiency rare unless totally absent from diet or PN solution	• Central nervous system abnormalities • Hyperirritability • Hallucinations • Manganese deposition in basal ganglia • Nephritis • Pancreatitis • Parkinson-like motor dysfunction	• Hepatobiliary disease • Long-term PN patients with biliary duct obstruction	No reliable biomarkers of status identified Toxicity: whole blood manganese correlates best to MRI results	AI: Male/Female 2.3/1.8 mg	60–100 mcg
Selenium	• Oxidative injury • Altered thyroid metabolism • Increased plasma glutathione • Altered biotransformation enzyme activity • Keshan disease – an endemic cardiomyopathy in areas of China • Cardiomyopathy/skeletal weakness	• PN without selenium • Selenium-poor soil • Statins interfere with selenoprotein synthesis • Decreased levels in trauma patients	• Nausea • Vomiting • Hair and nail loss • Tooth decay • Skin lesions • Irritability • Fatigue • Peripheral neuropathy	Excessive intake	Plasma/serum selenium reflects recent intake; erythrocyte concentration reflects long-term status Measurement of functional status: Plasma glutathione peroxidase	RDA: 55 mcg	20–60 mcg

| Zinc | • Scaling of skin
• Nasolabial seborrhea
• Poor wound healing
• Pressure ulcers
• Hypogeusia
• Hypogonadism
• Impaired night vision
• Anorexia
• Impaired immune function
• Impaired vitamin A status
• Hyposmia
• Alopecia
• Glucose intolerance
• Impaired hepatic function | • Inhibitors of zinc absorption (calcium, vitamins, milk proteins, phytic acid, alcohol, disease processes)
• At risk – elderly, alcoholics, postop patients, burn patients
• Malabsorption (intestinal bypass/resection)
• Renal disease
• Losses via wounds | • GI distress
• Impaired immune function
• Decreased high density lipoprotein levels | Excessive doses of zinc | Serum or plasma zinc Interpret values cautiously with inflammation and hypoalbuminemia | RDA: 11/8 mg Excess supplementation of zinc (20–250 mg/d) can contribute to copper deficiency | 2.5–5 mg |
| Iron | • Koilonychia
• Pale conjunctiva
• Pallor
• Fatigue
• Atrophic lingual papillae
• Tachycardia
• Poor capillary refilling
• Impaired behavioral/intellectual performance
• Impaired ability to maintain body temperature in cold environment
• Decreased resistance to infections | • Blood loss
• Celiac disease
• Crohn's disease
• Gastric/intestinal surgery
• Levels decrease with inflammation | • Damage to liver, heart, pancreas
• Skin pigmentation | • Excessive exposure or supplementation | • Testing absorption: measure serum iron 2–4 hr after 325 mg dose ferrous sulfate
• Decreased transferrin saturation and plasma iron, and increased plasma transferrin
• Continued depletion results in decreased serum ferritin (reflects tissue stores)
• Iron deficiency anemia confirmed by decreased mean corpuscular volume and decreased Hgb concentration | RDA: 19–50 years Male/Female 8/18 mg >50 years 8 mg | Not routinely added 25–50 mg/ month (without blood loss) Provide iron dextran in lipid-free PN |

TABLE 1.4

Conditions and Diseases That Contribute to Malnutrition and Nutrient Deficiencies

Surgical procedures: Bariatric surgery, GI surgery

Conditions: Anorexia nervosa, substance abuse, wounds/pressure ulcers

Diseases: Organ failure (heart, kidney, liver, pancreas)

Malabsorption: Steatorrhea, short bowel syndrome, fistula, inflammatory bowel disease, celiac disease, cystic fibrosis

1.4 NUTRITION DIAGNOSIS

The nutrition diagnosis focuses on the patient's primary nutrition-related problem, its signs and symptoms, and its etiology.[2,5] If a patient is malnourished, the nutrition diagnosis should clearly state the degree of malnutrition, the signs and symptoms noted, and the etiology of the development of malnutrition. A clearly written nutrition diagnosis sets the stage for the intervention. Note that the nutrition diagnosis is not a medical diagnosis. The NCP terminology may not be available for use in all outpatient and home care practices.

1.5 NUTRITION INTERVENTION

This is the primary reason for performing a nutrition assessment. The clinician must identify what can be done, if anything, to improve or stabilize the patient's nutritional status and identify the patient's nutrition education needs. The nutrition care plan should be communicated with the healthcare team, the patient, and the patient's caregivers. The plan should be directed at correcting nutrient deficits, promoting nutrition literacy, and improving functional capacity and quality of life. The nutrition intervention should have a measurable goal that can be monitored by the healthcare team.

1.6 MONITORING AND EVALUATION

An intervention is not a static action. The clinical impact of the intervention as well as the patient's understanding, adherence and tolerance of the regimen must be monitored in order to determine if the intervention will be effective, and if not, to change the intervention to obtain the desired results. Ongoing evaluation helps to achieve outcomes that are beneficial to the patient. This requires communication among healthcare providers, the patient, the patient's caregivers, and the RDN.

1.7 CONCLUSION

Interactions with individuals in the outpatient setting run the gambit from diet instruction for weight loss to managing home nutrition support for a patient with severe malabsorption. Regardless of the patient population, the healthcare provider should utilize an organized approach to information gathering and problem identification and prioritization. Nutrition assessment is the foundation on which the nutritional care of the patient rests. A thorough review of the patient's metabolic systems, nutrient intake, physical appearance, and functional capabilities enables the clinician to develop a nutrition intervention to maintain or improve the patient's nutritional status and quality of life. The identification of malnutrition is an integral part of the nutrition assessment. Treat a nutrition deficit with a nutrition intervention. The nutritional issues have to be identified so that the clinician knows when to institute a nutrition intervention. Communication within the healthcare team and with the patient and their caregiver is essential to monitoring the plan so that it can be adjusted as needed. The nutritional well-being of the patient is the responsibility of the entire team.[28]

REFERENCES

1. Malnutrition Quality Improvement Initiative (MQii)—Toolkit. http://malnutritionquality.org/mqii-toolkit.html. Accessed June 9, 2020.
2. Skipper A, Coltman A, Tomesko J, et al. Adult malnutration (undernutrition) screening: an evidence analysis center systematic review. *J Acad Nutr Diet.* 2020;120(4):669–708.
3. Lacey K, Pritchett E. Nutrition care process and model ADA adopts road map to quality care and outcomes management. *J Am Diet Assoc.* 2003;103(8):1061–1072.
4. Brantley SL, Russell MK, Mogensen KM, et al. American society for parenteral and enteral nutrition and academy of nutrition and dietetics: Revised 2014 standards of practice and standards of professional performance for registered dietitian nutritionists (competent, proficient, and expert) in nutrition support. *Nutr Clin Pract.* 2014;29(6): 792–828.
5. Durfee SM, Adams SC, Arthur E, et al. A.S.P.E.N. Standards for nutrition support: Home and alternate site. *Nutr Clin Pract.* 2014;29(4):542–555.
6. Academy Quality Management Committee. Academy of Nutrition and Dietetics: Revised 2017 standards of practice in nutrition care and standards of professional performance for registered dietitian nutritionists. *J Acad Nutr Diet.* 2018;118:132–140.
7. White JW, Guenter P, Jensen G, et al. Consensus statement: Academy of Nutrition and Dietetics and American Society for Parenteral and Enteral Nutrition: Characteristics recommended for the identification and documentation of adult malnutrition (undernutrition). *JPEN J Parenter Enteral Nutr.* 2012;36(3):275–283.
8. Nicolo M, Compher CW, Still C, et al. Feasibility of accessing data in hospitalized patients to support diagnosis of malnutrition by the Academy—A.S.P.E.N. malnutrition consensus recommended clinical characteristics. *JPEN J Parenter Enteral Nutr.* 2014;38(8):954–959.
9. Fuhrman MP, Charney P, Mueller C. Hepatic proteins and nutrition assessment. *J Am Diet Assoc.* 2004;104:1258–1264.
10. Fuhrman MP. Nutrition screening and assessment in home nutrition support. In: Ireton-Jones C, DeLegge MH, eds. *Handbook of Home Nutrition Support.* Sudbury, MA: Jones & Bartlett Publishers. 2007:27–57.
11. National Institutes of Health. Clinical guidelines on the identification and treatment of overweight and obesity in adults – the evidence report. *Obes Res.* 1998;6 (suppl 2);51S–209S.
12. Lefton JC. Anthropometric measurements. In: Charney P, Malone AM, eds. *ADA Pocket Guide to Nutrition Assessment,* 3rd edition. Chicago, IL: Academy of Nutrition and Dietetics. 2016.

13. Centers for Disease Control and Prevention. *Body Mass Index: Considerations for Practitioners*. www.cdc.gov/obesity/downloads/BMIforPractitioners.pdf. Accessed June 9, 2020.
14. Metropolitan Life Insurance Company. Statistical Bulletin. January–June, 1983.
15. National Center for Health Statistics. Plan and Operation of the Health and Nutrition Examination Survey, United States, 1976–1980 (Part A—Development, Plan and Operation) Vital and Health Statistics. Series 1, No. 15. DHEW Publ. No. (PHS) 81–1317. Washington, DC: US Government Printing Office. 1981.
16. Hamwi GJ. Changing dietary concepts. In: Danowski TS, ed. *Diabetes Mellitus: Diagnosis and Treatment*, Vol 1. New York: American Diabetes Association, Inc. 1964:73–78.
17. Osterkamp LK. Current perspective on assessment of human body proportions of relevance to amputees. *J Am Diet Assoc*. 1995;95(2):215–218.
18. Peiffer SC, Blust P, Leyson JF. Nutritional assessment of the spinal cord injured patient. *J Am Diet Assoc*. 1981;78(5):501–505.
19. McCann L, ed. *Pocket Guide to Nutrition Assessment of the Patient with Kidney Disease*, 5th edition. New York, NY: National Kidney Foundation. 2015.
20. Karnofsky DA, Burchenal JH. The clinical evaluation of chemotherapeutic agents in cancer. In: *Evaluation of Chemotherapeutic Agents*. New York: Columbia University Press. 1949:191.
21. National Institute on Aging. *Assessing Physical Performance in the Older Patient*. www.nia.nih.gov/research/labs/leps/short-physical-performance-battery-sppb Accessed June 9, 2020.
22. Treacy D, Hassett L. The short physical performance battery. *J Physiother*. 2018;64:61.
23. Frankenfield D, Rowe WA, Smith JS, et al. Validation of several established equations for resting metabolic rate in obese and nonobese people. *J Am Diet Assoc*. 2003;103(9):1152–1159.
24. Malone A, Russell M. Nutrient requirements. In: Charney P, Malone AM, eds. *ADA Pocket Guide to Nutrition Assessment*. 3rd edition. Chicago, IL: Academy of Nutrition and Dietetics. 2016.
25. Peterson S. Nutrition-focused physical assessment. In: Charney P, Malone AM, eds. *ADA Pocket Guide to Nutrition Assessment*. 3rd edition. Chicago, IL: Academy of Nutrition and Dietetics. 2016.
26. Morrison SG. Clinical nutrition physical examination. *Support Line*. 1997;19(2):16–18.
27. Mordarski B, Wolff J. *Nutrition Focused Physical Exam Pocket Guide*, 2nd edition. Chicago IL: Academy of Nutrition and Dietetics. 2018.
28. Tappenden KA, Quatrara B, Parkhurst ML, et al. Critical role of nutrition in improving quality of care: an interdisciplinary call to action to address adult hospital malnutrition. *JPEN J Parenter Enteral Nutr*. 2013;37(4):482–497.

2 Gastrointestinal Tests and Procedures

Khushboo Gala, Allyson Stout,
and Endashaw Omer

2.1 INTRODUCTION

When a patient presents with nutritional disorders, there are several tests and procedures that can be done to help establish diagnosis and plan ongoing nutritional intervention and disease management. All clinicians working with these patients should have a basic understanding of the tests that may have been done or should be performed to determine and maintain an optimal treatment plan. This chapter will review the most common procedures utilized in evaluating gastrointestinal dysfunction.

The Following Procedures and Tests Are Discussed in This Chapter

1. Esophagogastroduodenoscopy (EGD)
2. Enteroscopy
3. Capsule Endoscopy
4. Sigmoidoscopy/Colonoscopy
5. Endoscopic Ultrasound
6. Endoscopic Retrograde Cholangiopancreatography (EECP)
7. Modified Barium Swallowing Study (MBSS)
8. Esophagram
9. High-Resolution Manometry
10. Functional Lumen Imaging Probe
11. Gastric Emptying Scintigraphy
12. SmartPill™
13. Ambulatory pH Testing
14. Hydrogen Breath Testing
15. Enteral Access

2.2 ESOPHAGOGASTRODUODENOSCOPY (EGD)

An esophagogastroduodenoscopy (EGD) is a procedure that examines the esophagus, stomach, and first portion of the duodenum (small intestine) using an endoscope. It is a well-tolerated procedure. It is widely utilized as a diagnostic and therapeutic tool. The popularity of EGDs as a diagnostic and therapeutic tool is rising, with a 50% increase in EGD utilization observed among Medicare recipients

DOI: 10.1201/9780429322570-2

from 2000 to 2010 [1]. In a patient with nutritional disorders, an EGD can be a very useful diagnostic aid when used appropriately.

2.2.1 INDICATIONS

The indications for EGD in patients, with relevance to nutritional disorders include, but are not limited to:

- Iron deficiency
- Abdominal pain, especially symptoms that persist despite an appropriate trial of therapy
- Dysphagia or odynophagia
- Weight loss
- Persistent vomiting of unknown cause
- Chronic diarrhea or malabsorption
- Assess small bowel bacterial overgrowth (SIBO)
- Unintentional weight loss

In patients with severe anorexia and weight loss, EGD may also be used for placement of feeding tubes (e.g., nasojejunal tube, percutaneous endoscopic gastrostomy [PEG], direct percutaneous endoscopic jejunostomy [DPEJ]).

2.2.2 CONTRAINDICATIONS

The absolute contraindications for EGD include:

- Perforated bowel
- Toxic megacolon
- Peritonitis

Some relative contraindications for EGD are:

- Coagulopathy, severe thrombocytopenia, or impaired platelet function
- Severe neutropenia
- Increased risk of perforation including connective tissue disorders, recent bowel surgery, or bowel obstruction

2.2.3 PRE-PROCEDURE PREPARATION

Routine EGDs in the United States are performed in the outpatient setting with patients under sedation. Emergent or urgent procedures may be done at the hospital bedside or in an endoscopy suite. Preparation for elective EGD, as is indicated for most patients with nutritional disorders, involves a period of fasting, with a minimum of 2 hours after ingestion of clear liquids, 6 hours after ingestion of light meals, and 8 hours of fasting after regular meal [2]. Most medications are continued before the procedure, with the exception of anti-thrombotic agents. The duration of discontinuing anti-thrombotic agents prior to the procedure depends on the class of the agent and has been elaborated in the American Society for Gastrointestinal Endoscopy practice guidelines [3].

2.2.4   PRE-PROCEDURE ANTIBIOTICS

The use of antibiotics prior to performing an EGD is no longer recommended except in PEG tube placement. Antibiotics covering cutaneous sources of bacterial infection such as intravenous cefazolin being administered 30 minutes before the procedure has been shown to decrease rate of peristomal infection [4].

2.2.5   BRIEF DESCRIPTION OF PROCEDURE

An EGD is performed using a gastroscope, which is 9–10 mm in diameter for a standard adult scope and 5 mm for a pediatric scope. The gastroscope also has an instrument channel, through which various accessories including biopsy forceps and polypectomy snares can be inserted. During an EGD, examination of the mucosal surfaces of the esophagus and esophagogastric junction, stomach, and duodenum up to the third portion is performed. Biopsies may be obtained from suspicious sites as well as routine biopsies from designated sites.

EGD is employed for both diagnostic and therapeutic purposes. Mucosal abnormalities, strictures, masses, etc. can be inspected. Targeted and random biopsies can be obtained to help in establishing diagnosis, as in celiac disease.

Common therapeutic functions include:

- Polypectomy
- Dilation of strictures
- Stent placement
- Removal of foreign bodies
- Treatment of GI bleeding with hemoclip, injection, banding, coagulation, and sclerotherapy
- Endoscopic therapy dysplasia or early cancer
- Closure of gastrocutaneous fistulas

2.2.6   COMPLICATIONS

The documented adverse event rates are 1 in 200 to 1 in 10,000, and mortality rates range from none to 1 in 2000 [5]. The majority of the complications are cardiopulmonary adverse events related to sedation and analgesia. Other complications include infections and transient bacteremia, bleeding, and perforation. Procedures performed during EGDs, like dilations, polypectomy, percutaneous endoscopic enteral access, and endoluminal therapy, carry their own complications; however, EGDs are still considered low-risk procedures and are well tolerated.

2.3   ENTEROSCOPY

An extension of EGD that helps evaluate the small bowel is push enteroscopy. This examines that part of the small bowel that is 50 to 150 cm distal to the ligament of Treitz. Newer techniques like deep small bowel enteroscopy (double or single balloon enteroscopy) permit evaluation of the small bowel by using insertion techniques that pleat the small bowel onto an overtube. The advantage of using enteroscopy over capsule endoscopy is that along with visualization, there is also capability for interventional therapy.

2.4   CAPSULE ENDOSCOPY

Video capsule endoscopy is a procedure that helps to visualize the GI tract by transmitting images wirelessly from a disposable capsule to a data recorder worn by the patient. There are multiple small bowel capsules (PillCam SB, EndoCapsule, MiRo capsule, and CapsoCam), one esophageal capsule (PillCam ESO), and a colonic capsule (PillCam Colon) available. Capsule endoscopy is a diagnostic procedure only, with no therapeutic capabilities. It is used to visualize the mucosal surface of the GI tract.

2.4.1   INDICATIONS

The indications for capsule endoscopy include:

- Evaluation of obscure GI bleeding and/or iron deficiency anemia in a patient in whom upper and lower endoscopy have not identified a cause
- Evaluation of the small bowel in patients with known or suspected Crohn's disease
- Screening and surveillance of the small bowel in patients with inherited polyposis syndromes
- Suspected small intestinal pathology, like tumors or malabsorptive syndromes

2.4.2   CONTRAINDICATIONS

Contraindications to capsule endoscopy include, but are not limited to:

- Patients who cannot cooperate with swallowing of the capsule or who may inadvertently damage the equipment
- Swallowing disorders or dysmotility
- Strictures, fistulae, or bowel obstruction
- Patients with defibrillators or pacemakers (except CapsoCam)
- Pregnancy

2.4.3   PRE-PROCEDURE PREPARATION

Preparation for a capsule endoscopy is similar to that for a colonoscopy. It includes being on a clear liquid diet the day prior to the procedure with an overnight period of fasting. The use of a bowel preparation the night before the procedure is recommended by some societies. Some centers also use prokinetic agents such as metoclopramide and erythromycin, and anti-foaming agents such as simethicone.

2.4.4 BRIEF DESCRIPTION OF PROCEDURE

The patient is provided with a sensor belt which gathers the capsule's transmitted images, and then told to swallow the capsule with water in an upright position. In some cases, the capsule may be placed in the stomach or duodenum endoscopically using a device (AdvanCE capsule endoscopy delivery device).

2.4.5 COMPLICATIONS

Capsule endoscopy is one of the safest procedures for endoscopic visualization. The largest risk is retention of the capsule within the GI tract, in which case it is recommended to obtain a plain abdominal radiograph to confirm passage if the capsule is not seen in the cecum.

2.5 COLONOSCOPY/SIGMOIDOSCOPY

Colonoscopy is a procedure that examines the rectum, colon, and a portion of the terminal ileum using an endoscope. Sigmoidoscopy reaches from the rectum up to the splenic flexure, allowing visualization of the left side of the colon only. These are increasingly popular, with over 3.3 million outpatient colonoscopies being performed annually in the United States [1]. They allow evaluation of large bowel pathology and offer therapeutic interventions when needed.

2.5.1 INDICATIONS

Indications for colonoscopy include [6]:

- Evaluation of an abnormality on an imaging study
- Evaluation of GI bleeding
- Presence of fecal occult blood
- Unexplained iron deficiency anemia
- Screening and surveillance for colon neoplasia
- Evaluation of patients with chronic inflammatory bowel disease of the colon, since more precise diagnosis, or determination of the extent of activity of disease will influence management
- Clinically significant diarrhea of unexplained origin
- Colonic decompression as in acute colonic pseudo-obstruction

2.5.2 CONTRAINDICATIONS

Colonoscopy and sigmoidoscopy are contraindicated in the following situations [7]:

- Severe coagulopathy, severe thrombocytopenia, severe neutropenia
- Highly uncooperative or agitated patients, including patients who refuse the required colonic preparation

- Tense ascites or severe abdominal distention
- Peritonitis, bowel perforation, or colonic necrosis
- Toxic megacolon and fulminant colitis
- Acute diverticulitis and diverticular abscess

2.5.3   PRE-PROCEDURE PREPARATION

Prior to elective colonoscopy, a low-residue diet, or clear liquids for at least one day is recommended. The duration of discontinuing anti-thrombotic agents prior to the procedure depends on the class of the agent and has been elaborated in the American Society for Gastrointestinal Endoscopy practice guidelines [3]. Per the American Society of Anesthesiologists guidelines, preparation for elective procedure involves a period of fasting, with a minimum of 2 hours after ingestion of clear liquids and 6 hours after ingestion of light meals and 8 hours after regular meal [2]. Because the risk of infection related to routine diagnostic or therapeutic colonoscopy is low, antibiotic prophylaxis is not recommended for colonoscopy. Lastly, good bowel preparation is critical for colonoscopy because the diagnostic accuracy and therapeutic safety of colonoscopy depends on it. Specific bowel regimens depend on the practice and provider preference, however the ASGE recommends split-dose regimens for all patients with a portion of the preparation taken within 3 to 8 hours of the procedure to enhance colonic cleansing and patient tolerance [8].

2.5.4   BRIEF DESCRIPTION OF PROCEDURE

The patient is positioned in the left lateral decubitus position. The first step is inspection of the perianal region and digital rectal examination. A colonoscope is then inserted into the rectum with air insufflation, suctioning of residual fluid, and pulling back of the colonoscope to enable visualization. Examination of the large bowel up to the terminal ileum is performed, and other interventions like polypectomy, treatment of bleeding lesions, and dilations may also be performed.

Along with evaluation of the large bowel, the following therapeutic interventions can be performed:

- Treatment of bleeding lesions (e.g., vascular malformation, ulceration, neoplasia, and polypectomy site)
- Foreign body removal
- Excision or ablation of lesions
- Decompression of acute megacolon or sigmoid volvulus
- Balloon dilation of stenotic lesions (e.g., anastomotic strictures)
- Palliative treatment of stenosing or bleeding neoplasms (e.g., laser, electro-coagulation, stenting)

2.5.5   COMPLICATIONS

Colonoscopies are generally safe, with a low rate of complications (severe complications have been found at a rate of 2.8 per 1000 examinations [9]). Common complications including perforation, bleeding, infection, and complications related to anesthesia.

2.6 ENDOSCOPIC ULTRASOUND

Endoscopic ultrasound (EUS) is an endoscopic examination that uses a type of endoscope that contains an ultrasound transducer in order to evaluate the upper and lower GI tract. It is especially useful to evaluate the mediastinum as well as the pancreas, which may be a concern in patients with nutritional disorders. The use of fine needle aspiration (FNA) and fine needle biopsy (FNB) along with EUS provides valuable pathological information for sites that are not otherwise easily accessible.

2.6.1 INDICATIONS

The indications for performing EUS include [10, 11]:

- Tumor staging of the GI tract, pancreas, bile ducts, and mediastinum
- Evaluating abnormalities of and sampling tissue of lesions within or adjacent to the GI tract wall
- Evaluation of abnormalities of the pancreas and biliary tree

2.6.2 CONTRAINDICATIONS

Contraindications to EUS are similar to those described for EGDs (see previous).

2.6.3 PRE-PROCEDURE PREPARATION

The pre-procedure preparation for EUS is similar to those described for EGDs (see previous). The ASGE recommends use of antibiotics before EUS-FNA of mediastinal cysts and advises against administration of prophylactic antibiotics before EUS-FNA of pancreatic and peripancreatic cystic lesions [11]. For EUS performed in the lower GI tract, bowel preparation similar to colonoscopy is used (see the following).

2.6.4 BRIEF DESCRIPTION OF PROCEDURE

EUS is performed similar to EGDs, and the endoscope is advanced to emit sound waves which create a precise image of surrounding tissue, including the mediastinum, stomach, small intestine, pancreas, bile ducts, lymph nodes, and liver. When the target structure is identified, a biopsy or FNA can be taken. It can also be used in the lower GI tract when advanced through the rectum.

EUS guided interventions include:

- Placement of radiologic (fiducial) markers into tumors within or adjacent to the wall of the GI tract
- Treatment of symptomatic pseudocysts by creating an enteral-cyst communication
- Providing access into the bile ducts or pancreatic duct, either independently or as an adjunct to ERCP
- Celiac plexus block or neurolysis

2.6.5 COMPLICATIONS

Complications for EUS and FNA are rare. Many complications are similar to those of EGDs; therapeutic procedures may have their own small risk of complications, including pancreatitis for those undergoing pancreatic biopsy.

2.7 ENDOSCOPIC RETROGRADE CHOLANGIOPANCREATOGRAPHY (ERCP)

ERCP is an advanced technique that combines the use of endoscopy and fluoroscopy to evaluate the biliary or pancreatic ductal systems. A specialized side-viewing upper endoscope is guided into the duodenum, allowing for instruments and contrast to be passed into the bile and pancreatic ducts, permitting their radiologic visualization, and allowing for a variety of therapeutic interventions. Due to advances in cross-sectional imaging and advent of EUS, ERCP is rarely done for diagnostic purposes.

2.7.1 INDICATIONS

The indications for ERCP as are follows [12]:

- Suspected biliary obstruction with or without jaundice
- Pancreatic duct stricture
- Pancreatic duct leak (e.g., necrotizing pancreatitis), pseudocyst
- Manometric evaluation of the sphincter of Oddi

2.7.2 CONTRAINDICATIONS

Contraindications to EUS are similar to those described for EGDs (see previous). In addition, coagulopathies and active pancreatitis are relative contraindications.

2.7.3 PRE-PROCEDURE PREPARATION

ERCPs are performed with sedation both in the outpatient and inpatient settings. If an intervention is anticipated, coagulation studies and a complete blood count should be ordered. Coagulation studies are also recommended for patients with active bleeding, a known or suspected bleeding disorder (including a history of abnormal bleeding), an increased risk of bleeding due to medication use (e.g., ongoing anticoagulant use, prolonged antibiotic use), or other conditions associated with acquired coagulopathies. The duration of discontinuing anti-thrombotic agents prior to the procedure depends on the class of the agent and has been elaborated in the American Society for Gastrointestinal Endoscopy practice guidelines [3]. Per the American Society of Anesthesiologists guidelines, preparation for elective procedure involves a period of fasting, with a minimum of 2 hours after ingestion of clear liquids, 6 hours after ingestion of light meals, and 8 hours of regular diet [2].

2.7.4 PRE-PROCEDURE ANTIBIOTICS

Pre-procedure antibiotics for ERCP are recommended for known or suspected biliary obstruction in which complete relief of the obstruction is not anticipated, or in patients undergoing immunosuppression after liver transplantation, patients with active bacterial cholangitis, patients with pancreatic pseudocysts, or in any patients with additional concerns about the risk of infection [13].

2.7.5 BRIEF DESCRIPTION OF PROCEDURE

The initial procedure is similar to an EGD. After advancing the endoscope into the duodenum, the Ampulla of Vater is visualized and a cannula is inserted into it. Radiocontrast is injected into the bile ducts and/or pancreatic duct, and the entire system is visualized fluoroscopically. When needed, sphincterotomy may be performed by a sphincterotome. Procedures like stent insertion, stone removal, and cyst drainages may be performed.

2.7.6 THERAPEUTIC INTERVENTIONS

ERCP is not used as a diagnostic procedure anymore due to advances in cross-sectional imaging, advent of EUS, and high risk of complications. However, it is widely used as therapeutic procedure as in the following:

- Biliary sphincterotomy
- Stent placement across benign or malignant strictures, fistulae, postoperative bile leak, or in high-risk patients with large unremovable common duct stones
- Dilation of ductal strictures and balloon dilation of the papilla
- Nasobiliary drain placement
- Pancreatic pseudocyst drainage, stent of pancreatic duct leak
- Ampullectomy of adenomatous neoplasms of the major papilla
- Facilitation of cholangioscopy and/or pancreatoscopy

2.7.7 COMPLICATIONS

ERCP poses a higher potential for serious complications than any other standard endoscopic technique [14]. Complications include pancreatitis (most common), bleeding, sepsis, and perforation. These are in addition to complications related to anesthesia.

2.8 MODIFIED BARIUM SWALLOWING STUDY (MBSS)

The MBSS, also known as a video fluoroscopic swallow study, is a noninvasive, contrast-enhanced radiographic study to evaluate anatomy and swallowing physiology. It provides both anatomical and functional information. It analyzes swallowing through three phases: oral, pharyngeal, and upper esophagus.

2.8.1 INDICATIONS

The most common indication for an MBSS is dysphagia. Patients are usually evaluated prior to an MBSS by a speech-language pathologist (SLP) with a bedside swallow study. If appropriate after the clinical evaluation, the patient is referred for an MBSS.

Patients may also be directly sent for an MBSS, including new tracheostomy placements and those for whom it is necessary to rule out an esophageal leak.

2.8.2 CONTRAINDICATIONS

The contraindications to an MBSS are similar to those for an esophagram (see following).

2.8.3 PRE-PROCEDURE PREPARATION

Routine MBSSs in the United States are performed both in the inpatient and outpatient settings with very little preparation. Patients may be asked to maintain a period of fasting for 2–6 hours.

2.8.4 BRIEF DESCRIPTION OF PROCEDURE

Patients are presented with a series of the barium products, from thin to thick in consistency, and from a lower volume to higher volume; specifically, 5 mL thin liquid, graduating to 15 mL thin liquid, then a single sip from a cup or straw, then continuous sips from a cup or straw, progressing similarly to nectar, to honey, to pudding, and finally, to a cookie dipped in pudding. Radiographic images are taken while swallowing, using a lateral and AP view, and interpreted in real time by both the SLP and the radiologist. If a disorder is identified during the study, the SLP can implement a compensatory posture or maneuver to attempt to change the swallowing dynamics on the next swallow of the same volume/consistency.

2.8.5 COMPLICATIONS

Complications after an MBSS are very rare and include hypersensitivity of barium and aspiration.

2.9 ESOPHAGRAM

The (barium) esophagram is a noninvasive, contrast-enhanced radiographic study to evaluate the upper gastrointestinal tract. It can assist in diagnosis of both structural and functional issues [15]. It provides anatomical information (including diverticula, strictures, ulcers, polyps, masses) and helps evaluate swallowing function and esophageal motility. When esophageal perforation or tracheoesophageal fistula is suspected, Gastrografin is used instead of barium as a contrast agent to reduce risk of chemical pneumonitis.

2.9.1 INDICATIONS

The indications for a barium esophagram mainly include patients with symptoms of dysphagia or dysmotility.

2.9.2 CONTRAINDICATIONS

The contraindications to a barium esophagram include:

- Patients who cannot swallow and/or protect their airway
- Suspected esophageal perforation (Gastrografin can be used)
- Suspected acute, chemical esophageal injury
- Barium allergy

2.9.3 PRE-PROCEDURE PREPARATION

Routine esophagrams in the United States are performed in the outpatient setting with very little preparation. Patients may be asked to maintain a period of fasting for 2–6 hours.

2.9.4 BRIEF DESCRIPTION OF PROCEDURE

The test is performed by having the patient swallow approximately 3–7 oz of barium contrast while undergoing X-ray or fluoroscopy, a continuous X-ray beam. The radiologist will then evaluate the imaging to determine any structural abnormalities of the esophagus. The test is considered abnormal if reflux, tertiary contractions, retention of barium in the esophagus, or other abnormalities are observed. In a timed barium esophagram, images will be obtained at specific intervals after the patient swallows the barium. The physician will evaluate the height and width of the barium column to assess the esophageal emptying. For most individuals, if the barium has not emptied from the esophagus in one minute, then further tests are warranted to characterize the dysmotility.

2.9.5 COMPLICATIONS

Esophagrams are generally very well-tolerated procedures. Rare complications include:

- Nausea and emesis (commonly within 30 mins of procedure)
- Hypersensitivity to barium
- Aspiration
- Extravasation into mediastinum

2.10 HIGH-RESOLUTION MANOMETRY

High-resolution manometry (HRM) is used for the evaluation of esophageal motility disorders. HRM is indicated in patients with dysphagia, gastroesophageal reflux disease prior to anti-reflux surgery, and other cases with suspected dysmotility. It uses 36 longitudinally distributed sensors to conduct simultaneous pressure readings within both sphincters and the esophageal body. Measurements like the integrated relaxation pressure (assesses esophageal-gastric junction relaxation with swallowing), the distal contractile integral (assesses distal esophageal contraction), and the distal latency (assesses premature distal esophageal contraction) help to identify dysmotility. HRM is an outpatient procedure performed without sedation.

2.11   FUNCTIONAL LUMEN IMAGING PROBE (FLIP)

Functional Lumen Imaging Probe (FLIP) is a new addition to the gamut of tests available for motility evaluation. It is indicated in patients with achalasia, GERD, upper esophageal sphincter function, esophageal motility, gastroparesis, and anorectal dysmotility. It uses high-resolution impedance planimetry to evaluate the functional geometry and cross-sectional area/pressure relationship (i.e., distensibility) [16]. This has been used in the evaluation of the esophageal sphincters and body, the pyloric and anal sphincters. The device is a catheter with a balloon mounted on the distal end, which is placed across the lower esophageal sphincter or pylorus and then used to conduct sequential measurements of cross-sectional area and pressure. FLIP is an advanced procedure indicated only in a few cases with complex disease or to monitor improvement with interventions. FLIP is an outpatient procedure usually performed under sedation.

2.12   GASTRIC EMPTYING SCINTIGRAPHY

This is a test used for evaluating delayed gastric transit and gastroparesis. Standard tests involve the use of a solid and/or a liquid nutrient meal containing radioisotope. Some centers utilize real eggs or omelets with higher fat content to test for gastroparesis. Imaging is performed immediately after and at 1, 2, and 4 hours following ingestion. Using the standard egg meal, delayed gastric emptying is defined as gastric retention of >10% at 4 hours and/or >60% at 2 hours [17]. Optimal gastric emptying tests show good correlation between the delayed gastric emptying and symptoms.

2.13   SMARTPILL™

The SmartPill™ motility testing system uses a capsule that measures pressure, pH, transit time, and temperature as it passes through the entire gastrointestinal tract. It provides information including gastric emptying time, colonic transit time, whole gut transit time, and pressure patterns from the antrum and duodenum. These newer technologies are the future for motility testing.

2.14   AMBULATORY pH TESTING

Ambulatory pH testing is used in the diagnosis of gastroesophageal reflux disease (GERD). There are two types of testing available: 24-hour pH monitoring using a trans-nasal catheter and the 48- or 96-hour wireless BRAVO® capsule test. Both provide valuable ambulatory pH monitoring information.

2.14.1 INDICATIONS

pH testing is specifically indicated in patients with proton pump inhibitor (PPI)-refractory GERD, which is defined as persistent symptoms after 4-week standard dosage and 8-week high-dosage PPI therapy. However, in patients with alarm features (i.e., new-onset dyspepsia at age greater than 60, dysphagia, odynophagia, weight loss, bleeding, anemia, persistent vomiting), a trial of PPI therapy is not necessary and the work-up should directly proceed to early endoscopy.

2.14.2 CONTRAINDICATIONS

The contraindications for 24-hour pH monitoring include:

- History of nasal surgery or trauma
- History of underlying bleeding diathesis or concurrent use of anticoagulants

The contraindications for the wireless BRAVO capsule include:

- Pregnancy patients
- History of underlying bleeding diathesis or concurrent use of anticoagulants
- Known esophageal strictures, varices, diverticula
- Known severe esophagitis with intestinal metaplasia

2.14.3 PRE-PROCEDURE PREPARATION

Patients should be instructed to be fasting for 4–6 hours before procedure. In most cases, patients are asked to stop any anti-reflux therapy before the test, as follows:

- PPI therapy: 7 days prior to procedure
- H2 receptor blocker therapy: 2 days prior to procedure
- Antacids: 6 hours prior to procedure

In cases in which the patient has a known history of refractory GERD and the indication for pH testing is to diagnose weakly acidic (non-acid) reflux, PPI therapy may be continued.

2.14.4 BRIEF DESCRIPTION OF PROCEDURE

In the 24-hour catheter-based testing, a probe is placed trans-nasally into the esophagus and taped to the side of the face. The pH sensors are positioned 5 cm above the lower esophageal sphincter (LES), and impedance measurements are taken for 24 hours.

For a 48- or 96-hour BRAVO capsule test, a small pH capsule is attached to the esophageal wall 6 cm above the lower esophageal sphincter guided by endoscopy or manometry catheter to determine the distance of LES. The capsule naturally falls off the wall of the esophagus and is eliminated via feces.

Both tests have recording devices and the patient needs to record symptoms.

2.14.5 COMPLICATIONS

Ambulatory pH monitoring is a low risk procedure; however, it carries a small risk of nasal trauma (catheter-based testing), or capsule retention (BRAVO testing).

2.15 HYDROGEN BREATH TESTING

Hydrogen breath testing is utilized to diagnose small intestinal bacterial overgrowth (SIBO) and carbohydrate malabsorption by measuring the gases produced in the intestine, which are then diffused into the systemic circulation and expired through the lungs. Patients will be asked to limit starches and sugars the day prior to testing and fast for 8 to 12 hours. Antibiotics should be avoided for 4 weeks prior to testing and certain medications may be held. For the test, the patient will ingest carbohydrates, primarily glucose or lactulose, and breath samples will be obtained every 15 minutes for up to 3 hours and hydrogen concentration measured. A rise of greater than or equal to 20 parts per million from baseline in hydrogen by 90 minutes is considered to suggest the presence of SIBO. Breath testing is a simple and safe method to identify patients with SIBO.

2.16 ENTERAL ACCESS

In patients who need long-term enteral feeding, the use of more permanent enteral feeding tubes has become common. These include percutaneous endoscopic gastrostomy (PEG), direct percutaneous endoscopic jejunostomy (DPEJ), and trans-gastric jejunostomy tube (PEG-J).

A PEG tube is a flexible feeding tube placed through the abdominal wall and into the stomach.

A DPEJ tube is a flexible feeding tube placed through the abdominal wall and into the jejunum.

A PEG-J is a PEG tube with a trans-gastric jejunostomy tube, through which a jejunal extension tube allows post-pyloric feeding.

2.16.1 INDICATIONS

Permanent enteral feeding tubes are indicated in patients requiring enteral feeding for more than 4 to 5 weeks.

Usually, PEG or gastrostomy or G tubes are the initial feeding tube of choice. Use of a PEJ or PEG-J may be indicated instead of PEG in the following cases:

- In patients who have upper gastrointestinal dysmotility, in which case tethering a PEG tube to the anterior abdominal wall can potentially worsen gastroesophageal reflux
- In patients who cannot tolerate gastrostomy feeds

2.16.2 PRE-PROCEDURE PREPARATION

Patients should be instructed to be fasting as for other endoscopic procedures. Most medications are continued before the procedure, with the exception of anti-thrombotic agents (duration depending on class of drug).

2.16.3 BRIEF DESCRIPTION OF PROCEDURE

PEG, DPEJ, and PEG-Js are placed endoscopically using procedural sedation or anesthesia. The endoscope is passed through the mouth into the stomach (PEG) or small bowel (DPEJ) to identify proper position for the feeding tube guided by transillumination of scope light through the abdominal wall, finger indentation, and needle aspiration. Then a small incision is made on the abdominal wall for placement of the feeding tube. The PEG can be converted to PEG-J either by passing smaller caliber J-extension (two-piece PEG-J) through the PEG or a single-piece PEG-J which has gastric and jejunal ports which can be used for venting and feeding, respectively. Feeding can be started 4 hours after placement of the tube.

2.16.4 COMPLICATIONS

Complications of enteral tube placement include:

- Pain at the tube site
- Leakage of stomach contents around the tube site
- Dislodgment or malfunction of the tube
- Infection of the tube site
- Aspiration (more commonly with PEG tubes)
- Bleeding
- Perforation

2.17 CONCLUSION

The number and technology of available GI tests and procedures is rapidly evolving. These should be selected appropriately, using suitable inputs from the gastroenterologist. When used in the correct clinical context, they can aid greatly in the diagnosis and management of nutritional disorders.

REFERENCES

1. Peery AF, Dellon ES, Lund J, Crockett SD, McGowan CE, Bulsiewicz WJ, Gangarosa LM, Thiny MT, Stizenberg K, Morgan DR, et al. Burden of gastrointestinal disease in the United States: 2012 update. Gastroenterology. 2012;143(5):1179–87 e3.
2. Practice guidelines for preoperative fasting and the use of pharmacologic agents to reduce the risk of pulmonary aspiration: Application to healthy patients undergoing elective procedures: An updated report by the American Society of Anesthesiologists task force on preoperative fasting and the use of pharmacologic agents to reduce the risk of pulmonary aspiration. Anesthesiology. 2017;126(3):376–93.
3. Committee ASOP, Acosta RD, Abraham NS, Chandrasekhara V, Chathadi KV, Early DS, Eloubeidi MA, Evans JA, Faulx AL, Fisher DA, et al. The management of antithrombotic agents for patients undergoing GI endoscopy. Gastrointest Endosc. 2016;83(1):3–16.
4. Lipp A, Lusardi G. Systemic antimicrobial prophylaxis for percutaneous endoscopic gastrostomy. Cochrane Database Syst Rev. 2006(4):CD005571.
5. Committee ASOP, Ben-Menachem T, Decker GA, Early DS, Evans J, Fanelli RD, Fisher DA, Fisher L, Fukami N, Hwang JH, et al. Adverse events of upper GI endoscopy. Gastrointest Endosc. 2012;76(4):707–18.

6. Rex DK, Schoenfeld PS, Cohen J, Pike IM, Adler DG, Fennerty MB, Lieb JG, 2nd, Park WG, Rizk MK, Sawhney MS, et al. Quality indicators for colonoscopy. Am J Gastroenterol. 2015;110(1):72–90.

7. Cappell MS, Friedel D. The role of sigmoidoscopy and colonoscopy in the diagnosis and management of lower gastrointestinal disorders: Technique, indications, and contraindications. Med Clin North Am. 2002;86(6):1217–52.

8. Committee ASOP, Saltzman JR, Cash BD, Pasha SF, Early DS, Muthusamy VR, Khashab MA, Chathadi KV, Fanelli RD, Chandrasekhara V, et al. Bowel preparation before colonoscopy. Gastrointest Endosc. 2015;81(4):781–94.

9. Whitlock EP, Lin JS, Liles E, Beil TL, Fu R. Screening for colorectal cancer: A targeted, updated systematic review for the U.S. preventive services task force. Ann Intern Med. 2008;149(9):638–58.

10. Dumonceau JM, Polkowski M, Larghi A, Vilmann P, Giovannini M, Frossard JL, Heresbach D, Pujol B, Fernandez-Esparrach G, Vazquez-Sequeiros E, et al. Indications, results, and clinical impact of endoscopic ultrasound (EUS)-guided sampling in gastroenterology: European society of gastrointestinal endoscopy (ESGE) clinical guideline. Endoscopy. 2011;43(10):897–912.

11. Coe SG, Raimondo M, Woodward TA, Gross SA, Gill KR, Jamil LH, Al-Haddad M, Heckman MG, Crook JE, Diehl NN, et al. Quality in EUS: An assessment of baseline compliance and performance improvement by using the American Society for Gastrointestinal Endoscopy—American College of Gastroenterology Quality Indicators. Gastrointest Endosc. 2009;69(2):195–201.

12. Baron TH, Petersen BT, Mergener K, Chak A, Cohen J, Deal SE, Hoffinan B, Jacobson BC, Petrini JL, Safdi MA, et al. Quality indicators for endoscopic retrograde cholangiopancreatography. Am J Gastroenterol. 2006;101(4):892–7.

13. Alkhatib AA, Hilden K, Adler DG. Comorbidities, sphincterotomy, and balloon dilation predict post-ERCP adverse events in PSC patients: Operator experience is protective. Dig Dis Sci. 2011;56(12):3685–8.

14. Committee ASOP, Chandrasekhara V, Khashab MA, Muthusamy VR, Acosta RD, Agrawal D, Bruining DH, Eloubeidi MA, Fanelli RD, Faulx AL, et al. Adverse events associated with ERCP. Gastrointest Endosc. 2017;85(1):32–47.

15. Baker ME. Role of the barium esophagram in antireflux surgery. Gastroenterol Hepatol (N Y). 2014;10(10):677–9.

16. Carlson DA. Functional lumen imaging probe: The FLIP side of esophageal disease. Curr Opin Gastroenterol. 2016;32(4):310–8.

17. Tougas G, Eaker EY, Abell TL, Abrahamsson H, Boivin M, Chen J, Hocking MP, Quigley EM, Koch KL, Tokayer AZ, et al. Assessment of gastric emptying using a low fat meal: Establishment of international control values. Am J Gastroenterol. 2000;95(6):1456–62.

3 Digestion and Absorption

Matthew Kaspar

3.1 INTRODUCTION

Digestion and absorption of nutrients are accomplished by a number of organ systems working in concert to mechanically and chemically alter ingested exogenous substances into forms that can be utilized by the body. This assimilation of nutrients into the body is primarily performed by the gastrointestinal (GI) system and occurs through three distinct processes: (i) movement of food throughout the GI tract; (ii) mechanical and chemical digestion of food; and (iii) absorption of nutrients.

3.2 DIGESTION

Digestion is a form of catabolism whereby the complex chemical structures found in whole foods are broken down into small molecules that can be absorbed across the intestinal mucosa. Digestion occurs when food is moved through the digestive system. It begins in the mouth and continues, in one form or another, until ingested products exit the body as stool.

Digestion can be categorized as two basic types: mechanical and chemical.

3.2.1 MECHANICAL DIGESTION

Mechanical digestion is a purely physical process, whereby food is broken into smaller pieces by motion and force without significant chemical alteration. The resulting increase in mobility allows movement through the GI tract, and increased surface area of individual particles facilitates the processes of chemical digestion. In the mouth, mastication and tongue movements help break food into smaller pieces and mix food with saliva. Once a sufficient texture has been achieved, this slippery mass of partially digested food particles is then swallowed as a bolus.

The mechanical breakdown of food continues in the stomach. Muscular contractions of the stomach, primarily in the antrum, mash, mix, slosh, and propel food to further break it apart and expose more of its surface area to gastric acid. This creates chyme, an acidic, semiliquid material consisting of a mixture of gastric acid, digestive enzymes, and food particles no larger than 3 mm. Chyme is passed, in metered doses, from the stomach to the small intestine. There, it is subjected to two different types of muscular contractions: peristalsis and segmentation. Peristalsis is characterized by waves of smooth muscle contraction, which propel food forward

DOI: 10.1201/9780429322570-3

through the small bowel. In segmentation, *non-peristaltic* contractions isolate portions of the small bowel, forming temporary "sausage link" type segments that allow chyme to slosh food back and forth to promote mixing of the chyme and facilitate contact between all portions of enteric contents and the mucosal surface of the small intestine.

3.2.2 Chemical Digestion

Chemical digestion is the biochemical process by which macromolecules in food are transformed into smaller molecules that can be absorbed across the intestinal mucosa and transported to cells throughout the body. Substances in food that must be chemically digested include carbohydrates, proteins, lipids, and micronutrients. Carbohydrates must be broken down into simple sugars; proteins into small peptides and individual amino acids; lipids into fatty acids and glycerol; and some micronutrients, such as vitamins and trace elements, must be converted into a form suitable for transport across the intestinal mucosa. These processes are performed with the help of many different digestive enzymes. These enzymes are secreted by specialized exocrine glands (primarily the salivary gland and exocrine pancreas) or by the mucosal layer of various segments of the GI tract.

3.2.2.1 Absorption of Macronutrients

Almost all the components of food are completely broken down to their simplest units by the time they have transited the first 25 cm of the small intestine. By the time enteric contents have reached the proximal jejunum, proteins, carbohydrates, and lipids have been digested into amino acids, monosaccharides, and emulsified components of triglycerides, respectively. Additionally, micronutrients (vitamins, minerals, trace elements) have been converted into absorbable forms.

The absorptive capacity of the alimentary canal is immense. Each day, the alimentary canal processes up to 10 L of food, liquids, and GI secretions. Of these 10 L, approximately 2 L enter the large intestine and less than 200 mL are excreted as stool. The small intestine is presented with approximately 9–10 L of fluid to absorb daily, of which 2 L are dietary fluid and 7–8 L are secretions. Almost all ingested food, 80% of electrolytes, and 90% of water are absorbed in the small intestine. Although the entire small intestine is involved in the absorption of water and lipids, most absorption of fats, carbohydrates, and proteins occurs in the proximal jejunum. The architecture of the small intestinal mucosa and villi maximizes the potential surface area for absorption. The absorptive area of the small intestine is greater than 200 square meters, which is approximately the same area as a tennis court. The large surface area is achieved by the plicae circulares, villi, and microvilli. The stomach, on the other hand, does not have the same surface area. The only substances that are absorbed in the stomach in appreciable amounts are alcohol and aspirin (water is also absorbed here to some degree). By the time chyme reaches the large intestine, it has been essentially reduced to indigestible food residue (mainly plant fibers such as cellulose), waste products, water, and millions of bacteria.

3.3   CARBOHYDRATE DIGESTION AND ABSORPTION

Carbohydrates are classified according to the number of monomers they contain. Broadly, they can be considered as simple sugars (monosaccharides and disaccharides) or complex sugars (polysaccharides). All carbohydrates must be digested into one of three monosaccharides (glucose, galactose, or fructose) in order to be absorbed across the intestinal mucosa.

The chemical digestion of starches begins in the mouth with salivary amylase, which facilitates the conversion of long-chain carbohydrates into smaller sugars via cleavage of α-1,4 linkages within molecules of amylose and amylopectin. Salivary amylases are most active within a relatively neutral pH range, and as such, their action is impeded once the food bolus is acidified by gastric acid. Salivary amylase is responsible for ~30–40% of carbohydrate digestion.

In the small intestine of adults, pancreatic amylase does the "heavy lifting" for starch and carbohydrate digestion, because bonds between constituent sugars in carbohydrate molecules are hydrolyzed by pancreatic α-amylase to form the oligosaccharides maltose, maltotriose, and α-dextrins. Brush border enzymes are then responsible for further digestion of the oligosaccharides, breaking off one glucose unit at a time. Three brush border enzymes hydrolyze sucrose, lactose, and maltose into monosaccharides (Figure 3.1).

Sucrase splits sucrose into one molecule of fructose and one molecule of glucose. Maltase breaks down maltose and maltotriose into two and three glucose molecules, respectively. Lactase breaks down lactose into one molecule of glucose and one molecule of galactose. Insufficiency of any of these brush border enzymes can lead to maldigestion and malabsorption of the target sugar, leading to symptoms such as gas, bloating, and diarrhea.

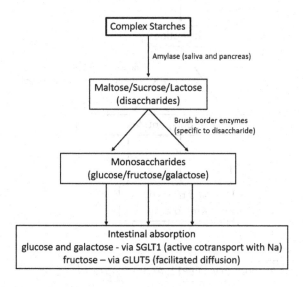

FIGURE 3.1   Carbohydrate digestion and absorption.

Carbohydrates are rapidly absorbed in the form of monosaccharides before reaching the terminal ileum. The small intestine absorbs monosaccharides at an estimated rate of 120 g/hour. Glucose and galactose are transported into the epithelial cells by common protein carriers via secondary active transport (sodium-glucose transporters [SGLT 1]). The monosaccharides leave these cells via facilitated diffusion and enter the capillaries through intercellular clefts. Fructose is unique in that it is absorbed and transported by facilitated diffusion alone via the GLUT5 transporter.

Carbohydrates that cannot be digested by the processes above are often called "fiber." These complex starches, such as cellulose, are passed relatively unaltered into the colon where they are digested in variable degrees by colonic bacteria. These products of bacterial digestion are primarily excreted as waste. However, some of these, primarily short-chain fatty acids (SCFAs), are absorbed by colonic enterocytes where they can be utilized as a source of "salvage" energy.

3.4 PROTEIN DIGESTION AND ABSORPTION

Proteins are polymers composed of amino acids linked by peptide bonds to form long chains. These complex molecules must be reduced to their constituent amino acids or di- and tripeptides in order to be absorbed. Digestion of protein starts in the stomach, where HCl and pepsin break proteins into smaller polypeptides. In the small intestine, endopeptidases (trypsin, chymotrypsin, elastase) hydrolyze internal polypeptide bonds (Figure 3.2).

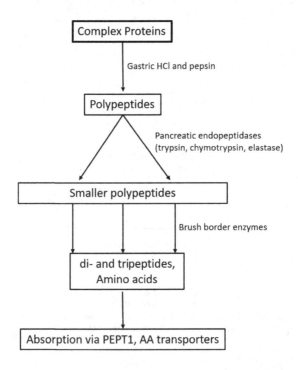

FIGURE 3.2 Protein digestion and absorption.

Pancreatic carboxypeptidases (the exopeptidases) hydrolyze the carboxy terminal and the amino terminal amino acids of the polypeptides. Finally, brush border enzymes such as aminopeptidase and dipeptidase further break down two- and three-peptide chains. Peptidase activity is highly sensitive to the ambient pH. For example, gastric pepsin requires a highly acidic environment, while pancreatic and small bowel enzymes are degraded in an acidic environment and rely on effective neutralization of gastric chyme by pancreatic bicarbonate and bile to function.

Products of protein digestion are absorbed with great affinity by specialized transporters in the proximal small bowel. Most of these are linked to the active transport of sodium. Short chains of two amino acids (dipeptides) or three amino acids (tripeptides) are transported actively via the PEPT1 transporter, while amino acids are absorbed by specialized transporters with varying affinities for each amino acid. However, after they enter the absorptive epithelial cells, all absorbed peptides (mono/di/tri) are broken down into their constituent amino acids before leaving the cell and entering the capillary blood.

Bacteria in the colon digest some of the remaining protein producing urea, which produces ammonia that is absorbed and transported to the liver. Nearly all the protein in stool comprises cellular or bacterial debris.

3.5 LIPID DIGESTION AND ABSORPTION

The most common dietary lipids are triglycerides, which include a glycerol molecule bound to three fatty acid chains. Relatively smaller amounts of dietary cholesterol and phospholipids are also consumed.

The three enzymes responsible for lipid digestion are lingual lipase, gastric lipase, and pancreatic lipase. The contribution of gastric lipase is small, but lingual lipase in adults hydrolyzes up to 30% of dietary fat. However, because the pancreas is the only consequential source of lipase, the majority of fat digestion occurs in the duodenum by pancreatic lipase. Pancreatic lipase, as well as bile secreted by the liver, breaks down each triglyceride into two free fatty acids and a monoglyceride. The resulting free fatty acids are classified according to the length of their carbon chains. SCFAs have less than 10–12 carbons in length and long-chain fatty acids have >12 carbons (Figure 3.3).

SCFA are relatively water soluble and can enter the absorptive cells (enterocytes) directly. Despite being hydrophobic, the small size of SCFAs enables them to be absorbed by enterocytes via simple diffusion and then take the same path as monosaccharides and amino acids into the blood capillary of a villus.

By contrast, the large and hydrophobic long-chain fatty acids and monoacylglycerides are not so easily suspended in the watery intestinal chyme. Bile salts and lecithin resolve this issue by enclosing them in a micelle, a tiny sphere with polar (hydrophilic) ends facing the aqueous environment and hydrophobic tails turned to the interior, creating a receptive environment for the long-chain fatty acids. The core also includes cholesterol and fat-soluble vitamins. Without micelles, lipids would sit on the surface of chyme and never come in contact with the absorptive surfaces of the epithelial cells. Micelles can easily squeeze between microvilli and get very near the luminal cell surface. At this point, lipid substances exit the micelle and are absorbed via simple diffusion.

The free fatty acids and monoacylglycerides that enter the epithelial cells are reincorporated into triglycerides. The triglycerides are mixed with phospholipids and

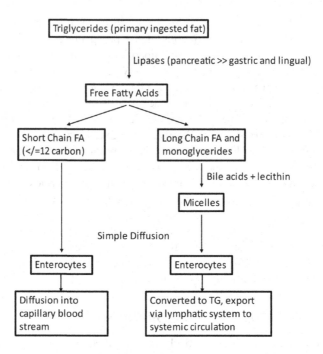

FIGURE 3.3   Fat digestion and absorption.

cholesterol and surrounded with a protein coat. This new complex, called a chylomicron, is a water-soluble lipoprotein. After being processed by the Golgi appara-
tus, chylomicrons are released from the cell. Too big to pass through the basement
membranes of blood capillaries, chylomicrons instead enter the large pores of lacteals. The lacteals come together to form the lymphatic vessels. The chylomicrons
are transported in the lymphatic vessels and empty through the thoracic duct into
the subclavian vein of the circulatory system. Once in the bloodstream, the enzyme
lipoprotein lipase breaks down the triglycerides of the chylomicrons into free fatty
acids and glycerol. These breakdown products then pass through capillary walls to
be used for energy by cells or stored in adipose tissue as fat. Liver cells combine the
remaining chylomicron remnants with proteins, forming lipoproteins that transport
cholesterol in the blood.

3.6   DIGESTION AND ABSORPTION OF MICRONUTRIENTS

Table 3.1 summarizes the absorption sites for micronutrients as well as additional
organs required for absorption/digestion.

3.7   WATER AND ELECTROLYTE ABSORPTION

Fluid absorption from the small and large bowel functions with 98% efficiency,
allowing only 100 to 200 mL to be excreted each day in the stool. This efficiency is
achieved by the unique tissue, cellular, and molecular architecture of the small and

TABLE 3.1

Anatomic Site	Micronutrients Absorbed	Additional Organs Required
Stomach	None significant	
Duodenum	• Calcium • Iron • Selected B vitamins (1, 2, 3, 5, 6) • Folate • Riboflavin • Fat-soluble vitamins • Trace metals	Pancreas
Jejunum	• Water-soluble vitamins • Fat-soluble vitamins • Trace elements	Pancreas
Ileum	• Vitamin B12	Salivary glands, stomach, pancreas
Colon	• Sodium, chloride, potassium • Vitamin K • Biotin	

large intestine in combination with regulatory mechanisms that include endocrine and paracrine hormones, neurotransmitters, immunomodulators, and luminal factors. When the balance is disturbed, as occurs with an enteric infection for example, electrolyte and water wasting (diarrhea) ensues.

All intestinal segments from the duodenum to the distal colon have mechanisms for transepithelial fluid movement, supported by a varied array of transporters encountered within them. For example, glucose- and amino acid-coupled transporters in the jejunum are well suited for absorption of large volumes of nutrients and water, but the cecum, proximal colon, and distal colon exhibit distinctly different transporters, with electrogenic Na^+ absorption in the distal colon accomplishing the final fluid extraction to prepare feces for excretion.

The paracellular space and junctional complexes between cells define the barrier function of epithelia. Epithelia with a low transepithelial voltage and low resistance are considered leaky, and those that exhibit a high transepithelial voltage and high resistance are considered tight. The tight junctions in villi have higher resistance than those in crypts, and transepithelial resistance increases in a cephalocaudal direction. Water movement across the epithelium can follow 4 routes: (1) diffusion through the lipid bilayer, or via proteins including (2) water channels, (3) uniporters, and (4) cotransporters. These include the apical Na^+-glucose transporter (SGLT), the urea transporter, and the Na^+/K^+-$2Cl^-$ cotransporter 1 (NKCC1).

In response to a meal, water is mostly absorbed by passive water permeability in combination with transport through SGLT1 and amino acid transporters on the apical membrane and exits the basolateral membrane via GLUT2 and the K^+-Cl^- cotransporter. Water movement across the intestine occurs under both isotonic conditions, when luminal and serosal osmolarity are 300 mOsm and when the luminal osmolarity increases in the upper small intestine in response to a meal. The classic explanation is that basolateral exit of glucose creates a hypertonic compartment in the paracellular space, thereby generating an osmotic gradient for fluid entry from the lumen. Transport across SGLT1 is electrogenic (2 Na^+ to 1 glucose) and transports galactose, but not fructose.

Osmolality is an important factor in patients receiving enteral nutrition. Compared with simple sugars, complex carbohydrates provide a significant number of calories with minimal osmolality. Similarly, absorption of dipeptides and tripeptides instead of single amino acids reduces intestinal osmolality. This balance between calories and osmolality becomes clinically relevant in effectively designing appropriate tube-feeding regimens and feeding patients with short bowel syndrome (SBS) or intestinal failure. Osmolality is also important in designing second-generation oral rehydration therapy (ORT) formulations; by replacing glucose with complex carbohydrates like rice, intestinal absorption is further stimulated by creating a hypotonic luminal environment, thereby enhancing water absorption.

Electrolyte and water absorption continue in the colon. The colon has a large reserve absorptive capacity for electrolytes and water, estimated to be 3 to 4 L/day of isotonic salt solution. Preservation of even part of the colon can reduce fecal electrolyte and water losses significantly in patients with SBS. Comparing patients with a jejunocolic anastomosis versus end jejunostomy, the latter group is less likely to require nutrition support.

4 Irritable Bowel Syndrome

Carol Ireton-Jones

4.1 INTRODUCTION

Irritable bowel syndrome, a functional gastrointestinal disorder, presents with multiple symptoms. The pathophysiology of IBS as well as current treatment options will be described; specifically, nutrition management with a FODMAP elimination diet. Implications of the low FODMAP diet in treatment of other GI disorders will be explored.

Irritable bowel syndrome (IBS) is a functional gastrointestinal (GI) disorder that involves abdominal pain and cramping, as well as changes in bowel movements (1). The Rome Foundation Global Study of Functional Gastrointestinal Disorders noted the prevalence of IBS ranges from 1.1 to 45% worldwide (2). Although more specifically, it has been estimated that 10–15% of adults in Europe and North America suffer from IBS/IBS symptoms (1). There is a greater prevalence in women. A diagnosis of IBS is based on the 2016 Rome IV criteria defining IBS as "a functional bowel disorder in which recurrent abdominal pain is associated with defecation or a change in bowel habits" (3–5) (https://theromefoundation.org/rome-iv/rome-iv-criteria/). The presence of disordered bowel habits is typical (i.e., constipation, diarrhea, or a mix of constipation and diarrhea), as are symptoms of abdominal bloating/distension occurring over at least 6 months and not less than 3 months (3–5). There are three IBS subtypes that include IBS-C (constipation), IBS-D (diarrhea), and IBS-M (mixed constipation and diarrhea) (5, 6). Typically, the diagnosis is made after other diagnoses such as celiac disease and inflammatory bowel disease that have been ruled out but pain and symptoms continue (5, 7). However, it should be noted that IBS or IBS-like symptoms may be observed in patients with other GI disorders such as celiac disease, IBD, and colitis (8, 9). Updated and revised medical information on diagnosis, structure, and interaction of "disorders of gut–brain interactions" are being further studied with an anticipated Rome V publication in 2026 (https://theromefoundation.org/rome-iv/rome-v/).

4.2 PATHOPHYSIOLOGY OF IRRITABLE BOWEL SYNDROME

IBS presentation of symptoms and their severity greatly varies from patient to patient. The symptoms include constipation, diarrhea, abdominal pain, bloating, gas, and urgency often without a known abnormal pathology (5, 10, 11). Patients also report that over time, symptoms can change and cross subgroups such as initially being

DOI: 10.1201/9780429322570-4

IBS-C and constipation-predominant to IBS-M that would also include diarrhea (7). Bloating, defined as the sensation of abdominal fullness and distention, resulting in an increase in abdominal girth, has been reported by more than 80% of patients with IBS; however, it is not reported by all (12). Symptoms also differ by gender with females reporting abdominal pain and constipation more often than males who report diarrhea (11, 13). In the United States, 5.9 million prescriptions annually are written for the treatment of IBS symptoms, with direct and indirect costs exceeding $20 billion, including missed work and increased physician visits (5, 14). Therefore, treatment requires an individualized approach.

It is thought that several separate gastrointestinal disorders may be universally called IBS, which accounts for the differences observed in symptoms, etiology, and pathophysiology (5, 15, 16). In the past, physicians treating IBS focused on abnormalities in GI motility, visceral sensation, brain–gut interactions, and psychosocial factors; however, none of these modalities accounted for symptoms in all IBS patients. Additional research has shown that an altered gut immune activation, diet, stress, and the intestinal and colonic microenvironment differ in patients with IBS and should be a consideration in the treatment provided (5, 16–18).

4.3   MANAGEMENT OF IRRITABLE BOWEL SYNDROME

Management of IBS begins with a diagnosis, typically provided by the gastroenterologist after listening to the patients' symptoms. "Red flag" signs which are not indictive of IBS alone include acute weight loss, fever, and blood in the stool (11). Often patients have had a protracted road to diagnosis of IBS and IBS is a diagnosis of exclusion, so a full diagnostic work-up including radiologic and endoscopic testing, comprehensive patient history, complete physical exam, and baseline laboratory tests is warranted (11). Upper endoscopy with biopsies for celiac disease, colonoscopy, and possibly a small bowel series may be done. Based on reported symptoms, testing for small intestinal bacterial overgrowth (SIBO) may also be indicated (19).

Management of IBS initially may be to utilize over-the-counter medications to resolve diarrhea or constipation, although this is most often when full testing has not been done and is early in the diagnostic process (5, 11). This includes the use of antidiarrheals, probiotics, and antispasmodics for diarrhea, and the use of fiber supplements and laxatives for constipation (11). If symptoms readily resolve and do not return, then no further action is required. However, in many IBS patients, symptoms have been present from months to years and diagnosis has been hard to determine. In patients such as these, management of symptoms with a specialized nutrition program is now being used as the first line of treatment (20).

4.4   NUTRITION INTERVENTIONS

The majority of patients with IBS report that food triggers symptoms; up to 90% restrict one or more types of food to help alleviate symptoms and symptom severity (21). Food intolerances and food sensitivity are frequently reported in patients with

IBS (5, 10). Through assessment of the commonly reported food intolerances, it was originally hypothesized that certain categories of foods cause an increase in susceptibility to Crohn's disease (22). This supposition further extended into the role of these food components in functional bowel disorders such as IBS. Foods identified to be associated with these symptoms are high in fermentable oligosaccharides, disaccharides, monosaccharides, and polyols which are carbohydrates that are poorly absorbed by the small intestine, are molecularly small and osmotically active, and are rapidly fermented by bacteria (16, 23). The GI effects from consumption of these foods results in excessive intestinal fluid, increased gas production, bowel distention, and bloating resulting in abdominal pain and diarrhea (16, 21, 23–25). The fermentation rate of these molecules is determined by the length of the carbohydrate chain (23). Foods can be classified within categories such as those with excess fructose (like some fruits), lactose-containing, oligosaccharides (e.g., fiber and beans), and polyol-containing foods.

Monash University in Australia coined a term for these foods as Fermentable, Oligosaccharides, Disaccharides, Monosaccharides, and Polyols known as FODMAPs (23, 26). Numerous studies have confirmed the biological feasibility and well-defined modes of action of these carbohydrates with evidence-based and efficacious diet interventions (20, 23, 26–28).

4.5 THE FODMAP ELIMINATION DIET

The FODMAP diet is a 3-phase diet plan of an initial elimination phase of all high-FODMAP foods for a specific period of time; then "phase 2" with a methodical and gradual reintroduction of eliminated, higher-FODMAP foods to determine tolerance based on symptoms; and finally "phase 3" or the personalization of the diet for each individual (10, 16, 20, 25, 28–30).

Foods high in FODMAPs that are more likely to cause GI distress are listed in Table 4.1.

The elimination of all high-FODMAP foods followed by reintroduction of these foods allows an individual to determine what specific foods cause the most distress, allowing for an individualized approach. It is important to note that the foods noted as high-FODMAP seem to "change" based on the resources used. This is because research into the FODMAP content of foods is ongoing and therefore data will change (11, 16). The Monash FODMAP app is an excellent tool for determining high-FODMAP foods and updated regularly. It also has foods from various countries that have been analyzed in the Monash lab (www.med.monash.edu.au/cecs/gastro/fodmap/iphone-app.html). The FODMAP elimination diet implemented by a skilled dietitian trained on the FODMAP diet principles and nuances has been identified as first-line therapy in managing IBS (10, 21, 27, 30, 31).

The ACG Clinical Guidelines on the Management of IBS states, "We recommend a limited trial of a low FODMAP diet in patients with IBS to improve global symptoms" (31). This is a conditional recommendation with very low quality of evidence related to the "complexity of the low FODMAP diet, combined with the potential for nutritional deficiencies, and the time and resources required to provide

TABLE 4.1
Food Groups Containing Higher FODMAP Foods

Food Group – FODMAP	High FODMAP-Containing Foods
Meat, Fish, Poultry, Oils (no FODMAPs) Moderate to lower fat	Marinated meats, processed meats (e.g., sausages, salami)
Dairy (Lactose – Disaccharide)	Milk (skim or whole), buttermilk, evaporated milk, ice cream, gelato, cottage cheese, custard, yogurt, American cheese, cream cheese, ricotta cheese (>1 T), Kefir, A2 Milk
Fruits (Fructose – Monosaccharides primarily, may contain polyols)	Nectarines, watermelon, plum, pomegranate ->1/3 c, prunes, dates; pears (pear juice), apples (apple juice, apple cider), blackberries, stone fruit – apricots, peaches, cherries, >1/2 c coconut, avocado >1/8
Cereals and Grains Fructoligosaccharides (FOS) (Fructans) *Note that some gluten-free flours contain FODMAPs	Wheat, barley, rye, wheat bran, almond meal, coconut or spelt flour, couscous, amaranth, buckwheat kernels Fiber: Inulin/FOS/Chicory root extract
Vegetables (Contain polyols, fructans, and galacto-oligosacccharides (GOS))	Jerusalem and globe artichokes, asparagus, brussels sprouts, cabbage (savoy), cauliflower, fennel (bulb), snow peas, sugar snap peas, mushrooms Garlic, leek, onion (1 T white onion is okay), shallot, white part of green onion, onion/garlic powder (foods containing garlic/onion) Pinto beans, kidney beans, lima beans, split peas, soybeans, pistachios, cashews, limit almonds (10 nuts)
Other	Molasses, agave, honey, high fructose corn syrup, ketchup, commercial salad dressing Balsamic vinegar – sparingly (2 T) Tahini paste – 1 T, Worcestershire sauce – 2 T Ingredients added to low-sugar or sugar-free foods for sweetness: Isomalt, sorbitol, xylitol, mannitol Oat milk, soy products such as soymilk

Source: Derived from FODMAP resources including the FODMAP app developed by Monash University. Dept. of Gastroenterology, Central Clinical School, Melbourne, Victoria, Australia. FODMAP composition of foods is continually being researched and updates may not be reflected on these pages.

proper counseling on the 3 phases of the plan, and it requires the services of a properly trained GI dietitian." Training is available for dietitians worldwide who would like to acquire expertise in this therapy through online training and mentoring by experts in the area, such as that from Monash University (www.monashfodmap.com/online-training/dietitian-course/). Understanding the carbohydrate components of the diet and how these affect digestion and symptom management is important.

4.6 OLIGOSACCHARIDES (FRUCTANS OR GALACTANS)

Fructans are linear-branched fructose polymers and naturally occurring carbohydrates that are found in onions, garlic, artichokes, some fruits, and cereals (23). Wheat is one of the main sources of fructans in the American diet. Inulin and fructo-oligosaccharides (FOS) are commercially used as fiber additives (20). Fructans, especially in patients with IBS, are not absorbed in the intestine and, as a result, reach the colon undigested and are fermented into gas and short-chain fatty acids (SCFAs) (21, 26). Galactans are naturally found in legumes, lentils, chickpeas, and red kidney beans, and function similar to fructans (21). Humans lack the enzyme needed to digest and absorb galactans, so galactans are rapidly fermented in the small intestine and produce gas (21). In the absence of IBS or GI compromise, fructans provide a readily available source of fiber to many people and therefore, when these are eliminated, other sources of fiber should be encouraged. Soluble fibers and those derived from psyllium husk are well tolerated in IBS. In addition, the modification of the fructan intake specifically affects prebiotic foods (including FOS) and therefore changes the microbiota (5, 16, 32). It is not clear if that is a negative effect.

4.7 DISACCHARIDES

Lactose is a disaccharide found in dairy products from cows, sheep, and goats (20). For the body to completely digest a lactose molecule, the enzyme lactase is needed. The enzyme lactase breaks down the disaccharide into a monosaccharide, glucose, and galactose molecule, which can then be absorbed. Malabsorption of lactose is common and can be confirmed with a hydrogen breath test; a lactose tolerance test may also be indicated (23, 33). Typically, lactose intolerance is dose-dependent; therefore small amounts of lactose may be well-tolerated. Lactose intolerance is not synonymous with dairy intolerance which indicates a whey or casein (protein) allergy. Avoidance of lactose-containing foods usually resolves symptoms if lactose intolerance is present, precluding the need for the breath hydrogen test in most cases.

4.8 MONOSACCHARIDES

Fructose is a monosaccharide found in fruit, honey, and high fructose corn syrup (1, 20). Food manufacturing in the United States is using more high fructose corn syrup and it is the main ingredient in a wide variety of foods and beverages, causing the overall consumption of fructose in the American diet to be on the rise. Two pathways are involved in the absorption of fructose: GLUT-2, which cotransports fructose with glucose via facilitated diffusion (the preferred high-capacity pathway) and GLUT-5 carrier-mediated diffusion, which is used and needed when an abundance of fructose is absorbed at once (16, 23, 27). Problems with digestion arise when fructose is present in excess of glucose and free fructose is in the intestinal lumen awaiting transport, causing limited absorption, and colonic fermentation (16). The average American consumes 55 g of fructose daily; however, most healthy adults can only absorb 15–25 g (26). To test a person's ability to completely absorb a fructose load, a hydrogen breath test is performed using a moderately high amount of fructose (35 g); however, if limiting high-fructose foods improves symptoms, a fructose malabsorption test is necessary only for confirmation (16).

4.9 POLYOLS

Polyols are a group of sugar alcohols naturally found in foods such as apples, pears, and mushrooms, and in polydextrose and isomalt (16, 23, 34.) They are also found in sugar substitutes including sorbitol, mannitol, maltitol, xylitol, and erythritol (34). Polyol consumption can cause laxative effects when consumed in excess because of slow and inadequate absorption in the small intestine (34). Only about one-third of polyols consumed are absorbed (27). They have an osmotic effect in the small intestine and are also fermented in the colon, resulting in GI distress (23, 34).

4.10 IMPLEMENTING THE FODMAP ELIMINATION DIET

There are three phases in the FODMAP elimination diet. The first phase (called the elimination phase) involves limiting or eliminating high-FODMAP foods from the diet for a period of 3–6 weeks. Often, patients see an improvement in symptoms within 2 weeks but elimination for 3–6 weeks allows for improvement in understanding which foods actually cause symptoms when these are added back. When counseling on the elimination phase of the diet, it is important to provide as many low-FODMAP food choices as possible. In the second phase (called the reintroduction or "challenge" phase), higher-FODMAP foods in each category (fructose, lactose, etc.) are added back into the diet in a methodical and organized way to identify symptoms associated with a particular food or class of foods (35). During the challenge phase, it is suggested to have the patient add back the foods they "missed" to determine the level of tolerance for favorite foods. It is during this "trial-and-error" time that the patient will understand the triggers of the FODMAP food and know which foods will cause symptoms. It is important to remember that although the high-FODMAP foods are associated with increased symptoms that may cause pain or discomfort, these are not food allergies and therefore will not cause a reaction such as anaphylaxis. During both phases of the FODMAP elimination diet, the expertise and support of a registered dietitian/nutritionist (RDN) to explain the diet as well as help with meal planning to avoid the potential for nutrient deficiencies is essential. The FODMAP diet is not a cure for IBS but a way of managing symptoms. The goal of the FODMAP elimination diet is to manage high-FODMAP food intake to allow a variety of food and nutrient intake, as tolerated. Foods that cause symptoms can be eliminated or limited.

Evidence has repeatedly shown that the low-FODMAP diet provides symptom relief for patients with IBS (5, 10, 20, 31). The effects on the GI tract of these foods and the relief of symptoms are reproducible and well documented. In a study of ostomy output in 12 individuals without IBS, consumption of a FODMAP diet showed increased weight and water content as well as ingested FODMAP materials with high-FODMAP intake still contained in the ostomy effluent (36). This did not occur with a low-FODMAP intake, demonstrating that the consumption of foods high in FODMAPs does have an osmotic effect and increases the amount of malabsorbed food particles. Following a low-FODMAP diet for 21 days has been shown to decrease the total intestinal bacteria and also significantly reduce prebiotic bacteria, including Bifidobacteria, and butyrate-producing bacteria (37). The reduction of total bacteria while following a low-FODMAP diet supports a theory that IBS symptoms may be due to bacterial overgrowth of the small intestine and that correction of this overgrowth can lead to symptom relief (20). A low-FODMAP diet does affect gut microbiota composition; however, the long-term implications of this are not yet known (37).

Overall, the current research shows that patients with IBS following a low-FODMAP diet see an improvement in GI symptom severity, particularly with abdominal pain, bloating, and flatulence. To date, there is no validated and reliable tool to assess gastrointestinal symptoms in relation to the phases of the FODMAP elimination diet in IBS patients. A valid and reliable tool to assess GI symptoms and their severity is needed. A new GI symptom assessment (GSS) tool specifically designed for IBS patients was used to assess symptoms prior to the low-FODMAP diet initiation and after following the diet for approximately one month (38). Although only a pilot study of 18 patients, the GSS confirmed changes in symptom severity between the two assessments as scored by the patients. The GSS not only provided feedback for the RDN but also for the patients to be able to see the magnitude of improvement they had experienced.

The FODMAP elimination diet is not the only component of the nutrition management of IBS; additional strategies should be addressed as well (11, 16). Carbonated beverages, chewing gum, and eating too may quickly result in gas and cause discomfort; so, these should be limited or avoided. Large meals may cause cramping and diarrhea; therefore, small meals, eaten more often (4–6 times per day) may improve IBS symptom management. Because a high-fat diet can slow down motility, a lower-fat diet may be better tolerated. Insoluble fiber is limited in the low-FODMAP diet; therefore, the importance of adding soluble fiber should be addressed to meet daily fiber needs.

4.11   OTHER FACTORS IN IBS MANAGEMENT

Nutrition assessment is an important component of the initial nutrition plan that should be completed by the dietitian prior to initiating the low-FODMAP diet (11) (see Chapter 1). Nutrition assessment should include a review of symptoms, presence of other diagnoses, and physical assessment; current medication history should also be evaluated.

Concomitant diagnoses should be managed as well, such as celiac disease, diabetes, or IBD. Previous diet interventions, history of intake, and non-traditional therapies should be evaluated because there is an increased incidence of disordered eating for patients suffering from GI disorders (39). Orthorexia is an obsessive and unsafe focus on foods perceived as healthy with patients at higher risk for this disorder when following diets specifically for digestive issues/intolerances (39). In this case a "simplified" or less restrictive approach to diet modification may be most beneficial.

Anxiety and stress are often confounding factors in IBS symptom occurrence and management. Medications including antianxiety, antispasmodics, laxatives, and antidiarrheal mediations may be a part of the treatment plan (11). Incorporation of the low-FODMAP diet with the medications may allow for discontinuation of the medications over time. Antianxiety medications play a role in the gut–brain connection and may be a valuable concomitant therapy (11, 16). Yoga was found to be equally as effective as the low-FODMAP diet in relieving symptoms in one study and can certainly be incorporated in overall IBS management (40). Stress reduction may take the form of meditation, acupuncture, or exercise – for example, walking, aerobic exercise, strength training. Exercise has been shown to improve GI motility, and adequate sleep can also improve the outcome.

Gut-directed psychotherapy has been found to be effective in improving symptom management for managing IBS provided by specially trained psychotherapists (41–43). A number of techniques may be employed in therapy to help reduce stress and feelings of anxiety.

Herbal therapies have been used in IBS and many of them have evidence-based data to support their use (11, 16). For example, iberogast and peppermint oil may help to improve global symptoms and reduce abdominal pain (16). Probiotics are currently being studied for application in IBS although data is variable and the most recent ACG Guidelines do not recommend probiotics for IBS management (19, 44).

Although not a symptom of IBS, small intestine bacterial overgrowth (SIBO) may be experienced by patients with IBS since it is associated with abdominal pain and diarrhea and motility changes in the GI tract (19). SIBO happens when bacteria from the large intestine enter the small intestine for reasons such as lack of an ileocecal valve, impaired motility, and long-term usage of PPIs. It remains unclear if the changes in motility affect the bacteria or the bacteria cause motility changes in the GI tract because the origin of SIBO in IBS is not fully understood. Current treatment for SIBO is with antibiotics; empiric treatment with antibiotics is commonly used even without breath testing although breath testing has been recommended by the ACG (19). The goal of the antibiotic therapy is to eliminate the excessive bacteria in the small intestine. During antibiotic therapy, probiotic therapy is not recommended. There is not a specific diet recommendation for SIBO (although many can be found on the Internet); however, the low-FODMAP diet has been suggested due to the decrease in symptoms from reducing fermentable products in the GI tract.

Another point to consider in management of IBS-like symptoms, such as bloating, gas, and diarrhea, that are not fully managed by therapies for IBS, is the presence of sucrase-isomaltase deficiency (45, 46). Congenital Sucrase-Isomaltase Deficiency (CSID) or Sucrase-Isomaltase Deficiency (SID) when found in adulthood is caused by genetic mutations in the SI gene which affects sucrose and disaccharide digestion and may cause symptoms similar to IBS (46). The diagnosis of CSID/SID is made through a carbon-13 (13C-sucrose) breath test, symptom development with sucrose ingestion, or endoscopic biopsy. Although rare, clinicians should consider this evaluation in refractory IBS cases (47).

IBS is considered a diagnosis of exclusion and diagnosis may be made based on the symptoms. The evidence for improvement in symptoms and therefore the function and quality of life in IBS confirms the implementation of the FODMAP elimination diet as a primary component of treatment. The goal of the elimination diet is firstly to avoid higher-FODMAP foods to reduce or eliminate symptoms over a period of time; secondly to reintroduce higher-FODMAP foods in a methodical manner to determine the foods that cause symptoms; and finally to liberalize or "personalize" the diet as much as possible. The dietitian plays a pivotal role in suggesting alternative foods and assuring nutrient needs are met initially and in the successful reintroduction and personalization of the nutrition plan. IBS requires a comprehensive management plan that centers on nutrition but incorporates other modalities as well.

REFERENCES

1. Lacy BE, Patel NK. Rome criteria, and a diagnostic approach to irritable bowel syndrome. J. Clin. Med. 2017;6:99. doi: 10.3390/jcm6110099 www.mdpi.com/journal/jcm).
2. Sperber AD, Bangdiwala SI, Drossman DA, et al. Worldwide prevalence and burden of functional gastrointestinal disorders, results of Rome Foundation global study. Gastroenterology. 2021 Jan;160(1):99–114.e3. doi: 10.1053/j.gastro.2020.04.014.
3. Schmulson MJ, Drossman D. What is new in Rome IV. J Neurogastroenterol Motil 2017 30;23(2):151–163.
4. Definition of Irritable Bowel Syndrome. Rome Foundation website. www.romecriteria. org/criteria/).
5. Chey WD, Kurlander J, Eswaran S. Irritable bowel syndrome: A clinical review. JAMA. 2015;313(9):949–958.
6. Engsbro AL, Simren M, Bytzer P. Short term stability of subtypes in the irritable bowel syndrome: Prospective evaluation using the Rome III classification. Aliment Pharmacol Ther. 2012;35(3):350–359.
7. Spiegel BM, Farid M, Esrailian E, Talley K, Chang L. Is irritable bowel syndrome a diagnosis of exclusion? A survey of primary care providers, gastroenterologists and IBS experts. Am J Reference on IBS and other GI diseases Gastroenterol. 2010;105(4):848–858.
8. Barros LL, Farias AQ, Rezaaie. Gastrointestinal motility and absorptive disorders in patients with inflammatory bowel diseases: Prevalence, diagnosis and treatment. World J Gastroenterol. 2019 August 21; 25(31): 4414–4426.
9. Testa A, Imperatore N, Rispo A, et al. Beyond irritable bowel syndrome: The efficacy of the low fodmap diet for improving symptoms in inflammatory bowel diseases and celiac disease. Dig Dis. 2018;36(4):271–280. doi: 10.1159/000489487. Epub 2018 May 15. PMID: 29763907.
10. Ireton-Jones C. Outcomes of nutrition intervention in IBS: Use of a symptom assessment tool. J Acad Nutr Diet. 2014;114(9):A27.
11. Ireton-Jones C, Weisberg MF. Management of irritable bowel syndrome: Physician-dietitian collaboration. Nutr Clin Pract. 2020 Oct;35(5):826–834. doi: 10.1002/ncp. 10567. Epub 2020 Aug 12. PMID: 32786046.
12. Ringel Y, Williams RE, Kalilani L, Cook SF. Prevalence, characteristics and impact of bloating symptoms in patients with irritable bowel syndrome. Clin Gastroenterol Hepatol. 2009;7(1):68–72.
13. Lovell RM, Ford AC. Effect of gender on prevalence of irritable bowel syndrome in the community: Systematic review and meta-analysis. Am J Gastroenterol. 2012;107(7): 991–1000.
14. Wolf WA, Kiraly LN, Ireton-Jones C. Incorporating FODMAP dietary restrictions: Help or hype? Current Nutrition Reports, published online July 11, 2015.
15. Ng QX, Soh AYS, Loke W, Lim DY, Yeo WS. The role of inflammation in irritable bowel syndrome (IBS). J Inflamm Res. 2018 Sep 21;11:345–349. doi: 10.2147/JIR.S174982. PMID: 30288077; PMCID: PMC6159811.

16. Matarese L, Mullin G, Roland B et al. The irritable bowel syndrome – Contemporary management strategies. J Parenter Enteral Nutr. 2014;38:781–799.

17. Holtmann G, Shah A, Morrison M. Pathophysiology of functional gastrointestinal disorders: A holistic overview. Dig Dis. 2017;35 Suppl 1:5–13. doi: 10.1159/000485409. Epub 2018 Feb 8. PMID: 29421808.

18. Weaver KR, Melkus GD, Henderson WA. Irritable bowel syndrome. Am J Nurs. 2017 Jun;117(6):48–55. doi: 10.1097/01.NAJ.0000520253.57459.01. PMID: 28541989; PMCID: PMC5453305.

19. Pimentel M, Saad RJ, Long MD, Rao SSC. ACG clinical guideline: Small intestinal bacterial overgrowth. Am J Gastroenterol. 2020;115:165–178.

20. Mansueto P, Seidita A, D'Alcamo A, et al. Role of FODMAPs in patients with irritable bowel syndrome: A review. Nutr Clin Pract. 2015;30(5):665–682.

21. Hayes PA, Fraher MH, Quigley EM. Irritable bowel syndrome: The role of food in the pathogenesis and management. Gastroenterol Hepatol (NY). 2014;10(3):164–174.

22. Gibson PR, Shepherd SJ. Personal view: Food for thought – Western lifestyle and susceptibility to Crohn's disease. The FODMAP hypothesis. Aliment Pharmacol Ther. 2005;21:1399–1409.

23. Gibson PR, Shepherd SJ. Evidence based dietary management of functional gastrointestinal symptoms: The FODMAP approach. J Gastroenterol Hepatol. 2010;25:252–258.

24. Bellini M, Tonarelli S, Mumolo MG, et al. Low fermentable oligo-, di- and mono-saccharides and polyols (FODMAPs) or gluten free diet: What is best for irritable bowel syndrome? Nutrients. 2020 Nov 1;12(11):3368. doi: 10.3390/nu12113368. PMID: 33139629; PMCID: PMC7692077.

25. Poortmans P, Kindt S. Diagnostic approach to chronic diarrhoea and recent insights in treatment of functional diarrhoea including irritable bowel syndrome. Acta Gastroenterol Belg. 2020 Jul–Sep;83(3):461–474. PMID: 33094595.1.

26. Khan MA, Nusrat S, Khan MI, et al. Low FODMAP diet for irritable bowel syndrome: Is it ready for prime time? Dig Dis Sci. 2015;60(5):1169–1177.

27. Gibson PR, Shepherd SJ. Food choice as a key management strategy of functional gastrointestinal symptoms. Am J Gastroenterol. 2012;107:657–666.

28. Shepherd SJ, Lomer MC, Gibson PR. Short-chain carbohydrates and functional gastrointestinal disorders. Am J Gastroenterol. 2013;108(5):707–717.

29. Halmos EP, Power VA, Shepherd SJ, et al. A diet low in FODMAPs reduces symptoms of irritable bowel syndrome. Gastroenterology. 2014;146(1):67–75 e65.

30. Ireton-Jones C. The low FODMAP diet: Fundamental therapy in the treatment of irritable bowel syndrome. Curr Opin Clin Nutr Metab Care. 2017;20(5):414–419.

31. Lacy BE, Pimentel M, Brenner DM, et al. ACG clinical guideline: Management of irritable bowel syndrome. Am J Gastroenterol. 2021 Jan 1;116(1):17–44.

32. van Lanen AS, de Bree A, Greyling A. Efficacy of a low-FODMAP diet in adult irritable bowel syndrome: A systematic review and meta-analysis. Eur J Nutr. 2021 Sep;60(6):3505–3522. doi: 10.1007/s00394-020-02473-0. Epub 2021 Feb 14. Erratum in: Eur J Nutr. 2021 Jun 28; PMID: 33585949; PMCID: PMC8354978.

33. Variu P, Gede N, Szakacs Z, et al. Lactose intolerance but not lactose maldigestion is more frequent in patients with irritable bowel syndrome than in healthy controls: A meta-analysis. Neurogastroenterol Motil. 2019;31(5):e13527.

34. Lenhart A, Chey WD. A systematic review of the effects of polyols on gastrointestinal health and irritable bowel syndrome. Adv Nutr. 2017 Jul 14;8(4):587–596. doi: 10.3945/an.117.015560. PMID: 28710145; PMCID: PMC5508768.

35. Vakil N. Dietary fermentable oligosaccharides, disaccharides, monosaccharides, and polyols (FODMAPs) and gastrointestinal disease. Nutr Clin Pract. 2018 Aug;33(4):468–475. doi: 10.1002/ncp.10108. Epub 2018 Jun 5. PMID: 29870082.

36. Barrett JS, Gearry RB, Muir JG, et al. Dietary poorly absorbed, short chain carbohydrates increase delivery of water and fermentable substrate to the proximal colon. Aliment Pharmacol Ther. 2010;31:874–882.
37. Halmos EP, Christophersen CT, Bird AR, et al. Diets that differ in their FODMAP content alter the colonic luminal microenvironment. Gut. 2015;64(1):93–100.
38. Heffernan-Swingle E, Radler D, Marcus A, et al. Change in self-reported gastrointestinal symptom severity and frequency following a registered dietitian counseling session for the management of irritable bowel syndrome. J Acad Nutr and Diet. 2016;116(9) Suppl: A74.
39. Tuck CJ, Sultan N, Tonkovic M, Biesiekierski JR. Orthorexia nervosa is a concern in gastroenterology: A scoping review. Neurogastroenterol Motil. 2022 Aug;34(8):e14427. doi: 10.1111/nmo.14427. Epub 2022 Jul 10. PMID: 35811419.
40. D'Silva A, MacQueen G, Nasser Y, et al. Yoga as a therapy for irritable bowel syndrome. Dig Dis Sci. 2019 Dec 12. doi: 10.1007/s10620-019-05989-6. [Epub ahead of print].
41. Lindfors P, Unge P, Arvidsson P, et al. Effects of gut-directed hypnotherapy on IBS in different clinical settings – results from two randomized, controlled trials. Am J Gastroenterol. 2012;107:276–285.
42. Peters SL, Muir JG, Gibson PR. Review article: Gut-directed hypnotherapy in the management of irritable bowel disease and inflammatory bowel disease. Aliment Pharmacol Ther. 2015 Jun;41(11):1104–1115.
43. Vasant DH, Whorwell PJ. Gut-focused hypnotherapy for functional gastrointestinal disorders: Evidence-base, practical aspects, and the Manchester protocol. Neurogastroenterol Motil. 2019;(31): [Epub ahead of print].
44. Su GL, Ko, CW, Bercik P, et al. AGA clinical practice guidelines on the role of probiotics in the management of gastrointestinal disorders. Gastroenterology. 2020. https://doi.org/10.1053/j.gastro.2020.05.059.
45. Henström M, Diekmann L, Bonfiglio F, et al. Functional variants in the sucrase-isomaltase gene associate with increased risk of irritable bowel syndrome. Gut. 2018; 67(2):263–270.
46. Garcia-Etxebarria K, Zheng T, Bonfiglio F, et al. Increased prevalence of rare sucrase-isomaltase pathogenic variants in irritable bowel syndrome patients. Clin Gastroenterol Hepatol. 2018;16(10):1673–1676.
47. Kim SB, Calmet FH, Garrido J, Garcia-Buitrago MT, Moshiree B. Sucrase-isomaltase deficiency as a potential masquerader in irritable bowel syndrome. Dig Dis Sci. 2020 Feb;65(2):534–540. doi: 10.1007/s10620-019-05780-7. Epub 2019 Sep 6. PMID: 31493040.

5 Inflammatory Bowel Disease

Neha D. Shah and Berkeley Limketkai

5.1 INTRODUCTION

Inflammatory bowel diseases (IBDs) are chronic inflammatory conditions of the gastrointestinal tract that includes Crohn's disease (CD) and ulcerative colitis (UC). The most common sites of inflammation in CD are the terminal ileum and cecum, although it can affect any segment of the gastrointestinal tract from the mouth to the anus.[1] CD may present with patchy areas of transmural inflammation and occasionally a "cobblestone" appearance along the intestinal mucosa. These phenomena can lead to the development of oral ulcers, abdominal pain, diarrhea, increased frequency of bowel movements, urgency, strictures, fistulas, and abscesses. Unlike CD, inflammation in UC is superficial and limited to the colon, although it may rarely affect the terminal ileum.[2] Inflammation with ulceration begins in the rectum and extends continuously (without patchiness) more proximally in two-thirds of patients. Similarly to CD, patients with UC may present with abdominal pain, diarrhea, and urgency although bloody diarrhea is more common with UC. Extraintestinal manifestations of inflammation can also arise in both CD and UC, such as uveitis, joint pain, primary sclerosing cholangitis, and skin lesions.

The highest incidence of IBD has been found in North America (CD: 20.2 per 100,000 person-years; UC: 19.2 per 100,000 person-years) and Europe (CD: 12.7 per 100,000 person-years; UC: 24.3 per 100,000 person-years).[3] Similarly, the highest prevalence of IBD has been found in North America (CD: 319 per 100,000 persons; UC: 249 per 100,000 persons) and Europe (CD: 322 per 100,000 persons; UC: 505 per 100,000 persons). For unclear reasons, the incidence and prevalence of IBD have been increasing worldwide, including in regions where IBD has not historically been commonly found. As the underlying hypothesized etiology of IBD is felt to result from the complex interplay between susceptible genes, the immune system, the host microbiome, and environment, researchers suspect changes in environmental triggers to have led to the increase in the incidence of IBD. Environmental factors that are considered to increase the risk of developing IBD are smoking, diet, drugs, geography, and stress.[4] Antibiotics, especially if given early in life, may also increase the risk of developing IBD.[5]

There has also been increased interest in the role of the microbiome in affecting IBD pathogenesis and severity.[5] The gut microbiota in patients with IBD tend to have reduced species diversity and a markedly distinct composition.[6] Unlike healthy intestines where *Firmicutes* and *Bacteroidetes phyla* predominate and contribute to the production of epithelial metabolic substrates, the microbiota in CD is characterized by a relative lack of *Firmicutes* and *Bacteroidetes* and an overrepresentation

DOI: 10.1201/9780429322570-5

of enterobacteria; in UC, there is a reduction of *Clostridioides* and an increase in *Escherichia coli*.[7] IBD patients appear to have an increase in mucosa-associated *E. coli* in both the ileum and colon, and their presence in granulomas suggests a pathogenic role.[8] Moreover, patients with CD were found to have an alteration in bacterial carbohydrate metabolism, and bacterial–host interactions in their ileum.[9]

5.2   ROLE OF DIET IN IBD

The potential role of diet for the treatment of IBD is based on the premises that (1) the diet can strongly influence the gut microbiota, which itself has been implicated in IBD pathogenesis[10]; and (2) certain foods may be pro- or anti-inflammatory.

Dietary fiber is an indigestible carbohydrate, a polysaccharide, found only in plant-based foods of whole grains, fruits, vegetables, and legumes. High intake of fiber in the form of fruits and vegetables may reduce the risk of CD, but not of UC. In a recent study, adult patients in remission with CD showed to have reduced risk of flares with a high-fiber intake than those patients who limited high-fiber foods.[11] The same study found no associations between patients with UC flares and fiber intake. As such, the global shift to a diet high in fat and sugar has been hypothesized as a culprit in the development of dysbiosis and increase in the worldwide incidence of IBD.[12, 13] In studies in which mice are fed a high-fat and high-carbohydrate diet, there was a resulting increase in *Firmicutes* and a decrease in *Bacteroidetes*.[14, 15] A meta-analysis of observational data also found a positive association between CD and a high intake of fat, polyunsaturated fatty acids, and n-6 polyunsaturated fatty acids (PUFAs).[16] On the other hand, a diet high in fruit and fiber, which has beneficial effects on the microbiome, seemed to be protective.[17] Children in Burkina Faso, Africa who are reared on a high-fiber, plant-based diet exhibit a vastly different gastrointestinal microbial community than children in Europe whose calories come from diets richer in sugar, fat, and protein.[12] In parallel, there is a very low incidence of IBD in Africa and a high incidence in Europe.[18] Although the cause and effect has not been proven, animal models have shown a causal role for diet-induced changes of gut microbes in the development of the disease.[19]

Short-chain fatty acids (SCFAs) are produced by fermentation of non-digestible carbohydrates via a subset of anaerobic bacteria in the human colon (primarily in the cecum and colon).[20] The SCFA butyrate has been shown to improve the intestinal defense mechanism by restoring mucosal integrity, stimulating MUC2 (mucin gene expression), in which its protein products are often altered in IBD, and modulating the expression of an antimicrobial peptide, cathelicidin.[21, 22] Early studies have also found that butyrate inhibits interleukin (IL)-12 production by stimulating monocytes, enhances IL-10 production, and inhibits IL-2.[23] A study performed using discordant twin pairs – one healthy and the other with CD – found differences in their ability to process carbohydrates.[24] The enzyme pathways involved in complex carbohydrate metabolism, which results in the production of SCFAs, were diminished in the twin with CD. Pathways involved in mucin degradation were also decreased in those with CD.

Besides the effects on the gut microbiome, the diet and its metabolites can exert pro- or anti-inflammatory properties. An earlier systematic review showed that a high consumption of n-6 fatty acids and meats is implicated with both CD and UC.[17] Foods high in n-6 PUFAs promote arachidonic acid metabolism and an increase in the production of the pro-inflammatory leukotrienes.[25] By contrast, n-3 PUFAs possess anti-inflammatory properties. Eskimos in Greenland, who are consumers of large amounts of n-3 PUFAs in fish oils, appear to have a low prevalence of IBD.[26, 27]

Patients often believe that IBD is caused by or can be cured by diet. The Internet is replete with dietary advice and many individuals may follow fairly restrictive diets. The European Society of Parenteral and Enteral Nutrition (ESPEN) published guidelines for nutrition management of IBD and overall, there is no specific diet recommended for IBD since the evidence is limited in efficacy of diet to induce or maintain remission.[28] Modifications to the diet are often recommended to alleviate symptoms in an active flare; however, every individual is different, and the tolerance may differ as well. A healthy and varied diet is recommended for all patients with IBD during remission, which includes fruits, vegetables, meat, olive oil, fish, and fiber.[29] In presence of intestinal stenosis, insoluble fiber is to be restricted.

5.3   MALNUTRITION IN IBD

Malnutrition is found in 65–75% in CD and 18–62% in UC.[30] Malnutrition in IBD is also associated with increased hospitalizations, length of stay, utilization of healthcare resources, and mortality rates.[31] The impact of malnutrition is based on the segment(s) of the bowel that is involved, duration of disease, and severity of disease activity. A main contributor to malnutrition in IBD is decreased nutritional intake.[30] Patients may limit or avoid intake of specific foods due to aggravation of symptoms such as nausea, abdominal pain, vomiting, and diarrhea in setting of active disease activity. Food avoidance patterns are more common in active flares than remission.[32] Other contributors include alterations in digestive and absorptive processes, presence of fistula(e), hypertrophy of villi, blind loops, bacterial overgrowth, bile salt malabsorption, medications, and protein-losing enteropathy.[28, 30] Sarcopenia, which involves a deterioration in muscle mass and strength, has also been associated with malnutrition in IBD.[30] A reduction in physical activity has also been seen with increased disease activity.[33] The barriers to physical activity in IBD were pain, fatigue, and sense of urgency. Quality of life related to physical and mental health has been shown to be significantly reduced in IBD patients with malnutrition.[34]

5.4   MICRONUTRIENT DEFICIENCIES IN IBD

Micronutrient deficiencies can arise in IBD in the setting of inflammation, malabsorption, and fistula output.[35] Medications can also interfere with absorption of micronutrients. Decreased nutritional intake and unintentional weight loss can further increase the risk of deficiencies. Deficiencies have also been shown to be present in patients who are in remission.[36] Due to risk, patients should be routinely screened for deficiencies. Micronutrients can be negative or positive acute phase reactants, and therefore, it is important to factor in that serum levels for micronutrients may elevate or reduce in setting of an inflammatory process.[37]

Anemia is the most common complication of IBD, and therefore, screening for anemia must be done routinely in IBD. Anemia may arise from a deficiency in iron, folate, or vitamin B12, with iron deficiency being the most common contributor.[38] Anemia of chronic disease can also arise due to inflammation. To screen for anemia, a complete blood count, ferritin, and C-reactive protein levels should be obtained to assist with interpretation. Ferritin levels can be elevated in an inflammatory process and levels less than 100 μg/L can be considered to be reflective of iron deficiency anemia. If mild iron deficiency anemia is present, iron supplementation is recommended with the goal of utilizing oral iron therapy initially. Intravenous iron should be considered in patients with active disease and with an intolerance to oral iron. Serum calcium and 25-hydroxy vitamin D levels should be routinely monitored in patients in active flares or who have utilized steroids in treatment. Supplementation should commence if needed to reduce risk of osteopenia and osteoporosis. Dual-energy X-ray absorptiometry (DXA) should be done to rule out osteopenia and/or osteoporosis. There is a risk for vitamin B12 deficiency when more than 60 cm of the terminal ileum has been removed in a surgical resection, which disrupts sites of vitamin B12 absorption.[39] Vitamin B12 supplementation should be administered when needed.

5.5 NUTRITION SCREENING

ESPEN has set recommendations that all patients with IBD should undergo screening for malnutrition in a timely manner to allow appropriate utilization of interventions for treatment.[28] Although there are various screening tools available, the three-step Malnutrition Universal Screening Tool (MUST) has been utilized to screen for malnutrition in IBD. The tool has already been validated in several patient populations, including medical, surgical, and oncology patients, and has been shown to predict mortality and length of stay of a hospital admission.[40] One study has shown that the MUST tool correlated with disease activity in CD.[41] Further studies are needed for UC. The tool assigns a score each to the BMI, to the percentage of weight loss, and to the effect of acute disease. The total score can range from 0, which indicates low risk, or 1 for medium risk, or greater than 2, which indicates high risk for malnutrition.

TABLE 5.1
Malnutrition Universal Screening Tool (MUST)

Step	Criteria	Score
Step I: Body Mass Index Score	BMI >20 and BMI >30	0
	BMI 18.5–20	1
	BMI <18.5	2
Step II: Weight Loss Score	Weight loss <5% in the past 3–6 months	0
	Weight loss 5–10% in the past 3–6 months	1
	Weight loss >10% in the past 3–6 months	2
Step III: Acute Disease Effect Store	Patient is feeling acutely ill and with poor intake of diet	2
	None	0

Add all the scores
Low Risk of Malnutrition = 0
Medium Risk of Malnutrition = 1
High Risk of Malnutrition = >2

Patients can easily use the tool to self-screen for malnutrition in IBD outpatient clinics.[42,43] The results from the self-screen were found to correlate to results obtained from the screen by providers.

5.6   NUTRITION ASSESSMENT

All patients screened to have or at risk for malnutrition should be referred to a registered dietitian specializing in IBD for a formal nutrition assessment.[28] The Academy of Nutrition and Dietetics (AND) defines nutrition assessment as a systematic process to gather, verify, and interpret data to assist with determining the cause of nutrition-relevant concerns.[44] A nutrition assessment encompasses a multidimensional evaluation of elements of patient history (medical, surgical, social), changes in anthropometrics (e.g., weight loss), findings from a nutrition-focused physical examination (e.g., loss of muscle mass), alterations in laboratory measurements (e.g., electrolytes, inflammatory markers, micronutrients), diagnostic tests (e.g., colonoscopy for disease activity), and a food/nutrition history (e.g., food intolerances, intake from each food group for adequacy).

The patient's goals and readiness to change are also factored into the nutrition assessment.

TABLE 5.2
Nutrition Assessment in IBD

Patient History	Demographics
	• Age
	• Sex
	• Language
	• Profession
	• Education
	Medical history
	• Signs/symptoms (e.g., GI symptoms, fatigue)
	• Medical history
	• Surgical history
	Social history
	• Socioeconomic status
	• Family and friend support
	• Housing status and environment
	• Psychological well-being
	• Quality of life
	Medication history
	• Prescription medications
	• Over-the-counter medications
	• Micronutrient supplements
	• Fiber supplements
	• Herbal supplements
	• Prebiotics and probiotics

TABLE 5.2 (*Continued*)
Nutrition Assessment in IBD

Anthropometrics	% Weight Change for Nutritional Significance
	% Weight Change = *Usual Body Weight – Current Body Weight* × *100/Usual Body Weight*
	Nutritional significance:
	• 2% weight change in 1 week
	• 5% weight change in 1 month
	• 7.5% weight change in 3 months
	• 10% weight change in 6 months
	Body mass index (BMI)
	• <18: Underweight
	• 19–25: Normal
	• 25–29: Overweight
	• 30–40: Obese
	• >40: Morbidly obese
Nutrition-Focused Physical Examination	Evaluate the following areas for physical appearance and note abnormalities:
	• Head
	• Hair
	• Eyes
	• Nose
	• Mouth
	• Nails
	• Skin
	• Musculoskeletal
Biochemical Data, Tests, and Procedures	• Complete metabolic panel
	• Micronutrient labs
	• Fecal calprotectin
	• Intake and output
	• Dual-energy X-ray absorptiometry
Food and Nutrition History	Food/fluid intake
	• Oral diet
	• Enteral or parenteral nutrition (if applicable)
	• Food allergies
	• Food intolerances
	• Intake from each food group (macronutrient and micronutrient intake)
	• Fluid intake
	• Food textures
	• Size, timing, and frequency of meals
	Nutrition-related beliefs
	• Source of information
	• Level and accuracy
	Food access
	• Ability to purchase food
	• Ability to prepare food
	Physical activity level
	• Types and frequency of aerobic activity
	• Types and frequency of muscle strengthening activity

Once the nutrition assessment is completed, a nutrition plan of care is developed to address goals and issues established from the assessment to aid in optimizing nutritional status. Nutrition education is provided to address any knowledge deficits (e.g., role of diet in IBD, foods and their portions to counteract symptoms, fluids to optimize hydration). Nutrition counseling is provided to address barriers to readiness to change that may interfere with implementation of the plan of care. Ongoing nutrition monitoring is indicated to modify the plan of care based on progress.

Energy requirements in IBD are similar to those of the general population[28]; however, caloric requirements should be individualized based on nutrition goals. Longitudinal studies are not available; however, a cross-sectional study showed that patients with an active disease did have an increase in the resting energy expenditure (REE), along with the disease location.[45] Disease severity is usually associated with exudative protein losses and loss of muscle mass. Protein requirements are increased to 1.2–1.5 gram/kg with active disease activity.[28] Once in remission, protein requirements are 1 gram/kg and are similar to those of the general population. If a patient has an increased fistula output, they may require an increased protein intake up to 1.5–2.0 gram/kg: however, there are no randomized studies assessing protein needs in this patient population.

5.7 DIETS OF INTEREST IN IBD

Diet should be individualized for each patient based on presence of nutritional impairments, severity of symptoms and level of disease activity. The claims and evidence should be discussed with the patient as well as the risks and benefits to assist with making an informed decision.

5.7.1 LOW FIBER DIET

Various types of fiber exist in the diet and its role in health is determined by the characteristic of the fiber. The primary characteristics of fiber are solubility, fermentability, and viscosity.[46] The Institute of Medicine has set Dietary Reference Intakes (DRI) for daily fiber intake for only healthy individuals, including infants, children, adolescents, and adults.[47] The guidelines do not set parameters for fiber intake in chronic disease. For a low-fiber diet, the type and amount of fiber to include is not clear from the literature. Some studies on the low-fiber diet established a daily intake of 10 grams of fiber.[48] However, the type of restricted fiber has not been included in the discussions. The diet will often restrict whole grains, beans, raw vegetables, nuts, fruit, and vegetable skins.

In IBD, the diet has been used to reduce stool output and frequency of bowel movements during active flares. There are minimal studies at this time.

5.7.2 LOW RESIDUE DIET

The term residue has been described in the literature in various ways. Earlier animal studies described residue as the presence of stool appearing after ingestion of foods and fluids as well as any food or fluid increasing the volume of stool.[49] In addition, crude fiber that consists of cellulose, hemicellulose, and lignin was referred to as residue. Since there are varying descriptions of residues, the low-residue diet may restrict non-fiber foods (e.g., dairy) in addition to fiber. Because there is no single description of residue available to assist with defining parameters for intake, AND removed the low-residue diet from the Nutrition Care Manual.[50]

The diet has been often utilized to reduce stool volume and frequency during active flares in IBD. The studies are also very limited overall. A study of 71 adult patients with active CD found no difference in outcomes related to surgery, hospitalizations, and partial obstruction between patients who stayed on the low-residue diet (elimination of whole grains, beans, lentils, fruits, vegetables, and nuts) and those who transitioned from the low-residue diet to a diet without restrictions.[51] Limiting residue in the form of fiber may not be needed due to positive tolerance to an unrestricted diet.

5.7.3 Low FODMAP Diet

FODMAPs (Fermentable Oligosaccharides, Disaccharides, Monosaccharides, and Polyols) refer to a cluster of short-chain fermentable carbohydrates and consists of the fructans, galactans, lactose, fructose, and polyols.[52] Not all carbohydrates are considered to be FODMAPs. Fructans and galactans are the oligosaccharides that are indigestible by humans and are found in wheat, garlic, onion, and beans. Lactose is a disaccharide of two monosaccharides glucose and galactose and found only in dairy. Fructose is a monosaccharide and is found in fruits, honey, and agave nectar. Polyols are the sugar alcohols and are found in stone fruits and artificial sweeteners. Osmotic activity is increased in the small bowel with presence of excess FODMAPs there, resulting in a constellation of symptoms, including abdominal pain, altered bowel habits, gas, or bloating. FODMAPs may also endure bacterial fermentation in the colon, resulting in production of excess gas.

There are three phases of the low FODMAP diet: elimination, reintroduction, and personalization. FODMAPs are categorized into three groups: low, moderate, and high FODMAPs. Consumption of FODMAPs is permitted; however, excess intake of FODMAPS is not. The elimination phase removes all high FODMAPs from the diet over 2–6 weeks. Consumption of low and moderate FODMAPs in appropriate portions is allowed. The reintroduction phase allows a trial of high-FODMAP foods to be brought back into the diet over 6–8 weeks to help identify threshold of tolerance to specific FODMAPs. The low-FODMAP diet continues during this phase concurrently. The personalization phase involves tailoring portions for all FODMAPs for tolerance to help expand variety in the diet.

The low-FODMAP diet has been primarily utilized in the treatment of irritable bowel syndrome (IBS) in which the studies have shown the diet to be effective in reducing functional symptoms associated with IBS. Functional symptoms may include abdominal pain, diarrhea, gas, bloating, and cramping. Given that symptoms are similar between IBS and IBD, there is interest in use of the low FODMAP diet in IBD. A study of 89 adult IBD patients (28 CD, 61 UC) in clinical remission or with mild-to-moderate active IBD with functional symptoms similar to IBS showed reduction in symptoms with the diet.[53] Another study evaluated patients with quiescent IBD that had symptoms associated with IBS and found that fructans worsened functional symptoms in patients with IBD whereas galactans and sorbitol did not.[54] The American Gastroenterological Association (AGA) has set guidelines which include a recommendation that the low FODMAP diet can be used as an option to assist with reducing functional symptoms in IBD.[55] Although studies have shown that the diet may aid in decreasing functional symptoms in IBD, it is not known at this time whether the diet can assist with reducing inflammation.

5.7.4 SPECIFIC CARBOHYDRATE DIET

The Specific Carbohydrate Diet (SCD) focuses on eliminating certain types of carbohydrates from the diet, all the disaccharides, oligosaccharides, and polysaccharides. The diet was initially utilized by Dr. Sidney Hass in the 1920s to treat celiac disease. Later in the 1950s, Elaine Gottschall, a Canadian biochemist, had her young 8-year-old daughter with ulcerative colitis follow the diet in hopes to treat it. After her daughter had a resolution of symptoms with the diet, she later wrote of the diet in her book *Breaking the Vicious Cycle* to outline the phases of the diet and provided recipes that can be used to help implement the diet.[56] The diet has set claims that inflammation and injury to the gastrointestinal tract can result from bacterial fermentation of poorly digested disaccharides, oligosaccharides, and polysaccharides and, therefore, these carbohydrates must be eliminated from the diet altogether to allow the gastrointestinal tract to heal. All grains, high lactose dairy, starchy vegetables, and foods sweetened with sucrose are not allowed on the diet. The only carbohydrates allowed in the diet are monosaccharides because monosaccharides do not require digestion prior to absorption. Foods of meat, poultry, fish, eggs, lactose-free dairy, fresh fruits, non-starchy vegetables, and honey are permitted for consumption. While symptoms persist, the diet is to be followed for one year and then once symptoms resolve, the diet is to be followed for another year. Reintroduction of other foods can proceed afterwards. If symptoms arise again, then the diet should be resumed until symptoms resolve.

The small studies have primarily evaluated the SCD diet in pediatric patients with Crohn's disease. The influence of the diet on mucosal healing was assessed in an earlier prospective study of nine pediatric patients with active CD. After following the diet for 12 weeks, all patients experienced clinical remission and showed significant improvements in mucosal healing based on findings from capsule endoscopy.[57] The diet continued to be followed up to 52 weeks by seven patients in which two patients maintained mucosal healing. Additional studies in pediatric patients with CD on the diet retrospectively showed a reduction in laboratory markers of inflammation.[58, 59] The studies are less robust in adults. An online survey completed by 417 adult patients with IBD (47% CD, 43% UC, and 10% indeterminate colitis) experienced improvement in abdominal pain and diarrhea after following the SCD diet for 2 months (33%).[60] The reduction in symptoms was sustained after following the diet for 12 months (42%). Further studies are needed to evaluate the usefulness of the diet on mucosal healing.

5.7.5 MEDITERRANEAN DIET

The Mediterranean diet is mainly a plant-based diet rich in fiber, phytonutrients, and unsaturated fats (mono- and polyunsaturated fats).[61] The diet encourages daily intake of beans, lentils, nuts, whole grains, fruits, and vegetables. Although fish is allowed for consumption as a source of animal protein, the consumption of meat, eggs, and dairy is to be reduced since these foods have higher amounts of saturated fat. Consumption of concentrated sweets is also less. Olive oil is the primary oil used. The diet also includes guidelines for how often the food groups should be consumed for daily or weekly consumption.

The use of the Mediterranean diet is of interest in IBD to reduce inflammation due to its abundance in nutrients deemed anti-inflammatory. A recent prospective study showed that adherence to the diet was associated with a lower risk of developing CD. Further studies are needed.[62]

5.8 NUTRITION SUPPORT IN IBD

5.8.1 ENTERAL NUTRITION

Enteral nutrition (EN) can be considered as an alternative treatment modality to immunosuppressive medications to induce remission in CD. Although the mechanism of action is not yet clear, EN has been proposed to aid in mucosal healing in CD by altering the microbiome, reducing intestinal permeability, restoring epithelial barrier function, and decreasing inflammatory cytokines in CD.[63] In children and adolescents with active CD, EN should be considered as first-line therapy.[28] Although EN can also be considered for adults, the therapy is not often offered to adults due to concern of adherence.

EN in the form of polymeric enteral formulas can be given as oral nutrition supplements (ONS) or can be administered through a feeding tube in CD. A recent Cochrane review suggests no differences in efficacy of inducing remission with polymeric, semi-elemental, or elemental formulas;[64] therefore, for palatability, polymeric formulas are recommended to give to patients for consumption. Patients who require long-term EN previously have done well with percutaneous gastrostomy (PEG) and jejunostomy (PEJ) feeding tubes, despite concerns that placement of the feeding tube would result in fistula formation.[65]

EN traditionally has been utilized as exclusive enteral nutrition (EEN) whereby EN meets 100% of nutrition needs. EEN is usually given for a duration of 4–6 weeks before oral diet is commenced again.[66] Earlier studies have shown that both pediatric and adult patients with CD without immunosuppressive medications on EN achieved mucosal healing and had a reduction in inflammatory cytokines.[67, 68] EEN may reduce the indication for surgery in CD patients that have strictures. A study that had patients do EEN prior to surgery found that compared to controls, patients on EEN had a significant decrease in C-reactive protein levels, duration of surgery, and reduced risk of postoperative abscess and/or anastomotic leak.[69]

Because EEN requires complete avoidance of oral diet, partial enteral nutrition (PEN) can also be considered when EN is used to supplement oral diet. A recent study compared tolerance and sustained remission with EEN to PEN in supplementation to a whole food diet in pediatric patients with active CD for 12 weeks.[70] The diet, the Crohn's Disease Exclusion Diet (CDED), eliminates foods that were thought to potentially alter the microbiome, intestinal barrier, and intestinal immunity. The EN formula used was Modulen (Nestle Science). Patients were randomly assigned into two groups: EEN for 6 weeks and then to an unrestricted diet with 25% PEN for another 6 weeks; or CDED with 50% PEN for 6 weeks and then CDED with 25% PEN for another 6 weeks. Compared to EEN, the patients tolerated the CDED in combination with PEN better and achieved remission with being free of corticosteroid use sooner. Reductions in fecal calprotectin and C-reactive protein levels were seen as well.

5.8.2 PARENTERAL NUTRITION

Parenteral nutrition (PN) has been traditionally used in IBD to serve as a sole source of nutrition to allow bowel rest in the midst of a flare. The purpose of bowel rest is to eliminate interactions of nutrients from the oral diet that could be potentially inflammatory to the bowel.[71] The studies are limited with this practice. In an earlier study, no differences were found in the rate of surgical interventions in UC patients, while PN patients with CD colitis on bowel rest showed a reduction.[72] In another earlier study that placed CD patients on PN for bowel rest, or on EN or on PN along with an oral diet, no differences were found in one-year remission rates between all the patients.[73] PN is overall indicated when the patient is not able to consume sufficient intake from oral diet and EN is not medically feasible to assist with meeting caloric needs. PN can be considered in combination with EN if the patient is able to tolerate EN, but not able to use EN to meet greater than 60% of caloric needs.[28] Patients with short bowel syndrome, high output stomas, and proximal fistulas will have impaired digestion and absorption of oral nutrients and are then likely candidates for PN, even for the long term. Lack of enteral access also serves as an indication for PN in patients that have obstructive bowel, and a feeding tube is not able to be placed beyond the obstruction. Perioperative PN can be used in patients who are severely malnourished prior to surgery.[74]

5.9 CONCLUSION

Nutrition care plays a pivotal role for patients with IBD, in active flares as well as in remission. New and innovative therapies for optimizing the microbiome and the diet continue to be the focus. There is no specific diet to induce or maintain remission in IBD because the evidence is limited.[28] In a flare, diet can be modified to reduce symptoms that arise with active disease. Tolerance can vary from person to person and therefore diet is individualized. EN can be considered for active CD. PN can be considered if EN is contraindicated. In remission, a diet filled with variety is recommended, which includes all the food groups for fruits, vegetables, meat, olive oil, fish, and fiber.

REFERENCES

1. Baumgart DC, Sandborn WJ. Crohn's disease. *Lancet.* 2012;380(9853):1590–1605.
2. Ungaro, R, Mehandru, S, Allen PB, Peyrin-Biroulet L, Colombel, JF. Ulcerative colitis. *Lancet.* 2017;389(10080):1756–1770.
3. Molodecky NA, Soon S, Rabi DM, et al. Increasing incidence and prevalence of the inflammatory bowel diseases with time, based on systematic review. *Gastroenterology.* 2012;142(1):46–54.
4. Loftus Jr EV. Clinical epidemiology of inflammatory bowel disease: Incidence, prevalence, and environmental influences. *Gastroenterology.* 2004;126(6):1504–1517.
5. Shaw SY, Blanchard JF, Bernstein CN. Association between the use of antibiotics and new diagnoses of Crohn's disease and ulcerative colitis. *Am J Gastroenterol.* 2011;106(12):2133–2142.
6. Sokol H, Lay C, Seksik P, Tannock GW. Analysis of bacterial bowel communities of IBD patients: What has it revealed? *Inflamm Bowel Dis.* 2008;14(6):858–867.
7. Martinez C, Antolin M, Santos J, et al. Unstable composition of the fecal microbiota in ulcerative colitis during clinical remission. *Am J Gastroenterol.* 2008;103(3):643–648.
8. Ryan P, Kelly RG, Lee G, et al. Bacterial DNA within granulomas of patients with Crohn's disease – detection by laser capture microdissection and PCR. *Am J Gastroenterol.* 2004;99(8):1539–1543.
9. Erickson AR, Cantarel BL, Lamendella R, et al. Integrated metagenomics/metaproteomics reveals human host-microbiota signatures of Crohn's disease. *PloS One.* 2012;7(11):e49138.
10. Sonnenburg ED, Sonnenburg JL. Starving our microbial self: The deleterious consequences of a diet deficient in microbiota-accessible carbohydrates. *Cell Metab.* 2014;20(5):779–786.
11. Brotherton CS, Martin CA, Long MD, Kappelman MD, Sandler RS. Avoidance of fiber is associated with greater risk of Crohn's disease flare in a 6-month period. *Clin Gastroenterol Hepatol.* 2016;14(8):1130–1136.
12. De Filippo C, Cavalieri D, Di Paola M, et al. Impact of diet in shaping gut microbiota revealed by a comparative study in children from Europe and rural Africa. *Proc Natl Acad Sci.* 2010;107(33):14691–14696.
13. Ng SC, Tang W, Ching JY, et al. Incidence and phenotype of inflammatory bowel disease based on results from the Asia-Pacific Crohn's and colitis epidemiology study. *Gastroenterology.* 2013;145(1):158–165.
14. Turnbaugh PJ, Bäckhed F, Fulton L, Gordon JI. Diet-induced obesity is linked to marked but reversible alterations in the mouse distal gut microbiome. *Cell Host Microbe.* 2008;3(4):213–223.
15. Zhang C, Zhang M, Wang S, et al. Interactions between gut microbiota, host genetics and diet relevant to development of metabolic syndromes in mice. *ISME J.* 2010;4(2):232–241.
16. Donnellan CF, Yann LH, Lal S. Nutritional management of Crohn's disease. *Ther Adv Gastroenterol.* 2013;6(3):231–242.
17. Hou JK, Abraham B, El-Serag H. Dietary intake, and risk of developing inflammatory bowel disease: A systematic review of the literature. *Am J Gastroenterol.* 2011;106(4):563–573.
18. Lakatos L, Lakatos PL. Changes in the epidemiology of inflammatory bowel diseases. *Orv Hetil.* 2007;148(5):223–228.
19. Leone VA, Cham CM, Chang EB. Diet, gut microbes, and genetics in immune function: Can we leverage our current knowledge to achieve better outcomes in inflammatory bowel diseases? *Curr Opin Immunol.* 2014;31:16–23.

20. Wong JM, De Souza R, Kendall CW, Emam A, Jenkins DJ. Colonic health: Fermentation and short chain fatty acids. *J Clin Gastroenterol.* 2006;40(3):235–243.
21. Willemsen L, Koetsier M, Van Deventer S, Van Tol E. Short chain fatty acids stimulate epithelial mucin 2 expression through differential effects on prostaglandin E1 and E2 production by intestinal myofibroblasts. *Gut.* 2003;52(10):1442–1447.
22. Moehle C, Ackermann N, Langmann T, et al. Aberrant intestinal expression, and allelic variants of mucin genes associated with inflammatory bowel disease. *J Mol Med.* 2006;84(12):1055–1066.
23. Säemann MD, Böhmig GA, Österreicher CH, et al. Anti-inflammatory effects of sodium butyrate on human monocytes: Potent inhibition of IL-12 and up-regulation of IL-10 production. *FASEB J.* 2000;14(15):2380–2382.
24. Eaton SB, Konner M, Shostak M. Stone agers in the fast lane: Chronic degenerative diseases in evolutionary perspective. *Am J Med.* 1988;84(4):739–749.
25. Jeffery N, Newsholme E, Calder P. Level of polyunsaturated fatty acids and the n-6 to n-3 polyunsaturated fatty acid ratio in the rat diet alter serum lipid levels and lymphocyte functions. *Prostaglandins Leukot Essent Fatty Acids.* 1997;57(2):149–160.
26. Kromann N, Green A. Epidemiological studies in the Upernavik district, Greenland: incidence of some chronic diseases 1950–1974. *Acta Med Scand.* 1980;208(1-6):401–406.
27. Bang H, Dyerberg J, Sinclair HM. The composition of the Eskimo food in northwestern Greenland. *Am J Clin Nutr.* 1980;33(12):2657–2661.
28. Bischoff SC, Bager, P, Escher J, et al. ESPEN guideline: Clinical nutrition in inflammatory bowel disease. *Clin Nutr.* 2023;42(3):352–379.
29. Lucendo AJ, De Rezende LC. Importance of nutrition in inflammatory bowel disease. *World J Gastroenterol WJG.* 2009;15(17):2081.
30. Scaldaferri F, Pizzoferrato M, Lopetuso LR, et al. Nutrition and IBD: Malnutrition and/or sarcopenia? A practical guide. *Gastroenterol Res Pract.* 2017;2017.
31. Nguyen GC, Munsell M, Harris ML. Nationwide prevalence and prognostic significance of clinically diagnosable protein-calorie malnutrition in hospitalized inflammatory bowel disease patients. *Inflamm Bowel Dis.* 2008;14(8):1105–1111.
32. Marsh A, Kinneally J, Robertson T, Lord A, Young A, Radford – Smith G. Food avoidance in outpatients with inflammatory bowel disease – who, what and why. *Clin Nutr ESPEN.* 2019;31:10–16.
33. Tew GA, Jones K, Mikocka-Walus A. Physical activity habits, limitations, and predictors in people with inflammatory bowel disease: A large cross-sectional online survey. *Inflamm Bowel Dis.* 2016;22(12):2933–2942.
34. Pulley J, Todd A, Flatley C, Begun J. Malnutrition, and quality of life among adult inflammatory bowel disease patients. *JGH Open.* 2020;4(3):454–460.
35. Hwang C, Ross V, Mahadevan U. Micronutrient deficiencies in inflammatory bowel disease: From A to zinc. *Inflamm Bowel Dis.* 2012;18(10):1961–1981.
36. Filippi J, Al-Jaouni R, Wiroth J-B, Hébuterne X, Schneider SM. Nutritional deficiencies in patients with Crohn's disease in remission. *Inflamm Bowel Dis.* 2006;12(3):185–191.
37. Tomkins A. Assessing micronutrient status in the presence of inflammation. *J Nutr.* 2003;133(5):1649S–1655S.
38. Patel D, Trivedi C, Khan N. Management of anemia in patients with inflammatory bowel disease (IBD). *Curr Treat Options Gastroenterol.* 2018;16(1):112–128.
39. Yakut M, Üstün Y, Kabaçam G, Soykan I. Serum vitamin B12 and folate status in patients with inflammatory bowel diseases. *Eur J Intern Med.* 2010;21(4):320–323.
40. Stratton RJ, Hackston A, Longmore D, et al. Malnutrition in hospital outpatients and inpatients: Prevalence, concurrent validity, and ease of use of the 'malnutrition universal screening tool' ('MUST') for adults. *Br J Nutr.* 2004;92(5):799–808.
41. Rahman A, Williams P, Sandhu A, Mosli M. Malnutrition universal screening tool (MUST) scores predicts disease activity in patients with Crohn's disease. *Can J Nutr.* 2016;1:1–5.

42. Keetarut K, Zacharopoulou-Otapasidou S, Bloom S, Majumdar A, Patel P. An evaluation of the feasibility and validity of a patient-administered malnutrition universal screening tool ('MUST') compared to healthcare professional screening in an inflammatory bowel disease (IBD) outpatient clinic. *J Hum Nutr Diet.* 2017;30(6):737–745.

43. Sandhu A, Mosli M, Yan B, et al. Self-screening for malnutrition risk in outpatient inflammatory bowel disease patients using the malnutrition universal screening tool (MUST). *J Parenter Enter Nutr.* 2016;40(4):507–510.

44. Lacey K, Pritchett E. Nutrition care process and model: ADA adopts road map to quality care and outcomes management. *J Am Diet Assoc.* 2003;103(8):1061–1072.

45. Gong J, Zuo L, Guo Z, et al. Impact of disease activity on resting energy expenditure and body composition in adult Crohn's disease: A prospective longitudinal assessment. *J Parenter Enter Nutr.* 2015;39(6):713–718.

46. Gill SK, Rossi, M, Bajka, B, Whelan, K. Dietary fibre in gastrointestinal health and disease. *Nat Rev Gastroenterol Hepatol.* 2021;18(2):101–116.

47. Lupton JR, Brooks J, Butte N, Caballero B, Flatt J, Fried S. Dietary reference intakes for energy, carbohydrate, fiber, fat, fatty acids, cholesterol, protein, and amino acids. *Natl Acad Press Wash DC USA.* 2002;5:589–768.

48. Lijoi D, Ferrero S, Mistrangelo E, et al. Bowel preparation before laparoscopic gynaecological surgery in benign conditions using a 1-week low fibre diet: A surgeon blind, randomized and controlled trial. *Arch Gynecol Obstet.* 2009;280(5):713–718.

49. Hosoi K, Alvarez WC, Mann FC. Intestinal absorption: A search for a low residue diet. *Arch Intern Med.* 1928;41(1):112–126.

50. Cunningham E. Are low-residue diets still applicable? *J Acad Nutr Diet.* 2012;112(6): 960.

51. Levenstein S, Prantera C, Luzi C, D'ubaldi A. Low residue, or normal diet in Crohn's disease: A prospective controlled study in Italian patients. *Gut.* 1985;26(10):989–993.

52. Gibson PR, Shepherd SJ. Evidence-based dietary management of functional gastrointestinal symptoms: The FODMAP approach. *J Gastroenterol Hepatol.* 2010;25(2):252–258.

53. Pedersen N, Ankersen DV, Felding M, et al. Low-FODMAP diet reduces irritable bowel symptoms in patients with inflammatory bowel disease. *World J Gastroenterol.* 2017;23(18):3356.

54. Cox SR, Prince AC, Myers CE, et al. Fermentable carbohydrates [FODMAPs] exacerbate functional gastrointestinal symptoms in patients with inflammatory bowel disease: A randomised, double-blind, placebo-controlled, cross-over, re-challenge trial. *J Crohns Colitis.* 2017;11(12):1420–1429.

55. Colombel J-F, Shin A, Gibson PR. AGA clinical practice update on functional gastrointestinal symptoms in patients with inflammatory bowel disease: Expert review. *Clin Gastroenterol Hepatol.* 2019;17(3):380–390.

56. Gottschall E, Gottschall EG. *Breaking the Vicious Cycle: Intestinal Health through Diet.* Kirkton, Ontario: Kirkton Press; 1994.

57. Cohen SA, Gold BD, Oliva S, et al. Clinical and mucosal improvement with specific carbohydrate diet in pediatric Crohn disease. *J Pediatr Gastroenterol Nutr.* 2014; 59(4):516–521.

58. Obih C, Wahbeh G, Lee D, et al. Specific carbohydrate diet for pediatric inflammatory bowel disease in clinical practice within an academic IBD center. *Nutrition.* 2016;32(4):418–425.

59. Burgis JC, Nguyen K, Park K, Cox K. Response to strict and liberalized specific carbohydrate diet in pediatric Crohn's disease. *World J Gastroenterol.* 2016;22(6):2111.

60. Suskind DL, Wahbeh G, Cohen SA, et al. Patients perceive clinical benefit with the specific carbohydrate diet for inflammatory bowel disease. *Dig Dis Sci.* 2016;61(11): 3255–3260.

61. Davis C, Bryan J, Hodgson J, Murphy K. Definition of the Mediterranean diet: A literature review. *Nutrients.* 2015;7(11):9139–9153.

62. Khalili H, Håkansson N, Chan SS, et al. Adherence to a Mediterranean diet is associated with a lower risk of later-onset Crohn's disease: Results from two large prospective cohort studies. *Gut.* Published online 2020.
63. Alhagamhmad MH. Enteral nutrition in the management of Crohn's disease: Reviewing mechanisms of actions and highlighting potential venues for enhancing the efficacy. *Nutr Clin Pract.* 2018;33(4):483–492.
64. Narula N, Dhillon A, Zhang D, Sherlock ME, Tondeur M, Zachos M. Enteral nutritional therapy for induction of remission in Crohn's disease. *Cochrane Database Syst Rev.* 2018;(4).
65. Anstee QM, Forbes A. The safe use of percutaneous gastrostomy for enteral nutrition in patients with Crohn's disease. *Eur J Gastroenterol Hepatol.* 2000;12(10):1089–1093.
66. Wall CL, Day AS, Gearry RB. Use of exclusive enteral nutrition in adults with Crohn's disease: A review. *World J Gastroenterol WJG.* 2013;19(43):7652.
67. Fell J, Paintin M, Arnaud-Battandier F, et al. Mucosal healing, and a fall in mucosal pro-inflammatory cytokine mRNA induced by a specific oral polymeric diet in paediatric Crohn's disease. *Aliment Pharmacol Ther.* 2000;14(3):281–290.
68. Yamamoto T, Nakahigashi M, Umegae S, Kitagawa T, Matsumoto K. Impact of elemental diet on mucosal inflammation in patients with active Crohn's disease: Cytokine production and endoscopic and histological findings. *Inflamm Bowel Dis.* 2005;11(6):580–588.
69. Heerasing N, Thompson B, Hendy P, et al. Exclusive enteral nutrition provides an effective bridge to safer interval elective surgery for adults with Crohn's disease. *Aliment Pharmacol Ther.* 2017;45(5):660–669.
70. Levine A, Wine E, Assa A, et al. Crohn's disease exclusion diet plus partial enteral nutrition induces sustained remission in a randomized controlled trial. *Gastroenterology.* 2019;157(2):440–450.
71. Triantafillidis JK, Papalois AE. The role of total parenteral nutrition in inflammatory bowel disease: Current aspects. *Scand J Gastroenterol.* 2013;49(1):3–14.
72. McIntyre P, Powell-Tuck J, Wood S, et al. Controlled trial of bowel rest in the treatment of severe acute colitis. *Gut.* 1986;27(5):481–485.
73. Greenberg G, Fleming C, Jeejeebhoy K, Rosenberg I, Sales D, Tremaine W. Controlled trial of bowel rest and nutritional support in the management of Crohn's disease. *Gut.* 1988;29(10):1309–1315.
74. Schwartz E. Perioperative parenteral nutrition in adults with inflammatory bowel disease: A review of the literature. *Nutr Clin Pract.* 2016;31(2):159–170.

6 Chronic Constipation and Diarrhea

Lisa D. Lin and Nancee Jaffe

6.1 INTRODUCTION

Chronic constipation and chronic diarrhea are common disorders that can significantly impact an individual's quality of life. Because benefits usually outweigh risks, dietary interventions should be first-line treatments for individuals with mild-to-moderate symptoms and can also be important adjunctive therapy for patients with severe symptoms. Dietary therapy can help normalize bowel habits through its effects on stool consistency, fecal mass, intestinal transit times, or changes in the microbiome.

Causes of chronic constipation or diarrhea can be organic or functional. For organic causes, treatment focuses on addressing the underlying disease pathophysiology. For those with functional features, nutritional interventions can play an important role. This chapter will focus on evidence-based dietary management for chronic functional constipation and diarrhea in adults, although the principles can also be applied to other disorders with symptoms of constipation and diarrhea (Table 6.1). Nutritional therapy for irritable bowel syndrome (IBS) is discussed in chapter 4.

6.2 CHRONIC CONSTIPATION

The definition for constipation varies, but the Rome IV definition for functional constipation is widely used (Table 6.2).[1]

Constipation can be acute (lasting <1 week) or chronic (lasting ≥3 months). Primary constipation (e.g., functional constipation) is the most common form and stems from primary disturbances, such as diet or lifestyle, or a disorder of colonic motility or rectal emptying. Primary constipation can be categorized as normal transit constipation, slow transit constipation, or rectal evacuation disorders (e.g., dyssynergic defecation).[2] Secondary constipation can be caused by medications, local colon pathologies (e.g., colon cancer), or organic diseases (e.g., hypothyroidism).[2]

6.2.1 FIBER

"Dietary fiber" is defined as non-digestible carbohydrates and lignin that are intrinsic and intact in plants.[3] Examples include foods such as whole grains, legumes, vegetables, and fruits. Another class of fiber called "functional fiber" (e.g., psyllium husk) is defined as isolated non-digestible carbohydrates extracted from foods that have beneficial physiological effects in humans. "Synthetic fiber" is an artificial polymer, such as methylcellulose and calcium polycarbophil.[4] "Total fiber" is defined as the

DOI: 10.1201/9780429322570-6

TABLE 6.1

Summary of Recommendations for Dietary Treatment of Functional Constipation and Diarrhea

	Functional Constipation	Functional Diarrhea
Higher Level of Evidence	High-fiber diet ≥25–30 g/day	FODMAP elimination and reintroduction under dietitian guidance
	Increase foods that have high-insoluble fiber (grains, vegetables, fruits especially 2 kiwis/day or prunes)	Avoid or minimize coffee or other dietary triggers
	Use psyllium husk supplementation	Use psyllium husk supplementation
	Choose a coarse particle fiber supplement	Use non-psyllium soluble fiber (e.g., wheat dextrin, guar gum)
Lower Level of Evidence	Use insoluble fiber supplement	Low-fat diet
	Use probiotics	

TABLE 6.2

Rome IV Diagnostic Criteria for Functional Constipation and Functional Diarrhea

Functional Constipation*

Must include ≥2 of the following:
- Straining during >1/4 (25%) of defecations
- Lumpy or hard stools (Bristol Stool Form Scale 1–2) >1/4 (25%) of defecations
- Sensation of incomplete evacuation >1/4 (25%) of defecations
- Sensation of anorectal obstruction/blockage >1/4 (25%) of defecations
- Manual maneuvers to facilitate >1/4 (25%) of defecations (e.g., digital evacuation, support of the pelvic floor)
- Fewer than 3 spontaneous bowel movements per week
- Loose stools are rarely present without the use of laxatives
- Insufficient criteria for irritable bowel syndrome

Functional Diarrhea*
- Loose or watery stools, without predominant abdominal pain or bothersome bloating, occurring in >25% of stools
- Insufficient criteria for irritable bowel syndrome

* Criteria fulfilled for the last 3 months with symptom onset at least 6 months prior to diagnosis.

sum of dietary fiber, functional fiber, and synthetic fiber.[5] Different fibers exert varying effects on bowel habits depending on their solubility, viscosity, particle size, and fermentability (Tables 6.3 and 6.4).

Soluble fibers dissolve in water, while insoluble fibers do not. Soluble fibers are usually more easily fermented by colonic bacteria and can be viscous or non-viscous.[6] Generally, soluble fibers also have more water-holding capacity than

TABLE 6.3
Fiber Supplements and Their Characteristics

	Solubility	Viscosity	Fermentability	Coarse Particle Available
Psyllium Husk (e.g., Metamucil, Konsyl)	✓	✓	✗	✓^
Wheat Dextrin (e.g., Benefiber)	✓	✗	✓	✗
Inulin	✓	✗	✓	✗
Guar Gum (e.g., Sunfiber)	✓	✓	✓	✗
Corn Fiber (e.g., FiberCel)	✓	✗	✓	✗
Acacia Fiber (e.g., Heather's)	✓	✗	✓	✗
Polydextrose (e.g., Fiber Well)	✓	✗	✓	✗
Wheat Bran	✗	✗	✗	✓^
Methylcellulose (e.g., Citrucel)	✓*	✓*	✗	✗
Calcium Polycarbophil (e.g, FiberCon)	✓	✗	?	✗

^ Whole = coarse particles; Powder = fine particles.
* Chemically treated to be soluble and viscous.

TABLE 6.4
Fiber by Type

Dietary Fiber	Functional Fiber	Synthetic Fiber
Whole Grains	Psyllium Husk	Calcium Polycarbophil
Vegetables	Wheat Dextrin	Methylcellulose
Fruits	Guar Gum	
Beans/Legumes	Acacia Fiber	
Nuts	Polydextrose	
Seeds	Inulin	
	Corn Fiber	

insoluble fiber. In contrast, insoluble fibers are either poorly or not fermentable; because they do not dissolve in water, they are non-viscous by definition. Soluble fibers generally slow gastrointestinal (GI) transit whereas insoluble fibers accelerate GI transit.[5,7]

Viscosity refers to the ability of some fibers to thicken in consistency when hydrated. A more viscous fiber slows down the rate of fecal passage through the GI tract. A soluble fiber that has high water-holding capacity and increased viscosity can result in a stool-normalizing effect with correction or prevention of both constipation and diarrhea.[6]

Particle size and shape of fiber can also affect the GI transit time and fiber fermentation. Large coarse particles have a laxative effect by causing mechanical irritation that results in secretion of mucus and water, leading to larger and softer stools and faster transit times through the colon. In contrast, small smooth particles do not have this laxative effect.[8] The fermentation rate of fiber is also directly related to its surface area. The smaller the fiber particle, the more surface area there is for bacteria to come into direct contact with, leading to an increased rate of fermentation.[7]

Fiber, after resisting enzymatic digestion in the small intestine, can be fermented by colonic bacteria to produce end products, including short-chain fatty acids and gases.[5, 6, 9] Fibers can be classified as fermentable or non-fermentable. In order to have a laxative effect via mechanical irritation of colon and the capacity to hold water, fiber must resist bacterial fermentation to remain intact and present throughout the colon.[4]

6.2.2   OUTDATED PRACTICE: DRINK MORE WATER OR FLUID

Although it is touted in popular culture that an increase in water or fluid intake can treat constipation, there is no high-quality evidence to support this claim in an individual who is not dehydrated. Multiple studies have found the drinking volume to be similar between constipated individuals and non-constipated controls.[10–13] Three studies have examined whether drinking more fluid can treat constipation and have yielded conflicting results. In one study with 118 constipated children randomized to one of three groups (increased daily water intake by 50%, additional hyperosmolar liquids such as juices, or no change), there were no differences in stool frequency, consistency, or ease of defecation.[14] In another study with 117 constipated adults placed on a diet with 25 g/day of fiber and randomized to either fluid intake *ad libitum* (resulting in 1.1 L/day of water) or 2 L/day of mineral water, the mineral water group had increased stool frequency and decreased laxative use, but this was confounded by the presence of magnesium and other ions in the mineral water that may have acted as a light laxative.[15] A third study included 11 healthy patients who ingested wheat bran supplements with or without an extra 600 mL of fluid; there was no effect from the use of additional water.[16] Current evidence does not support increase of fluid intake to treat constipation unless there is evidence of dehydration or to increase fluid intake with fiber supplementation.[5, 17]

6.2.3   RECOMMENDATION: INGEST A HIGH-FIBER DIET

Low-fiber intake has been associated with constipation.[18–20] In a large prospective cohort study with 62,036 adult women, including 3,327 with constipation, it was observed that women with a median intake of 20 g of fiber/day had a 36% lower prevalence of constipation compared with women who ingested 7 g of fiber/day.[20] On the other hand, this association has not been consistently demonstrated. In a large cross-sectional study using the National Health and Nutrition Examination Surveys data from 2005–2008, which included 10,914 adult men and women, there was no association found between low-fiber intake and constipation.[21] Overall, more studies have shown an association between low-fiber intake and constipation. While a low-fiber diet is not always the cause of constipation, it can be a contributing factor.

Most guidelines recommend a high-fiber diet of at least 25–30 g/day for patients with constipation or 14 g per 1,000 kcal/day.[2, 22, 23] The average American ingests only 15 g/day of dietary fiber.[22] Dietary fiber increases stool bulk and frequency and decreases consistency in healthy people, but the evidence for dietary fiber's effect in constipated individuals is limited.[17] Generally, increased fiber intake is recommended for treatment of mild-to-moderate constipation. However, increased fiber intake may worsen symptoms in a subgroup of patients with more severe constipation due to slow transit or disordered defecation.[5, 17] Fiber should be introduced starting at a low dosage and gradually increased to minimize potential side effects of bloating, distention, flatulence, and cramping.[24]

6.2.4 RECOMMENDATION: INCREASE FIBER-RICH FOODS

Fiber-rich foods generally have a mix of soluble and insoluble fibers (Table 6.5).[6] For constipation, one should choose foods that have more insoluble fiber. A systematic review evaluating the effects of dietary fiber from cereals, fruits, and vegetables in healthy individuals demonstrated that cereal and vegetable fiber resulted in similarly increased fecal weight, which was higher than that from fruit fiber.[25] Fruit fiber tends to be more fermentable and soluble than those from vegetables or cereals.

TABLE 6.5
Fiber-Rich Foods by Solubility

	Predominantly Soluble Fiber	Predominately Insoluble Fiber
Fruits	Apples without skin	Apples with skin
	Apricots	Blackberries
	Avocado	Blueberries
	Banana	Cherries
	Oranges/Citrus (without membrane)	Pear with skin
	Peaches	Raspberries
	Plums	Strawberries
	Watermelon	
Vegetables	Asparagus	Bell peppers
	Broccoli	Beets
	Brussels sprouts	Celery
	Carrots	Corn
	Eggplant (without skin)	Kale
	Green beans	Mushrooms
	Potato (without skin)	Okra
	Onion	Tomato
	Pumpkin	Peas
	Zucchini	Turnips
Grains	Refined pasta	Whole grain pasta
	White rice	Brown/Wild rice
	Oats	Most whole grains
Nuts and Seeds		All varieties
Beans and Legumes		All varieties

This study also showed that in healthy individuals with a slower whole gut transit time of ≥48 hours, each gram of increased dietary fiber reduced the transit time by 30 minutes, regardless of the food fiber type. When the transit time is already <48 hours, additional dietary fiber did not change the transit time.[25] A meta-analysis of 20 small randomized controlled trials showed that wheat bran increased stool weight and decreased transit time in healthy controls and constipated patients, but the constipated patients still had lower stool output and slower transit times than controls, with or without wheat bran.[26] Overall, based on limited data, increasing fiber-rich foods in the form of whole grains, vegetables, and fruits is encouraged for constipated patients, with grain and vegetable fibers being potentially more effective than fruit fibers.

Dried plums (prunes) and prune juice have also traditionally been used for treatment of constipation. The laxative effects of prunes are thought to be due to the presence of sugar alcohol sorbitol, polyphenols, and fiber, which also exist in prune juice.[27, 28] In a single-blind randomized cross-over study in which 40 constipated patients received either prunes (50 g or about 6 prunes twice daily) or psyllium (1 tablespoon twice daily) for 3 weeks, prunes resulted in a greater increase in the number of complete spontaneous bowel movements and improvement in stool consistency when compared to psyllium.[28] This result was similar to those in other small studies using prune juice.[27, 29] However, prunes also contain fructan sugars, which are highly fermentable, potentially causing adverse effects of gas and bloating.

Kiwi fruit (*Actinidia deliciosa* or "Hayward" variety) has also been shown to significantly improve constipation by increasing stool frequency and decreasing colonic transit time.[30, 31] One study gave 33 constipated patients and 20 healthy volunteers two kiwi fruits daily and showed that the constipated patients had significantly more weekly complete spontaneous bowel movements, improved colonic transit time, and fewer days of laxative use.[30] Similarly, another study with 54 patients with constipation-predominant IBS compared with 16 healthy individuals, both given 2 kiwi fruits daily, found that kiwi fruit significantly improved weekly defecation frequency and decreased colonic transit time in the constipated patients.[31] The mechanism of action for kiwi fruit's effect on constipation is incompletely understood but is thought to be due to the fruit's fiber content, potential influence on the microbiome, and the presence of enzyme actinidin's effect on GI motility.[32]

6.2.5 RECOMMENDATION: CONSIDER ADDING FIBER SUPPLEMENTATION TO DIETARY FIBERS

The evidence for supplemental fiber's efficacy for constipation is mixed, partly due to studies using different fiber types and variable study designs. These studies have been limited by small sample sizes, short duration of therapy, and lack of validated outcome measures.[33, 34] Despite heterogeneity among available data, soluble fiber, especially psyllium, has been shown to be effective in chronic constipation.[24, 35] The largest randomized controlled trial with 201 constipated patients showed that when compared with placebo, psyllium significantly improved global symptoms and straining.[36] In two smaller studies, psyllium use was associated with a significant improvement in bowel movement frequency, stool consistency, pain on defecation,[37] and "normalization of evacuation."[38] Other studies comparing psyllium with other laxatives, such as lactulose or docusate, also showed a significant improvement in stool frequency or consistency with psyllium, although these studies were limited by poor quality.[39, 40] Overall, there is moderate evidence to support the use of soluble fiber, especially psyllium, in chronic idiopathic constipation.[24, 35]

The benefit of insoluble fiber and synthetic fiber on chronic idiopathic constipation is less clear. There have been three randomized controlled trials done with wheat bran.[41–43] The highest quality trial of the three was a crossover randomized placebo-controlled study that showed no significant difference in the improvement of stool frequency or consistency, although the trial was limited by a small sample size with only 24 patients.[41] One study that compared methylcellulose with psyllium in constipated individuals over 10 days found no differences in stool frequency, consistency, or ease of defecation between the two groups.[44]

The use of fiber is overall safe.[33] One study reported more abdominal pain in the psyllium group than placebo but no difference in bloating or cramping,[37] while other studies have noted more GI side effects of bloating and flatulence with fiber.[24, 33, 35] To minimize these potential side effects, fiber should be initiated at a low dose of 3–4 g/day (e.g., 1 teaspoon of psyllium) and increased weekly by 3–4 g/day or at a rate tolerable to the patient up to a goal dose of 10–15 g/day or until desired stool consistency and frequency is achieved.[8]

In summary, low- to intermediate-quality randomized controlled trials show psyllium improves stool frequency and consistency.[33] There are not enough data on non-psyllium soluble fiber, insoluble fiber, and synthetic fiber to support recommending them for chronic constipation.[24, 33, 35] Given the available evidence, psyllium should be attempted first for treatment of chronic constipation. If soluble fiber has not been effective for the patient, then insoluble or synthetic fiber can be tried.

6.2.6 RECOMMENDATION: CONSIDER USING A COARSER FIBER

Coarser or larger fiber particle sizes are more effective in decreasing transit time than finer fiber particle sizes.[45, 46] One study with 24 young adult men demonstrated that supplementation with coarse bran resulted in shorter mean colonic transit time and higher fecal moisture content than supplementation with finely ground bran, although no significant differences in stool frequency were seen.[45] Another study with 18 healthy adults showed that daily ingestion of plastic cut to larger bran-like flakes resulted in shorter gut transit time than smaller plastic granules.[47] One study done on 12 healthy men given either daily coarse wheat bran or plastic particles of same size showed that both types of supplementation similarly increased fecal mass and decreased the whole gut transit time when compared with their normal diet.[46]

6.2.7 PROBIOTICS

In a systematic review and meta-analysis which included 3 randomized controlled trials, probiotics appeared to have beneficial effects on chronic idiopathic constipation by increasing stool frequency.[48] The largest trial in this review had 135 women treated with fermented milk containing *Bifidobacterium lactis* DN-173010, resulting in increased stool frequency and consistency compared with placebo.[49] In another trial with 70 constipated patients, a probiotic beverage containing *Lactobacillus casei* Shirota given for 4 weeks improved constipation severity and stool consistency.[50] Outside this meta-analysis, a randomized placebo-controlled trial with 40 adults with functional constipation found that *Lactobacillus reuteri* (DSM 17938) increased stool frequency but not consistency.[51] In another randomized controlled trial, *Escherichia coli* Nissle 1917 significantly increased stool frequency compared with placebo.[52] Therefore, probiotics may be effective in patients with mild-to-moderate functional constipation, although it is not clear which specific bacterial strain or composition is ideal and the efficacy of probiotics have not been studied in comparison with fiber supplementation.[5]

6.3   CHRONIC DIARRHEA

Diarrhea is defined by the World Health Organization as the passage of ≥3 loose or liquid stools per day, or more frequently than is normal for the individual,[53] although some call frequent defecation with normal consistency "pseudodiarrhea."[54] Diarrhea can be acute (<2 weeks) or chronic (>4 weeks). For functional diarrhea, the Rome IV definition is frequently used (Table 6.1).[1]

The content of food ingested can affect GI motility. For example, dietary fat entering the duodenum activates the gastrocolic reflex, which can lead to fecal urgency and bowel movements soon after meals.[55] Solid food also slows gastric and small bowel transit compared with liquid solution.[56] Changes in GI motility can affect stool consistency because accelerated transit of food chemicals through the gut can result in insufficient time for absorption, which can lead to diarrhea.[55]

Effects from food digestion can be broken down into multiple categories. There are substances that cause diarrhea even in a normal gut when ingested in sufficient quantities (e.g., fructose). There are foods that cause diarrhea due to an underlying condition (e.g., lactose intolerance due to lactase deficiency). There are organic gut alterations that limit digestion or absorption of nutrients, which then result in diarrhea (e.g., short bowel syndrome). There are also idiosyncratic food intolerances.[54] It is important to note that food malabsorption is different from food intolerance (see Chapter 9).

6.3.1   RECOMMENDATION: TRIAL OF ELIMINATING OSMOTICALLY ACTIVE SUGARS

Fermentable oligo-, di-, monosaccharides, and polyols (FODMAPs) are a group of fermentable carbohydrates that include fructans, galactooligosaccharides, disaccharides (e.g., lactose), monosaccharides (e.g., fructose), and polyols (e.g., sorbitol, xylitol).[57] These carbohydrates are poorly absorbed in the small intestine, resulting in delivery of excess substrate to the colon, and therefore act as highly osmotic substances that may cause an influx of water into the colon and result in diarrhea.[55,58] Fructose and polyols predominantly increase small bowel water content, while fructans and galactooligosaccharides largely increase gas production.[59, 60] Lactose increases both small bowel water content and gas production.[61] Most studies on efficacy of a low-FODMAP diet have been done in IBS patients with a focus on outcomes of abdominal pain and bloating, but a reduction in FODMAP consumption should theoretically reduce symptoms of diarrhea as well.[62] A low-FODMAP diet is not meant to be permanent and if patients have significant symptom improvement while on a low-FODMAP diet, they should undergo a challenge phase with reintroduction of specific FODMAPs according to tolerance.[62]

Lactose is a commonly malabsorbed carbohydrate, making lactose intolerance a common cause of diarrhea.[63, 64] All mammals need lactase activity in the intestinal tract to digest and absorb lactose in infancy, and the prevalence of lactase persistence varies by ethnicity.[55, 65] Symptoms depend on both the amount of lactase enzyme activity remaining and on the amount of lactose consumed.[55] Milk that has been treated to hydrolyze lactose can reduce symptoms. Ingestion of lactase tablets with lactose-containing food is usually less successful due to poor mixing and incomplete hydrolysis of lactose.[55]

When the amount of fructose ingested exceeds the small bowel's absorptive capacity, malabsorption and diarrhea can occur.[66] The threshold dose of fructose ingestion that causes GI symptoms is still unclear, because fructose absorption varies depending on the way fructose is ingested, such as whether it is consumed with solid food or the ratio between glucose and fructose within a food.[66, 67] Therefore, the amount of fructose reduction to result in improvement of diarrhea needs to be individualized.

Humans do not have active transporters for sugar alcohols such as sorbitol, mannitol, and xylitol, but intake of up to 10 g/day may be well tolerated by most people via absorption by passive diffusion.[55] Therefore, excess ingestion of these sugar alcohols, which are common sweeteners in "sugar-free" products (e.g., candies, chewing gums, mints) and can exist in medications, may also lead to a malabsorptive diarrhea.[68] Sorbitol and mannitol also naturally exist in some vegetables, fruits, and fruit juices.[55]

Patients with non-celiac gluten sensitivity have a negative celiac workup but may experience diarrhea, bloating, and extraintestinal symptoms that improve after gluten elimination. There is controversy over whether it is the actual gluten protein in wheat, barley, and rye or the fructan sugar found in the grains that causes these symptoms. Previous studies involving gluten restriction have either not been done to evaluate chronic diarrhea or have not shown a significant change in diarrhea with or without gluten.[69–71]

6.3.2   Recommendation: Trial of Low-Fat Diet

Dietary fat is one of the main activators of the gastrocolic response, which can be exaggerated in some individuals and lead to diarrhea. Dietary fat is also hydrolyzed into long-chain fatty acids; if malabsorbed by the small intestine, either due to mucosal disease or ingestion above the intestinal absorptive capacity, long-chain fatty acids will enter the colon in excess and cause a laxative effect.[55] Most fat is absorbed in the jejunum and fat entering the lower ileum will trigger the ileal brake, which inhibits gastric emptying and proximal small bowel transit. Patients with substantial ileal resections may lack this mechanism, which then results in increased amounts of unabsorbed nutrients to enter the colon after meals, resulting in diarrhea.[55] Although a significant proportion of IBS patients report sensitivity to dietary fat, there have been no studies evaluating the efficacy of a low-fat diet in treating diarrhea in either patients with IBS or functional diarrhea.[72] A low-fat diet can be considered in patients with reported sensitivity to fatty foods or in patients with prior ileal resection.

6.3.3   Recommendation: Avoid Other Potential Dietary Triggers

Coffee is commonly thought to stimulate bowel function and carry a laxative effect, although the data supporting this are limited. One survey study found that 60% of healthy participants reported that coffee may stimulate a bowel movement.[73] Coffee has not been shown to increase small intestinal secretion and transit speed,[74] although one study demonstrated an increase in rectosigmoid motor activity within 4 minutes of drinking black coffee, either caffeinated or decaffeinated, in healthy volunteers who reported that coffee caused a desire to defecate.[75] Another study demonstrated both caffeinated and decaffeinated coffee increased colonic activity comparable to a high-calorie meal.[73] Based on current evidence, coffee can potentially induce bowel movements by increasing colonic motor activity and should be moderated or avoided in patients reporting sensitivity to it.

6.3.4   Recommendation: Consider Soluble Fiber Supplementation

Some soluble fibers have high water-holding capacity and viscosity and can form a gel consistency; it is therefore thought to treat diarrhea by improving stool consistency and slowing GI transit.[76] One randomized crossover study with 8 healthy volunteers given lactulose three times daily with or without psyllium showed that psyllium significantly delayed gastric and colonic transit, but did not change small bowel transit time.[77] Another small study with 9 participants with induced diarrhea showed that psyllium, but not calcium polycarbophil or wheat bran, improved stool consistency and increased fecal viscosity in a dose-dependent manner.[78] One study with 183 patients with chronic diarrhea showed that psyllium ingestion reduced stool looseness again in a dose-dependent manner without changing water content.[79] Most other studies evaluating fiber's effects on diarrhea were done in adults on enteral nutrition. A meta-analysis analyzing 26 studies showed that soluble fiber significantly reduced diarrhea by 53% in patients receiving enteral nutrition.[80]

6.3.5   Probiotics

Although probiotics have shown efficacy for prevention and treatment of certain types of acute diarrhea, such as antibiotic-associated diarrhea or infectious diarrhea, there has been sparse high-quality evidence studying its efficacy in chronic diarrhea.[81] Therefore, no specific recommendations regarding probiotic use for chronic diarrhea can be made at this time.

6.4   NOVEL APPROACHES

Fiber has long been known to improve constipation in patients, although it has not been adequately emphasized in practice. In addition to merely increasing fiber intake, the type (i.e., soluble fibers) and size (i.e., coarser or larger particles) of fiber are important for improving constipation. For diarrhea, use of soluble fiber, reduction of osmotically active sugars, trial of a low-fat diet, and avoidance of dietary triggers such as coffee are some nutritional treatment strategies to consider. Probiotics have been explored for constipation and diarrhea, although their benefit is yet unclear.

6.5 INCORRECT/OUTDATED PRACTICES

For chronic constipation, fluid intake does not appear to be a significant contributor. The current evidence does not support the recommendation of drinking more water or fluids as a sole treatment for constipation. While increasing intake of fiber can help, the use of insoluble and synthetic fibers are not as effective as soluble fibers, such as psyllium. For chronic diarrhea, routine food allergy testing is not recommended.

PRACTICE PEARLS

For chronic constipation

- Recommending more fluid intake in an individual who is not dehydrated is unnecessary.
- Recommend a high-fiber diet with at least 25–30 g of fiber/day or 14 g/1,000 kcal/day.
- Consider offering patients 2 kiwis/day. Consider recommending up to 6 prunes twice daily but this can worsen bloating.
- If encouraging fiber supplementation, recommend a soluble fiber such as psyllium husk. Recommend coarse husk form to encourage mechanical irritation.
- Do not recommend probiotics as first-line therapy due to limited data.

For chronic diarrhea

- Food allergy testing should only be considered in adults who have other allergic features, such as hives, upper respiratory symptoms, or abnormal labs.
- Consider trial elimination of osmotically active sugars, such as lactose, fructose, and polyols under the guidance of an expert dietitian.
- Evidence does not support the recommendation of a gluten-free diet to treat chronic diarrhea.
- Trial of low-fat diet can be considered in patients with reported sensitivity to fatty foods or with prior ileal resection as second-line therapy due to limited data.
- Limit coffee intake in patients with reported sensitivity or if drunk in excess.
- If encouraging fiber supplementation, recommend a soluble fiber such as psyllium husk. Recommend the fine particle form.
- Do not recommend probiotics as first-line therapy for chronic diarrhea due to limited data.

REFERENCES

1. Mearin F, Lacy BE, Chang L, et al. Bowel disorders. *Gastroenterology*. Feb 18, 2016;150(6):1393–407. doi:10.1053/j.gastro.2016.02.031.
2. Camilleri M, Ford AC, Mawe GM, et al. Chronic constipation. *Nat Rev Dis Primers*. Dec 14, 2017;3:17095. doi:10.1038/nrdp.2017.95.
3. Institute of Medicine Panel on the Definition of Dietary Fiber and the Standing Committee on the Scientific Evaluation of Dietary Reference I. *Dietary Reference Intakes Proposed Definition of Dietary Fiber*. National Academies Press (US) Copyright 2001 by the National Academy of Sciences. All rights reserved. 2001.
4. McRorie JW, Jr., McKeown NM. Understanding the physics of functional fibers in the gastrointestinal tract: An evidence-based approach to resolving enduring misconceptions about insoluble and soluble fiber. *J Acad Nutr Diet*. Feb 2017;117(2):251–64. doi:10.1016/j.jand.2016.09.021.
5. Fernandez-Banares F. Nutritional care of the patient with constipation. *Best Pract Res Clin Gastroenterol*. 2006;20(3):575–87. doi:10.1016/j.bpg.2005.11.002.
6. McRorie JW, Jr. Evidence-based approach to fiber supplements and clinically meaningful health benefits, part 1: What to look for and how to recommend an effective fiber therapy. *Nutr Today*. Mar 2015;50(2):82–9. doi:10.1097/nt.0000000000000082.
7. Mudgil D, Barak S. Composition, properties and health benefits of indigestible carbohydrate polymers as dietary fiber: A review. *Int J Biol Macromol*. Oct 2013;61:1–6. doi:10.1016/j.ijbiomac.2013.06.044.
8. McRorie JW, Jr. Evidence-based approach to fiber supplements and clinically meaningful health benefits, part 2: What to look for and how to recommend an effective fiber therapy. *Nutr Today*. Mar 2015;50(2):90–7. doi:10.1097/nt.0000000000000089.
9. Cummings JH, Macfarlane GT, Englyst HN. Prebiotic digestion and fermentation. *Am J Clin Nutr*. Feb 2001;73(2 Suppl):415s–20s. doi:10.1093/ajcn/73.2.415s.
10. Preston DM, Lennard-Jones JE. Severe chronic constipation of young women: 'Idiopathic slow transit constipation'. *Gut*. Jan 1986;27(1):41–8. doi:10.1136/gut.27.1.41.
11. Anderson AS. Dietary factors in the aetiology and treatment of constipation during pregnancy. *Br J Obstet Gynaecol*. Mar 1986;93(3):245–9. doi:10.1111/j.1471-0528.1986.tb07901.x.
12. Towers AL, Burgio KL, Locher JL, Merkel IS, Safaeian M, Wald A. Constipation in the elderly: Influence of dietary, psychological, and physiological factors. *J Am Geriatr Soc*. Jul 1994;42(7):701–6. doi:10.1111/j.1532-5415.1994.tb06527.x.
13. Lindeman RD, Romero LJ, Liang HC, Baumgartner RN, Koehler KM, Garry PJ. Do elderly persons need to be encouraged to drink more fluids? *J Gerontol a Biol Sci Med Sci*. Jul 2000;55(7):M361–5. doi:10.1093/gerona/55.7.m361.
14. Young RJ, Beerman LE, Vanderhoof JA. Increasing oral fluids in chronic constipation in children. *Gastroenterol Nurs*. Jul–Aug 1998;21(4):156–61. doi:10.1097/00001610-199807000-00002.
15. Anti M, Pignataro G, Armuzzi A, et al. Water supplementation enhances the effect of high-fiber diet on stool frequency and laxative consumption in adult patients with functional constipation. *Hepatogastroenterology*. May–Jun 1998;45(21):727–32.
16. Ziegenhagen DJ, Tewinkel G, Kruis W, Herrmann F. Adding more fluid to wheat bran has no significant effects on intestinal functions of healthy subjects. *J Clin Gastroenterol*. Oct 1991;13(5):525–30. doi:10.1097/00004836-199110000-00010.
17. Muller-Lissner SA, Kamm MA, Scarpignato C, Wald A. Myths and misconceptions about chronic constipation. *Am J Gastroenterol*. Jan 2005;100(1):232–42. doi:10.1111/j.1572-0241.2005.40885.x.
18. Sandler RS, Jordan MC, Shelton BJ. Demographic and dietary determinants of constipation in the US population. *Am J Public Health*. Feb 1990;80(2):185–9. doi:10.2105/ajph.80.2.185.

19. Roma E, Adamidis D, Nikolara R, Constantopoulos A, Messaritakis J. Diet and chronic constipation in children: The role of fiber. *J Pediatr Gastroenterol Nutr.* Feb 1999;28(2):169–74. doi:10.1097/00005176-199902000-00015.

20. Dukas L, Willett WC, Giovannucci EL. Association between physical activity, fiber intake, and other lifestyle variables and constipation in a study of women. *Am J Gastroenterol.* Aug 2003;98(8):1790–6. doi:10.1111/j.1572-0241.2003.07591.x.

21. Markland AD, Palsson O, Goode PS, Burgio KL, Busby-Whitehead J, Whitehead WE. Association of low dietary intake of fiber and liquids with constipation: Evidence from the national health and nutrition examination survey. *Am J Gastroenterol.* May 2013;108(5):796–803. doi:10.1038/ajg.2013.73.

22. Trumbo P, Schlicker S, Yates AA, Poos M. Dietary reference intakes for energy, carbohydrate, fiber, fat, fatty acids, cholesterol, protein and amino acids. *J Am Diet Assoc.* Nov 2002;102(11):1621–30. doi:10.1016/s0002-8223(02)90346-9.

23. Dahl WJ, Stewart ML. Position of the academy of nutrition and dietetics: Health implications of dietary fiber. *J Acad Nutr Diet.* Nov 2015;115(11):1861–70. doi:10.1016/j.jand.2015.09.003.

24. Ford AC, Moayyedi P, Lacy BE, et al. American college of gastroenterology monograph on the management of irritable bowel syndrome and chronic idiopathic constipation. *Am J Gastroenterol.* Aug 2014;109 Suppl 1:S2–26; quiz S27. doi:10.1038/ajg.2014.187.

25. de Vries J, Birkett A, Hulshof T, Verbeke K, Gibes K. Effects of cereal, fruit and vegetable fibers on human fecal weight and transit time: A comprehensive review of intervention trials. *Nutrients.* Mar 2, 2016;8(3):130. doi:10.3390/nu8030130.

26. Muller-Lissner SA. Effect of wheat bran on weight of stool and gastrointestinal transit time: A meta analysis. *Br Med J (Clin Res Ed).* Feb 27 1988;296(6622):615–17. doi:10.1136/bmj.296.6622.615.

27. Piirainen L, Peuhkuri K, Backstrom K, Korpela R, Salminen S. Prune juice has a mild laxative effect in adults with certain gastrointestinal symptoms. *Nutrition Res.* 2007;27:511–13.

28. Attaluri A, Donahoe R, Valestin J, Brown K, Rao SS. Randomised clinical trial: Dried plums (prunes) vs. psyllium for constipation. *Aliment Pharmacol Ther.* Apr 2011;33(7):822–8. doi:10.1111/j.1365-2036.2011.04594.x.

29. Cheskin LJ, Kamal N, Crowell MD, Schuster MM, Whitehead WE. Mechanisms of constipation in older persons and effects of fiber compared with placebo. *J Am Geriatr Soc.* Jun 1995;43(6):666–9. doi:10.1111/j.1532-5415.1995.tb07203.x.

30. Chan AO, Leung G, Tong T, Wong NY. Increasing dietary fiber intake in terms of kiwifruit improves constipation in Chinese patients. *World J Gastroenterol.* Sep 21, 2007;13(35):4771–5. doi:10.3748/wjg.v13.i35.4771.

31. Chang CC, Lin YT, Lu YT, Liu YS, Liu JF. Kiwifruit improves bowel function in patients with irritable bowel syndrome with constipation. *Asia Pac J Clin Nutr.* 2010;19(4):451–7.

32. Drummond L, Gearry RB. Kiwifruit modulation of gastrointestinal motility. *Adv Food Nutr Res.* 2013;68:219–32. doi:10.1016/b978-0-12-394294-4.00012-2.

33. Brandt LJ, Prather CM, Quigley EM, Schiller LR, Schoenfeld P, Talley NJ. Systematic review on the management of chronic constipation in North America. *Am J Gastroenterol.* 2005;100 Suppl 1:S5–S21. doi:10.1111/j.1572-0241.2005.50613_2.x.

34. Eswaran S, Muir J, Chey WD. Fiber and functional gastrointestinal disorders. *Am J Gastroenterol.* May 2013;108(5):718–27. doi:10.1038/ajg.2013.63.

35. Suares NC, Ford AC. Systematic review: The effects of fibre in the management of chronic idiopathic constipation. *Aliment Pharmacol Ther.* Apr 2011;33(8):895–901. doi:10.1111/j.1365-2036.2011.04602.x.

36. Fenn GC, Wilkinson PD, Lee CE, Akbar FA. A general practice study of the efficacy of Regulan in functional constipation. *Br J Clin Pract.* May 1986;40(5):192–7.

37. Ashraf W, Park F, Lof J, Quigley EM. Effects of psyllium therapy on stool characteristics, colon transit and anorectal function in chronic idiopathic constipation. *Aliment Pharmacol Ther.* Dec 1995;9(6):639–47. doi:10.1111/j.1365-2036.1995.tb00433.x.

38. Nunes F, Nunes C, Levis E. A double-blind trial of a celandine, Aloe vera and psyllium laxative preparation in adult patients with constipation. *Rev Bras Med.* 2005;62:352–7.

39. Dettmar PW, Sykes J. A multi-centre, general practice comparison of ispaghula husk with lactulose and other laxatives in the treatment of simple constipation. *Curr Med Res Opin.* 1998;14(4):227–33. doi:10.1185/03007999809113363.

40. Rouse M, Chapman N, Mahapatra M, Grillage M, Atkinson SN, Prescott P. An open, randomised, parallel group study of lactulose versus ispaghula in the treatment of chronic constipation in adults. *Br J Clin Pract.* Spring 1991;45(1):28–30.

41. Badiali D, Corazziari E, Habib FI, et al. Effect of wheat bran in treatment of chronic nonorganic constipation. A double-blind controlled trial. *Dig Dis Sci.* Feb 1995;40(2):349–56. doi:10.1007/bf02065421.

42. Anderson AS, Whichelow MJ. Constipation during pregnancy: Dietary fibre intake and the effect of fibre supplementation. *Hum Nutr Appl Nutr.* Jun 1985;39(3):202–7.

43. Graham DY, Moser SE, Estes MK. The effect of bran on bowel function in constipation. *Am J Gastroenterol.* Sep 1982;77(9):599–603.

44. Hamilton JW, Wagner J, Burdick BB, Bass P. Clinical evaluation of methylcellulose as a bulk laxative. *Dig Dis Sci.* Aug 1988;33(8):993–8. doi:10.1007/bf01535996.

45. Heller SN, Hackler LR, Rivers JM, et al. Dietary fiber: The effect of particle size of wheat bran on colonic function in young adult men. *Am J Clin Nutr.* Aug 1980;33(8):1734–44. doi:10.1093/ajcn/33.8.1734.

46. Tomlin J, Read NW. Laxative properties of indigestible plastic particles. *Bmj.* Nov 5, 1988;297(6657):1175–6. doi:10.1136/bmj.297.6657.1175.

47. Lewis SJ, Heaton KW. Roughage revisited: The effect on intestinal function of inert plastic particles of different sizes and shape. *Dig Dis Sci.* Apr 1999;44(4):744–8. doi:10.1023/a:1026613909403.

48. Ford AC, Quigley EM, Lacy BE, et al. Efficacy of prebiotics, probiotics, and synbiotics in irritable bowel syndrome and chronic idiopathic constipation: Systematic review and meta-analysis. *Am J Gastroenterol.* Oct 2014;109(10):1547–61; quiz 1546, 1562. doi:10.1038/ajg.2014.202.

49. Yang YX, He M, Hu G, et al. Effect of a fermented milk containing *Bifidobacterium lactis* DN-173010 on Chinese constipated women. *World J Gastroenterol.* Oct 28, 2008;14(40):6237–43. doi:10.3748/wjg.14.6237.

50. Koebnick C, Wagner I, Leitzmann P, Stern U, Zunft HJ. Probiotic beverage containing *Lactobacillus casei* Shirota improves gastrointestinal symptoms in patients with chronic constipation. *Can J Gastroenterol.* Nov 2003;17(11):655–9. doi:10.1155/2003/654907.

51. Ojetti V, Ianiro G, Tortora A, et al. The effect of Lactobacillus reuteri supplementation in adults with chronic functional constipation: A randomized, double-blind, placebo-controlled trial. *J Gastrointestin Liver Dis.* Dec 2014;23(4):387–91. doi:10.15403/jgld.2014.1121.234.elr.

52. Mollenbrink M, Bruckschen E. [Treatment of chronic constipation with physiologic *Escherichia coli* bacteria. Results of a clinical study of the effectiveness and tolerance of microbiological therapy with the *E. coli* Nissle 1917 strain (Mutaflor)]. *Med Klin (Munich).* Nov 15, 1994;89(11):587–93. Behandlung der chronischen Obstipation mit physiologischen Escherichia-coli-Bakterien. Ergebnisse einer klinischen Studie zur Wirksamkeit und Vertraglichkeit der mikrobiologischen Therapie mit dem E.-coli-Stamm Nissle 1917 (Mutaflor).

53. WHO. Diarrhoeal disease. Accessed March 16, 2020. www.who.int/news-room/fact-sheets/detail/diarrhoeal-disease.

54. Schiller LR, Pardi DS, Sellin JH. Chronic diarrhea: Diagnosis and management. *Clin Gastroenterol Hepatol*. Feb 2017;15(2):182–93.e3. doi:10.1016/j.cgh.2016.07.028.
55. Schiller LR. Nutrition management of chronic diarrhea and malabsorption. *Nutr Clin Pract*. Feb 2006;21(1):34–9. doi:10.1177/011542650602100134.
56. Camilleri M, Brown ML, Malagelada JR. Impaired transit of chyme in chronic intestinal pseudoobstruction. Correction by cisapride. *Gastroenterology*. Sep 1986;91(3):619–26. doi:10.1016/0016-5085(86)90631-1.
57. Gibson PR, Shepherd SJ. Personal view: Food for thought – western lifestyle and susceptibility to Crohn's disease. The FODMAP hypothesis. *Aliment Pharmacol Ther*. Jun 15, 2005;21(12):1399–409. doi:10.1111/j.1365-2036.2005.02506.x.
58. Rao SS, Yu S, Fedewa A. Systematic review: Dietary fibre and FODMAP-restricted diet in the management of constipation and irritable bowel syndrome. *Aliment Pharmacol Ther*. Jun 2015;41(12):1256–70. doi:10.1111/apt.13167.
59. Murray K, Wilkinson-Smith V, Hoad C, et al. Differential effects of FODMAPs (fermentable oligo-, di-, mono-saccharides and polyols) on small and large intestinal contents in healthy subjects shown by MRI. *Am J Gastroenterol*. Jan 2014;109(1):110–19. doi:10.1038/ajg.2013.386.
60. Major G, Pritchard S, Murray K, et al. Colon hypersensitivity to distension, rather than excessive gas production, produces carbohydrate-related symptoms in individuals with irritable bowel syndrome. *Gastroenterology*. Jan 2017;152(1):124–33.e2. doi:10.1053/j.gastro.2016.09.062.
61. Staudacher HM, Whelan K. The low FODMAP diet: Recent advances in understanding its mechanisms and efficacy in IBS. *Gut*. Aug 2017;66(8):1517–27. doi:10.1136/gutjnl-2017-313750.
62. Hill P, Muir JG, Gibson PR. Controversies and recent developments of the low-FODMAP diet. *Gastroenterol Hepatol (N Y)*. Jan 2017;13(1):36–45.
63. Shaw AD, Davies GJ. Lactose intolerance: Problems in diagnosis and treatment. *J Clin Gastroenterol*. Apr 1999;28(3):208–16. doi:10.1097/00004836-199904000-00005.
64. Mattar R, de Campos Mazo DF, Carrilho FJ. Lactose intolerance: Diagnosis, genetic, and clinical factors. *Clin Exp Gastroenterol*. 2012;5:113–21. doi:10.2147/ceg.s32368.
65. Bayless TM, Brown E, Paige DM. Lactase non-persistence and lactose intolerance. *Curr Gastroenterol Rep*. May 2017;19(5):23. doi:10.1007/s11894-017-0558-9.
66. Wang XJ, Camilleri M, Vanner S, Tuck C. Review article: Biological mechanisms for symptom causation by individual FODMAP subgroups – the case for a more personalised approach to dietary restriction. *Aliment Pharmacol Ther*. Sep 2019;50(5):517–29. doi:10.1111/apt.15419.
67. Tuck CJ, Ross LA, Gibson PR, Barrett JS, Muir JG. Adding glucose to food and solutions to enhance fructose absorption is not effective in preventing fructose-induced functional gastrointestinal symptoms: Randomised controlled trials in patients with fructose malabsorption. *J Hum Nutr Diet*. Feb 2017;30(1):73–82. doi:10.1111/jhn.12409.
68. Fernandez-Banares F, Esteve M, Viver JM. Fructose-sorbitol malabsorption. *Curr Gastroenterol Rep*. Oct 2009;11(5):368–74. doi:10.1007/s11894-009-0056-9.
69. Kamal A, Pimentel M. Influence of dietary restriction on irritable bowel syndrome. *Am J Gastroenterol*. Feb 2019;114(2):212–20. doi:10.1038/s41395-018-0241-2.
70. Biesiekierski JR, Peters SL, Newnham ED, Rosella O, Muir JG, Gibson PR. No effects of gluten in patients with self-reported non-celiac gluten sensitivity after dietary reduction of fermentable, poorly absorbed, short-chain carbohydrates. *Gastroenterology*. Aug 2013;145(2):320–8.e1–3. doi:10.1053/j.gastro.2013.04.051.
71. Skodje GI, Sarna VK, Minelle IH, et al. Fructan, rather than gluten, induces symptoms in patients with self-reported non-celiac gluten sensitivity. *Gastroenterology*. Feb 2018;154(3):529–39.e2. doi:10.1053/j.gastro.2017.10.040.

72. Cozma-Petrut A, Loghin F, Miere D, Dumitrascu DL. Diet in irritable bowel syndrome: What to recommend, not what to forbid to patients! *World J Gastroenterol*. Jun 7, 2017;23(21):3771–83. doi:10.3748/wjg.v23.i21.3771.

73. Rao SS, Welcher K, Zimmerman B, Stumbo P. Is coffee a colonic stimulant? *Eur J Gastroenterol Hepatol*. Feb 1998;10(2):113–18. doi:10.1097/00042737-199802000-00003.

74. Boekema PJ, Samsom M, van Berge Henegouwen GP, Smout AJ. Coffee and gastrointestinal function: Facts and fiction. A review. *Scand J Gastroenterol Suppl*. 1999;230:35–9. doi:10.1080/003655299750025525.

75. Brown SR, Cann PA, Read NW. Effect of coffee on distal colon function. *Gut*. Apr 1990;31(4):450–3. doi:10.1136/gut.31.4.450.

76. Generoso SV, Lages PC, Correia M. Fiber, prebiotics, and diarrhea: What, why, when and how. *Curr Opin Clin Nutr Metab Care*. Sep 2016;19(5):388–93. doi:10.1097/mco.0000000000000311.

77. Washington N, Harris M, Mussellwhite A, Spiller RC. Moderation of lactulose-induced diarrhea by psyllium: Effects on motility and fermentation. *Am J Clin Nutr*. Feb 1998;67(2):317–21. doi:10.1093/ajcn/67.2.237.

78. Eherer AJ, Santa Ana CA, Porter J, Fordtran JS. Effect of psyllium, calcium polycarbophil, and wheat bran on secretory diarrhea induced by phenolphthalein. *Gastroenterology*. Apr 1993;104(4):1007–12. doi:10.1016/0016-5085(93)90267-g.

79. Wenzl HH, Fine KD, Schiller LR, Fordtran JS. Determinants of decreased fecal consistency in patients with diarrhea. *Gastroenterology*. Jun 1995;108(6):1729–38. doi:10.1016/0016-5085(95)90134-5.

80. Kamarul Zaman M, Chin KF, Rai V, Majid HA. Fiber and prebiotic supplementation in enteral nutrition: A systematic review and meta-analysis. *World J Gastroenterol*. May 7, 2015;21(17):5372–81. doi:10.3748/wjg.v21.i17.5372.

81. Koretz RL. Probiotics in gastroenterology: How pro is the evidence in adults? *Am J Gastroenterol*. Aug 2018;113(8):1125–36. doi:10.1038/s41395-018-0138-0.

7 Celiac Disease

Taylor Stauble and Stephen A. McClave

7.1 PREVALENCE, PRESENTATION, AND LONG-TERM COMPLICATIONS OF CELIAC DISEASE

Celiac disease (CD) is defined as a chronic small intestinal immune-mediated enteropathy precipitated by exposure to dietary gluten in genetically predisposed individuals (an autoimmune disorder). Gluten is a complex of water-insoluble proteins (gliadins and glutenins) from wheat, but proteins in rye, barley, triticale, Kamut, and spelt show similar immunogenic properties and can elicit a similar response.

The prevalence of CD is estimated to be 1:100 births in genetically susceptible individuals, with a nationwide prevalence 0.7–1.0% of the US population. CD may be grossly underdiagnosed, though, since it is estimated that less than 10–15% of current CD cases are formally diagnosed in this country. CD is 4.0–4.5 times more prevalent than it was 50 years ago, suggesting the emergence of some sort of CD "epidemic." While the exact causes of such an epidemic are not known, the increasing prevalence may be related to dietary grains with increased gluten, more wheat in diets worldwide, other environmental factors, or changes in the collective intestinal microbiota.[1]

The classical form of CD on presentation is less prevalent now. The average age of CD at the time of diagnosis is in fifth decade. Many patients are overweight on initial evaluation. While the sero-prevalence between male and female is equal, the diagnosis is made much more frequently in females than males. Alternative presentations are being increasingly recognized. In a large case series of 770 patients diagnosed with CD, classical symptoms of CD were seen in 34% on initial evaluation with diarrhea, steatorrhea, weight loss, or growth failure.[2] Non-classical symptoms, on the other hand, were seen in 66% of CD patients on initial presentation, which included bloating (20%), elevated liver enzymes (29%), aphthous stomatitis (18%), anemia (34%), alternating bowel habits (15%), gastroesophageal reflux disease (12%), osteopenia/osteoporosis (52%), constipation (13%), and recurrent miscarriages (12%). Additional but more atypical symptoms on initial presentation included ataxia, behavioral abnormalities, depression, epilepsy, hypotonia, dermatitis herpeteformis, infertility, pubertal delay, and defects in tooth enamel. Irritable bowel-type symptoms were seen on presentation in over a third of patients.[2]

The diagnosis of CD is made by serologic testing and small bowel biopsy done at the time of upper endoscopy. Damage from the disease is most intense in the proximal small bowel or duodenum. The Marsh Classification grades the disease severity by duodenal mucosal biopsy over a range of 0–3, based on increased epithelial

DOI: 10.1201/9780429322570-7

lymphocyte infiltration, crypt hyperplasia, and villous atrophy. The serologic diagnosis is confirmed by positive anti-tissue transglutaminase antibody (TTG Ab). This is the single most important, most specific antibody test for CD. It is also the one antibody to follow to document adherence once a CD patient is placed on a gluten-free diet (TTG Ab levels should normalize in 1–2 years with dietary compliance). One problem to remember is that 5–10% of patients with CD are IgA deficient, so either both IgG and IgA antibodies for TTG must be ordered, or IgA TTG with a total IgA level confirmation. Anti-endomysial antibody (EMA) and Antigliadin antibody (AGA) are also available and should be positive in CD, but getting these levels in addition to the anti-TTG Ab does not substantially improve the sensitivity for making the diagnosis and is more likely to introduce false positives when the TTG Ab is negative. In children under the age of 3 years, the TTG Ab may be falsely negative, so an IgA and IgG deamidated gliaden peptide (DGP) should be obtained instead to confirm the diagnosis. Genetic testing is more helpful in excluding CD than for confirming the diagnosis. Two markers, HLA DQ2 and DQ8, are associated with increased risk for CD, but their presence does not alone confirm the diagnosis (patients can have one or both markers positive and not have CD). The absence of the two markers, however, excludes CD (but not non-celiac gluten sensitivity).

Several long-term complications are seen with undiagnosed CD, a point which emphasizes the importance of dietary compliance. Bone health may be compromised, since CD is associated with decreased bone mineral density in adolescents and children (which improves after 1 year with dietary restrictions). An increased incidence of non-Hodgkin's lymphoma is seen in CD, and following a strict gluten-free diet (GFD) for 5 years may be protective. Reproductive function may be diminished, with sexual dysfunction and low sperm quality in men and delayed menarche, increased amenorrhea, and early menopause in women. But most importantly, there is long-term mortality risk. Epidemiologic evidence describes increased mortality rates in adults with undiagnosed CD, and again, a GFD may be protective. While strict adherence to a GFD is associated with no increase in mortality, poor compliance is associated with a two-fold increase and noncompliance with a six-fold increase in mortality.[3]

7.2   NON-CELIAC GLUTEN SENSITIVITY

One of the difficulties in making an accurate diagnosis of CD in a patient on presentation is the overlap of symptoms that can occur over a wide spectrum of disease that extends from CD to Non-Celiac Gluten Sensitivity (NCGS) to Irritable Bowel Syndrome (IBS). NCGS is a diagnosis of exclusion in a patient who presents with symptoms identical to CD (made worse by gluten in the diet), but has negative serology (TTG Ab), normal duodenal biopsies, and resolution of symptoms on a gluten-free diet. In comparison to patients with confirmed CD, patients with NCGS are half as likely to have malabsorption, a family member with CD, or a personal history of autoimmune disorders, and a third as likely to have micronutrient deficiencies.[4] A true IgE-mediated wheat allergy is less common, but must be excluded in a patient with similar symptoms in whom CD has been excluded.

7.3   GLUTEN-FREE DIET IN THE HEALTHY INDIVIDUAL

Problems with experimentation, self-diagnosis, and interpretation of the response to initiation of a GFD create confusion and misleading presumptions for the general public. The placebo response to a GFD in patients with IBS is over 70%. Gluten is hard to digest, increases stool volume, and often eliminates other dietary factors. Potentially other mechanisms may explain the benefit from a GFD, such as a sensitivity to factors other than gluten or even grains. The positive predictive value (the likelihood of confirming a true diagnosis of CD) of symptomatic improvement after gluten withdrawal is only 36% in one study.[5] And patients with CD are more likely to complain of IBS-type symptoms compared with healthy controls.

Over two-thirds of those who eat gluten-free foods do so because they believe a GFD is healthier, one quarter believe it will help with weight loss, and another 10% are convinced it will reduce inflammation and help fight depression.[6] In a survey of people who considered themselves to have gluten sensitivity, only 25% met criteria for a diagnosis of CD. Most initiated a GFD without excluding CD, and 25% reported that their symptoms were poorly controlled despite avoiding gluten-containing foods. In these patients, other dietary intolerances were eventually documented for fermentable oligo-, di-, monosaccharides and polyols (FODMAPs), and caffeine.[6] Traditional use of a GFD is appropriate for CD, gluten intolerance/sensitivity, and wheat allergies. But the lay press have suggested more non-traditional uses that have little evidentiary support and may be inappropriate:

- Autism, behavioral disorders – Scientific trials, no improvement
- Inflammatory Bowel Disease (IBD), Multiple Sclerosis, Rheumatoid Arthritis – No evidence
- Athletes – No scientific evidence
- Weight control – Weight loss only if caloric intake is lowered
- Healthier diet – GFD has higher carbohydrate and fat content, fewer nutrients, greater expense

A self-diagnosis based solely on symptomatic response to a GFD can be a problem if the patient does in fact have true CD. Such an individual is much less likely to get appropriate follow-up and to maintain strict adherence to a GFD. Compliance tends to be higher when the patient has symptoms in response to gluten ingestion, the diagnosis is made at a young age, there is participation in support groups, the diagnosis is biopsy-proven, there is follow-up with medical professionals, and there is ready availability of gluten-free foods. Clear-cut outcome benefits are seen from compliance with a GFD, which include minimizing damage to the intestine, lowering risk of developing gastrointestinal cancers, increasing quality of life, raising life expectancy, and reducing healthcare costs.

7.4   NUTRITION INTERVENTION

The diet management of celiac disease includes the elimination of wheat, rye, barley, and contaminated oats. It is important to note that many alternative names may be used for gluten. Learning to read labels with confidence is key to managing celiac disease. CD patients should know the hidden sources of gluten in foods which otherwise would be unsuspected.[7, 8]

Foods likely to contain gluten:

- Soups, gravies, and sauces (thickeners)
- Salad dressings (thickening agents, soy sauce, and seasonings are often added)
- Seasonings (look for the full list of ingredients vs. a generalized seasoning ingredient)
- Soy sauce (unless listed as GF tamari)
- Granola bars (contaminated oats)
- Candy, gum, and snack foods
- Casseroles and/or cheesy potatoes in which flour is likely used
- Bouillon cubes
- Meat and fish alternatives (artificial crab, veggie burgers, pre-made meats)
- Ice cream, including those with cookies and/or candy (look for those with minimal ingredients. Often, the least expensive options contain additional fillers that have gluten)
- Continuously re-check labels (items that may have been GF previously could experience a change in the manufacturing process or be reformulated)
- Communion wafers
- Omelets or eggs at restaurants may contain pancake batter

A surprising number of foods can serve as hidden sources of gluten. Oats are naturally gluten-free (GF), but may be packaged in a gluten-containing facility or grown next to wheat. Only consume certified GF oats. Tricky ingredients may include but are not limited to hydrolyzed vegetable protein, hydrolyzed wheat protein, modified starch or simply starch (without the source, such as corn listed), soy sauce, maltodextrin, malt flavoring (made from barley), or vinegar. The CD patient should know all forms of wheat (e.g., spelt). Wheat-free does not mean gluten-free. If unsure of the ingredients and not labeled "gluten-free," it is best to avoid consuming. The safest options include fresh and whole foods, such as plain chicken and non-processed fruits and vegetables. With more ingredients, the likelihood of gluten-containing additives is increased. Choose dedicated fryers. Foods fried in the same oil as gluten-containing items, such as battered chicken, are not safe for those with CD. This contact likely contains more than the recommended 20 ppm and can cause an effect. Kitchen cross-contamination can occur easily. Avoid sharing toasters, cutting boards, baking pans, and utensils (flour sifters). Avoid shared condiments and spreads, such as peanut butter jars and dips, since the same utensil may be used on gluten-containing foods when dipped. Phone apps to help determine if a product contains gluten can be helpful. Learning to read labels and looking for certified GF products is best.

Alcohol can be a key source of gluten. Choose certified GF spirits. Be mindful of malt liquor or malt flavorings. Choose certified GF beers. Be aware of beers from which gluten has been removed or which tests below 20 ppm. Gluten can add up when more than one beverage is consumed. Wine is naturally GF. Medications and supplements often contain gluten as well. Only consume those certified GF. Do not rely on the pharmacy to determine if a specific medication is certified GF. It is unlikely that the pharmacist or technician will understand all gluten additives and their system may miss ingredients beyond wheat. The CD patient should call the drug company and/ or look up the medication ingredient list on the manufacturer's website. Do not rely on the physician to know if the drug is certified GF. The CD patient must become an expert in GF medications!

There are many non-traditional sources of gluten. Makeup such as lipstick and lip balm will inevitably be digested and must be GF. Those patients with dermatitis herpetiformis and those with skin sensitivities will want to avoid gluten in their skin products, including lotions, shampoo, soap, etc. Look for naturally GF skin and makeup products. Patients who are thumb-suckers or nail-biters should consider products on their hands, such as lotion. Even toothpaste, cooking spray, and kissing may cause exposure to gluten! This may seem silly, but kissing someone drinking beer containing gluten is a form of cross-contamination. Also, ensure the lip products worn by that other person are GF.

How cooking and eating is organized at home may be a big factor in a patient's ability to adhere to a GFD and avoid inadvertent contamination. For a gluten-free home, one should have two sets of cooking items, GF and non-GF (e.g., toasters, baking items, utensils). CD patients should dispose of aged cutting boards and utensils that have cracks where gluten can remain. If the CD patient is the only person in the home on a GF diet, they should learn to cook and become the chef! If the patient relies on someone to cook the GF meals, make sure that person has a clear understanding of the patient's medical condition and is an expert with the diet. The patient must place the trust of their health in the hands of these other persons. Consider whether the family will all be GF or will cook separate meals.

Tips for dining at restaurants:

- Avoid shared fryers.
- Avoid cooking surfaces shared with gluten containing items, e.g., pizza ovens.
- Visit restaurants with GF menus.
- Call ahead and speak to the manager. Do this even when someone else makes the reservation.
- Tell your waiter/waitress you have CD at the start of your visit. If the staff seems questionable on their view of GF items, politely ask for the manager.
- If there is not a GF menu, ask to speak to the manager or chef to explain options.
- Ask questions. Are the fryers shared? Is the cooking surface thoroughly cleaned or dedicated GF?
- When in doubt, the CD patient should go with their instincts. If one is uncertain whether the restaurants options are safe, select another place to dine out. It's not worth the risk.
- The CD patient should be mindful of where they are dining. While it is not always the case, an upscale restaurant with a chef may be more inclined to understand celiac disease than a fast-food facility.
- Avoid buffets and salad bars, since cross-contamination greatly increases.

Tips for parties and events:

- Eat before. This is key when the CD patient is uncertain of the foods being served.
- Ask the hostess well in advance of the event about the food options and explain individual intolerance to gluten. It can be uncomfortable for the GF person and the hostess to ask at the time of the event.
- The CD patient may want to bring a dish, or several if desired. One can count on these to be GF.
- Snack on whole vegetables, fruits, and cheeses.
- Eating beforehand can decrease the uneasy feeling of requiring a GF diet. It is too easy to focus on those foods which should not be eaten, when the CD patient is hungry.
- If there are minimal foods to eat, the CD patient should try not to let it affect their experience. If necessary to not stand out, grab a plate with items that should not be eaten to draw less attention and/or make the host comfortable. This is only one moment in time. The CD patient can eat after the event, where they know the foods are safe.
- Children with CD should bring GF foods to all events, especially those who are younger and may not understand why their diet is different. Also, these same patients should bring a GF dessert, so they do not feel left out.

Support for the CD patient and a GF lifestyle cannot be overstated. It is important to work with a registered dietitian (RD) to help manage CD. The RD can assist with education regarding reading food labels and disease management, including physician and lab check-ups. Find a gastroenterologist who specializes in CD. The CD patient should work with the gastrocntcrologist for repeat biopsies and annual lab work. While a GFD is the primary intervention for CD, it is important to follow up with the gastroenterologist to ensure that the intestinal mucosa has healed and remains healthy. Obviously, the CD patient should avoid cheating on a GFD. Foods that are not GF will affect the overall outcome of the person with CD. While the person may or may not experience immediate outward symptoms with meals or foods containing gluten (e.g., non-dedicated fryers, one beer, non-GF dessert), the adverse effects on health and the body's physiologic response will eventually be evident. The body recognizes these ingredients as foreign and will only result in further damage. It is essential to remain on a GFD for life. The patient with CD should focus on the foods they CAN have versus those they cannot. One's attitude toward a GFD will go a long way in achieving long-term health!

REFERENCES

1. Rubio-Tapia A, Ludvigsson JF, Brantner TL, Murray JA, Everhart JE. The Prevalence of Celiac Disease in the United States. Am J Gastroent 2012;107(10):1538–44. doi: 10.1038/ajg.2012.219.
2. Volta U, Caio G, Stanghellini V, de Giorgio R. The Changing Clinical Profile of Celiac Disease: A 15 Year Experience (1998–2012) in an Italian Referral Center. BMC Gastroenterology 2014;14:194–202.

3. Ludvigsson JF, Rubio-Tapia A, van Dyke CT, et al. Increasing Incidence of Celiac Disease in a North American Population. Am J Gastroenterol 2013 May;108(5):818–24.

4. Carroccio A, Mansueto P, Iacono G, et al. Non-Celiac Wheat Sensitivity Diagnosed by Double-Blind Placebo-Controlled Challenge: Exploring a New Clinical Entity. Amer J Gastro 2012;107:1898–907.

5. Campanella J, Biagi F, Bianchi PI, Zanellati G, Marchese A, Corazza GR. Clinical Response to Gluten Withdrawal Is Not an Indicator of Coeliac Disease. Scand J Gastroenterol 2008;43:1311–14.

6. Biesiekierski JR. Characterization of Adults with a Self-Diagnosis of Nonceliac Gluten Sensitivity. Nutr Clin Pract 2014;29:504–9.

7. Celiac Disease Foundation. Sources of Gluten, 2020. https://celiac.org/gluten-free-living/what-is-gluten/sources-of-gluten/.

8. Healthy Lifestyle. Nutrition and Healthy Eating. Gluten Free Diet. Mayo Clinic, 2019. www.mayoclinic.org/healthy-lifestyle/nutrition-and-healthy-eating/in-depth/gluten-free-diet/art-20048530.

8 Gastroparesis

Carol Ireton-Jones and Lucian Panait

8.1 INTRODUCTION

Gastroparesis is a chronic neuromuscular dysfunction characterized by delayed gastric emptying of solid food in the absence of a mechanical obstruction. It may be secondary to diabetes, postsurgical (intentional division of the vagi nerves such in gastric resections for ulcer, or inadvertent injury in hiatal hernia repairs), or idiopathic (unknown etiology thought to be related to a viral illness, autoimmune disease etc.) (1). It is generally regarded as a debilitating and incurable disease. The main goals of treatment are to alleviate symptoms and improve quality of life, while preventing nutritional deficiencies and maintaining adequate weight (2).

Symptoms of gastroparesis are often non-specific and require a thorough history. Typical complaints include nausea and vomiting, early satiety and bloating, and epigastric pain, which may be experienced by patients in varying degrees. Other symptomatology includes heartburn, loss of appetite, and weight loss, or, in acute exacerbation, patients may present with episodes of severe dehydration or diabetic ketoacidosis, requiring hospital admission. The Gastroparesis Cardinal Symptom Index is a useful tool both in the initial and subsequent visits and helps assess response to treatment (3). Differential diagnoses of gastroparesis include conditions such as functional dyspepsia, cyclic vomiting syndrome, median arcuate ligament syndrome, irritable bowel syndrome, peptic ulcer disease, gastric outlet obstruction, neoplasm, superior mesentery artery syndrome, etc. (4, 5). It is also important to distinguish isolated gastroparesis from global gastrointestinal tract dysmotility conditions.

Once mechanical obstruction has been ruled out by endoscopy and other imaging studies, the gold standard test for diagnosis of gastroparesis is the 4-hour solid phase gastric emptying scintigraphy, also known as gastric emptying study (GES) (1). This nuclear medicine test assesses the gastric emptying in response to ingestion of a radiolabeled meal. Retention of food in the stomach is calculated at different time intervals, with a confirmatory test being represented by >10% retention at 4 hours. Other diagnostic modalities are represented by antroduodenal manometry, stable isotope labeled breath test, wireless motility capsule, impedance planimetry, gastric barostat, and so on; however, their use is not widely spread and is often limited to specialized centers (6).

The first line of treatment is represented by diet and lifestyle modifications which are described in the next section. Diet modifications are advised in all patients with gastroparesis and should continue even after a surgical intervention. Eating small portions and avoiding foods rich in fat content may help improve symptoms. Liquids and low-residue foods are better tolerated than solids and foods with high-fiber content. In patients with diabetes, good blood glucose control with a target HbA1c < 7% leads to reduced symptom severity (1, 2, 4).

DOI: 10.1201/9780429322570-8

8.2 NUTRITION INTERVENTIONS

Malnutrition and weight loss may occur over time if gastroparesis is not diagnosed and treated appropriately (2). People with gastroparesis may present with vitamin and mineral deficiencies as well as weight loss (2). A thorough nutrition assessment with a detailed evaluation of food intake should be completed prior to planning nutrition intervention. Depending on the time it takes for gastric emptying, food intake may be minimally affected or severely limited requiring enteral or parenteral nutrition support. Nutrition is the primary therapy in gastroparesis because of the effect of the gastric dysmotility in allowing nutrients to pass into the small intestine for normal digestion and absorption. Nutrition management is of utmost importance and a key treatment related to the severity of gastroparesis as well as other underlying conditions such as diabetes, Ehlers-Danlos syndrome, postural orthostatic tachycardia syndrome (POTS), or cyclic vomiting syndrome (4). As with any gastrointestinal (GI) disease, nutrition assessment and interventions must be individualized and specifically for gastroparesis, therapy should concentrate on enhancing gastric emptying. Although there is no specific diet for gastroparesis, the fundamental components of nutrition therapy include (2, 4):

1. Eating small meals 5–7 times per day
2. Avoiding high-fat foods or greasy foods which may further slow gastric emptying
3. If diabetic, maintaining diabetic diet recommendations to manage blood glucose control
4. Avoiding fibrous foods such as raw fruits and vegetables and insoluble fibers
5. Chewing food well
6. Drinking fluids between meals and not at meals to avoid filling up the stomach
7. Sitting up while eating and at least 1–2 hours after a meal to allow gravity to assist with gastric emptying

Often the patient has begun to consume small meals due to their feeling of fullness even prior to diagnosis. The smaller meals or small meals with snacks should also include the additional tenets of the GP diet which include avoiding high-fat foods or greasy foods such as fried foods, fatty meats, and creamed products as well as higher-fiber foods such as raw fruits and vegetables that may be associated with the development of a bezoar. Higher-fat and higher-fiber foods are poorly tolerated since these increase satiety and decrease motility (1, 2, 4, 7). Spicy and highly acidic foods as well as carbonated beverages may also be poorly tolerated.

In addition, time of day may affect the severity of GP with some individuals able to tolerate more "solid" food at certain times of the day. Ground or pureed foods may be helpful and better tolerated. Dehydration may occur if oral fluid is limited; therefore, strategies to avoid dehydration such as goal setting for fluid and food intake is recommended.

Some gastroparesis nutrition references separate the diet into phases or stages as follows: Phase/Stage 1 – liquid; Phase/Stage 2 – soft; and Phase/Stage 3 – long term, regular-modified diet (8). There is no data to support phasing or stages of diet; however, depending on the person and their current status, any one of the diet manipulations may be used. A liquid diet contains liquid or pureed and strained foods that are the consistency of liquid. A soft diet can be quite ambiguous but consists of foods with more structure and consistency than those in a liquid diet. Either of these may be interspersed in the daily or weekly diet of a person with GP.

Particle size of foods is related to gastric emptying rate. In diabetics, this further relates to postprandial glucose levels (9). In a study by Olausson, et al., meals of small particle size and large particle size were compared in normal subjects and individuals with diabetic gastroparesis (10). Two identical meals of 100 g meat (beef), 40 g pasta, 150 g carrots, and 5 g oil were used. The small particle meal consisted of minced and baked beef with the pasta and carrots cooked and mixed in a food processor with additional oil. The large particle meal had roast beef, cooked pasta, and grated raw carrots with oil. Gastric lag phase 120 minutes from ingestion of the meal was measured radiographically in both groups comparing small particle meals and large particle meals. In the healthy subjects the retention of food in the stomach was significantly less after the small particle meal versus the large particle meal. Similarly, the retention of food in the stomach was significantly less in those with diabetic gastroparesis. Although this was a small study of only 7 people per group, the data are helpful in managing food intake and glucose control for individuals with gastroparesis, specifically those with diabetes. Modifying food texture, which may mean modification to near-liquid consistency, allows for most foods to be consumed. A summary of nutrition management techniques is found in Table 8.1.

8.3   MEDICATIONS

Medications can be used to treat GP, but these are limited in scope to those that stimulate muscle contractions to allow for an improvement in gastric emptying (1, 2, 4, 5). Various medications are used when diet and lifestyle modifications are ineffective. The two main categories are prokinetic/promotility agent (e.g., Metoclopramide, Domperidone, Erythromycin), which influence gastric emptying; and anti-emetic agents (e.g., serotonin 5-HT3 receptor antagonists, antihistamines, phenothiazines, low-dose tricyclic antidepressants, etc.), which do not have an influence on the gastric emptying but help with nausea and vomiting symptoms (11). For example, prucalopride (a third-generation, highly selective 5-hydroxytryptamine 4 [5-HT4] receptor agonist) formulated for the treatment of functional constipation may be useful in gastroparesis (12).

8.4   SURGICAL INTERVENTIONS

Surgical interventions are reserved for patients with severe cases of gastroparesis who are not responding to medical management (2, 4). Most of these procedures can be performed in minimally invasive fashion (laparoscopic or robotic).

Gastric electrical stimulation with an implanted gastric neurostimulator, or gastric "pacemaker," is a treatment option that requires specialized expertise and

TABLE 8.1

Summary of Strategies for Gastroparesis

- Try to consume 3–4 small meals and add 2–3 snacks per day.
- Low-fiber foods should be better tolerated – instead of raw, fresh fruits and veggies, use well-cooked fruits and vegetables.
- Fat slows movement in the GI tract so select lower-fat foods. Some fat is good and adds taste – just use small amounts at one time. Avoid fried or fatty foods.
- Some fibrous fruits and vegetables, such as oranges and broccoli, may be difficult to digest and form bezoars.
- Some people find that liquids are easier to pass through the stomach. Try soups (with pureed veggies and meats) and pureed foods. Oral nutrition supplements may be used or homemade recipes.
- Sit up while eating and for 1–2 hours after – let gravity do the work.
- Try gentle exercise after eating such as going for a walk.
- Manage blood glucose to avoid hyperglycemia.

Gastroparesis care may include management of:
- Nausea, vomiting
- Motility augmentation
- Pain
- Stress and other symptoms through counseling, acupressure, biofeedback, and hypnotherapy

Mild gastroparesis: Nutrition, glucose control, and anti-emetic therapy

Moderate gastroparesis: As stated earlier, consider prokinetics, stress reduction, counseling, pain management if needed

Severe gastroparesis: As stated earlier, may need more than one anti-emetic, prokinetics, nutrition support (jejunal tube feeding), pain management, surgical intervention

Source: Courtesy of Good Nutrition for Good Living.

management (3). Gastric electrical stimulation involves delivery of low-amplitude/ high-frequency electrical impulses to the anterior wall of the antrum by a battery implanted in the subcutaneous tissues. These impulses alter the afferent vagal conduction and alleviate nausea and vomiting symptoms. They do not accelerate gastric emptying. The procedure tends to be more effective in patients with diabetic gastroparesis and those whose predominant symptoms are nausea/vomiting (versus bloating/ fullness). Most patients do not obtain immediate relief with insertion of the stimulator and several sequential adjustments of current amplitude, frequency, and time on/off are required over the course of weeks or months post-procedure in order to achieve adequate clinical response.

Pyloric interventions are meant to decrease the resistance to gastric emptying. Endoscopic pyloric injection of botulinum toxin is employed by some physicians for temporary relaxation of the pylorus muscle, either for relief of gastroparesis-related symptoms or to assess the anticipated response prior to pyloroplasty. Even though some patients report symptomatic improvement, this therapy did not show effectiveness in clinical trials when compared with sham procedure and is not recommended by specialized societies (13).

Pyloroplasty is a gastric drainage procedure, which results in accelerated gastric emptying. It involves longitudinal division of the pylorus sphincter and reconstruction of the wound created in transverse fashion, thus resulting in widening of the gastric outlet. The procedure is effective in patients with predominant symptoms of bloating and fullness, and those with idiopathic gastroparesis. In patients with severe disease, pyloroplasty and gastric electrical stimulation can be performed either sequentially or concomitantly.

Peroral endoscopic pyloromyotomy (G-POEM, POP) is an emerging endoscopic option in which partial division of the pyloric wall (muscularis and serosal layers) is performed endoscopically through a short submucosal tunnel in the antrum with the goal to minimize resistance to food passage that may be related to pylorospasm. Initial clinical studies showed effectiveness similar to pyloroplasty (14).

Subtotal gastrectomy is rarely used as a first-line procedure for gastroparesis. It is generally reserved for patients who failed other surgical options and involves resection of the majority of the dysfunctional stomach with Roux-en-Y reconstruction between the remaining small pouch and jejunum.

A special consideration is the management of gastroparesis in the setting of morbid obesity. Many patients with obesity also suffer from diabetes, and lack of control of this disease may further worsen the symptoms of gastroparesis. Strong consideration for bariatric surgery should be given in these cases. Although emerging data with the use of laparoscopic sleeve gastrectomy with or without pyloroplasty is promising, the most commonly accepted treatment option in this population is the laparoscopic gastric bypass with Roux-en-Y reconstruction (15). However, the dysfunctional remnant stomach may still lead to persistence of symptoms after the procedure, even if food bypasses it. If that is the case, remnant gastrectomy will be beneficial.

8.5 NUTRITION SUPPORT

Some individuals with gastroparesis cannot tolerate a normal or even texture-modified intake and require an alternative method of nutrition (2, 4). Enteral nutrition is sometimes required in patients with severe gastroparesis and malnutrition, either as a temporary measure in preparation for other surgical intervention or more rarely as a permanent means of nutritional support. Since the stomach is dysfunctional in these patients, the preferred route is the jejunum, either as a jejunostomy tube or as a gastro-jejunostomy tube (with a gastric port for venting and a jejunal port for feeding). Enteral nutrition is usually well tolerated as long as the feeding tube is placed through the pylorus and into the small intestine. A venting gastrostomy tube may also be needed to allow gastric secretions to empty (1). This may require a specialized tube placement. Chapter 18 describes enteral nutrition for both children and adults. Occasionally, the GP is associated with further intestinal dysmotility and therefore, enteral nutrition is not tolerated. In these cases, parenteral nutrition (Chapter 20) is required to maintain nutrition status. Close monitoring and expert nutrition care are important for successful management of gastroparesis to avoid malnutrition and maintain health.

REFERENCES

1. Camilleri M, Parkman HP, Shafi MA, Abell TL, Gerson L. American college of gastro-enterology. Clinical guideline: management of gastroparesis. Am J Gastroenterol. 2013 Jan;108(1):18–37.
2. Liu N, Abell T. Gastroparesis updates on pathogenesis and management. Gut Liver. 2017;11(5):579–89.
3. Revicki DA, Speck RM, Lavoie S, et al. The American Neurogastroenterology and Motility Society gastroparesis cardinal symptom index—daily diary (ANMS GCSI-DD): Psychometric evaluation in patients with idiopathic or diabetic gastroparesis. Neurogas-troenterol Motil. 2019 Apr;31(4):e13553.
4. Usai-Satta P, Bellini M, Morelli O, et al. Gastroparesis: New insights into an old disease. World J Gastroenterol. 2020 May 21; 26(19): 2333–48.
5. Velanovich V. Expert commentary: Algorithm for the treatment of gastroparesis. In: Grams J, Perry K, Tavakkoli A (eds) The SAGES manual of foregut surgery. Springer Nature Switzerland AG, Cham, 2019.
6. Cline M, Rouphael C. Diagnostic evaluation of gastroparesis. In: Ibele A, Gould J (eds) Gastroparesis. Springer, Cham, 2020.
7. Parkman HP. Idiopathic gastroparesis. Gastroenterol Clin North Am. 2015 Mar; 44(1):59–68.
8. www.mngi.com/conditions/dietary-needs accessed 8.30.21.
9. Olausson EA, Störsrud S, Grundin H, et al. A small particle size diet reduces upper gas-trointestinal symptoms in patients with diabetic gastroparesis: A randomized controlled trial. Am J Gastroenterol. 2014 Mar;109(3):375–85.
10. Olausson EA, Alpsten M, Larsson A, et al. Small particle size of a solid meal increases gastric emptying and late postprandial glycemic response in diabetic subject with gast-roparesis. Diabetes Res Clin Pract. 2008;80:231–7.
11. Bielefeldt K, McKenzie P, Fang JC. Medical management of gastroparesis. In: Ibele A, Gould J (eds) Gastroparesis. Springer, Cham, 2020.
12. Hong JT. Current opinion on prucalopride in gastroparesis and chronic constipation treatment: A focus on patient selection and safety. Ther Clin Risk Manag. 2021 Jun 8;17:601–15.
13. Camilleri M, Parkman HP, Shafi MA, Abell TL, Gerson L. American College of Gastro-enterology. Clinical guideline: Management of gastroparesis. Am J Gastroenterol. 2013 Jan;108(1):18–37; quiz 38.
14. Rodriguez J, Strong AT, Haskins IN, et al. Per-oral pyloromyotomy (POP) for medically refractory gastroparesis: Short term results from the first 100 patients at a high volume center. Ann Surg. 2018;268:421–30.
15. Zihni AM, Dunst CM, Swanstrom LL. Surgical management for gastroparesis. Gastro-intest Endosc Clin N Am. 2019;29:85–95.

9 Short Bowel Syndrome, Malabsorption, Small Intestinal Bacterial Overgrowth

Carol Ireton-Jones

9.1 SHORT BOWEL SYNDROME

Short bowel syndrome (SBS) is defined as insufficient functional intestinal mass necessary to digest and absorb nutrients and fluids to maintain protein, energy, and micronutrient balance (1). In children, SBS is also associated with poor growth and development (2). The loss of intestinal function may also occur due to massive bowel resection, bowel obstruction, dysmotility, congenital gastrointestinal defects, or loss of absorptive capacity as a consequence of disease or treatment such as radiation enteritis (3). Intestinal failure (IF) has been described by a consensus of experts to be a state of "inability to maintain protein-energy, fluid, electrolyte or micronutrient balance" (4). The European Society for Parenteral and Enteral Nutrition has defined intestinal failure as "the reduction of gut function below the minimum necessary for the absorption of macronutrients and/or water and electrolytes, such that intravenous supplementation is required to maintain health and/or growth" (5). SBS may be due to the physical loss of the intestine or due to functional impairment. Children may be born with a congenital malformation such as gastroschisis or may experience necrotizing enterocolitis or volvulus (2). Adults may experience SBS for reasons including resection from malignancies or Crohn's disease, radiation enteritis, volvulus, or trauma (3, 6). In adults as well as in neonates and children, the degree of malabsorption and metabolic complications occurring in SBS depend on the site and extent of intestinal resection or dysfunction (3, 7, 8). The length of the small intestine along with presence or absence and length of remaining colon may be used to categorize IF/SBS as well as to estimate the level of dependence on alternative means of nutrition support, including enteral or parenteral nutrition (3, 6, 7). Oral or enteral intake may be inadequate because of significant malabsorption due to the loss of surface area or function of the small intestine.

9.1.1 INTESTINAL FAILURE

There are three types of intestinal failure (IF) which can be used to define and categorize treatment and nutrition intervention (3). Type 1 is considered a transient state

DOI: 10.1201/9780429322570-9

of intestinal function disruption for which parenteral nutrition (PN) support may be required; however, the IF is temporary and fully reverses. Examples include an ileus after abdominal surgery or trauma until enteral nutrition can be established. Type 2 IF happens with severe illness such as major surgery, burns, or radiation enteritis, for which nutrition support is required for a prolonged period of time related to recovery of intestinal function. This may progress to Type 3 IF. When the IF is persistent and becomes chronic IF, it is considered Type 3 and will require long-term PN support. Motility disorders (i.e., chronic intestinal pseudo-obstruction), significant intestinal surgical resection, congenital disorders, and progression of Type 2 IF are common diagnoses. Short bowel syndrome is the most common cause of Type 3 IF whether surgical or functional (3).

9.1.2 DIGESTION AND ABSORPTION

An understanding of GI anatomy is important in the nutrition care and management of SBS. The duodenum, jejunum, and ileum have roles in the digestion and absorption of individual nutrients (macro- and micronutrients) as well as fluids and electrolytes. In addition, the presence of the ileocecal valve and the amount of colon in continuity affect nutrient absorption, especially related to transit time. Digestion begins in the mouth not only with mastication but also with the presence of saliva, which provides moisture for swallowing and contains amylase that begins the breakdown of starches and fats (9). Food is swallowed and makes its way into the stomach. The stomach has been described as "pouchlike" and acts as a container not only to hold food for passage into the small intestine but also to begin the breakdown of food into chyme through mechanical and chemical digestion (9). Gastric acid as well as enzymes in the stomach begin the digestion of macronutrients. The chyme or partially digested food passes through the stomach through the pyloric sphincter and into the first part of the small intestine or duodenum. The small intestine length consists of the duodenum, jejunum, and ileum (in order) and is approximately 6 m or 20 ft long (9). In the duodenum, most chemical digestion occurs due to hormonal release of digestive enzymes from the gallbladder and pancreas. Carbohydrates, protein, and fats are broken down into monosaccharides, amino acids, and fatty acids, respectively (6). The jejunum is where the most significant portion of absorption of nutrients takes place; and finally, in the ileum, vitamins (and specifically vitamin B12), electrolytes, and any nutrients not absorbed in the jejunum occurs (6, 9). The interior of the small intestine is made up of millions of villi with an absorptive surface area of approximately 30 m^2 (10). The colon or large intestine receives any undigested food as well as water and electrolytes from the small intestine. An additional 2 m^2 of an absorptive surface area is found in the large intestine (colon). Very little nutrition absorption occurs in the colon in normal digestion and absorption although the absorption of water and electrolytes as well as compression of food contents for excretion are extremely important and can be a delicate balance in some GI disorders. Short-chain fatty acids such as butyrate may be absorbed in the colon and account for caloric intake, especially in patients with SBS (9).

9.1.3 NUTRITION INTERVENTION

Nutrition care for SBS, which includes Type 3 IF, is complex, multi-factorial, and ongoing as the patient recovers and the intestine adapts. With SBS the length and function of the small intestine and the presence and length/function of the large intestine are important as well (1, 3, 6, 7). Various estimates have been proposed related to the type of nutrition therapy required and the length of a small bowel remaining. At least initially, parenteral nutrition (PN) is utilized to provide total nutrients for patients with SBS (3, 6). Medical and surgical therapies may be utilized to improve the absorptive capacity (3, 4, 6, 7). The function of the remaining GI anatomy and an intact ileocecal valve will further influence the absorption of nutrients and the toleration of nutrition therapy (3, 6, 7).

The indication for PN in adults and children with SBS is similar, in that PN will support nutrition needs when absorption is nonexistent or minimal. PN will provide carbohydrate in the form of dextrose, fat in the form of lipid, and protein as amino acids, plus sterile water to account for fluid needs as well as age- and need-specific vitamins, minerals, and electrolytes (see Chapter 19). In neonates and pediatric patients, calorie and protein needs are much higher than for adults (8). In addition, higher levels of dextrose in milligrams per kilogram and specialized amino acid solutions are used in the pediatric population receiving PN (8). Patients with SBS and those with IF 2 or IF 3 may need long-term or lifetime PN which is received at home and called home parenteral nutrition or HPN. Vascular access via the central venous route allows higher concentrations of the macronutrients with specialized vascular access devices appropriate for long-term HPN (see Chapter 20). Because SBS patients are likely to receive HPN, pristine care of their central line is crucial for avoidance of central line-associated bloodstream infection (CLABSI), a potential complication of long-term HPN. Optimizing the HPN formulation providing adequate macronutrients/micronutrients/fluid as well as vitamins, trace elements, and managing electrolytes is essential. Management of PN and home PN in the adult is included in Chapter 19 of this book. For more information on management of PN and home PN in pediatric patients, refer to the ESPGHAN/ESPEN/ESPR/CSPEN guidelines on pediatric parenteral nutrition and other references (11–13).

With SBS, the period of time after resection or injury mucosal hyperplasia occurs in the remaining small bowel resulting in improved nutrient absorption is the adaptation phase (3, 6). This adaptation phase happens almost immediately and lasts several months but usually reaches its peak level within 2 years (6, 7, 14). While PN is most often required early on with SBS, enteral (tube) feeding may be used depending on the remaining GI anatomy and function (see Chapters 3, 18). Enteral or oral nutrition is encouraged in adult SBS patients and pediatric patients because of the potential trophic effects on the GI lumen. In pediatric patients, enteral feeding may be used even if it is in very small amounts to provide some energy and also to enhance gut function and adaptation. When an enteral (tube) feeding is used, an elemental or semielemental formula may be better tolerated due to the diminished capacity for digestion of intact nutrients and therefore the absorption of nutrients in this form (see Chapter 18).

For many years, people with SBS requiring HPN either were told not to eat or later to eat whatever they could. Since the early work of Wilmore and colleagues, it has been shown that what is consumed can make a difference in absorption and fluid management (7, 15). The diet for SBS has become more sophisticated as management of SBS has evolved (6, 7, 15). Understanding the remaining GI anatomy – length of a small bowel, presence and amount of the colon, and presence or absence of the ileocecal valve – forms the basis for oral diet recommendations. The oral diet may be "for pleasure only," partial nutrient intake, or consumed with the goal of transitioning completely to an oral diet. In general, oral diet recommendations are (3, 6, 7, 15):

- Consume small meals 5–6 times per day.
- Minimize simple carbohydrates (sugars) and maximize complex carbohydrate intake.
- Certain carbohydrates may be less well tolerated with SBS including lactose as well as FODMAP-containing foods (see Chapter 4).
- If the ileum has been removed and a full or partial colon is present, evaluate for potential restriction of oxalate intake to prevent kidney stones from forming.
- Fat should provide about 20%–30% of total calories. Fat malabsorption may be present if the ileum has been resected.
- Protein intake should be maintained at 20%–25% of total calories. Protein supplements may be necessary.
- Fiber should be provided primarily as a soluble fiber.
- For patients not receiving HPN, a multivitamin supplement should be taken daily, and additional specific micronutrients may be required.

Adequate fluid intake should be maintained to prevent dehydration to avoid deleterious effects on kidney function. To assure fluid homeostasis, intake should equal the output. Output may be affected by ostomy output, diarrhea, vomiting, or fever, and excess fluid loss should be accounted for in calculating the required intake. Because of the GI anatomy in SBS, water may not be adequately absorbed because it requires an active transporter for osmosis to occur. Therefore, fluids with added sodium and a small amount of glucose will facilitate the absorption of the fluid and prevent or treat dehydration. Beverages that are appropriate to provide this hydration are called oral rehydration solutions or ORS. An ORS should have sodium in levels of 70–90 mEq (equal to about ¾ to 7/8 tsp NaCl or table salt), in 1 L, a small amount of glucose, or a simple sugar (28–30 g/L) to assist with the facilitation of the sodium into the lumen and should be isotonic or hypoosmolar (diluted) so that it is easily absorbed by a compromised GI tract. The WHO originated the ORS to treat the dehydration of diarrhea as seen in third-world countries. The WHO recipe for ORS and other recipes may be found at https://cdn.ymaws.com/oley.org/resource/resmgr/ors_recipes/ORS_recipes_handout.pdf. Commercial ORS beverages include Pedialyte© (requires added sodium to meet 70–90 mEq sodium content), Jianas Brothers (Amazon.com), DripDrop© (www.dripdrop.com), and Ceralyte© (www.ceralyte.com). ORS does taste salty and can be flavored with a small amount of fruit juice (1/2 cup to 1 L of water) or a sugar-free taste enhancer. These should be sipped over several hours rather than consumed in a large amount at one time.

9.1.4 Other Considerations

Symptoms associated with SBS include diarrhea, vomiting, and dysmotility due to the multitude of functional and anatomical changes that may arise. Medications may be used to treat symptoms such as anti-diarrheal medications and anti-nausea medications (oral and intravenous), as well as modifications to oral/enteral intake (3, 15, 16). Note that higher than normal doses may be necessary to reach therapeutic levels. Surgical strategies to modify bowel length may be considered in adult and pediatric SBS/IF Type 3 patients to effect absorptive capacity or transit time.

For patients with dysmotility, small intestinal bacterial overgrowth (SIBO) may be present and require occasional to regular antibiotic therapy. This will be discussed in more detail later in this chapter and Chapter 10.

An important and targeted pharmacologic therapy for the management of SBS is teduglutide a GLP-2 analog used to enhance the villus height in the small intestine and therefore improve absorption of nutrients and fluids (3, 17, 18). Phase III clinical trials with teduglutide have demonstrated ~20% reductions in need for HPN or IV fluids in adults with SBS/IF which has been deemed clinically meaningful (17). A meta-analysis has further confirmed the effectiveness of teduglutide for HPN reduction and further that this benefit increases up to 1 year from the initiation of treatment (18). Recent findings show that the presence of the colon in continuity was a positive predictor for weaning which might be expected given the ability of the colon to absorb short-chain fatty acids and fluid (18). Currently, Gattex® (teduglitide a GLP-2 analog for injection) is FDA approved for treatment of SBS in adults.

Liver abnormalities – gallstones, biliary sludge, cholestasis, steatohepatitis – and liver failure are potential complications of long-term HPN. Intestinal failure-associated liver disease (IFALD) is liver dysfunction associated with a non-functioning or poorly functioning small intestine. IFALD has been associated with PN since Type 3 IF is an indication for long-term HPN; however, it is now known that there are multiple associated factors in the development of liver abnormalities (19). Optimizing the HPN formulation in macro- and micronutrient content, especially the type and amount of ILE, avoiding over-feeding, cycling HPN, encouraging oral/enteral nutrition, and preventing CLABSI may help prevent IFALD.

The nutrition interventions in SBS require careful and close monitoring, preferably by a team of nutrition professionals including the physician, nurse, pharmacist, and registered dietitian/nutritionist (RDN). The RDN with an expertise in SBS management can assist the patient and family whether pediatric or adult – in whatever therapy they may be receiving, from PN to oral to a combination of therapies. There is much more information available on management of SBS and nutrition support and should be reviewed for further understanding of this diagnosis.

9.2 MALABSORPTION

Most digestion of macronutrients occurs in the small intestine with tiny amounts beginning in the mouth with chewing as well as the production of a few enzymes primarily for carbohydrates and some fat. Nutrients are absorbed mainly by the small intestine but also fluid and some nutrients from the large intestinal mucosa via both passive and active mechanisms (20). This includes macronutrients (fats, carbohydrates, and lipids) as well as micronutrients (vitamins, minerals, fluids, and electrolytes). The gall bladder and pancreas are responsible for producing enzymes for the digestion of fats, starches, and proteins. In normal absorption, most dietary lipid is absorbed in the proximal two-thirds of the jejunum facilitated by pancreatic lipase (20). While protein digestion begins in the stomach, proteases largely act in the small intestine. When absorption is interrupted due to disease, illness, or surgical resection affecting absorptive capacity, malabsorption and concomitant nutritional deficiencies can occur. Any disease process that affects the function of the pancreas will affect digestion and therefore absorption. Examples of diagnoses include chronic pancreatitis, cystic fibrosis, pancreatic tumors, or resections resulting in pancreatic insufficiency or inborn errors of metabolism. Exocrine pancreatic insufficiency (EPI) is becoming better recognized as a cause of malabsorption due to inadequate pancreatic secretion (21). To recognize malabsorption, the first place a clinician may start is with the signs and symptoms an individual may exhibit. Malabsorption may cause weight loss and nutrient loss. Signs and symptoms of malnutrition may also exist. In fact, weight loss may be less severe than the nutrient loss/deficiency and lead to additional problems such as inability to see or walk, or even cognitive dysfunction. Other symptoms that may occur include steatorrhea, abdominal distension, gas, decreased appetite, or alternatively increased appetite with little weight gain.

Diarrhea is often a symptom found with malabsorption. This may be caused by enzyme deficiency such as in lactose intolerance, excessive sugar alcohol as with sorbitol, bile salt, or pancreatic insufficiency (20, 21). Chronic diarrhea, lasting for several weeks, should be evaluated. Secretory diarrhea in which there are increased secretions into the bowel with or without nutrients entering the bowel can be caused by bile acid malabsorption, microscopic colitis, post-surgical malabsorption, and radiation enteritis. Because this is associated with increased output, limiting intake for 24 hours can help determine the type of diarrhea which will in turn help determine the strategy for treatment. IBS may also be associated with diarrhea; however, unless severe, it is less likely to cause significant malabsorption such as seen with diarrhea associated with inflammatory bowel disease (see Chapter 5). FODMAPs may be associated with diarrhea and therefore limiting certain carbohydrate-containing foods, including sugar alcohols and excess fructose (see Chapter 4), may be helpful. Carbohydrate malabsorption is more likely to cause osmotic diarrhea while steatorrhea may be seen in celiac disease and EPI. Congenital sucrase-isomaltase deficiency (CSID) is a genetic alteration of the enzyme sucrase-isomaltase which causes symptoms including gas, bloating, and diarrhea (23). While it is "congenital" it may not be recognized in adulthood due to lack of a definitive diagnosis (see Chapter 4). *Clostridioides difficile* (*C. diff*) or a parasite may also be a cause for chronic diarrhea and should be evaluated thoroughly and treated succinctly. Vomiting may be present in malabsorption and may indicate decreased motility or blockage which tends to be related to anatomic changes or abnormalities.

9.2.1 Nutrition Intervention

Treatment for malabsorption requires a thorough medical and nutrition evaluation as does excessive or chronic diarrhea. The medical and nutrition assessment should investigate suspicion for macro- and micronutrient deficiencies that may develop (see Chapter 1). Once the cause for the malabsorption is established a plan for treatment and repletion can begin. In the cause of EPI or pancreatic insufficiency, pancreatic enzymes can be taken prior to each meal or snack (21) for lifelong therapy. For patients with IBS who have limited carbohydrate intolerances due to functional GI symptoms, enzyme therapy is being developed specific to disaccharidases, inulinases, and alphagalactosidases (24). There is an enzyme replacement therapy for CSID which can help with sucrase insufficiency; however, with isomaltase insufficiency as well, changes to diet must be implemented (23). For someone with pancreatic insufficiency, these enzymes would not be adequate to improve digestion and absorption. Enteral nutrition products for oral intake or tube feeding have been developed that are specific for patients (pediatric and adults) with absorptive challenges (see Chapter 18). If there is insufficient absorptive capacity, parenteral nutrition support may be necessary to provide macro- and micronutrients – short-term or lifetime (see Chapter 19).

9.3   SMALL INTESTINAL BACTERIAL OVERGROWTH

Small intestinal bacterial overgrowth (SIBO) is defined as an excessive number of bacteria present in the small intestine which is associated with symptoms including gas, bloating, abdominal pain, and diarrhea (25, 26). Chapter 10 provides a more complete review of SIBO; however, its prevalence in malabsorption and SBS warrants attention here. SIBO appears to be more prevalent in women, older individuals, and people with motility disorders (27). The ileocecal valve which is a "sphincter muscle" between the ileum and the cecum (distal small intestine and proximal large intestine), as well as the effect of peristalsis, should minimize the flow of bacteria from the large intestine into the small intestine. In cases of an absent or resected ileocecal valve, dysmotility and the use of proton pump inhibitors may be associated with an increased incidence of SIBO (25). In addition, conditions such as IBS, IBD, and SBS may be associated with an increased incidence of SIBO (28). Although the presence of symptoms may be adequate to empirically treat a patient, the American College of Gastroenterology recommends breath testing to diagnose SIBO (28, 29). While a GI aspirate to assess the bacterial content may be the gold standard, breath testing can be used to determine the presence of SIBO with varying levels of sensitivity and specificity (25).

Treatment of SIBO, once diagnosed or empiric treatment, is to relieve symptoms by destroying the excessive (overgrowth) bacteria present in the small bowel with antibiotic therapy (25, 28). Rifaximin is a non-systemic antibiotic that has been successfully used for the treatment of SIBO; however, some patients' insurance coverage may not reimburse for the drug, making it inaccessible (25, 28–30). Alternative systemic antibiotics may be used to treat SIBO although these are not as well studied specific to SIBO (28). Probiotic and herbal agents have not proven to be effective in treatment for SIBO (25). SIBO is not a chronic condition although patients may experience a recurrence of SIBO up to 9 months after treatment (25). If SIBO continues to be present, a GI aspirate to determine the bacteria present and treat with an antibiotic sensitive to the bacteria is warranted. For patients with extreme dysmotility, SBS, or an ineffective ileocecal valve, other considerations such as a prokinetic agent or regular/cyclical antibiotic therapy may be necessary (25).

9.3.1 Nutrition Intervention

There is no nutrition intervention for SIBO although many have been purported without any scientific validity (27, 28). An elemental diet has been proposed as a therapy for SIBO along with antibiotic therapy (31). The goal is to provide little fuel for the bacteria to feed on in the small intestine and therefore decrease activity and symptoms. In PubMed there is no published study that has evaluated the clinical efficacy of an elemental diet on management of SIBO. The use of the low-FODMAP diet has been proposed for use in patients who have SIBO to decrease the effects of the symptoms (28, 32). While this has been reviewed, it remains hypothetical; however, given the symptoms associated with SIBO, the symptom management based on the low-FOD-MAP diet may be helpful. Most importantly, assessing for adequate intake, food aversions, and orthorexia is an important part of the overall nutrition care plan (28). In addition, patients with SIBO may reach out to non-licensed or scientifically unsound providers who provide supplements and therapies which have no clinical basis. An empathetic but science-based approach to nutrition care is important.

REFERENCES

1. Massironi S, Cavalcoli F, Rausa E, Invernizzi P, Braga M, Vecchi M. Understanding Short Bowel Syndrome: Current Status and Future Perspectives. Dig Liver Dis. 2020 Mar;52(3):253–261. Doi: 10.1016/j.dld.2019.11.013. Epub 2019 Dec 28. PMID: 31892505.
2. Lauro A, Lacaille F. Short Bowel Syndrome in Children and Adults: From Rehabilitation to Transplantation. Expert Rev Gastroenterol Hepatol. 2019 Jan;13(1):55–70. Doi: 10.1080/17474124.2019.1541736. Epub 2018 Oct 31. PMID: 30791840.
3. Bielawska B, Allard JP. Parenteral Nutrition and Intestinal Failure. Nutrients. 2017 May 6;9(5):466. Doi: 10.3390/nu9050466. PMID: 28481229; PMCID: PMC 5452196.
4. O'Keefe SJD, Buchman AL, Fishbein TM, Jeejeebhoy KN, Jeppesen PB, Shaffer J. Short Bowel Syndrome and Intestinal Failure: Consensus Definitions and Overview. Clin Gastroenterol Hepatol. 2006;4(1):6–10.
5. Pironi L, Arends J, Baxter J, et al. ESPEN Endorsed Recommendations. Definition and Classification of Intestinal Failure in Adults: Home Artificial Nutrition and Chronic Intestinal Failure; Acute Intestinal Failure Special Interest Groups of ESPEN. Clin Nutr. 2015;34(2):171–180.
6. Wall EA. An Overview of Short Bowel Syndrome Management: Adherence, Adaptation and Practical Recommendations. J Acad Nutr Diet. 2013;113:1200–1208.
7. Matarese LE. Short Bowel Syndrome. In: Gastrointestinal and Liver Disease: Nutrition Desk Reference. Mullin G, Matarese L, Palmer M (Eds.). Boca Raton, FL: CRC Press; 2012:35–49.
8. Gattini D, Roberts AJ, Wales PW, Beath SV, Evans HM, Hind J, Mercer D, Wong T, Yap J, Belza C, Huysentruyt K, Avitzur Y. Trends in Pediatric Intestinal Failure: A Multicenter, Multinational Study. J Pediatr. 2021 Oct;237:16–23.e4. doi: 10.1016/j.jpeds.2021.06.025. Epub 2021 Jun 18. PMID: 34153281.
9. van Ongen M, Mullin GE. Major Components of the Gastrointestinal System and Their Role in Digestion. In: Gastrointestinal and Liver Disease: Nutrition Desk Reference. Mullin G, Matarese L, Palmer M (Eds.). Boca Raton, FL: CRC Press; 2012:1–8.
10. Helander HF, Fändriks L. Surface Area of the Digestive Tract – Revisited. Scand J Gastroenterol. 2014;49(6):681–689.

11. Mihatsch WA, Braegger C, Bronsky J, et al. ESPGHAN/ESPEN/ESPR/CSPEN Guidelines on Pediatric Parenteral Nutrition. Clin Nutr. 2018 Dec;37(6 Pt B):2303–2305. Doi: 10.1016/j.clnu.2018.05.029. Epub 2018 Jun 7. PMID: 30471662.

12. Krasaelap A, Kovacic K, Goday PS. Nutrition Management in Pediatric Gastrointestinal Motility Disorders. Nutr Clin Pract. 2020 Apr;35(2):265–272. Doi: 10.1002/ncp.10319. Epub 2019 Jul 18. PMID: 31321821.

13. Goulet O, Abi Nader E, Pigneur B, Lambe C. Short Bowel Syndrome as the Leading Cause of Intestinal Failure in Early Life: Some Insights into the Management. Pediatr Gastroenterol Hepatol Nutr. 2019 Jul;22(4):303–329. Doi: 10.5223/pghn.2019.22.4.303. Epub 2019 Jun 27. PMID: 31338307; PMCID: PMC6629594.

14. Billiauws L, Thomas M, Le Beyec-Le Bihan J, Joly F. Intestinal Adaptation in Short Bowel Syndrome. What Is New? Nutr Hosp. 2018 May 17;35(3):731–737. English. Doi: 10.20960/nh.1952. PMID: 29974785.

15. Matarese LE, Harvin G. Nutritional Care for Patients with Intestinal Failure. Gastroenterol Clin North Am. 2021 Mar;50(1):201–216. Doi: 10.1016/j.gtc.2020.10.004. Epub 2021 Jan 7. PMID: 33518165.

16. Kumpf V. Challenges and Obstacles of Long-Term Parenteral Nutrition. Nutri Clin Pract. 2019;34(2):196–203.

17. Iyer KR, Kunecki M, Boullata JI, Fujioka K, Joly F, Gabe S, Pape UF, Schneider SM, Virgili Casas MN, Ziegler TR, Li B, Youssef NN, Jeppesen PB. Independence from Parenteral Nutrition and Intravenous Fluid Support During Treatment with Teduglutide Among Patients with Intestinal Failure Associated with Short Bowel Syndrome. JPEN J Parenter Enteral Nutr. 2017 Aug;41(6):946–951. Doi: 10.1177/0148607116680791. Epub 2016 Nov 23. PMID: 27875291; PMCID: PMC5639959.

18. Bioletto F, D'Eusebio C, Merlo FD, Aimasso U, Ossola M, Pellegrini M, Ponzo V, Chiarotto A, De Francesco A, Ghigo E, Bo S. Efficacy of Teduglutide for Parenteral Support Reduction in Patients with Short Bowel Syndrome: A Systematic Review and Meta-Analysis. Nutrients. 2022 Feb 14;14(4):796. Doi: 10.3390/nu14040796. PMID: 35215445; PMCID: PMC8880479.

19. Mundi M, et al. Management of Parenteral Nutrition in Hospitalized Adult Patients. JPEN. 2017;41(4):535–549.

20. Montoro-Huguet MA, Belloc B, Domínguez-Cajal M. Small and Large Intestine (I): Malabsorption of Nutrients. Nutrients. 2021 Apr 11;13(4):1254. Doi: 10.3390/nu13041254. PMID: 33920345; PMCID: PMC8070135.

21. Diéguez-Castillo C, Jiménez-Luna C, Prados J, Martín-Ruiz JL, Caba O. State of the Art in Exocrine Pancreatic Insufficiency. Medicina (Kaunas). 2020 Oct 7;56(10):523. Doi: 10.3390/medicina56100523. PMID: 33036352; PMCID: PMC7599987.

22. Burgers K, Lindberg B, Bevis ZJ. Chronic Diarrhea in Adults: Evaluation and Differential Diagnosis. Am Fam Physician. 2020 Apr 15;101(8):472–480. PMID: 32293842.

23. Smith H, Romero B, Flood E, Boney A. The Patient Journey to Diagnosis and Treatment of Congenital Sucrase-Isomaltase Deficiency. Qual Life Res. 2021 Aug;30(8):2329–2338. Doi: 10.1007/s11136-021-02819-z. Epub 2021 Mar 27. PMID: 33772704; PMCID: PMC8298246.

24. Singh PK, Kumar V, Yadav R, Shukla P. Bioengineering for Microbial Inulinases: Trends and Applications. Curr Protein Pept Sci. 2017;18(9):966–972. Doi: 10.2174/138920371 8666161122112251. PMID: 27875964.

25. Rao SSC, Bhagatwala J. Small Intestinal Bacterial Overgrowth: Clinical Features and Therapeutic Management. Clin Transl Gastroenterol. 2019 Oct;10(10):e00078. Doi: 10.14309/ctg.0000000000000078. PMID: 31584459; PMCID: PMC6884350.

26. Ghoshal UC, Sachdeva S, Ghoshal U, et al. Asian-Pacific Consensus on Small Intestinal Bacterial Overgrowth in Gastrointestinal Disorders: An Initiative of the Indian Neurogastroenterology and Motility Association. Indian J Gastroenterol. 2022 Oct 10:1–25. Doi: 10.1007/s12664-022-01292-x. Epub ahead of print. PMID: 36214973; PMCID: PMC9549446.

27. Posserud I, Stotzer PO, Björnsson ES, et al. Small Intestinal Bacterial Overgrowth in Patients with Irritable Bowel Syndrome. Gut. 2007;56:802–808.

28. Ireton-Jones C, Weisberg MF. Management of Irritable Bowel Syndrome: Physician-Dietitian Collaboration. Nutr Clin Pract. 2020 Oct;35(5):826–834. Doi: 10.1002/ncp.10567. Epub 2020 Aug 12. PMID: 32786046.

29. Quigley EMM, Murray JA, Pimentel M. AGA Clinical Practice Update on Small Intestinal Bacterial Overgrowth: Expert Review. Gastroenterology. 2020 Oct;159(4):1526–1532. Doi: 10.1053/j.gastro.2020.06.090. Epub 2020 Jul 15. PMID: 32679220.

30. Cottreau J, Baker SF, DuPont HL, Garey KW. Rifaximin: A Nonsystemic Rifamycin Antibiotic for Gastrointestinal Infections. Expert Rev Anti Infect Ther. 2010 Jul;8(7):747–760. Doi: 10.1586/eri.10.58. PMID: 20586560.

31. Rezaie A, Pimentel M, Rao SS. How to Test and Treat Small Intestinal Bacterial Overgrowth: An Evidence-Based Approach. Curr Gastroenterol Rep. 2016 Feb;18(2):8. Doi: 10.1007/s11894-015-0482-9. PMID: 26780631.

32. Wielgosz-Grochowska JP, Domanski N, Drywień ME. Efficacy of an Irritable Bowel Syndrome Diet in the Treatment of Small Intestinal Bacterial Overgrowth: A Narrative Review. Nutrients. 2022 Aug 17;14(16):3382. Doi: 10.3390/nu14163382. PMID: 36014888; PMCID: PMC9412469.

10 Small Intestinal Bacterial Overgrowth

Sujithra Velayuthan, Thomas J. Sferra, and Senthilkumar Sankararaman

10.1 INTRODUCTION

Small intestinal bacterial overgrowth (SIBO) corresponds to the excessive growth of inherent small intestinal flora or the growth of colonic type flora in the small intestine, causing symptoms as a result of early bacterial fermentation, malabsorption, and inflammation (1, 2).

In physiological conditions, the concentration and diversity of microbiota vary in different regions of gastrointestinal (GI) tract (Figure 10.1). The number of bacteria in the human GI tract increases in the cephalocaudal direction (3). The microbiota of the upper small intestine is more representative of the oropharyngeal flora, comprising mostly gram-positive aerobes and facultative anaerobes, and may have some *Enterobacteriaceae* similar to the colonic flora (2, 4). In a normal state of health, the jejunal fluid contains less than 10^3 CFU/mL (5).

The distal part of the ileum is a transitional zone between the small bowel and the colon. The microbial density at the ileocecal valve is approximately 10^6 to 10^8 CFU/mL (2, 6, 7). In the caudal region of the GI tract, the concentration of bacteria increases progressively, reaching up to 10^{12} CFU/mL in the colon (5). The composition of the flora in the ileum is predominantly gram-negative aerobic and some anaerobic bacteria whereas it is mostly anaerobic bacteria in the colon (8). The colonic microbiome is involved in many physiologic processes. The commensal colonic microbial bacteria have enzymatic mechanisms to metabolize indigestible components of the diet such as pectin, inulin, and cellulose by fermentation (as anaerobic environment prevails in the colon) into short-chain fatty acids (acetate, butyrate, and propionate) and gases such as hydrogen, carbon dioxide, and methane (6). The commensal gut microbiome establishes a symbiotic relationship with the host and also offers many other advantages to the host, such as prevention of pathogenic bacterial proliferation, synthesis of vitamins including vitamin K and folate, enhancement of the mucosal immunity, and stimulation of neuropeptide secretion (2, 9). Short-chain fatty acids produced by the flora nourish the colonic epithelium and help to maintain intestinal mucosal homeostasis. The microbiota also metabolizes some prodrugs to release active drugs as in the case of sulfasalazine (8). Dysbiosis is a term referring to any change in the composition of the resident commensal microbiota compared to the microbiota noted in healthy individuals (10).

DOI: 10.1201/9780429322570-10

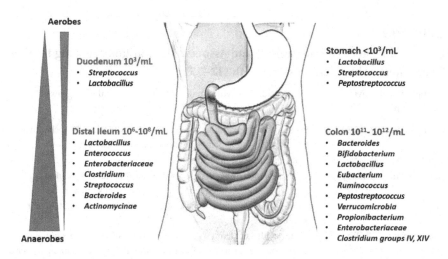

Aerobes

Duodenum 10³/mL
* *Streptococcus*
* *Lactobacillus*

Distal Ileum 10⁶-10⁸/mL
* *Lactobacillus*
* *Enterococcus*
* *Enterobacteriaceae*
* *Clostridium*
* *Streptococcus*
* *Bacteroides*
* *Actinomycinae*

Anaerobes

Stomach <10³/mL
* *Lactobacillus*
* *Streptococcus*
* *Peptostreptococcus*

Colon 10¹¹- 10¹²/mL
* *Bacteroides*
* *Bifidobacterium*
* *Lactobacillus*
* *Eubacterium*
* *Ruminococcus*
* *Peptostreptococcus*
* *Verrucomicrobia*
* *Propionibacterium*
* *Enterobacteriaceae*
* *Clostridium groups IV, XIV*

FIGURE 10.1 Distribution of gut microbiota – bacterial counts CFU/mL.

TABLE 10.1

Natural Protective Mechanisms against Small Intestinal Bacterial Overgrowth

Factor	Mechanism
Gastric acid	Antibacterial action
Bile acids	Antibacterial action
Pancreatic enzymes	Antibacterial action
Small bowel motility	Periodic sweeping (phase III contractions of migrating motor complexes, MMC) of the intestinal contents making colonization difficult
Ileocecal valve	Acts as a physical barrier preventing entry of colonic bacteria into small intestine
Mucosal immunity	Secretory IgA and non-IgA antibodies, T cells, defensins, and an intact mucosal layer contribute to the mucosal defense and epithelial integrity

10.2 PATHOGENESIS OF SIBO

The homeostasis of the gut microflora is maintained by several factors (Table 10.1). The proximal region of the small intestine is kept relatively sterile by the interplay of gastric acid, bile acids, pancreatic enzymes, intestinal motility, mucosal immunity, and an intact ileocecal valve (2, 5, 6). The normal small bowel anatomy and uninterrupted flow of the GI contents in the antegrade direction are essential to maintain the physiological composition of the microbiome. Disruptions in these protective factors such as decreased gastric acidity, reduced pancreaticobiliary secretions, disorders of intestinal motility, altered intestinal anatomy, and decreased mucosal immunological defense mechanisms may result in SIBO (2) (Table 10.2). In SIBO, the overgrowth of bacteria is mostly the colonic type of bacteria, which consists mostly of coliforms and anaerobic species (2, 11).

TABLE 10.2
Disrupted Protective Mechanisms and Associated Conditions Leading to Small Intestinal Bacterial Overgrowth (12–15)

Disrupted Protective Mechanism*	Conditions with Small Intestinal Bacterial Overgrowth
Gastric acid production	Achlorhydria (surgical, atrophic, or autoimmune gastritis), hypochlorhydria resulting from proton pump inhibitors or atrophic gastritis
Pancreatic enzyme secretion	Chronic pancreatitis, cystic fibrosis
Gastrointestinal anatomy	Surgical resection of the ileocecal valve, small bowel diverticulosis, surgically fashioned blind loops, strictures (Crohn's disease, radiation enteritis), enterocolonic fistulas, small bowel narrowing due to tumors, and adhesions
Small intestinal motility	Diabetes mellitus enteropathy, scleroderma, chronic intestinal pseudo-obstruction, chronic usage of medications interfering with motility such as opioids, anticholinergics
Mucosal immunity	Common variable immune deficiency, IgA deficiency, chronic and severe malnutrition, acquired immune deficiency syndrome

* In many conditions such as cirrhosis, old age, chronic pancreatitis, celiac disease, nonalcoholic fatty liver disease, and immunodeficient states, the disrupted protective mechanisms can be multifactorial or the exact mechanisms may be unknown.

Decreased gastric acid production from the use of proton pump inhibitors (PPIs) has been associated with an increase in the incidence of SIBO (16). Despite this, the impact of PPI use on the small intestinal microbiota remains elusive. A study by Weitsman et al. utilizing microbial deep sequencing examined the incidence of SIBO in subjects with and without PPI use (17). Participants underwent upper endoscopy and SIBO was diagnosed based on culture methods. The incidence of SIBO was not different between the two groups, and there was no difference in the microbial composition or diversity.

Alteration in the anatomy of the GI tract that leads to stagnation of the intestinal contents such as strictures (radiation, surgical, or Crohn's disease), blind loops, and diverticulae predisposes to SIBO. Surgical resection of the ileocecal valve promotes bacterial overgrowth in the small intestine (7, 8).

Phase III contractions of the migrating motor complex (MMC), which are intense phasic and tonic contractions, help in the antegrade propagation of intestinal contents along with bacteria from the stomach or proximal small bowel into the colon (11, 18, 19). Disruption of this intestinal housekeeping mechanism either in primary endogenous GI dysmotility syndromes (chronic intestinal pseudo-obstruction) or secondary to underlying conditions such as generalized neuropathies or myopathies promote bacterial colonization (11, 20, 21). In addition, medications such as opioids and anticholinergics slow down intestinal motility, enhancing the development of SIBO (11). The aforementioned factors could act alone or in combination leading to the pathogenesis of SIBO. In a prospective study using wireless motility capsules, patients with SIBO were shown to have decreased ileocecal junction pressure, increased small bowel transit time, and increased intestinal pH when compared with the control population without SIBO (18). Disruption of mucosal immunity and increased mucosal permeability in immunodeficiency states are found to be associated with enhanced jejunal bacterial growth (22). Bacterial overgrowth is common in immunodeficiency states regardless of the type of immunodeficiency and the jejunal bacterial density is increased in children with immunodeficiency conditions.

10.3 PREVALENCE AND CONDITIONS ASSOCIATED WITH SIBO

The exact prevalence of SIBO is unknown due to the lack of consensus in definition, diagnostic criteria, and testing methods (23). Similarly, SIBO has vague and heterogeneous presentations and its symptoms often overlap with other conditions such as irritable bowel syndrome (IBS) or celiac disease, which makes defining the epidemiology challenging (2, 23). Old age is associated with a higher prevalence of SIBO and this is likely due to increased association with achlorhydria and dysmotility with increasing age (24). In addition, SIBO is more prevalent in women.

SIBO is studied extensively in association with IBS and the reported prevalence of SIBO in IBS patients ranges from 8–84% with a pooled prevalence of 38% (25). Other gastrointestinal conditions with a reported high prevalence of SIBO include celiac disease (55%), cirrhosis (50–60%), intestinal failure (50%), chronic pancreatitis (36%), and Crohn's disease (33%) (26–30). In Crohn's disease, the presence of prior surgeries and fibrostenosing disease increase the risk of SIBO (30, 31). Similarly, patients with Roux-en-Y gastric bypass and other blind loop procedures and GI surgeries are also associated with an increased prevalence of SIBO.

Conditions resulting in dysmotility such as hypothyroidism, Parkinson's disease, scleroderma, myotonic dystrophy type 1, and long-standing diabetes mellitus (DM) have increased prevalence of SIBO (2). In adults with type 2 DM, orocecal transit time is significantly delayed in the SIBO population when compared to patients without SIBO (32). SIBO is also seen in association with many systemic conditions such as rosacea, cystic fibrosis (CF), fibromyalgia, restless leg syndrome, and multiple sclerosis, but the exact mechanisms by which SIBO develops in these conditions are not known (6, 11, 33).

Immunodeficiency states such as IgA deficiency, chronic variable immune deficiency (CVID), and acquired immune deficiency syndrome (AIDS) have an increased prevalence of SIBO. In addition to disruption of mucosal integrity, vagal dysfunction is also found to be associated with SIBO in AIDS-associated enteropathy (34). Patients with morbid obesity, metabolic syndrome, and nonalcoholic fatty liver disease (NAFLD) have an increased association with SIBO (35, 36). The overgrowth of bacteria in the small intestine may lead to changes in intestinal permeability via disruption of epithelial tight junctions (7, 33, 36–38). The resulting endotoxemia (gram-negative bacterial cell wall contains endotoxin which is made up of lipopolysaccharides) from SIBO leads to secretion of proinflammatory cytokines which potentially contributes to the development of NAFLD. Specifically, SIBO with gram-negative bacteria may contribute to NAFLD via multiple mechanisms such as enhanced insulin resistance, increased endogenous ethyl alcohol production, and deficiency of choline (39).

10.4 CLINICAL MANIFESTATIONS AND NUTRITIONAL CONSEQUENCES

Symptoms of SIBO are non-specific and result mainly from excessive fermentation of carbohydrates, bacterial consumption of nutrients, and malabsorption of macro- and micronutrients (40). Increased bacterial utilization of the unabsorbed carbohydrate results in increased gas and water production from fermentation (2). This increased gas formation results in bloating sensation, abdominal distension, and flatulence (2, 40). The other reported symptoms include belching, abdominal pain, abdominal discomfort, nausea, and loose stools.

In most instances, the symptoms are mild, but in some patients, severe manifestations such as weight loss, steatorrhea, and manifestations of macro- and micronutrient deficiencies may be noted (11, 41). The excessive bacterial load can deconjugate bile acids and disrupt its enterohepatic circulation, thereby limiting its availability for the absorption of fat and fat-soluble vitamins (2, 6, 40). The intestinal bacteria help with the production of folic acid, vitamin K, and vitamin B12 in the physiological state. Although few bacterial species produce vitamin B12, in SIBO, vitamin B12 deficiency may be noted due to overwhelming bacterial consumption and malabsorption of vitamin B12 (2, 39). Vitamin B12 deficiency results in macrocytic anemia, and neurological manifestations of peripheral neuropathy, such as weakness, sensory ataxia, and paresthesia (40). In extreme cases, vitamin D deficiency may lead to hypocalcemia resulting in tetany, vitamin A deficiency may manifest as night blindness, and vitamin E deficiency may result in peripheral neuropathy (6). Physical examination may reveal mild abdominal distension and borborygmi from excessive gassiness, but may also be normal. In severe cases, children are prone to growth retardation due to the malabsorptive nature of this condition (7).

The intestinal histology in SIBO is usually unaltered, and in some instances, epithelial damage with mucosal inflammation may be noted (6). The excessive bacterial growth with its metabolic products can cause inflammatory changes in the epithelium resulting in villous atrophy (6, 42). This villous atrophy leads to a reduction in absorptive surface and also can result in loss of disaccharidases (such as lactase deficiency), further contributing to malabsorption (23, 40). Additionally, the deconjugated bile acids, such as lithocholic acid, cause injury to the intestinal epithelium and cause diarrhea by secretomotor effect (2). While diarrhea is a common symptom of SIBO, patients with methanogenic archaea, *Methanaobrevibacter smithii*, may present with constipation since methane is shown to slow the intestinal transit (12, 43). The symptoms of SIBO also lead to reduced food intake, further limiting the availability of nutrients (2).

Fermentation of the unabsorbed carbohydrates in SIBO by some strains of colonic-type bacteria such as *Lactobacillus* and *Bifidobacterium* results in the formation of D-lactic acid (44). Humans cannot metabolize a large amount of D-lactic acid resulting in D-lactic acidosis-induced encephalopathy, which manifests as brain fogginess (44, 45). This brain fogginess is characterized by short-lived confusion, impairment of concentration, judgment, and memory, along with gait disturbance and slurred speech.

10.5 DIAGNOSIS

10.5.1 SMALL INTESTINAL FLUID ASPIRATION AND CULTURE

The diagnosis of SIBO is based on the concentration of bacterial flora from a jejunal aspirate. Historically, when these studies were done on patients with intestinal blind loops, a cutoff value of over 10^5 CFU/mL was considered diagnostic of SIBO (46). However, recent studies suggest the bacterial count from jejunal aspirates in normal subjects rarely exceeds 10^3 CFU/mL (23, 46). Thus, the definition based on the culture of duodenal/jejunal aspirate is debatable. The North American consensus published in 2017 recommends using $>10^3$ CFU/mL as the cutoff (11, 47). The duodenal or jejunal aspirate is collected during an endoscopic procedure. Care is taken to avoid oral flora contamination, and the aspirated fluid is submitted to the laboratory for quantitative culture (2). Aspirates growing more than 10^3 CFU/mL are considered positive (48). Even though this is considered the gold standard to diagnose SIBO, it is invasive and expensive. The utility of this testing is limited due to technical difficulties in reaching the jejunum, lack of standards for aspiration and culture techniques, and possible contamination with oropharyngeal flora (1). Additionally, the distribution of the bacterial overgrowth may not be uniform within the jejunum, leading to false-negative results when the sample is obtained from a non-representative region (sampling error). Fastidious bacteria requiring special culture techniques and longer incubation periods are difficult to culture using standard methods.

10.5.2 BREATH TEST

Hydrogen breath testing is a simple and cost-effective alternative to jejunal cultures in diagnosing SIBO and is widely utilized in clinical settings. The hydrogen breath test is based on the fact that the only source of hydrogen in the human body is from bacterial degradation (unique to prokaryotic metabolism) of carbohydrates in the GI tract (3, 11). Other gases produced by bacterial degradation include methane and hydrogen sulfide. These gases are readily absorbed into the circulation and eventually exhaled from the lungs. The concentration of these gases in exhaled air can be measured using gas chromatography. The currently available gas chromatography machines for routine clinical testing measure only hydrogen and methane. Analysis of methane in the exhaled gas is essential since some patients have predominantly methane-producing archaea. However, a smaller fraction of patients with SIBO may have predominantly hydrogen sulfide-producing bacteria and these patients are not detected with this test.

Glucose and lactulose are commonly used substrates for this test. In physiological states, glucose is entirely absorbed in the proximal small intestine and is not available for the colonic bacterial degradation. However, in patients with SIBO, bacteria in the proximal small bowel ferment the glucose before absorption from the intestinal lumen, producing the volatile gases. In addition, malabsorption associated with SIBO provides glucose substrate for the bacteria residing in distal small intestines. Lactulose, on the other hand, is a synthetic, non-absorbable, fermentable disaccharide.

TABLE 10.3

Preparations before the Breath Tests (21, 48, 49)

Entity	Stop Prior to Testing	Rationale
Antibiotics	4 weeks	False-negative result due to treatment of SIBO if present
Bismuth preparations	2–4 weeks	False-negative result due to suppression of SIBO if present
Prokinetics and Laxatives	1 week	False-positive result due to decreased intestinal transit time
Food	8–12 hours	False-positive result due to colonic bacterial fermentation of sugars consumed prior to testing
Smoking	Day of testing	False-positive result due to increased hydrogen and carbon dioxide in the exhaled breath
Exertion	During testing	False-negative result due to low exhaled hydrogen associated with hyperventilation
Non-absorbable carbohydrates (pasta, bread, fiber cereal, beans)	Avoid the day before testing	Affects baseline breath hydrogen making the test not interpretable

In SIBO, due to bacterial overgrowth in the small intestine, the lactulose is fermented before it reaches the colon and an early rise in hydrogen is observed.

The North American consensus statement outlines the standards for preparation, performance, and interpretation of breath tests (47). Factors that affect the interpretation of hydrogen breath tests such as antibiotics, laxatives, prokinetics, diet, smoking, and exercise are avoided prior to the testing as noted in Table 10.3.

Patients need to fast for 8–12 hours before the test. Baseline hydrogen and methane values are obtained before the patient ingests the substrate. Either glucose or lactulose is utilized as the substrate in breath testing for SIBO. Glucose is given at a dose of 75 grams and lactulose at 10 grams mixed with or followed by a cup of water (47). After ingestion of the sugar, methane and hydrogen values are measured every 15 minutes. At this time, the general consensus to diagnose SIBO is a rise in hydrogen value ≥20 parts per million (PPM) or methane value ≥10 PPM above baseline within 90 minutes of ingesting glucose or lactulose (11). The extent of rise in hydrogen correlates with symptom severity in patients with SIBO (13). The sensitivity and specificity of the glucose breath test are 20–93% and 30–86%, respectively, when compared with small bowel fluid culture (46). For the lactulose breath test, the sensitivity and specificity are 31–68% and 44–100%, respectively. Conflicting results exist in the literature regarding the influence of using prebiotics, probiotics, and PPI on breath tests (47). Thus, it is unclear if their use should be modified or discontinued prior to the study.

Even though this test is technically easy to perform, various factors can influence the test results. The orocecal transit time varies between subjects, more so when using lactulose as the substrate since lactulose is a laxative (1, 14). Therefore, a rise in hydrogen before 90 minutes may not be reliable in all patients. When using lactulose as a substrate, double hydrogen peaks may be noted in SIBO due to bacterial fermentation. Studies using lactulose breath test in combination with scintigraphy in SIBO have shown an early rise in hydrogen and methane before the arrival of lactulose in the cecum, which corresponds to bacterial degradation in the distal ileum and the higher rise may be seen minutes later, which correlates with colonic fermentation (50). However, double peaks are not uniformly noticed in all lactulose breath tests and they are not required to diagnose SIBO. Incorporating methane in the breath test increases the sensitivity of the testing. Up to 30% of patients with SIBO may harbor predominantly methane-producing archaea such as *Methanaobrevibacter smithii* (43). Thus, testing only for hydrogen in breath tests may lead to false-negative results (12, 43).

10.6 MANAGEMENT

The management of SIBO is effectively accomplished by correcting the underlying predisposing conditions whenever possible, controlling the bacterial overgrowth with antibiotic therapy, and optimizing the deranged nutritional status (5). In patients with chronic PPI use and other medications promoting SIBO such as anticholinergics and narcotics, every attempt should be made to wean and discontinue their usage. The management of underlying conditions that predispose to SIBO should be optimized. For example, in long-standing, poorly controlled diabetic enteropathy, controlling the blood sugar levels will enhance motility and improve symptoms of SIBO.

10.6.1 ANTIBIOTICS

Treatment with antibiotics has been shown to result in breath test normalization and relief of symptoms (41). Melchior et al. demonstrated the superiority of antibiotics over gas absorbents in treating flatus incontinence in patients suffering from SIBO (51). Both systemic and non-systemic antibiotics have been used to treat SIBO. Different systemic antibiotics such as amoxicillin-clavulanate, ciprofloxacin, doxycycline, metronidazole, norfloxacin, tetracycline, and trimethoprim-sulfamethoxazole are tried in the management of SIBO. Antibiotics are shown to be more efficacious than placebo in a meta-analysis (41). The breath test normalization rate with antibiotics was 51% when compared with placebo at 9.8% (41). Given the limitations of current testing methods, an empiric course of antibiotic treatment is often attempted (42). But the disadvantage of empiric treatment is an overuse of antibiotics in conditions that mimic SIBO (52).

Rifaximin is the most widely studied non-absorbable, broad-spectrum antibiotic for the management of SIBO. It is minimally absorbed and the concentration of the drug in the GI tract far exceeds the minimum inhibitory concentration needed to inhibit most pathogenic bacteria (53). Rifaximin is overall successful in eradicating SIBO in more than two-thirds of patients (53, 54). A meta-analysis comparing rifaximin with systemic antibiotics (chlortetracycline and metronidazole) showed superior efficacy of rifaximin (53). Rifaximin also confers eubiotic effects by increasing the resident bacteria such as *Lactobacillus* and *Bifidobacterium* (49, 55). Rifaximin is used in a dose range of 600–1600 mg/day and the treatment duration varies between 5 days and 4 weeks (53). Higher doses are found to be associated with better eradication rates (53). Rifaximin can be used in combination with other therapies to enhance its effectiveness. Combinations with mesalamine have been shown to be beneficial in specific groups such as patients with diverticulitis and Crohn's disease (56, 57). The addition of a prebiotic, hydrolyzed guar gum, to rifaximin was more efficient in eradicating SIBO than rifaximin alone (58). Rifaximin is generally well tolerated in SIBO, and a meta-analysis showed the overall adverse events at 4.6% (53). Rifaximin is also relatively more expensive than the commonly used systemic antibiotics.

In patients with SIBO due to methanogenic archaea, single antibiotic therapy may not be effective because these micro-organisms are resistant to many antibiotics. A combination of neomycin and rifaximin may be effective (59, 60).

Approximately 30–40% of the SIBO patients have persistence of symptoms after antibiotic treatment (60). For these non-responders, other coexisting conditions such as disaccharidase deficiency, pancreatic insufficiency, food intolerances, medication side effects, and an alternate diagnosis (such as functional dyspepsia and factitious disorders) should be considered (1). An overgrowth of fungal organisms, a process called small intestinal fungal overgrowth, can mimic symptoms of SIBO (61).

Recurrence of SIBO is reported in many studies. In one study, 44% of patients relapsed with an abnormal breath test within 9 months of initial antibiotic management (60). In 10% of these patients, recurrence was noted as early as 3 months. The noted risk factors for recurrence include old age, treatment with a PPI, and history of an appendectomy. There are no controlled studies to direct the management of recurrent SIBO and the current management approaches are based on clinical experience (23). In patients with underlying anatomic abnormalities, including intestinal blind loops and small bowel diverticula, the recurrence of SIBO is common. Prolonged courses of antibiotics or repeated antibiotic courses of 5–7 days per month are recommended for the management of recurrent SIBO. Risk of long-term antibiotic use, such as antibiotic resistance, *Clostridioides difficile* infection, cost, and intolerance of antibiotics should be borne in mind while choosing this approach (8). In patients with infrequent recurrences (defined by some as ≤3/year), repeating the same antibiotic regimen is recommended (62). For more frequent recurrences (>3/year), rotating antibiotics every 1–2 months is recommended for patients with high risk of SIBO.

10.6.2 PROKINETICS

Prokinetic agents such as 5-HT4 agonists (e.g., prucalopride, cisapride), dopamine antagonists (e.g., domperidone), and motilin receptor agonists (e.g., erythromycin, azithromycin) have been tried to treat bacterial stasis in conditions with dysmotility, which also may help in the prevention of SIBO recurrence (15). These agents can augment the phase III MMC complexes (63). However, there is a paucity of data supporting this phenomenon and some prokinetics such as cisapride are not available (due to untoward side effects) in the United States (5). In AIDS-associated autonomic neuropathy, pyridostigmine (acetylcholinesterase inhibitor) has been tried in enhancing intestinal motility, which reduces SIBO and SIBO-associated complications, such as bacterial translocation and increased inflammatory markers (64). Similarly, in patients on long-term PPI, the risk of SIBO was reduced with concurrent use of prokinetics (65). Lubiprostone, by activating chloride-2 channels in the small bowel epithelium, increases small intestinal mucosal secretion, including mucus glycoprotein or mucin. Thus, in patients with chronic constipation, lubiprostone reduces SIBO by reducing the small bowel transit time (66).

10.7 NUTRITION AND OTHER NON-PHARMACOLOGICAL MANAGEMENT

Nutritional management plays a significant role in the management of SIBO. In addition to bacterial consumption of nutrients, the epithelial damage from toxic bacterial products also plays a part in nutrient malabsorption (2). Patients with SIBO require long-term nutritional surveillance (for both macro- and micronutrient deficiencies) and management since mucosal repair takes time (8, 56). Among the micronutrient deficiencies, vitamin B12, thiamin, nicotinamide, iron, and fat-soluble vitamins (A, D, and E) have been reported in SIBO (2, 67, 68).

An elemental diet, consisting of amino acids, is mostly absorbed in the first few feet of the intestines. It is speculated that an elemental diet reduces the amount of nutrients entering the distal small intestines, thereby depriving the bacteria of nutrients (69). In one study, an exclusive elemental diet for 15–21 days resulted in the normalization of the breath hydrogen excretion and improvement in clinical symptoms in the majority of patients with SIBO (69). However, adherence to this diet requires high patient motivation because these diets are unpalatable. Another dietary approach involves the reduction of fermentable products. Fermentable oligosaccharides, disaccharides, monosaccharides, and polyols (FODMAP) are short-chain carbohydrates that can be easily metabolized by small bowel bacteria. A low-FODMAP diet renders less substrate for the intestinal bacteria for fermentation and gas production and is found to improve symptoms in patients with IBS (70). However, the data available to recommend this diet for SIBO are sparse (1, 70). Other diets, such as biphasic, fast tract, and SIBO-specific diets have been utilized, and the literature on these diets is limited. The underlying principle of these diets is similar to the low-FODMAP diet (39). Prior to initiating the aforementioned restrictive diets, a referral to a registered dietitian will help patients to effectively balance the nutritional intake and prevent/improve both macro- and micronutrient deficiencies.

10.7.1 PROBIOTICS

Probiotics have been employed alone and in conjunction with antibiotics in the management of SIBO, but their exact role is unclear (71). Probiotics are perceived to act by fortifying intestinal barrier function and thereby modulating the intestinal inflammatory response (72). Probiotics carry out a competitive displacement of pathogenic organisms from the mucosal layer by outnumbering them and thereby limiting bacterial translocation (5, 73). They produce antibacterial substances (bacteriocin) and also help in modulating signaling between luminal bacteria, intestinal epithelium, and the mucosal immune system (5, 73, 74).

In a study evaluating the short-term efficacy of probiotics in patients with chronic liver disease, the symptoms of SIBO improved in the probiotic group when compared with the placebo group, although intestinal permeability did not change significantly between groups (75). In the probiotic group, the fecal excretion of three of the six administered probiotic species was significantly increased and no change was noted in the placebo group. Moreover, in the probiotic group, the reduction of SIBO followed a reduction in hydrogen-producing bacteria but not with the methane-producing microbiota.

A meta-analysis indicated that the use of probiotics was associated with a significantly higher eradication rate in SIBO and also effectively decreased abdominal pain scores (76). However, probiotic use was associated with a low but insignificant trend towards the prevention of SIBO. Although the use of probiotics is deemed safe, a study by Rao et al. evaluating patients with abdominal pain, gas, and bloating found an increased usage of probiotics and incidence of SIBO in patients with the brain fogginess when compared to patients without brain fogginess (44). This brain fogginess resolved after discontinuing probiotics and treating of SIBO with a course of antibiotics.

10.7.2 HERBAL REMEDIES

Herbal remedies are gaining popularity in SIBO, since they are considered natural and perceived to have fewer side effects, although more studies are required before recommending this management approach. An anecdotal case of successful management of SIBO using enteric-coated peppermint oil has been reported (77). A study involving IBS patients showed improved response to herbal remedies compared with rifaximin with respect to lactulose breath test normalization (33). The side effects were also less in the herbal groups compared to rifaximin in this study. The commercial herbal preparations (Dysbiocide®, FC-Cidal™, Candibactin-AR®, Candibactin-BR®) utilized in this study had more than one active ingredient. Similarly, herbal therapies used in complementary and alternative medical methods, such as traditional Chinese medicine and Ayurveda, are being explored in the management of SIBO (78, 79). Various mechanisms have been proposed for the action of herbs in SIBO including prokinetic and carminative actions and antimicrobial activity (80, 81). However, more studies are required to elucidate the safety and efficacy of the utility of herbal remedies in SIBO. IBS patients with positive lactulose breath tests showed greater test normalization with herbal remedies when compared with rifaximin (33). Side effects were also less in the herbal groups. There is nonetheless still limited evidence to suggest herbal remedies as a treatment for SIBO (33).

10.8 NOVEL APPROACHES

A novel orally ingested capsule device is being designed to measure hydrogen and carbon dioxide gases and sampling microbiota in different regions of the GI tract (1, 45). Current chromatography machines measure only hydrogen and methane but not hydrogen sulfide, leaving a few patients (who predominantly produce hydrogen sulfide) with symptoms of SIBO undiagnosed. Newer studies evaluating the utility of measuring hydrogen sulfide to improve the sensitivity of breath testing is under study (11). Measuring volatile substances in breath by mass spectrometry is another advancement in diagnosis of SIBO which is in early stages of development.

10.9 INCORRECT/OUTDATED PRACTICES

Serum markers, such as bile acids, folic acid, and cobalamin, were studied as surrogate markers for diagnosis of SIBO, but are not used any longer due to insufficient accuracy (8). Indirect methods to evaluate the bacterial activity, such as measuring urinary indican, cholyl-paraminobenzoic acid (cholyl-PABA), and 4-hydroxyphenylacetic acid, in SIBO were also employed in the past but fell out of favor (46). Similarly, breath tests utilizing D-xylose, ^{13}C-xylose, bile acids (radiolabeled ^{14}C or ^{13}C), and cholyglycine were outdated, given the lack of validity. There is also radiation hazard with ^{14}C materials and, hence, cannot be used in pregnant women and children.

10.10 CONCLUSION

SIBO is a common yet underrecognized condition with increased prevalence in subjects with underlying disease processes interfering with the normal anatomy, protective physiological mechanisms, and normal motility of the GI tract. The available diagnostic studies have their drawbacks and newer testing modalities are required to efficiently and confidently diagnose SIBO. At this time, the recommendation is to utilize glucose or lactulose breath testing to diagnose SIBO, which is comparable to the gold standard, the culture of duodenal or jejunal aspirates. Antibiotics and nutritional optimization, along with correction of the contributing factors whenever possible, remain the cornerstone in the management of SIBO. Further studies evaluating the role of specific diets and probiotics in the management of SIBO are needed.

PRACTICE PEARLS

- Symptoms of SIBO are non-specific and overlap with other GI disorders. Despite being known for a long time, there is lack of standardized methods for diagnosis and treatment of SIBO.
- The current gold standard method to diagnose SIBO is the culture of duodenal/jejunal aspirate showing more than 10^3 CFU/mL. However, indirect testing methods, such as lactulose or glucose breath testing, are widely used to diagnose SIBO due to less invasiveness and easy availability.
- The currently accepted mode of management is aimed at correcting the underlying conditions predisposing SIBO, decontamination using antibiotics, and correcting the nutritional deficiencies. Currently, there are no guidelines for the management of SIBO in the pediatric population.

- Probiotics and herbal remedies are found to be effective in small studies. More evidence is required to recommend these therapies for the management of SIBO.
- For recurrent SIBO, the culture of jejunal aspirate and treatment with appropriate antibiotics based on sensitivity pattern is recommended. In addition, the underlying and predisposing factors, such as medications (e.g., PPI and opioids), should be minimized. A careful search for an alternate diagnosis and other conditions with overlapping symptoms should be sought and treated accordingly for treatment failures.

REFERENCES

1. Rao SSC, Bhagatwala J. Small Intestinal Bacterial Overgrowth: Clinical Features and Therapeutic Management. Clin Transl Gastroenterol. 2019;10(10):e00078.
2. Adike A, DiBaise JK. Small Intestinal Bacterial Overgrowth: Nutritional Implications, Diagnosis, and Management. Gastroenterol Clin North Am. 2018;47(1):193–208.
3. Simren M, Stotzer PO. Use and Abuse of Hydrogen Breath Tests. Gut. 2006;55(3):297–303.
4. Sundin OH, Mendoza-Ladd A, Zeng M, Diaz-Arevalo D, Morales E, Fagan BM, et al. The Human Jejunum has an Endogenous Microbiota that Differs from Those in the Oral Cavity and Colon. BMC Microbiol. 2017;17(1):160.
5. Quigley EM, Quera R. Small Intestinal Bacterial Overgrowth: Roles of Antibiotics, Prebiotics, and Probiotics. Gastroenterology. 2006;130(2 Suppl 1):S78–90.
6. Gewecke K, Nannen-Ottens S. Bacterial Overgrowth: Nutrition as part of the Therapeutic Concept. Small Intestinal Bacterial Overgrowth (SIBO). Ernahrungs Umschau. 2017;64(4):67–73.
7. Avelar Rodriguez D, Ryan PM, Toro Monjaraz EM, Ramirez Mayans JA, Quigley EM. Small Intestinal Bacterial Overgrowth in Children: A State-of-the-Art Review. Front Pediatr. 2019;7:363.
8. Quigley EM, Abu-Shanab A. Small Intestinal Bacterial Overgrowth. Infect Dis Clin North Am. 2010;24(4):943-59, viii–ix.
9. Eckburg PB, Bik EM, Bernstein CN, Purdom E, Dethlefsen L, Sargent M, et al. Diversity of the Human Intestinal Microbial Flora. Science. 2005;308(5728):1635–8.
10. Petersen C, Round JL. Defining Dysbiosis and its Influence on Host Immunity and Disease. Cell Microbiol. 2014;16(7):1024–33.
11. Pimentel M, Saad RJ, Long MD, Rao SSC. ACG Clinical Guideline: Small Intestinal Bacterial Overgrowth. Am J Gastroenterol. 2020;115(2):165–78.
12. Kunkel D, Basseri RJ, Makhani MD, Chong K, Chang C, Pimentel M. Methane on Breath Testing is Associated with Constipation: A Systematic Review and Meta-analysis. Dig Dis Sci. 2011;56(6):1612–8.
13. George NS, Sankineni A, Parkman HP. Small Intestinal Bacterial Overgrowth in Gastroparesis. Dig Dis Sci. 2014;59(3):645–52.
14. Miller MA, Parkman HP, Urbain JL, Brown KL, Donahue DJ, Knight LC, et al. Comparison of Scintigraphy and Lactulose Breath Hydrogen Test for Assessment of Orocecal Transit: Lactulose Accelerates Small Bowel Transit. Dig Dis Sci. 1997;42(1):10–8.
15. Mulyadi YGR, Abdullah M, Shatri H. The Effect of Domperindone on Intestinal Motility and Bacterial Overgrowth in Patients with Liver Cirrhosis. Indones J Gastroenterol, Hepatol, Dig Endosc. 2012;13(3):130–5.

16. Su T, Lai S, Lee A, He X, Chen S. Meta-Analysis: Proton Pump Inhibitors Moderately Increase the Risk of Small Intestinal Bacterial Overgrowth. J Gastroenterol. 2018;53(1):27–36.
17. Weitsman S, Leite G, Celly S, Morales W, Sanchez M, Parodi G, et al. 979—A Large Scale Evaluation of the Small Intestinal Microbiome in Subjects on Proton Pump Inhibitors. Gastroenterology. 2019;156:206.
18. Chander Roland B, Mullin GE, Passi M, Zheng X, Salem A, Yolken R, et al. A Prospective Evaluation of Ileocecal Valve Dysfunction and Intestinal Motility Derangements in Small Intestinal Bacterial Overgrowth. Dig Dis Sci. 2017;62(12):3525–35.
19. Vantrappen G, Janssens J, Hellemans J, Ghoos Y. The Interdigestive Motor Complex of Normal Subjects and Patients with Bacterial Overgrowth of the Small Intestine. J Clin Invest. 1977;59(6):1158-66.
20. Stanghellini V, Cogliandro RF, De Giorgio R, Barbara G, Morselli-Labate AM, Cogliandro L, et al. Natural History of Chronic Idiopathic Intestinal Pseudo-Obstruction in Adults: A Single Center Study. Clin Gastroenterol Hepatol. 2005;3(5):449–58.
21. Di Nardo G, Di Lorenzo C, Lauro A, Stanghellini V, Thapar N, Karunaratne TB, et al. Chronic Intestinal Pseudo-Obstruction in Children and Adults: Diagnosis and Therapeutic Options. Neurogastroenterol Motil. 2017;29(1).
22. Pignata C, Budillon G, Monaco G, Nani E, Cuomo R, Parrilli G, et al. Jejunal Bacterial Overgrowth and Intestinal Permeability in Children with Immunodeficiency Syndromes. Gut. 1990;31(8):879–82.
23. Sachdev AH, Pimentel M. Gastrointestinal Bacterial Overgrowth: Pathogenesis and Clinical Significance. Ther Adv Chronic Dis. 2013;4(5):223–31.
24. Choung RS, Ruff KC, Malhotra A, Herrick L, Locke GR, 3rd, Harmsen WS, et al. Clinical Predictors of Small Intestinal Bacterial Overgrowth by Duodenal Aspirate Culture. Aliment Pharmacol Ther. 2011;33(9):1059–67.
25. Chen B, Kim JJ, Zhang Y, Du L, Dai N. Prevalence and Predictors of Small Intestinal Bacterial Overgrowth in Irritable Bowel Syndrome: A Systematic Review and Meta-analysis. J Gastroenterol. 2018;53(7):807–18.
26. Cole CR, Frem JC, Schmotzer B, Gewirtz AT, Meddings JB, Gold BD, et al. The Rate of Bloodstream Infection is High in Infants with Short Bowel Syndrome: Relationship with Small Bowel Bacterial Overgrowth, Enteral Feeding, and Inflammatory and Immune Responses. J Pediatr. 2010;156(6):941-7 e1.
27. Pande C, Kumar A, Sarin SK. Small-Intestinal Bacterial Overgrowth in Cirrhosis is Related to the Severity of Liver Disease. Aliment Pharmacol Ther. 2009;29(12):1273–81.
28. Rubio-Tapia A, Barton SH, Rosenblatt JE, Murray JA. Prevalence of Small Intestine Bacterial Overgrowth Diagnosed by Quantitative Culture of Intestinal Aspirate in Celiac Disease. J Clin Gastroenterol. 2009;43(2):157–61.
29. Capurso G, Signoretti M, Archibugi L, Stigliano S, Delle Fave G. Systematic Review and Meta-Analysis: Small Intestinal Bacterial Overgrowth in Chronic Pancreatitis. United European Gastroenterol J. 2016;4(5):697–705.
30. Ricci JERJ, Chebli LA, Ribeiro T, Castro ACS, Gaburri PD, Pace F, et al. Small-Intestinal Bacterial Overgrowth is Associated With Concurrent Intestinal Inflammation But Not With Systemic Inflammation in Crohn's Disease Patients. J Clin Gastroenterol. 2018;52(6):530-6.
31. Shah A, Morrison M, Burger D, Martin N, Rich J, Jones M, et al. Systematic Review with Meta-Analysis: The Prevalence of Small Intestinal Bacterial Overgrowth in Inflammatory Bowel Disease. Aliment Pharmacol Ther. 2019;49(6):624–35.
32. Rana SV, Malik A, Bhadada SK, Sachdeva N, Morya RK, Sharma G. Malabsorption, Orocecal Transit Time and Small Intestinal Bacterial Overgrowth in Type 2 Diabetic Patients: A Connection. Indian J Clin Biochem. 2017;32(1):84–9.

33. Chedid V, Dhalla S, Clarke JO, Roland BC, Dunbar KB, Koh J, et al. Herbal Therapy is Equivalent to Rifaximin for the Treatment of Small Intestinal Bacterial Overgrowth. Glob Adv Health Med. 2014;3(3):16–24.
34. Robinson-Papp J, Nmashie A, Pedowitz E, Benn EKT, George MC, Sharma S, et al. Vagal Dysfunction and Small Intestinal Bacterial Overgrowth: Novel Pathways to Chronic Inflammation in HIV. AIDS. 2018;32(9):1147–56.
35. Sabate JM, Jouet P, Harnois F, Mechler C, Msika S, Grossin M, et al. High Prevalence of Small Intestinal Bacterial Overgrowth in Patients with Morbid Obesity: A Contributor to Severe Hepatic Steatosis. Obes Surg. 2008;18(4):371–7.
36. Augustyn M, Grys I, Kukla M. Small Intestinal Bacterial Overgrowth and Nonalcoholic Fatty Liver Disease. Clin Exp Hepatol. 2019;5(1):1–10.
37. Wigg AJ, Roberts-Thomson IC, Dymock RB, McCarthy PJ, Grose RH, Cummins AG. The Role of Small Intestinal Bacterial Overgrowth, Intestinal Permeability, Endotoxaemia, and Tumour Necrosis Factor Alpha in the Pathogenesis of Non-Alcoholic Steatohepatitis. Gut. 2001;48(2):206–11.
38. Lauritano EC, Valenza V, Sparano L, Scarpellini E, Gabrielli M, Cazzato A, et al. Small Intestinal Bacterial Overgrowth and Intestinal Permeability. Scand J Gastroenterol. 2010;45(9):1131–2.
39. Ahuja AAN. Conventional, Complementary, and Controversial Approaches to Small Intestinal Bacterial Overgrowth. Pract Gastroenterol. 2018(Oct.):61.
40. Salem A, Roland B. Small Intestinal Bacterial Overgrowth (SIBO). J Gastrointestinal Dig Sys. 2014;4(5).
41. Shah SC, Day LW, Somsouk M, Sewell JL. Meta-analysis: Antibiotic Therapy for Small Intestinal Bacterial Overgrowth. Aliment Pharmacol Ther. 2013;38(8):925–34.
42. Kaufman SS, Loseke CA, Lupo JV, Young RJ, Murray ND, Pinch LW, et al. Influence Of Bacterial Overgrowth and Intestinal Inflammation on Duration of Parenteral Nutrition in Children with Short Bowel Syndrome. J Pediatr. 1997;131(3):356–61.
43. Saad RJ, Chey WD. Breath Testing for Small Intestinal Bacterial Overgrowth: Maximizing Test Accuracy. Clin Gastroenterol Hepatol. 2014;12(12):1964–72.
44. Rao SSC, Rehman A, Yu S, Andino NM. Brain Fogginess, Gas and Bloating: a Link Between SIBO, Probiotics and Metabolic Acidosis. Clin Transl Gastroenterol. 2018;9(6):162.
45. Uribarri J, Oh MS, Carroll HJ. D-Lactic Acidosis. A Review of Clinical Presentation, Biochemical Features, and Pathophysiologic Mechanisms. Medicine (Baltimore). 1998;77(2):73–82.
46. Khoshini R, Dai SC, Lezcano S, Pimentel M. A Systematic Review of Diagnostic Tests for Small Intestinal Bacterial Overgrowth. Dig Dis Sci. 2008;53(6):1443–54.
47. Rezaie A, Buresi M, Lembo A, Lin H, McCallum R, Rao S, et al. Hydrogen and Methane-Based Breath Testing in Gastrointestinal Disorders: The North American Consensus. Am J Gastroenterol. 2017;112(5):775–84.
48. Low K, Hwang L, Hua J, Zhu A, Morales W, Pimentel M. A Combination of Rifaximin and Neomycin is Most Effective in Treating Irritable Bowel Syndrome Patients with Methane On Lactulose Breath Test. J Clin Gastroenterol. 2010;44(8):547–50.
49. Maccaferri S, Vitali B, Klinder A, Kolida S, Ndagijimana M, Laghi L, et al. Rifaximin Modulates the Colonic Microbiota of Patients with Crohn's Disease: An in Vitro Approach Using a Continuous Culture Colonic Model System. J Antimicrob Chemother. 2010;65(12):2556–65.
50. Zhao J, Zheng X, Chu H, Zhao J, Cong Y, Fried M, et al. A Study of the Methodological and Clinical Validity of the Combined Lactulose Hydrogen Breath Test with Scintigraphic Oro-Cecal Transit Test for Diagnosing Small Intestinal Bacterial Overgrowth in IBS Patients. Neurogastroenterol Motil. 2014;26(6):794–802.
51. Melchior C, Gourcerol G, Bridoux V, Ducrotte P, Quinton JF, Leroi AM. Efficacy of Antibiotherapy for Treating Flatus Incontinence Associated with Small Intestinal Bacterial Overgrowth: A Pilot Randomized Trial. PLoS One. 2017;12(8):e0180835.

52. Rezaie A, Pimentel M, Rao SS. How to Test and Treat Small Intestinal Bacterial Overgrowth: An Evidence-Based Approach. Curr Gastroenterol Rep. 2016;18(2):8.
53. Gatta L, Scarpignato C. Systematic Review with Meta-Analysis: Rifaximin is Effective and Safe for the Treatment of Small Intestine Bacterial Overgrowth. Aliment Pharmacol Ther. 2017;45(5):604–16.
54. Parodi A, Paolino S, Greco A, Drago F, Mansi C, Rebora A, et al. Small Intestinal Bacterial Overgrowth in Rosacea: Clinical Effectiveness of its Eradication. Clin Gastroenterol Hepatol. 2008;6(7):759-64.
55. Ponziani FR, Zocco MA, D'Aversa F, Pompili M, Gasbarrini A. Eubiotic Properties of Rifaximin: Disruption of the Traditional Concepts in Gut Microbiota Modulation. World J Gastroenterol. 2017;23(25):4491-9.
56. Tursi A, Brandimarte G, Giorgetti GM, Elisei W. Assessment of Small Intestinal Bacterial Overgrowth in Uncomplicated Acute Diverticulitis of the Colon. World J Gastroenterol. 2005;11(18):2773-6.
57. Biancone L, Vernia P, Agostini D, Ferrieri A, Pallone F. Effect of Rifaximin on Intestinal Bacterial Overgrowth in Crohn's Disease as Assessed by the H2-Glucose Breath Test. Curr Med Res Opin. 2000;16(1):14–20.
58. Furnari M, Parodi A, Gemignani L, Giannini EG, Marenco S, Savarino E, et al. Clinical Trial: The Combination of Rifaximin with Partially Hydrolysed Guar Gum is More Effective Than Rifaximin Alone in Eradicating Small Intestinal Bacterial Overgrowth. Aliment Pharmacol Ther. 2010;32(8):1000–6.
59. Pimentel M, Chang C, Chua KS, Mirocha J, DiBaise J, Rao S, et al. Antibiotic Treatment of Constipation-Predominant Irritable Bowel Syndrome. Dig Dis Sci. 2014;59(6):1278-85.
60. Lauritano EC, Gabrielli M, Scarpellini E, Lupascu A, Novi M, Sottili S, et al. Small Intestinal Bacterial Overgrowth Recurrence After Antibiotic Therapy. Am J Gastroenterol. 2008;103(8):2031–5.
61. Erdogan A, Rao SS. Small Intestinal Fungal Overgrowth. Curr Gastroenterol Rep. 2015;17(4):16.
62. Krajicek EJ, Hansel SL. Small Intestinal Bacterial Overgrowth: A Primary Care Review. Mayo Clin Proc. 2016;91(12):1828–33.
63. Pittman N, Rawn SM, Wang M, Masetto A, Beattie KA, Larché M. Treatment of Small Intestinal Bacterial Overgrowth in Systemic Sclerosis: A Systematic Review. Rheumatology. 2018;57(10):1802–11.
64. Robinson-Papp J, Nmashie A, Pedowitz E, George MC, Sharma S, Murray J, et al. The Effect of Pyridostigmine on Small Intestinal Bacterial Overgrowth (SIBO) and Plasma Inflammatory Biomarkers in HIV-Associated Autonomic Neuropathies. J Neurovirol. 2019;25(4):551–9.
65. Revaiah PC, Kochhar R, Rana SV, Berry N, Ashat M, Dhaka N, et al. Risk of Small Intestinal Bacterial Overgrowth in Patients Receiving Proton Pump Inhibitors Versus Proton Pump Inhibitors Plus Prokinetics. JGH Open. 2018;2(2):47–53.
66. Sarosiek I, Bashashati M, Alvarez A, Hall M, Shankar N, Gomez Y, et al. Lubiprostone Accelerates Intestinal Transit and Alleviates Small Intestinal Bacterial Overgrowth in Patients With Chronic Constipation. Am J Med Sci. 2016;352(3):231–8.
67. DiBaise J. Nutritional Consequences of Small Intestinal Bacterial Overgrowth. Pract Gastroenterol. 2008;32(12):15–28.
68. Howard G, Xu H, Gupta A, Shin AS, Siwiec RM, Bohm M, et al. Mo1615 – Fat-Soluble Vitamins, B12, and Iron Deficiency in Patients with Coliform Small Intestinal Bacterial Overgrowth. Gastroenterology. 2019;156(6):S–802.
69. Pimentel M, Constantino T, Kong Y, Bajwa M, Rezaei A, Park S. Elemental Diet Pimentel. pdf. Dig Dis Sci. 2004;49(1):73–7.
70. Dionne J, Ford AC, Yuan Y, Chey WD, Lacy BE, Saito YA, et al. A Systematic Review and Meta-Analysis Evaluating the Efficacy of a Gluten-Free Diet and a Low

FODMAPs Diet in Treating Symptoms of Irritable Bowel Syndrome. Am J Gastroenterol. 2018;113(9):1290–300.

71. Garcia-Collinot G, Madrigal-Santillan EO, Martinez-Bencomo MA, Carranza-Muleiro RA, Jara LJ, Vera-Lastra O, et al. Effectiveness of Saccharomyces Boulardii and Metronidazole for Small Intestinal Bacterial Overgrowth in Systemic Sclerosis. Dig Dis Sci. 2020;65(4):1134–43.

72. Sadr-Azodi O, Orsini N, Andrén-Sandberg Å, Wolk A. Abdominal and Total Adiposity and the Risk of Acute Pancreatitis: A Population-Based Prospective Cohort Study. Am J Gastroenterol. 2013;108(1):133.

73. Dibaise JK, Young RJ, Vanderhoof JA. Enteric Microbial Flora, Bacterial Overgrowth, and Short Bowel Syndrome. Clin Gastroenterol Hepatol. 2006;4(1):11–20.

74. Hegarty JW, Guinane CM, Ross RP, Hill C, Cotter PD. Bacteriocin Production: A Relatively Unharnessed Probiotic Trait? F1000Res. 2016;5.

75. Kwak DS, Jun DW, Seo JG, Chung WS, Park SE, Lee KN, et al. Short-Term Probiotic Therapy Alleviates Small Intestinal Bacterial Overgrowth, but does not Improve Intestinal Permeability in Chronic Liver Disease. Eur J Gastroenterol Hepatol. 2014;26(12):1353–9.

76. Zhong C, Qu C, Wang B, Liang S, Zeng B. Probiotics for Preventing and Treating Small Intestinal Bacterial Overgrowth: A Meta-Analysis and Systematic Review of Current Evidence. J Clin Gastroenterol. 2017;51(4):300–11.

77. Logan AC, Beaulne TM. The Treatment of Small Intestinal Bacterial Overgrowth with Enteric-Coated Peppermint Oil: A Case Report. Altern Med Rev. 2002;7(5):410–7.

78. Bi Z, Zheng Y, Yuan J, Bian Z. The Efficacy and Potential Mechanisms of Chinese Herbal Medicine on Irritable Bowel Syndrome. Curr Pharm Des. 2017;23(34):5163–72.

79. Peterson CT, Sharma V, Uchitel S, Denniston K, Chopra D, Mills PJ, et al. Prebiotic Potential of Herbal Medicines Used in Digestive Health and Disease. J Altern Complement Med. 2018;24(7):656–65.

80. Yarnell E. Herbs for Upper Digestive Overgrowth of Flora. Alternative and Complementary Therapies. 2018;24(4):173–9.

81. Birdsall TC. Berberine: Therapeutic Potential of Alkaloid Found in Several Medicinal Plants. Altern Med Rev. 1997;2:94–103.

11 Nutrition Management of Eosinophilic Esophagitis

Gillian White

11.1 INTRODUCTION

Eosinophilic esophagitis (EoE) is a chronic disease that is isolated to the esophagus and uniquely allergen mediated. Its clinical and histological signatures are esophageal dysfunction stemming from inflammation driven by accumulation of eosinophils that can progress to fibrosis and stricture [1]. While there appears to be no increased risks for metastatic disease or morbidity, concern surrounding growing incidence and prevalence, burden of medical costs, and impaired quality of life are concerning [2]. Defining best practices for management of the condition has been difficult due in part to evolving diagnostic criteria, lack of standardization in treatment interventions and outcomes, complexity of dietary interventions, and invasive methods for histologic monitoring. Here we will examine the history of the disease, incidence and prevalence, pathology, clinical hallmarks, endoscopic features, and diagnostic pathways. In addition we will explore available options for treatment and specifically outline strategies to simplify dietary approaches for disease management.

11.2 INCIDENCE AND PREVALENCE

Prior to 1993, when eosinophilic esophagitis became a recognized clinical entity, there were only sparse case reports of the condition dating back to the 1970s [3–6]. Over the past three decades, EoE has emerged as the most prevalent eosinophilic gastrointestinal disorder and the second most common cause of dysphagia and chronic esophageal inflammation after gastroesophageal reflux disease (GERD) [7]. There is notable heterogeneity between studies evaluating epidemiology, namely regarding inclusion criteria dependent on how the disease was defined and whether or not endoscopies and biopsies were routinely performed. Despite this variance, all have demonstrated increasing rates of incidence and prevalence [5, 7–9]. It might be tempting to attribute this finding to increasing recognition and more frequent endoscopic evaluation; however, the increased rate of diagnosis outpaces that of increased biopsy [5, 10].

Most research in this area has been conducted in North America and Europe; there is sparse data available on epidemiology in areas where EoE has only more recently been identified, such as Asia, North Africa, and South America [5, 7]. Pooled incidence data from a recent meta-analysis indicates 7.2 per 100,000/year, and

DOI: 10.1201/9780429322570-11

prevalence of 28.1 per 100,000 inhabitance globally [7]. The United States reports similar incidence data and nearly double that in prevalence at 56.7 per 100,000 adults and 50,000 per 100,000 children [11]. Caucasian ethnicity, adults, and males have higher incidence and prevalence rates than that of other ethnic groups, children, and females, but this variance was only significant for gender and ethnicity [7]. Males are three times more likely to have EoE than females and as much as 90% of cases are of Caucasian descent [12]. Formerly a condition of obscurity, it now reflects incidence similar to that of inflammatory bowel disease in Europe, demonstrating mounting disease burden [7].

11.3 PATHOLOGY

One of the more compelling aspects of the disease is that it is an entirely unique form of allergy. Traditional allergies exist in terms of exaggerated immune response by immediate hypersensitivity reactions such as IgE or chronic autoimmune conditions propagated by antigen-specific T cells. A nuanced delayed hypersensitivity reaction driven by a T-helper cell (Th2) inflammatory cascade backs the pathogenesis of EoE [2, 13, 14]. Food allergens are predominant, though there are instances of aeroallergen [13, 15]. An important observation is that 50–80% of cases have concurrent atopic conditions, but it remains unproven that atopy predisposes to EoE [2, 15]. And while IgE food sensitization is more prominent in EoE compared to the general population, IgE antibodies are not directly involved in EoE manifestation. Interestingly, the development of EoE in 2.72% of individuals has occurred after undergoing sublingual immunotherapy for IgE food allergy. So there may as of yet be a connection of EoE to IgE through some switch-like mechanism [13, 15]. More recently, IgG4 antibodies have also been implicated and research in this area is ongoing [2, 13, 14].

11.4 RISK FACTORS

The pathway to disease is likely multifactorial involving inappropriate immune response to environmental factors due to genetic predisposition. As mentioned earlier, Caucasian males have significantly higher risk. As a whole, allergic disease is believed to have a genetic heritability of 50% and there is evidence that for EoE it is even higher. However, it does not follow classic Mendelian genetics since there are cases of EoE patients with an unaffected homozygote twin, as well as sporadic cases of EoE with no affected relatives. This speaks to environmental factors playing a role in disease onset [12]. The hygiene hypothesis and bacterial dysbiosis have been speculated. Factors elevating risk involving disruption of the gut microbiome include early antibiotic use or cesarean delivery; second-hand smoke exposure under the age of one is negatively correlated. There is sparse information regarding microbial populations within the esophagus, but recent findings demonstrate distinction in esophageal microbial colonization between EoE patients compared to healthy controls. In the future, signatures of esophageal microbial metabolomics could give way to biomarkers that serve a diagnostic purpose [2].

As for predisposing conditions, GERD may be implicated, but will be discussed in more detail later. Eradication of *Helicobacter pylori* (*H. pylori*) has been inversely associated with all allergic disease. To date, several studies have documented this independent negative correlation. This may speak to the hygiene hypothesis or possibly explain the ethnic preference in disease distribution. Another possible explanation may be shifts in allergic response with some evidence supporting *H. pylori* driving a T-helper type 1 (Th1) allergic response, which may protect against an EoE driving Th2 response. Robust prospective trials are warranted to provide further clarity into these insights [2, 14, 16].

11.5 DIAGNOSTICS

The short but eventful history of EoE as a recognized clinical entity gave way to rapid and ongoing evolution of disease understanding, diagnostic criteria, and treatments. Diagnostic guidelines were initially published in 2007, updated in 2013, and updated again in a recent international consensus. EoE is defined as symptoms of esophageal dysfunction, endoscopy, and biopsy that shows histologic findings of equal to or greater than 15 eosinophils/high power field (eos/hpf); and definitively diagnosed after evaluation proves no other significant cause of esophageal eosinophilia. Listed in Table 11.1 are conditions that can considerably contribute to esophageal eosinophilia. The majority are rare and distinctive from EoE with the exception of GERD [1, 2, 11].

11.6 GERD

GERD has particularly inspired controversy when EoE diagnostics are concerned. Formerly, GERD and EoE were considered entirely exclusive conditions [17, 18]. Normalization of esophageal eosinophilia following an 8-week PPI trial or pH

TABLE 11.1
Conditions with Corresponding Esophageal Eosinophilia

- Eosinophilic esophagitis
- Eosinophilic gastritis, gastroenteritis, or colitis
- Gastroesophageal reflux disease
- Achalasia
- Hypereosinophilic syndrome
- Crohn's disease
- Fungal or viral infections
- Connective tissue disorders
- Hypermobility syndrome
- Autoimmune disorders and vasculitides
- Pemphigus
- Hypersensitivity reactions to drugs
- Pill esophagitis
- Graft vs. host disease
- Mendelian disorders

---

monitoring was critical to distinguish GERD from EoE [19]. However, multiple studies demonstrated that clinical and histologic presentations of EoE with positive response to PPI did not always have clinical presentations consistent with GERD. Therefore, a new clinical entity called proton pump inhibitor-responsive esophageal eosinophilia (PPI-REE) was recognized [1, 18–21]. Later, it was also determined that PPI-REE was a subset of EoE because both conditions shared baseline clinical symptoms, endoscopic and histologic features, genetics, and concomitant atopic conditions [17, 18, 21]. It was also found that when taken off PPI therapy, PPI-REE normalized with standard treatments used in EoE, such as elimination diets and topical steroids. With consensus for removal of the required proton pump inhibitor (PPI) trial to diagnose EoE in 2017 emerging from the AGREE conference, a new diagnostic algorithm for EoE was determined, which removed PPIs as a diagnostic determinant, and made them a treatment option (Figure 11.1) [1, 22].

While EoE and GERD are distinct conditions, they can and do co-exist, and the relationship is very complex. Both conditions have the potential to cause secondary presentation of the other; chronic esophageal acid exposure from GERD can weaken esophageal barrier function and allow for allergen penetration and eosinophilic inflammation, and EoE can affect esophageal accommodation and motility, precipitating chronic reflux. Per in vitro data, PPI therapeutic properties are not limited to acid suppression, but have multiple modes of action, including antioxidant anti-inflammatory effects, downregulate allergic gene expression, and improved esophageal barrier function as a result of suppressing acid, which is known to impair esophageal mucosal integrity [1].

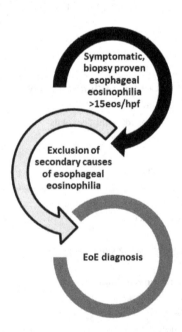

FIGURE 11.1 Updated diagnostic algorhythm for EoE.

11.7 CLINICAL PRESENTATION

Clinical presentation can differ between adult and pediatric cases. In infants and children, symptoms are nondescript, including vomiting, regurgitation, chest and abdominal pain, feeding difficulty (food refusal, stalled advances in food introduction, textural food aversion), and occasionally failure to thrive. Adolescents and adults will present with hallmark symptoms such as dysphagia and food impaction; they may also experience heartburn, odynophagia, and epigastric and chest pain that mimics gastroesophageal reflux disease [23, 24]. The differences in symptom presentation are attributed to advancement from inflammation to fibrosis over time, stressing the importance of early diagnosis and treatment [25]. The condition can remain undiagnosed for years despite significant anatomical changes to the esophagus due to the employment of various coping mechanisms. These include avoiding certain foods and textures such as meat or bread, use of fluids to wash down solids, and prolonged chewing to ease swallowing resulting in lengthier meal times [2, 24, 25]. Subjective scoring systems have been developed, but not validated for evaluating clinical presentation, such as the eosinophilic esophagitis activity index (EesAI) and Dysphagia Symptom Questionnaire (DSQ). Both were determined to be insufficient for detecting endoscopic, histologic, and overall remission [2]. Symptom resolution is an insufficient indicator of disease activity, and asymptomatic cases can occur [2, 13, 15, 26].

11.8 ENDOSCOPIC AND HISTOLOGIC ASSESSMENT

A number of endoscopic findings are associated with EoE, and increase likelihood of diagnosis. Visual findings by upper endoscopy include stenosis, strictures, narrow caliber esophagus, crepe paper esophagus, linear tears, furrows, lesions, edema, rings/Schatzki rings, esophageal mucosal tears from trachealization, and white exudates. Examples of these visual findings can be found in the references [2]. The EoE Endoscopic Reference Score (EREFS) is a validated classification system for EoE endoscopic findings, but lacks the sensitivity (15–48%) and overall predictive value for diagnostic purposes [25, 27]. In fact, 7–10% of patients with EoE will have a normal esophageal appearance when evaluated by endoscopy [28]. As with clinical presentation, there is variation in phenotype that is attributed to age and duration of disease. Pediatric or cases of more recent onset often demonstrate subtle endoscopic findings such as inflammation and edema, while adult or disease of long duration are more likely to have strictures and fibrosis [5].

As mentioned previously, the histologic signature of EoE is endoscopic biopsy findings of greater than 15 eosinophils per high-power field (>15 eos/HPF) in the absence of other treatable causes of eosinophilia [1]. Because the disease is not uniform but appears in scattered patches, a total of 2–4 biopsies should be obtained from the distal and proximal halves of the esophagus for a total of 6–9 biopsies [14, 29]. In addition, repeat endoscopies and biopsies to evaluate histology is mandatory to assess disease activity following treatment intervention. Histologic remission of peak eosinophil count to less than 15 cells/hpf is one of the treatment endpoints in EoE for the American College of Gastroenterology (ACG) as well as the European Society for Pediatric Gastroenterology Hepatology and Nutrition (ESPGHAN) [2, 23, 29].

11.9 PHARMACOLOGIC AND DIETARY TREATMENTS

Options for the treatment of EoE include the three Ds: drugs, diet, and dilation. Dietary interventions target the root cause of the condition, while pharmaceuticals and dilation address inflammatory consequences of the disease. Excluding dilation, Figure 11.2 depicts histologic comparison of all available treatment interventions [11]. We will examine each treatment option individually.

11.10 PROTON PUMP INHIBITORS

Histologic response of EoE to PPIs has been well documented in both pediatric and adult cases, with some variance between studies thought to be due to heterogeneity in evaluated populations and study design. Published reports show a pooled histologic response of 50–80% in children and adults [1, 13, 11]. Another review of 23 observational studies showed approximately one-third of PPI-treated cases had a positive histologic response, of note these findings were made using unweighted averages of the sample size [22]. Clinical response was less commonly studied and also plagued by heterogeneity, lacking utilization of validated screening tools. Symptom improvement ranged 23–82% [1]. Optimal PPI dosing to achieve remission is 1 mg/kg BID and maximal dosing of 30 mg lansoprazole BID or 40 mg omeprazole BID; other studies have reported lower initial and maintenance doses [1, 21, 30]. Identifying the lowest possible dose for maintenance therapy is prudent due to mounting evidence of adverse events associated with the therapy. These include kidney disease, hip fractures, pneumonia, hypomagnesemia, dementia, and small intestinal bacterial overgrowth [31, 32]. Long-term monitoring of clinical, endoscopic, and histologic features is advised because treatment response may be lost over time [1, 19].

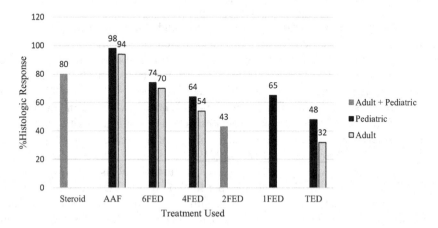

FIGURE 11.2 Histologic comparison of treatment.

Treatment response by percentage of histologic normalization in children and adults individually or combined depending on available data, adapted from recent literature review [11]. AAF: amino acid-based formula (elemental diet); 6FED: six-food elimination diet; 4FED: four-food elimination diet; 2FED: two-food elimination diet; 1FED: one-food elimination diet (has not yet been studied in adult populations); TED: targeted elimination diet.

11.11 TOPICAL GLUCOCORTICOSTEROIDS

To treat eosinophilic-predominant inflammation of EoE, topical steroids are recommended as a first-line pharmacologic therapy. While multiple studies have established that topical steroids can achieve statistically significant full or partial histologic remission in 57.8–82.1% of cases, it has had more variance in outcomes of clinical symptom improvement [23]. Heterogeneity between studies in clinical response may have to do with differences in screening tools used, short duration of the study and steroid administration, the subjective nature of symptom reporting, or the presence of fibrostenotic esophageal changes that may only respond to dilation. One meta-analysis did indicate superiority of budesonide over fluticasone in clinical response [23]. Administration of a budesonide steroid using an oral viscous solution may also be a more efficacious intervention in that it increases mucosal contact time [2]. Adequate long-term control of histologic response, as with PPI, is likely to be important in prevention of further tissue remodeling and stricture [23]. In one study, a 92% remission rate was attained with use of budesonide slurry and special instructions to take after meals and brushing teeth and waiting a duration of 2 hours before eating or drinking again [20]. Another review of 8 double-blind placebo-controlled studies showed that two-thirds of those treated with topical glucocorticosteroids achieved histologic remission as opposed to <15% of those receiving placebo [22]. Adverse outcomes of short-term steroid use in EoE include esophageal candidiasis in 4–26% of treated patients, which can effectively be treated by oral antifungal medication such as nystatin [23]. Possible long-term consequences of topical steroid use in EoE are osteoporosis or adrenal immunosuppression, risks of which have not been established by available research [22, 23]. It should be noted that the routine use of such medication is considered the standard of care for asthma in both children and adults [22].

11.12 ELEMENTAL DIETS

Evidence of food allergen implication in EoE was first demonstrated in a small pediatric cohort thought at that time to have refractory GERD. Twelve children completed the minimum 6-week dietary trial of elemental formula with the only other sustenance permitted being clear liquids, corn, or apples. All 12 subjects had resolved or improved clinical symptoms on elemental formula. Ten subjects underwent endoscopy and biopsy pre- and post-intervention and had a significant decrease from maximal esophageal intraepithelial eosinophil counts from 15–100 pre-intervention to 0–22 post-intervention. There was recurrence of symptoms in all patients following openly performed controlled reintroduction of standard food challenges [33]. There has been validation at multiple centers that diets free of intact proteins or peptides by means of amino acid-based formulas induce remission in most children and adult EoE sufferers [34, 35]. Of available dietary interventions, elemental diets have the highest efficacy in inducing histologic remission at 90–98% and similar effectiveness to steroids in improving symptoms in both children and adults [11, 36]. Of the dietary therapies, elemental formulas are the most restrictive but have the benefit of being nutritionally complete up until the age of 13, at which time additional micronutrient supplementation will be needed [11]. Issues with long-term adherence, such as cost, palatability, possible need of feeding tubes, and impediments to developing feeding skills, prevent the elemental diet from being considered as a first-line dietary therapy despite strong histologic response [24].

11.13 TARGETED ELIMINATION DIETS

The success of the elemental diet set the stage for the possibility of targeted elimination diets by means of food allergy testing to improve palatability and streamline therapy in EoE. There are acute hypersensitivity reactions to foods, known as food-specific IgE reactions, and are tested for by skin prick testing (SPT) or serum IgE testing. IgE sensitizations are reproducible and have a short onset, typically minutes to up to 4 hours; common symptoms include hives, eczema flares, angioedema, or anaphylaxis. There are also delayed hypersensitivity reactions that are reproducible, cell-mediated food reactions, which atopy patch testing is used to identify [38]. Molecular profiling has shown a T-helper type 2 (Th2) cytokine profile in EoE that helps to explain its concomitance with atopic disease such as asthma, allergic rhinitis, and dermatitis [38].

It appears that EoE represents a form of delayed hypersensitivity reaction to foods and not IgE. Emerging research has implicated IgG4 in the disease process, but further study is needed [39]. Interestingly, therapies for IgE desensitization, such as oral immunotherapy, have been linked with EoE onset, further indicating the unlikelihood of IgE reactions in EoE. Allergy testing to target foods for elimination is controversial, with no best testing method having been determined [24, 36–43]. While adult and pediatric subjects may test positive for food-specific IgE mediated allergens via skin prick, patch, or blood testing, elimination of these foods resulted in mixed symptom and histological response. Additionally, individuals negative for food allergy have still achieved remission through food elimination diets [25]. Reviews of recent research, most of which were single arm observational studies, found an overall efficacy ranging from 45–49% in allergen testing-directed elimination diets. Overall pediatric response of 48% is better than that found in adult-specific studies ranging from 26–35% [11, 22, 36]. These findings have led targeted elimination diets to fall out of favor.

11.14 EMPIRIC ELIMINATION DIETS

The limitations of elemental and targeted elimination diets discussed previously led to the evaluation of the blunt elimination of top primary allergens, regardless of individual allergy test results as a potential treatment. The six foods responsible for 90% of food allergies are milk, wheat, egg, soy, peanuts/tree nuts, and fish/shellfish. Initially, it was shown in children that removal of these allergens effectively established clinical and histologic remission of disease. This intervention came to be known as the 6-food elimination diet (6FED) [44, 45]. With known contrast in adults and children EoE phenotypes, it was uncertain if these differences indicated variance in pathophysiologic mechanisms that could affect treatment response. However, it was corroborated that the majority of adults did have improvements similar to pediatric cohorts in histologic, endoscopic, and symptomatic response to treatment with the 6FED; and there was return of all disease indicators with food reintroduction. Regarding differences in phenotype, there is a trend toward less likelihood of clinical improvement in those with more fibrotic anatomical changes

[46, 47]. A recent meta-analysis of pediatric and adult studies determined pooled efficacy of empiric elimination diets to be greater than 72.1 [11, 37]. There appears to be durability of disease control once allergen triggers are identified, with continued remission shown in different studies ranging from 1 to 3 years. However, as much as 10–30% of patients will not respond to an elemental or 6-food elimination diet [13]. Long-term compliance can be a barrier and may affect utilization as a maintenance therapy. Nonetheless, empiric elimination diets are classified as a first-line therapy for EoE; the American Academy of Allergy, Asthma, and Immunology is a wonderful resource for patient education materials [24]. Ultimately, elimination diets are best implemented with the expert guidance of a registered dietitian for prevention of nutrient deficiencies and improving adherence [11, 24, 48]. While it is important to note foods to be avoided and how to properly read a food label to help exclude allergens, it's even more important to emphasize what can be eaten, providing lists of acceptable foods and meal ideas that provide adequate overall nutrition. The framework for balanced meals should also be emphasized utilizing the My Plate guidelines (half plate produce, one-fourth fiber-rich starch, and one-fourth protein, milk substitutes or acceptable formula, and acceptable healthy fats). It's equally important to assess the patient's likes and dislikes to ensure there are sufficient available options to meet needs in light of preferences and restrictions. See Table 11.2 for a sample meal plan of the 6FED.

11.15 FOUR-FOOD, STEP-UP, AND SINGLE-FOOD ELIMINATION DIETS

Disadvantages of formerly discussed dietary interventions continue to be mitigated. Across multiple studies evaluating the 6FED, there have been 4 primary foods identified that trigger EoE. These are cow's milk (53–85%), wheat (27–60%), egg (5–36%), and soy (10–19%). Additionally, 65–85% of patients who have identified their food allergens after response to the 6FED have just 1 or 2 food triggers. These findings indicate that a potentially less restrictive and more effective approach could be utilized. The 4-food elimination diet (4FED) has proven itself in both adult and pediatric populations, with clinical symptom improvement in 36–91%, complete histologic response of 46–64%, and rescue with a 6FED of histologic non-responders has yielded up to another 29–31% remission rate. Some advantages of the 4FED are fewer restrictions, improved adherence, shortened intervention process, and a reduction in total number of endoscopies needed [11, 46, 49–53].

To further minimize restrictions and improve compliance of an elimination diet approach, a 2-food elimination diet (2FED) has been evaluated. Initially, dairy and wheat were excluded and non-responders were rescued with a step-up approach offering the 4FED, additionally restricting egg and soy, and then a 6FED further restricting peanuts/tree nuts, fish/shellfish if necessary. Overall remission rates were 43% of the 2FED, and 60% then 79% respectively of the step-up to 4FED and then 6FED. Compared to initiating therapy with the 6FED, a step-up approach can reduce endoscopic procedures by 20–25% and total diagnostic time by 35% [54]. About 65% of EoE patients have been found to only have a singular food allergen,

TABLE 11.2
6FED Sample Menu

Meal	Day 1	Day 2	Day 3	Day 4	Day 5
Breakfast	GF* toast, avocado, turkey bacon, salsa, mandarin orange, coffee or tea	Corn tortilla, black beans, sweet potato and mango salsa, coffee or tea	GF* oats mixed berries and chia seeds, glass of pea protein milk, coffee or tea	Smoothie: frozen banana, SunButter, flaxseed, pea protein milk, brown rice protein powder (optional)	GF* SF** DF*** NF† pancake or waffles, mixed berries, maple syrup, hemp milk, coffee or tea
Lunch	GF* bread, SunButter, jelly, carrots with hummus, and milk/soy milk alternative***	Corn, black beans, diced tomato, lettuce greens and avocado, black pepper, lemon juice and olive oil, tea or water	Corn or GF* tortilla, hummus, lunchmeat wrap, jicama and celery sticks, milk alternative***	GF* lentil soup, rice crackers topped with avocado and cilantro, milk alternative***	Shredded chicken, potatoes, green peas, grape tomatoes, carrots, tahini dressing, milk alternative***
Snack	Coconut yogurt	Roasted chickpeas	Rice cake with SunButter	Hummus and veggies	Fruit with SunButter
Dinner	Quinoa cooked in GF* broth, browned ground turkey, sautéed greens in olive oil, water or tea	Butternut squash, grilled chicken, spinach salad with olive oil and vinegar, water or tea	Chickpea or lentil pasta, ground turkey in marinara sauce, roasted broccoli, water or tea	Chicken stir fry with coconut aminos, brown rice, water or tea	Baked potato, pulled pork, GF* BBQ sauce, side salad with vinaigrette, water or tea

* GF=gluten-free, ** SF=soy-free, *** DF=dairy-free, calcium-enriched milk alternatives (hemp, pea, rice, coconut, quinoa, GF-oat), or amino acid-based formula (Neocate Junior, Elecare Junior, Neocate Splash, or E028 Splash), †NF=nut-free.

most commonly dairy at 88% [11]. Due to the predominance of milk-driven allergic response in EoE, some have proposed a single-food elimination diet. Milk elimination diets have only been looked at in three small pediatric studies, ranging in effect from 43–65% in inducing histologic remission [11, 15, 51].

11.16 PHASES OF ELIMINATION AND REINTRODUCTION

There is significant variance and no standardization in current allergen reintroduction protocols. The order of reintroduction as well as timing between reintroduction and endoscopy to check histology varies between studies and institutions. Initiation of empiric elimination diet of two, four, or six foods is observed for a minimum of 6 weeks before performing endoscopy and biopsy to evaluate remission status. If remission is achieved (<15 eos/hpf), reintroduction of potential allergens may commence. Some institutions opt to reintroduce allergens in ascending order of statistical likelihood of trigger potential, others by clinician and patient preference. Time between repeat endoscopy and biopsy following each individual allergen reintroduction can span 2–8 weeks depending on the study referenced, but typically a 6–8-week span is practiced [13, 20]. If EoE remains in remission, that food can remain in the diet while the next potential allergen is reintroduced and the process is repeated. If eosinophils return (biopsy of >15eos/hpf), that food is identified as an EoE allergen and permanently removed from the diet. After positively identifying an allergen, a washout period (returning to the allergen-free diet) may be observed; this can vary 4–8 weeks before the next potential allergen is introduced. Other institutions may forgo the washout period and immediately reintroduce the next potential allergen for 6–8 weeks, followed by EGD and biopsy, and so on and so forth through each reintroduction [47, 50, 52, 55].

11.17 DILATION

While not a means of treating root cause inflammation or normalizing histology in EoE, dilation has been proven safe and effective in treating dysphagia while demonstrating high rates of patient acceptance [56–61]. It should be considered as a second-line treatment in cases of stricture and small caliber esophagus when dysphagia or food impaction persist despite histologic normalization with anti-inflammatory treatment [60–63]. Dilation has shown symptom resolution of 18 months or longer [56]. Scarring and fibrosis common to this condition could place it at higher risk of complication from dilation such as perforation. However, it has been established that the chance of perforation in EoE is less than 2% when performed gradually [60, 63]. Repeat dilation may be needed over the course of a lifetime, but controlling inflammation by diet or steroid can lessen this necessity [64]. Should perforation occur, most cases will heal with conservative treatment, often involving inpatient monitoring and antibiotics. Subsequent dilation after perforation may be performed, but with heightened caution [17, 63, 65, 66]. Chest pain can be another benign complaint to warn patients of; this can last hours or days after dilation [60, 62]. For those with advanced fibro-stenotic changes, endoscopic dilation may be the only viable option for symptom resolution despite achieving histologic normalization with PPI, steroids, or diet therapy [56, 60].

11.18   NUTRIENT AND ADHERENCE CONCERNS

While diet therapy is the only treatment that tackles the root cause of EoE rather than treating the inflammatory consequences, it should not be undertaken without careful consideration and the aid of an EoE-knowledgeable dietitian. Medical nutrition therapy is a marriage of condition-specific, evidence-based interventions with an individual's current circumstances. Lifestyle, adherence potential, presence of family or other social support, and resource availability should all be considered when determining if treatment by elimination diet is appropriate on a case-by-case basis [11].

Elimination of entire food groups heightens potential for multiple nutrient deficiencies, malnutrition, and poor growth in children. This negative potential only grows more urgent and likely with each additional food group eliminated. A registered dietitian is instrumental in proper execution of these therapeutic dietary interventions to safeguard against macronutrient and micronutrient deficiencies. Individualized dietary interventions should include oral diet; allergen-free supplementation such as daily multivitamin, calcium, and vitamin D; and alternative nutrition support, such as enteral nutrition, as needed. Table 11.3 lists nutrients provided by each of the top 6 common allergens, and when eliminated, all nutrients of that

TABLE 11.3
Nutrients of Concern with Allergen Elimination

Milk	Wheat	Soy	Egg	Peanut/Tree Nut	Fish/Shellfish
Protein	Fiber	Protein	Protein	Protein	Protein
Fat	Iron	Fat	Fat	Fat	Fat
Calcium	Zinc	Calcium	Vitamin D	Fiber	Vitamin D
Vitamin D	Selenium	Iron	Selenium	Copper	Iron
Vitamin A	B1, Thiamin	Zinc	Vitamin A	Zinc	Zinc
B2, Riboflavin	B2, Riboflavin	B1, Thiamin	B5, Pantothenic Acid	Selenium	Copper
B5, Pantothenic Acid	B3, Niacin	B2, Riboflavin	B7, Biotin	Vitamin E	Selenium
B12, Cobalamin	B6, Pyridoxine	B3, Niacin	B12, Cobalamin	B3, Niacin	B12, Cobalamin
Iodine	B7, Biotin	B6, Pyridoxine	B2, Riboflavin	B9, Folate	Iodine
Potassium	B9, Folate	B9, Folate	Lutein	ALA Omega-3	EPA, DHA Omega-3

TABLE 11.4

Optimal Alternatives for Top Allergens

Milk	Wheat	Soy	Egg	Peanut/Tree Nut	Fish/ Shellfish
Pea Protein Beverage	*Amaranth*	*Other Beans and Legumes*	*Beans and Legumes* (not Soy)	*Seeds*	*Beans and Legumes* (not Soy)
Soy	*Millet*	Eggs	Soy	*Animal Meats*	*Animal Meats*
Almond Beverage + Pea Protein	*Teff*	*Animal Meats*	*Animal Meats*	Poultry	Poultry
Hemp Beverage + Pea Protein	*Quinoa*	Poultry	*Poultry*	Fish	Soy
Animal Meats	*Sorghum*	Fish	Fish	Shellfish	Egg
Poultry	*Buckwheat*	Shellfish	Shellfish	*Beans and Legumes* (not Soy)	Milk, Dairy
Fish	*Corn*	Milk, Dairy	Nuts	Soy	Nuts
Shellfish	*Gluten-Free Oats*	Nuts	*Seeds*	Avocado	Seeds
Nuts	*Wild or Brown Rice*	*Seeds*	Vegan Egg Substitutes	*Nut-Free Oils*	
Seeds	*Winter Squash*		Milk, Dairy		
Beans and Legumes (not Soy)	*Potatoes*	• Words in italics = allergen-free foods • Always check labels for potential allergens			

group must be adequately replaced by an appropriate allergen-free alternative listed in Table 11.4 [11, 24].

11.19 CONCLUSION

Nearly three decades have passed since the clinical distinction of EoE was made and multiple treatments have been identified over that time. While steroids and PPIs prove to be more of a band-aid to chronic inflammation management, diet therapies treat the root source but present significant nutrient risks. Great care must be taken with these patients and ideally patients should be monitored by a multidisciplinary team that includes a registered dietitian with allergy- or EoE-specific expertise when diet therapies are implemented. Future directions of research should include comparative head-to-head studies between drug and diet therapies as well as combination therapies. More research should also be directed at long-term studies on effectiveness of maintenance drug and diet therapies. Lastly, studies should target identification of biomarkers for diagnosis and disease monitoring, as well as less invasive office-based methods for evaluating histologic response that do not require endoscopy. Research in some of these areas is underway, but was outside the scope of this chapter to discuss.

REFERENCES

1. Dellon, E. S., et al. 2018. Updated international consensus diagnostic criteria for eosinophilic esophagitis: Proceedings of the AGREE conference. *Gastroenterol*, 155(4):1022–1033.
2. Chen, J. W., and Kao, J. Y. 2017. Eosinophilic esophagitis: Update on management and controversies. *BMJ*, 359.
3. Dobbins, J. W., Sheahan, D. G., and Behar, J. 1977. Eosinophilic gastroenteritis with esophageal involvement. *Gastroenterol*, 72:1312–1316.
4. Landres, R. T., Kuster, G. G., and Strum, W. B. 1978. Eosinophilic esophagitis in a patient with vigorous achalasia. *Gastroenterol*, 74:1298–1301.
5. Dellon, E. S., and Hirano, I. 2018. Epidemiology and natural history of eosinophilic esophagitis. *Gastroenterol*, 154(2):319–332.
6. Kim, H. P., and Dellon, E. S. 2018. An evolving approach to the diagnosis of eosinophilic esophagitis. *Gastroenterol Hepatol*, 14(6):358–366.
7. Arias, Á., et al. 2016. Systematic review with meta-analysis: The incidence and prevalence of eosinophilic oesophagitis in children and adults in population-based studies. *Aliment Pharmacol Ther*, 43:3–15.
8. Mansoor, E., and Cooper, S. G. 2016. The 2010–2015 prevalence of eosinophilic esophagitis in the United States: A population-based study. *Dig Dis Sci*, 61(10): 2928–2934.
9. Shaheen, N. J., et al. 2018. Natural history of eosinophilic esophagitis: A systematic review of epidemiology and disease course. *Dis Esophagus*, 31:1–14.
10. Dellon, E. S., et al. 2015. The increasing incidence and prevalence of eosinophilic oesophagitis outpaces changes in endoscopic and biopsy practice: National population-based estimates from Denmark. *Aliment Pharmacol Ther*, 41:662–670.
11. Bashaw, H., et al. 2020. Tutorial: Nutrition therapy in eosinophilic esophagitis – outcomes and deficiencies. *J Parenter Enteral Nutr*, 44:600–609.
12. Arias, A., et al. 2014. Efficacy of dietary interventions for inducing histologic remission in patients with eosinophilic esophagitis: A systematic review and meta-analysis. *Gastroenterol*, 146:1639–1648.
13. Kagalwalla, A. F., et al. 2011. Identification of specific food triggers responsible for inflammation in children with eosinophilic esophagitis successfully treated with empiric elimination diet. *J Pediatr Gastroenterol Nutr*, 53:145–149.
14. Gonsalves, N., et al. 2012. Elimination diet effectively treats eosinophilic esophagitis in adults: Food reintroduction identifies causative factors. *Gastroenterol*, 142:1451–1459.
15. Kavitt, R. T., et al. 2016. Randomized controlled trial comparing esophageal dilation to no dilation among adults with esophageal eosinophilia and dysphagia. *Dis Esophagus*, 29(8):983–991.
16. Holvoet, S., and Blanchard, C. 2014. Genetics and molecular mechanisms leading to eosinophilic esophagitis. *Revista Española De Enfermedades Digestivas*, 106(4):276–280.
17. Molina-Infante, J., et Al. 2017. Update on dietary therapy for eosinophilic esophagitis in children and adults. *Expert Rev Gastroenterol Hepatol*, 11(2):115–123.

18. Gómez-Aldana, A., et al. 2019. Eosinophilic esophagitis: Current concepts in diagnosis and treatment. *World J Gastroenterol*, 25(32):4598–4613.

19. Lucendo, A. J., et al. 2017. Guidelines on eosinophilic esophagitis: Evidence-based statements and recommendations for diagnosis and management in children and adults. *United Eu Gastroenterol J*, 5(3):335–358.

20. Shah, S. C., et al. 2019. Association between *Helicobactr pylori* exposure and decreased odds of eosinophilic esophagitis – a systematic review and meta-analysis. *Clin Gastroenterol Hepatol*, 17:2185–2198.

21. Dellon, E. S., et al. 2014. Markers of eosinophilic inflammation for diagnosis of eosinophilic esophagitis and proton pump inhibitor-responsive esophageal eosinophilia: A prospective study. *Clin Gastroenterol Hepatol*, 12:2015–2022.

22. Kia, L., and Hirano, I. 2015. Distinguishing GERD from eosinophilic oesophagitis: Concepts and controversies. *Nat Rev Gastroenterol Hepatol*, 12(7):379–386.

23. Lucendo, A. J., Arias, Á., and Molina-Infante, J. 2016. Efficacy of proton pump inhibitor drugs for inducing clinical and histologic remission in patients with symptomatic eosinophilic eosinophilia: A systematic review and meta-analysis. *Clin Gastroenterol Hepatol*, 14:13–22.

24. Philpott, H., et al. 2016. A prospective open clinical trial of proton pump inhibitor, elimination diet and/or budesonide for eosinophilic oesophagitis. *Aliment Pharmacol Thera*, 43:985–993.

25. Molina-Infante, J., Prados-Manzano, R., and Gonzalez-Cordero, P. L. 2016. The role of proton pump inhibitor therapy in the management of eosinophilic esophagitis. *Expert Rev Clin Immunol*, 12(9):945–952.

26. Hirano, I., et al. 2020. AGA institute and the joint task force on allergy-immunology practice parameters clinical guidelines for the management of eosinophilic esophagitis. *Gastroenterol*, 158:1776–1786.

27. Murali, A. R., et Al. 2016. Topical steroids in eosinophilic esophagitis: Systematic review and meta-analysis of placebo-controlled randomized clinical trials. *J Gastroenterol Hepatol*, 31:1111–1119.

28. Groetch, M., et al. 2017. Dietary therapy and nutrition management of eosinophilic esophagitis: A work group report of the American academy of allergy, asthma, and immunology. *J Allergy Clin Immunol Pract*, 5:312–324.

29. Miehlke, S. 2014. Clinical features of eosinophilic esophagitis. *Dig Dis*, 32:61–67.

30. Carr, S., Chan, E. S., and Watson, W. 2019. Correction to: Eosinophilic esophagitis. *Allergy Asthma Clin Immunol*, 15:22. https://doi.org/10.1186/s13223-019-0336-3.

31. Hirano, I., et al. 2013. Endoscopic assessment of the oesophageal features of eosinophilic oesophagitis: Validation of a novel classification and grading system. *Gut*, 62:489–495.

32. Dellon, E. S. 2012. Diagnosis and management of eosinophilic esophagitis. *Perspect Clin Gastroenterol Hepatol*, 10:1066–1078.

33. Dellon, E. S., et al. 2013. ACG clinical guideline: Evidenced based approach to the diagnosis and management of esophageal eosinophilia and eosinophilic esophagitis (EoE). *Am J Gastroenterol*, 108:679–692.

34. Gómez-Torrijos, E., et al. 2016. The efficacy of step-down therapy in adult patients with proton pump inhibitor-responsive oesophageal eosinophilia. *Aliment Pharmacol Ther*, 43:534–540.

35. Li, M., et al. 2019. Proton pump inhibitor use and risk of dementia: Systematic review and meta-analysis. *Medicine*, 98(7):1–8.

36. Wilkinson, J. M., Cozine, E. W., and Loftus, G. C. 2019. Gas, bloating, and belching: Approach to evaluation and management. *Am Fam Physician*, 99(5):301–309.

37. Kelly, K. J., et al. 1995. Eosinophilic esophagitis attributed to gastroesophageal reflux: Improvement with an amino acid-based formula. *Gastroenterol*, 109:1503–1512.

38. Markowitz, J. E., et al. 2003. Elemental diet is an effective treatment for eosinophilic esophagitis in children and adolescents. *Am J Gastroenterol*, 98:777–1782.
39. Peterson, K. A., et al. 2013. Elemental diet induces histologic response in adult eosinophilic esophagitis. *Am J Gastroenterol*, 108:759–766.
40. Aceves, S. S. 2014. Food allergy testing in eosinophilic esophagitis: What the gastroenterologist needs to know. *Clin Gastroenterol Hepatol*, 12(8):1216–1223.
41. Spergel, J., and Aceves, S. S. 2018. Allergic components of eosinophilic esophagitis. *J Allergy Clin Immunol*, 142(1):1–8.
42. O'shea, K., and Hogan, S. P. 2018. IgG4 in eosinophilic esophagitis: Perpetrator, accomplice, or bystander? *Ann Esophagus*, 1:14.
43. Anyane-Yeboa, A., Wang, W., and Kavitt, R. T. 2018. The role of allergy testing in eosinophilic esophagitis. *Gastroenterol Hepatol*, 14(8):463–469.
44. Philpott, H., et al. 2016. Allergy tests do not predict food triggers in adult patients with eosinophilic esophagitis. A comprehensive prospective study using five modalities. *Aliment Pharmacol Ther*, 44:223–233.
45. Spergel, J. M., et al. 2006. Predictive values for skin prick test and atopy patch test for eosinophilic esophagitis [Letter to the editor]. *J Allergy Clin Immunol*, 119(2):509–511.
46. Molina-Infante, J., et al. 2012. Selective elimination diet based on skin testing has suboptimal efficacy for adult eosinophilic esophagitis [Letter to the editor]. *J Allergy Clin Immunol*, 130(5):1200–1202.
47. Kagalwalla, A. F., et al. 2006. Effects of six-food elimination diet on clinical and histologic outcomes in eosinophilic esophagitis. *Clin Gastroenterol Hepatol*, 4:1097–1102.
48. Straumann, A., et Al. 2003. Natural history of primary eosinophilic esophagitis: A follow-up of 30 adult patients for up to 11.5 years. *Gastroenterol*, 125:1660–1669.
49. Reed, C. C., et al. 2017. Food elimination diets are effective for long-term treatment of adults with eosinophilic oesophagitis. *Aliment Pharmacol Ther*, 46:836–844.
50. Lucendo, A. J., et al. 2013. Empiric 6-food elimination diet induced and maintained prolonged remission in patients with adult eosinophilic esophagitis: A prospective study on the food cause of the disease. *J Allergy Clin Immunol*, 131:797–804.
51. Philpott, H., and Dellon, E. S. 2018. The role of maintenance therapy in eosinophilic esophagitis: Who, why, and how? *J Gastroenterol*, 53(2):165–171.
52. Molina-Infante, J., et al. 2014. Four-food group elimination diet for adult eosinophilic esophagitis: A prospective multicenter study. *J Allergy Clin Immunol*, 134(55):1093–1099.
53. Kagalwalla, A. F., et al. 2017. Efficacy of a 4-food elimination diet for children with eosinophilic esophagitis. *Clin Gastroenterol Hepatol*, 15:1698–1707.
54. Molina-Infante, J., et al. 2018. Step-up empiric elimination diet for pediatric and adult eosinophilic esophagitis: The 2–4–6 study. *J Allergy Clin Immunol*, 141(4):1365–1372.
55. Zhan, T., et al. 2018. Model to determine the optimal dietary elimination strategy for treatment of eosinophilic esophagitis. *Clin Gastroenterol Hepatol*, 16:1730–1737.
56. Chen, J. W., and Kao, J. Y. 2017. Eosinophilic esophagitis: Update on management and controversies. *BMJ*, 359.
57. González-Cervera, J., and Lucendo, A. J. 2016. Eosinophilic esophagitis: An evidence-based approach to therapy. *J Investig Allergol Clin Immunol*, 26(1):8–18.
58. Schoepfer, A. M., et al. 2010. Esophageal dilation in eosinophilic esophagitis: Effectiveness, safety, and impact on the underlying inflammation. *Am J Gastroenterol*, 105:1062–1070.
59. Morrow, J. B. et al. 2001. The ringed esophagus: Histological features of GERD. *Am J Gastroenterol*, 96:984–989.
60. Zimmerman, S. L., et al. 2005. Idiopathic eosinophilic esophagitis in adults: The ringed esophagus. *Radiol*, 236:159–165.
61. Alexander, J. A. 2014. Esophageal dilation in eosinophilic esophagitis. *Tech Gastrointest Endosc*, 16:26–31.

62. Dougherty, M., et al. 2017. Esophageal dilation with either bougie or balloon technique as a treatment for eosinophilic esophagitis: A systematic review and meta-analysis. *Gastrointest Endosc*, 86(4):581–591.
63. Lucendo, A. J., and Molina-Infante, J. 2018. Esophageal dilation in eosinophilic esophagitis: Risks, benefits, and when to do it. *Curr Opin Gastroenterol*, 34(4):226–232.
64. Runge, T. M., et al. 2017. Control of inflammation decreases the need for subsequent esophageal dilation in patients with eosinophilic esophagitis. *Dis Esophagus*, 30(7):1–7.
65. Lipka, S., Kumar, A., and Richter, J. E. 2018. Successful esophageal dilation of eosinophilic esophagitis (EoE) patients with a previous postdilation complication: Start low and go slow. *J Clin Gastroenterol*, 52(9):773–777.
66. Runge, T. M., et al. 2016. Outcomes of esophageal dilation in eosinophilic esophagitis: safety, efficacy, and persistence of the fibrostenotic phenotype. *Am J Gastroenterol*, 111(2):206–213.

12 Food Intolerances and IgE-Mediated Food Allergies

Senthilkumar Sankararaman, Aravind Thavamani, and Thomas J. Sferra

12.1 INTRODUCTION

Adverse reactions from food consumption is a common problem that can occur due to an underlying immune-based reaction (e.g., food allergies and celiac disease) or various non-immune mechanisms (i.e., food intolerances) (1, 2). Food sensitivity is an indistinct entity, which includes any symptom perceived to be related to food ingestion and hence this term may be subjected to wide range of usage and interpretation (3). When patients self-report a history of food allergies, they often misinterpret food intolerances or food sensitivities for food allergies. In food-intolerant conditions, the amount of food ingested directly correlates with the severity of symptoms, and exposure of food each time leads to reproducible symptoms. Food allergies are a heterogeneous group of disorders characterized by an adverse reaction resulting from a specific immune response to a food allergen (innocuous proteins in most individuals) (4). Allergic food reactions are often reproducible (5, 6). In contrast to food intolerance, in food allergies, even exposure to a small quantity of allergen can elicit a severe allergic reaction in an unpredictable fashion, more so on subsequent exposures (6).

12.2 FOOD INTOLERANCES

Food intolerances, reported in up to 20% of the population, often present with reproducible gastrointestinal (GI) symptoms (2). A classic example is lactose intolerance due to a deficiency of the digestive enzyme lactase, which leads to abdominal discomfort, gassiness, and bloating. Hydrogen breath tests are often utilized to diagnose lactose or fructose intolerances. Intolerance to fructose and fermentable oligo-, di-, and monosaccharides and polyols (FODMAPs) is commonly found in patients with functional GI disorders, such as irritable bowel syndrome (IBS) (2). Acute adverse food reactions also occur due to food contaminated with bacteria or toxins (e.g., aflatoxins) or due to high levels of histamine (e.g., scombroid poisoning, spoiled fish) (7). Moreover, when consumed in excess, the pharmacological effects of caffeine or tyramine (in tomatoes and cheese) often mimic allergic manifestations involving the skin or GI tract (5, 8). Improvement of GI symptoms with specific food avoidance

DOI: 10.1201/9780429322570-12

and reproducible symptoms upon food challenge are standard diagnostic methods to identify specific food intolerance.

Patients with food sensitivity often present with GI symptoms and may undergo blood tests, stool tests, and even endoscopy. Most are helpful for ruling out underlying organic diseases, such as celiac disease, eosinophilic GI diseases, *Helicobacter pylori* infection, and inflammatory bowel disease. In most instances, specific food sensitivities are poorly understood. Food-specific IgG testing is not recommended, since it is neither helpful to diagnose a possible adverse reaction to specific foods nor helpful in predicting future adverse reactions (9, 10). Presence of food-specific IgG is considered a marker of prior food exposure and tolerance to food, since positive results are expected in healthy individuals and it does not have any diagnostic or prognostic utility in clinical practice (3). However, limited evidence suggests that targeted food elimination based on food-specific IgG might benefit IBS (11).

12.3 FOOD ALLERGIES

Allergic reactions can be broadly classified as IgE-mediated, non-IgE-mediated, and combined IgE/non-IgE-mediated reactions (1, 12) (Figure 12.1).

This chapter will discuss IgE-mediated food allergies, while Chapter 13 will discuss non-IgE-mediated and mixed food allergies. Most food allergies first manifest during the first two years of life (8). The types of foods responsible for nearly 90% of food allergies in the United States are milk, eggs, nuts (peanuts and tree nuts), soy, wheat, fish, and shellfish (5, 8, 13) with milk as the most common allergen during infancy, peanut during early childhood, and seafood in adulthood (14).

Food allergies to specific foods, such as milk, soy, egg, and wheat, are more prevalent in the pediatric age group and these allergies often resolve (6, 15–17). On the contrary, allergic reactions to nuts (peanuts and tree nuts) and seafood (fish and shellfish) invariably persist for life (6, 15, 16). Shellfish allergy often appears in adulthood (18). The reasons for this spontaneous resolution occurring specifically in early life and only for some food allergens and not others are unclear (15, 16).

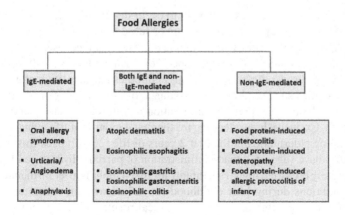

FIGURE 12.1 Classifications of food allergies.

12.4   EPIDEMIOLOGY

Food allergies are prevalent, particularly in the developed world (6). Epidemiological studies based on self-reported symptoms may overestimate the prevalence of food allergies, since most patients and caregivers tend to misinterpret food intolerances as a food allergy. Using allergen-specific IgE and age-based criteria in 8,203 subjects, the National Health and Nutrition Examination Survey (NHANES) 2005–2006 (19) Estimated the prevalence of food allergy to 4 foods (peanut, milk, egg, and shrimp) to be 2.5%, with increased prevalence noted in non-Hispanic blacks, males, and children (19).

Foods causing IgE-mediated food allergies vary in different regions of the world, depending on the prevailing dietary habits (6). In the Western world, milk, soy, peanuts, and seafood are the most common allergens. In Asia, seafood is the most common cause of food allergy (5, 20, 21). Disparities in the prevalence of food allergy among countries in the same geographical location have been reported (20, 22). For example, milk, egg, wheat, tree nuts, fish, and shellfish allergies were more prevalent in Northern Europe and the prevalence of soy and peanut allergies was higher in Western Europe (22). Similarly, wheat allergy was overall uncommon in most countries in Asia, but was the most common cause of anaphylaxis in Japan and Korea (20). In the United States, the Food Allergen Labeling and Consumer Protection Act (FALCPA) of 2004 mandates labeling of eight allergens (milk, eggs, fish, shellfish, tree nuts, peanuts, wheat, and soybeans) in all food products, dietary supplements, and infant formulas (13). In a given individual, the presence of one atopic disease increases the chance of the development of other atopic conditions (23). An increased prevalence of food allergies has been noted in patients with asthma, eczema, and allergic rhinitis. Infants with atopic dermatitis have an increased risk of developing IgE-mediated food allergic reactions and later asthma and allergic rhinitis. This concept is popularly referred to as the "atopic march" (6, 23).

12.5   PATHOGENESIS

Development of food allergies is thought to occur due to the failure to develop tolerance to food allergens upon initial exposure or subsequent loss of already established tolerance (24). For the majority of the atopic diseases, pathogenesis can be explained as the initial development of allergen-specific T helper type 2 (T_H2) response that later leads to the production of specific IgE antibodies and activation of granulocytes (23). Early studies suggested that the avoidance of dietary allergens during infancy and early childhood may prevent sensitization and development of food allergy in later life (25). Exclusive breast feeding for the first 4 months of life reduces the development of atopic dermatitis in the first 2 years of life (26). To back this hypothesis, some studies have suggested that administration of partially hydrolyzed formulas in non-exclusively breastfed high- risk infants for first 4 months after birth may decrease allergic conditions during later childhood (26, 27). However, concrete evidence is lacking to implement this in day-to-day clinical practice (26, 28). In the landmark LEAP (Learning Early about Peanut Allergy) randomized controlled trial (RCT), investigators demonstrated that early enteral introduction of peanuts could prevent peanut allergy in high-risk infants (29). In a similar RCT (EAT: Enquiring About Tolerance), early introduction of peanut and egg in infants decreased the prevalence of allergy to these foods, but there were no significant effects with early exposure of milk, sesame, fish, or wheat (30). Although the results of these studies are encouraging, the complex interaction of genetics, type of sensitization, and amount of exposure resulting in the development of individual food allergies remains unclear.

In 1989, Strachan proposed the "hygiene hypothesis" for the rising incidence of atopic allergies (31). This hypothesis proposed that increased standard of living, improved personal cleanliness, and the associated decrease in infectious diseases lead to a predisposition to atopic diseases (31). This hypothesis is relatively better explored in asthma but less clearly studied in the causation of food allergies (32). Also, the microbiome is increasingly recognized as one of the crucial factors influencing the development of food allergy. The mode of delivery at birth influences the microbiota of the infant and studies have found that Caesarean delivery is associated with an increase in prevalence of food allergies later in life (33). The use of prebiotics and probiotics to alter the body's response to food triggers is being investigated (34). When an extensively hydrolyzed formula was supplemented with the probiotic strain *Lactobacillus rhamnosus* GG, the acquisition of tolerance was expedited in infants with cow's milk allergy (35).

Recent studies suggest that non-oral routes (respiratory or cutaneous exposure of allergens) of sensitization have a role in food allergy. Skin sensitization to food antigens occurs, especially when there is epithelial barrier dysfunction as in atopic dermatitis. Similarly, food processing and methods of preparation have been explored as the trigger in the causality of food allergy (36). Immunomodulation through various dietary factors, such as vitamin D and omega-3 fatty acids, may play a protective role in the development of food allergies (25). Vitamin D participates in the development of immune tolerance, mucosal immunity, and gut integrity (37). Vitamin D deficiency has been associated in the pathogenesis of food allergy; in infancy, vitamin D deficiency is associated with three times higher incidence of peanut or egg allergy (6). In an observational study from Iceland, supplementation of fish oil during infancy reduced the development of both food sensitization and allergies to various food allergens (38). Allen et al. summarized the leading hypotheses of food allergies as "the 5 Ds: dry skin (atopic dermatitis), diet (tolerance vs. sensitization vs. allergy), dogs (microbiome), dribble (shared microbial exposure), and vitamin D" (39).

12.6   IgE-MEDIATED ALLERGIES

IgE-mediated allergies are rapidly occurring type 1 hypersensitivity reactions due to mast cell or basophil degranulation upon exposure to a triggering allergen (6, 8, 12). IgE-mediated food allergies manifest immediately from a few minutes to 1 to 2 hours after the ingestion of the food allergen (8, 40). An exception is the IgE-mediated reaction to mammalian meat, which has a delayed onset between 3 and 6 hours upon exposure. This unique reaction is to a carbohydrate antigen galactose-α-1,3-galactose (12).

IgE-mediated food allergies may manifest as oral allergy syndrome, urticaria, angioedema, and anaphylaxis (12, 41). IgE-based reactions are reproducible and are caused by food-specific IgE (8). A mild IgE-mediated reaction can progress to a more severe and potentially fatal anaphylactic reaction in an unpredictable fashion (6). The most common IgE-mediated manifestations involve cutaneous, GI, and respiratory systems. Severe reactions mostly include cardiovascular manifestations (12). Respiratory symptoms include difficulty breathing due to bronchoconstriction (6). Cutaneous manifestations are localized edema of the skin or mucus membranes and urticaria (12). GI manifestations include an oral tingling sensation, nausea, emesis, and abdominal pain (6).

12.6.1 ORAL ALLERGY SYNDROME

Oral allergy syndrome is an IgE-mediated allergy triggered by particular fruits and vegetables. Affected individuals usually have symptoms localized to the oral region affecting lips, mouth, and oropharynx. The symptoms usually are mild and self-limited and occasionally can be severe with angioedema. Given its mild nature, this form of allergy is often under-recognized. On exposure to the triggering foods, patients experience an oral itching and tingling sensation (1). This entity is more prevalent in adults, and symptoms usually start in the second decade of life (42). The most common food triggers include watermelon, banana, kiwi, and apple (1). This entity occurs as a result of the similarity between the antigenic epitopes of fruits and vegetables and the common pollens present in ragweed or birch (1). Patients with allergic rhinitis who are sensitized to pollen can develop symptoms due to an IgE response upon the ingestion of particular raw fruits or vegetables. Avoidance is recommended if the symptoms are bothersome for the patient, and management of allergic rhinitis with oral histamine therapy will help reduce the severity of the symptoms (1). If vegetables and certain fruits are cooked prior to ingestion, these symptoms are less pronounced.

12.6.2 URTICARIA AND ANGIOEDEMA

Acute urticaria and angioedema are the most common skin manifestations of food allergy and are usually mild. Acute urticaria and angioedema symptoms occur in up to one quarter of the US population (5, 12, 18). Food allergies are incriminated as one of the common causes of acute urticaria (hives), occurring more frequently than infections, medications, insect bites, or physical stressors (e.g., sunlight, cold, and pressure) (5, 12, 18). However, in chronic urticaria and angioedema (symptoms lasting more than 6 weeks), food allergies are often not the cause.

Urticaria appear as well circumscribed, pruritic, elevated, erythematous, blanchable, cutaneous wheals with a central pallor resulting from increased vascular permeability induced by vasoactive amines causing fluid extravasation into interstitial spaces in the superficial dermis (12). Angioedema occurs due to a similar mechanism deeper in the dermis and subcutaneous tissues and often accompanies urticaria. Angioedema is most often observed in areas with loose areolar tissues such as around the eyes, lips, oral cavity, larynx, distal extremities, and genitalia (12). In rare circumstances, angioedema can involve the alimentary tract mimicking an acute abdominal emergency such as pain, emesis, and loose stools (12, 18). In most instances, angioedema will resolve in 1–3 days (12). Milder symptoms, not involving the airway, are treated with antihistamines (H_1 receptor antagonists and possibly H_2 receptor antagonists). For severe symptoms and those involving the airway, epinephrine should be administered.

12.6.3 FOOD-INDUCED ANAPHYLAXIS

Anaphylaxis is an acute, often life-threatening immune reaction with the involvement of one or more organ systems. Food allergy is the most common etiology of anaphylaxis in the developed world. Milk, egg, and fish are common food triggers for anaphylaxis in children, and nuts and wheat in adults. Shrimp is common in all age groups (43). Anaphylactic reactions result from binding and cross-linking of cell-bound, allergen-specific IgE by the specific allergen (16, 21). In patients prone to anaphylaxis, allergen-specific IgE is produced when exposed to an allergen, which gets fixed to the high-affinity IgE receptors on mast cells and basophils (44). On subsequent exposure to the same allergen, the allergen-specific IgE molecules are cross-linked to form aggregates. This results in activation of mast cells and basophils with subsequent release of preformed mediators including histamine, tryptase, other inflammatory cytokines, and chemokines (44). This immune reaction occurs rapidly within 5–60 minutes of exposure to the offending allergen (21). In one fifth of the population with anaphylaxis, skin manifestations such as urticaria and pruritus may not be present and diagnosis can be easily missed (21). Anaphylaxis can present with life-threatening complications such as hypotension, cardiovascular collapse, arrhythmias, and respiratory failure (21). Prompt emergency treatment including immediate use of epinephrine and early access to emergency medical services is lifesaving (21).

12.7 DIAGNOSIS OF IgE-MEDIATED FOOD ALLERGIES

Skin prick testing (SPT) and IgE-based serum immunoglobulin testing are commonly used in the evaluation of allergen sensitization (patients may or may not have allergic manifestations to the tested food allergen) (45). SPTs are done by trained allergists who have the ability to handle emergency situations, such as anaphylaxis that can occur during testing (46). SPT is relatively inexpensive and provides immediate test results (47). For this test, the skin is pricked with a needle containing the allergen. If the subject is sensitized, the allergen interacts with the antigen-specific IgE attached to the cutaneous mast cells resulting in a wheal and flare response (6, 46). The SPT reaction is conventionally measured within 15 minutes (46). Generally, larger wheal size correlates with a diagnosis of food allergy rather than sensitization (15). When interpreted in the absence of a definite history of an incriminated food allergen, SPTs have a high negative predictive value (NPV) of approximately 90% (21). This high NPV value is useful to rule out allergic triggers when the history is not conclusive (46, 48). The positive predictive value (PPV) of SPT depends on the allergen, age of the patient, and size of the wheal (46, 48). Medications with antihistamine activity should be discontinued before the SPT to avoid a falsely negative test result.

In vitro extract-based testing for allergen-specific IgE in serum (sIgE) is utilized in patients who are unable to undergo SPT for many reasons, such as severe skin disease, inability to cooperate for testing, and inability to stop antihistamine medications (49). Serum IgE testing also helps in predicting reaction to oral food challenges (OFC). Overall, sIgE has high sensitivity but low specificity for food allergy. If sIgE levels are <50% PPV, an allergist may plan OFC to rule out the food allergy (49). Serial sIgE levels may be helpful to estimate the development of clinical tolerance. A newer immunoassay (ImmunoCAP immune-solid phase allergen chip or ImmunoCAP ISAC®) measures specific IgE to multiple allergens at the same time (47). While this new technique is more sensitive, it has the potential of over-diagnosing sensitization (49).

The basophil activation test (BAT) measures functional response to allergens by provoking an allergic reaction when an allergen binds the membrane IgE on basophils and mast cells, resulting in the degranulation of histamine and other mediators (4). Using flow cytometry, the surface activation markers can be measured on the allergen-activated basophils (4, 49). BAT has high specificity in diagnosing food allergy and is useful in differentiating truly allergic individuals from those who are only sensitized (4, 6, 49). Unlike conventional sIgE testing, which measures IgE to the whole food extract (with both allergenic and nonallergenic components), advanced testing such as molecular allergen analysis (MAA) identifies IgE bound to specific protein antigens in food (49). Another advanced technique is the epitope analysis. This test incorporates the analysis of the IgE-binding to specific segments of the allergen (epitopes). More data are needed for incorporating these newer techniques in routine clinical practice (49).

The gold standard for diagnosis of food allergy is the OFC, involving a double-blind, placebo-controlled challenge (45, 49). However, in clinical settings, single-blinded, or open challenge is often used. A food challenge is the administration of triggering food to establish if a patient has tolerance or allergy. Food is introduced in gradual, incremental doses to reduce the risk of anaphylaxis and also to find the lowest provoking dose (6). Also, many methods such as heat application (baking) reduce the allergenicity of some foods and are often employed in clinical practice (49). If no reaction is observed, then patients can be instructed to continue that challenged food at home regularly to pursue tolerance. Accurate diagnosis of food allergies (not sensitization of food allergens based on allergy testing) is vital to prevent the unnecessary elimination of foods (50). Because OFC is time-consuming and needs trained allergists, food allergy is often diagnosed by the combination of detailed history and allergy testing in clinical practice (4). Antigen specific-IgG levels, applied kinesiology, and cytotoxicity assays are not recommended in the diagnosis of food allergies (46, 49).

12.8 MANAGEMENT OF IGE-MEDIATED FOOD ALLERGIES

12.8.1 ALLERGEN AVOIDANCE

Currently, there is no definitive cure for food allergies (21, 51). Management is focused mainly on avoiding allergen ingestion and treating allergic reactions upon exposure to the food trigger (5, 12). In all patients with IgE-based anaphylactic reactions, self-administered epinephrine should be prescribed (8). Based on an allergy-focused detailed history, physical examination, and appropriate testing (either SPT and/ or sIgE), an elimination diet can be instituted (41). Because many food allergens are ubiquitous, allergen avoidance can be difficult, requiring patients and families to have a thorough education on reading labels and maintaining a nutritious diet. Especially since IgE-mediated diseases can be life-threatening, exposure to a food allergen by cross-contamination should be avoided (12). For school-age children, schools should follow a written safety action plan for the prevention of food allergy reactions. Efficient prevention of anaphylaxis includes meetings between parents and teachers with a discussion regarding possible food triggers, recognition of allergic reactions, and the treatment (12). Strict avoidance of food allergens is recommended for severe allergic reactions. This strict vigilance includes careful reading and interpretation of food labels, prevention of cross-contamination/cross-contact, and thorough education of the individuals who are involved in food preparation (21). Another means of allergen avoidance is the modification of the allergen in foods by heating with the goal of protein denaturation and subsequent elimination of its antigenicity. This is possible for a few foods, such as milk and eggs. However, this same principle does not apply to all allergens (e.g., peanuts).

12.8.2 Immunotherapy

Allergen immunotherapy is an allergen-specific treatment whereby the patient with an IgE-mediated allergy is administered small incremental amounts of the allergen. Whole food extracts of the specific allergens are utilized. Immunotherapy results in desensitization to a given allergenic food in most patients (52). This desensitization is a transient rise in the threshold for reactivity to that specific allergen (6). This may protect the individuals when an accidental exposure to the allergen occurs. This is achieved after many months of therapy and requires ongoing therapy (21). On the other hand, sustained unresponsiveness is the absence of a clinically evident reaction after exposure to the known food allergen after the active immunotherapy has been discontinued (21). This is acquired after a longer period of treatment and achieved by only a subset of patients undergoing immunotherapy (21).

The mechanism by which immunotherapy works is not completely understood. The desensitization acquired in immunotherapy may differ from a healthy state of immune tolerance (6). Oral tolerance is defined as the development of homeostatic, specific immunological non-responsiveness to antigens upon ingesting food (53). This response is natural and occurs early in life. Clinical tolerance produced by allergen immunotherapy may result in many responses such as reduced basophil reactivity, development of specific IgG4 and IgA, and decline in allergen-specific IgE in the serum (6, 16, 53, 54). In addition, immunotherapy is associated with selective omission of allergen-specific T_H2 cells and no major changes in the type 1 T helper (T_H1) and type 1 T regulatory (T_R1) cell populations. Instead of whole allergen extracts, short T lymphocyte epitope-based peptides of allergens have been utilized in successful desensitization (16). Unlike in natural tolerance, the duration of a sustained tolerance after immunotherapy is unknown.

Immunotherapy is administered via oral, sublingual, and epicutaneous routes (6, 21, 55). The differences of these forms of immunotherapy are detailed in Table 12.1.

TABLE 12.1

Different Routes of Available Immunotherapy

Route of Immunotherapy	Utilized Food Allergens	Comments
Oral	Nuts, milk, egg, wheat, fruits	• Adverse reactions such as anaphylaxis and gastrointestinal symptoms may happen • Most effective form of immunotherapy
Sublingual	Milk, certain nuts, fruits like kiwi	• Lower efficacy and lower risk of adverse reactions than oral immunotherapy • Oropharyngeal tingling reported • Unclear mechanism
Epicutaneous	Milk, peanut	• Not validated well • Unclear mechanism but has lower adverse reaction profile of all routes • Least effective compared with the other two

These newer modes of immunotherapies are much safer than the traditional subcutaneous immunotherapy (21, 54). The utility of immunotherapy is limited by the occurrence of allergic reactions during treatment and lack of persistent protection following therapy (8, 51, 52). IgE blockage with omalizumab during induction of oral immunotherapy has been shown to reduce side effects (56). Furthermore, Stranks et al. reported that omalizumab further reduced peanut- and Ara h 2 (peanut protein component that is the most frequent predictor of peanut allergy)-specific IgE antibodies and increased peanut- and Ara h 2-specific IgG4 antibodies (51).

Intramuscular epinephrine is the drug of choice for anaphylaxis and its timely use prevents mortality (21, 57). It has combined α and β sympathomimetic actions resulting in peripheral vasoconstriction, and causes an increase in cardiac output and bronchodilation (57). It also halts further release of inflammatory mediators from mast cells and basophils (57). Epinephrine can be self-administered using an auto-injector into the outer aspect of the mid-thigh (12). Medical management should focus on airway, breathing, and circulation (57). Hypotension requires fluid resuscitation and, if needed, additional vasopressor therapy (12). Epinephrine has a short half-life and often a second dose may be needed in 5–15 min (21). Epinephrine is still poorly utilized or under-prescribed in anaphylaxis despite its proven beneficial role (21). Biphasic reactions occur in 10% of patients (5, 12, 44). Therefore, patients should remain in observation for 4–6 hours or longer after the administration of a dose of epinephrine (5, 12, 44). A second dose of epinephrine may be required (12). Epinephrine should be administered as soon as possible within at least half an hour of the onset of symptoms (12, 21). Death due to anaphylaxis is associated with delayed usage of epinephrine (12). Glucocorticoids are often used in anaphylaxis, although there is no concrete evidence to support or oppose the use of corticosteroids in emergency management (44). For bronchospasm, supplemental oxygen and beta-agonist are recommended (12). Overall, medications such as antihistamines, steroids, and beta-agonists are adjunct medications and should never be used as first-line therapy (21). Medical alert devices (such as bracelets) with potential allergies listed could be life-saving for patients with food allergies (12, 21).

12.9 NOVEL APPROACHES

A variety of factors have been implicated for the prevention of food allergies. Exclusive breastfeeding for the first 4 months of life reduces the incidence of atopic dermatitis in the first 2 years of life (26). However, there are scarce data to substantiate the role of breastfeeding in either avoiding or delaying other types of food allergies (26). Consumption of common food allergens (milk, nuts, and wheat) by pregnant women appears to reduce the risk of allergy and asthma during childhood (58). Common allergenic complementary foods, such as eggs or fish, should not be indiscriminately avoided, either at the time of solid food introduction or by mothers during pregnancy or lactation (26, 39). Subsequent to the LEAP study, most guidelines recommend the introduction of peanut products in infants who are at high risk of developing peanut allergy (e.g., egg-allergic infants or infants with severe eczema) between 4 and 6 months of age under appropriate medical supervision (26, 59). In these high-risk infants, a negative allergic testing for peanut using SPT and/or sIgE is recommended before the challenge (26, 59). In infants with low risk of allergy, the American Academy of Pediatrics recommend introduction of all solids after 6 months of age in exclusively breastfed infants (26). The common allergenic complementary foods such as eggs and fish should not be indiscriminately avoided, either in infants at the time of solid food introduction or by mothers during pregnancy or lactation (26, 39).

12.10 INCORRECT/OUTDATED PRACTICES

Diagnosing food allergies mainly on the basis of self-reported history alone may lead to erroneous diagnosis and unnecessary dietary elimination with potential adverse health implications. All self-reported food allergies must be evaluated by an allergist with confirmation by OFC or allergic sensitization testing. Antigen specific-IgG levels, applied kinesiology, and cytotoxicity assays are not recommended in the diagnosis of food allergies (46, 49). Avoidance of common food allergens during pregnancy and during infancy is no longer recommended. Newer evidence supports introduction of allergenic foods in early life and continued consumption of common food allergens (milk, nuts, and wheat) by pregnant women, because they have been shown to reduce the risk of allergy and asthma during childhood.

PRACTICE PEARLS

- Due to overlapping symptoms, food intolerance and food sensitivity are often confused with food allergies.
- Patients with self-reported food allergy symptoms must be evaluated by a trained allergist and food allergy must be evaluated with allergic sensitization testing and confirmation.

- Routine use of serum IgE levels to diagnose food allergies is not recommended and testing for allergen-specific antibodies may be useful in identifying foods which potentially could trigger IgE-mediated allergic reactions.
- Epinephrine is life-saving for patients having anaphylactic reactions due to food allergens.

REFERENCES

1. Turnbull JL, Adams HN, Gorard DA. Review article: The diagnosis and management of food allergy and food intolerances. Aliment Pharmacol Ther. 2015;41(1):3–25.
2. Lomer MC. Review article: The aetiology, diagnosis, mechanisms and clinical evidence for food intolerance. Aliment Pharmacol Ther. 2015;41(3):262–75.
3. Lavine E. Blood testing for sensitivity, allergy or intolerance to food. Cmaj. 2012; 184(6):666–8.
4. Santos AF, Brough HA. Making the most of in vitro tests to diagnose food allergy. J Allergy Clin Immunol Pract. 2017;5(2):237–48.
5. Panel NI-SE, Boyce JA, Assa'ad A, Burks AW, Jones SM, Sampson HA, et al. Guidelines for the diagnosis and management of food allergy in the United States: Report of the NIAID-sponsored expert panel. J Allergy Clin Immunol. 2010;126(6 Suppl):S1–58.
6. Yu W, Freeland DMH, Nadeau KC. Food allergy: Immune mechanisms, diagnosis and immunotherapy. Nat Rev Immunol. 2016;16(12):751–65.
7. Hungerford JM. Scombroid poisoning: A review. Toxicon. 2010;56(2):231–43.
8. Cianferoni A. Non-IgE mediated food allergy. Curr Pediatr Rev. 2020;16(2):95–105.
9. Stapel SO, Asero R, Ballmer-Weber B, Knol E, Strobel S, Vieths S, et al. Testing for IgG4 against foods is not recommended as a diagnostic tool: EAACI task force report. Allergy. 2008;63(7):793–6.
10. Antico A, Pagani M, Vescovi PP, Bonadonna P, Senna G. Food-specific IgG4 lack diagnostic value in adult patients with chronic urticaria and other suspected allergy skin symptoms. Int Arch Allergy Immunol. 2011;155(1):52–6.
11. Atkinson W, Sheldon T, Shaath N, Whorwell P. Food elimination based on IgG antibodies in irritable bowel syndrome: A randomised controlled trial. Gut. 2004;53(10): 1459–64.
12. Davis CM, Kelso JM. Food allergy management. Immunol Allergy Clin North Am. 2018;38(1):53–64.
13. [Accessed on 3.28.2020]. Available from: www.fda.gov/food/food-allergensgluten-free-guidance-documents-regulatory-information/food-allergen-labeling-and-consumer-protection-act-2004-falcpa.
14. Willits EK, Park MA, Hartz MF, Schleck CD, Weaver AL, Joshi AY. Food allergy: A comprehensive population-based cohort study. Mayo Clin Proc. 2018;93(10):1423–30.
15. Savage J, Sicherer S, Wood R. The natural history of food allergy. J Allergy Clin Immunol Pract. 2016;4(2):196–203; quiz 4.
16. Prickett SR, Voskamp AL, Phan T, Dacumos-Hill A, Mannering SI, Rolland JM, et al. Ara h 1 CD4+ T cell epitope-based peptides: candidates for a peanut allergy therapeutic. Clin Exp Allergy. 2013;43(6):684–97.
17. Wood RA, Sicherer SH, Vickery BP, Jones SM, Liu AH, Fleischer DM, et al. The natural history of milk allergy in an observational cohort. J Allergy Clin Immunol. 2013;131(3):805–12.

18. Chafen JJS, Newberry S, Riedl M, Bravata DM, Maglione MA, Booth M, et al. Prevalence, natural history, diagnosis, and treatment of food allergy: A systematic review of the evidence. 2010. http://www.rand.org/pubs/working_papers/2010/RAND_WR757-1.pdf. Accessed May 29, 2023.

19. Liu AH, Jaramillo R, Sicherer SH, Wood RA, Bock SA, Burks AW, et al. National prevalence and risk factors for food allergy and relationship to asthma: Results from the national health and nutrition examination survey 2005–2006. J Allergy Clin Immunol. 2010;126(4):798–806 e13.

20. Lee AJ, Thalayasingam M, Lee BW. Food allergy in Asia: How does it compare? Asia Pac Allergy. 2013;3(1):3–14.

21. Jones SM, Burks AW. Food allergy. N Engl J Med. 2017;377(12):1168–76.

22. Nwaru BI, Hickstein L, Panesar SS, Roberts G, Muraro A, Sheikh A, et al. Prevalence of common food allergies in Europe: A systematic review and meta-analysis. Allergy. 2014;69(8):992–1007.

23. Hill DA, Spergel JM. The atopic march: Critical evidence and clinical relevance. Ann Allergy Asthma Immunol. 2018;120(2):131–7.

24. Iweala OI, Burks AW. Food allergy: Our evolving understanding of its pathogenesis, prevention, and treatment. Curr Allergy Asthma Rep. 2016;16(5):37.

25. Sicherer SH, Sampson HA. Food allergy: A review and update on epidemiology, pathogenesis, diagnosis, prevention, and management. J Allergy Clin Immunol. 2018;141(1):41–58.

26. Greer FR, Sicherer SH, Burks AW, Committee On N, Section On A, Immunology. The effects of early nutritional interventions on the development of atopic disease in infants and children: The role of maternal dietary restriction, breastfeeding, hydrolyzed formulas, and timing of introduction of allergenic complementary foods. Pediatrics. 2019;143(4).

27. Chafen JJ, Newberry SJ, Riedl MA, Bravata DM, Maglione M, Suttorp MJ, et al. Diagnosing and managing common food allergies: A systematic review. JAMA. 2010;303(18):1848–56.

28. Urashima M, Mezawa H, Okuyama M, Urashima T, Hirano D, Gocho N, et al. Primary prevention of cow's milk sensitization and food allergy by avoiding supplementation with cow's milk formula at birth: A randomized clinical trial. JAMA Pediatr. 2019;173(12):1137–45.

29. Du Toit G, Roberts G, Sayre PH, Bahnson HT, Radulovic S, Santos AF, et al. Randomized trial of peanut consumption in infants at risk for peanut allergy. N Engl J Med. 2015;372(9):803–13.

30. Perkin MR, Logan K, Tseng A, Raji B, Ayis S, Peacock J, et al. Randomized trial of introduction of allergenic foods in breast-fed infants. N Engl J Med. 2016;374(18):1733–43.

31. Strachan DP. Hay fever, hygiene, and household size. BMJ. 1989;299(6710):1259–60.

32. Gupta RS, Singh AM, Walkner M, Caruso D, Bryce PJ, Wang X, et al. Hygiene factors associated with childhood food allergy and asthma. Allergy Asthma Proc. 2016;37(6):e140–e6.

33. Marrs T, Bruce KD, Logan K, Rivett DW, Perkin MR, Lack G, et al. Is there an association between microbial exposure and food allergy? A systematic review. Pediatric Allergy and Immunology. 2013;24(4):311–20. E8.

34. Sharma G, Im SH. Probiotics as a potential immunomodulating pharmabiotics in allergic diseases: Current status and future prospects. Allergy Asthma Immunol Res. 2018;10(6):575–90.

35. Berni Canani R, Sangwan N, Stefka AT, Nocerino R, Paparo L, Aitoro R, et al. Lactobacillus rhamnosus GG-supplemented formula expands butyrate-producing bacterial strains in food allergic infants. ISME J. 2016;10(3):742–50.

36. Sicherer SH, Sampson HA. Food allergy: Epidemiology, pathogenesis, diagnosis, and treatment. J Allergy Clin Immunol. 2014;133(2):291–307; quiz 8.
37. Vassallo MF, Camargo Jr CA. Potential mechanisms for the hypothesized link between sunshine, vitamin D, and food allergy in children. J Allergy Clin Immunol. 2010;126(2):217–22.
38. Clausen M, Jonasson K, Keil T, Beyer K, Sigurdardottir ST. Fish oil in infancy protects against food allergy in Iceland—results from a birth cohort study. Allergy. 2018;73(6):1305–12.
39. Allen KJ, Koplin JJ. Prospects for prevention of food allergy. J Allergy Clin Immunol Pract. 2016;4(2):215–20.
40. D'Auria E, Abrahams M, Zuccotti GV, Venter C. Personalized nutrition approach in food allergy: Is it prime time yet? Nutrients. 2019;11(2).
41. Muraro A, Werfel T, Hoffmann-Sommergruber K, Roberts G, Beyer K, Bindslev-Jensen C, et al. EAACI food allergy and anaphylaxis guidelines: Diagnosis and management of food allergy. Allergy. 2014;69(8):1008–25.
42. Dunlop JH, Keet CA. Epidemiology of food allergy. Immunol Allergy Clin North Am. 2018;38(1):13–25.
43. Fernandes RA, Regateiro F, Pereira C, Faria E, Pita J, Todo-Bom A, et al. Anaphylaxis in a food allergy outpatient department: One-year review. Eur Ann Allergy Clin Immunol. 2018;50(2):81–8.
44. Liyanage CK, Galappatthy P, Seneviratne SL. Corticosteroids in management of anaphylaxis; A systematic review of evidence. Eur Ann Allergy Clin Immunol. 2017;49(5):196–207.
45. Hammond C, Lieberman JA. Unproven diagnostic tests for food allergy. Immunol Allergy Clin North Am. 2018;38(1):153–63.
46. Sampson HA, Aceves S, Bock SA, James J, Jones S, Lang D, et al. Food allergy: A practice parameter update—2014. J Allergy Clin Immunol. 2014;134(5):1016–25 e43.
47. Griffiths RLM, El-Shanawany T, Jolles SRA, Selwood C, Heaps AG, Carne EM, et al. Comparison of the performance of skin prick, ImmunoCAP, and ISAC tests in the diagnosis of patients with allergy. Int Arch Allergy Immunol. 2017;172(4):215–23.
48. Soares-Weiser K, Takwoingi Y, Panesar SS, Muraro A, Werfel T, Hoffmann-Sommergruber K, et al. The diagnosis of food allergy: A systematic review and meta-analysis. Allergy. 2014;69(1):76–86.
49. Gupta M, Cox A, Nowak-Węgrzyn A, Wang J. Diagnosis of food allergy. Immunol Allergy Clin North Am. 2018;38(1):39–52.
50. Mehta H, Groetch M, Wang J. Growth and nutritional concerns in children with food allergy. Curr Opin Allergy Clin Immunol. 2013;13(3):275–9.
51. Stranks AJ, Minnicozzi SC, Miller SJ, Burton OT, Logsdon SL, Spergel JM, et al. Immunoglobulin E blockade during food allergen ingestion enhances the induction of inhibitory immunoglobulin G antibodies. Ann Allergy Asthma Immunol. 2019;122(2):213–15.
52. Skripak JM, Nash SD, Rowley H, Brereton NH, Oh S, Hamilton RG, et al. A randomized, double-blind, placebo-controlled study of milk oral immunotherapy for cow's milk allergy. J Allergy Clin Immunol. 2008;122(6):1154–60.
53. Berin MC, Shreffler WG. Mechanisms underlying induction of tolerance to foods. Immunol Allergy Clin. 2016;36(1):87–102.
54. Varshney P, Jones SM, Scurlock AM, Perry TT, Kemper A, Steele P, et al. A randomized controlled study of peanut oral immunotherapy: Clinical desensitization and modulation of the allergic response. J Allergy Clin Immunol. 2011;127(3):654–60.
55. Dioszeghy V, Mondoulet L, Puteaux E, Dhelft V, Ligouis M, Plaquet C, et al. Differences in phenotype, homing properties and suppressive activities of regulatory T cells induced by epicutaneous, oral or sublingual immunotherapy in mice sensitized to peanut. Cell Mol Immunol. 2017;14(9):770–82.

56. MacGinnitie AJ, Rachid R, Gragg H, Little SV, Lakin P, Cianferoni A, et al. Omalizumab facilitates rapid oral desensitization for peanut allergy. J Allergy Clin Immunol. 2017;139(3):873–81 e8.
57. Anagnostou K, Turner PJ. Myths, facts and controversies in the diagnosis and management of anaphylaxis. Arch Dis Child. 2019;104(1):83–90.
58. Bunyavanich S, Rifas-Shiman SL, Platts-Mills TA, Workman L, Sordillo JE, Camargo CA, Jr., et al. Peanut, milk, and wheat intake during pregnancy is associated with reduced allergy and asthma in children. J Allergy Clin Immunol. 2014;133(5):1373–82.
59. Togias A, Cooper SF, Acebal ML, Assa'ad A, Baker JR, Beck LA, et al. Addendum guidelines for the prevention of peanut allergy in the United States: Report of the National Institute of Allergy And Infectious Diseases-sponsored expert panel. *Allergy Asthma Clin Immunol.* 2017;13(1):1.

13 Food Allergies Mediated Completely or Partially by Non-IgE Immune Mechanisms

Senthilkumar Sankararaman, Aravind Thavamani, and Thomas J. Sferra

13.1 INTRODUCTION

Allergic reactions to food can be broadly classified based upon their pathogenic mechanisms as IgE-mediated, non-IgE-mediated, and combined IgE/non-IgE-mediated reactions (Chapter 12 Figure 12.1). IgE-mediated allergies are rapidly occurring type 1 hypersensitivity reactions due to mast cell or basophil degranulation upon exposure to a triggering allergen (1, 2). In clinical practice, IgE-mediated food allergies are relatively easier to diagnose compared with the other types because they mostly manifest sooner (a few minutes to hours) after food allergen exposure and specific IgE-based diagnostic tests are available (3) (see Chapter 12). Unlike IgE-mediated allergies, non-IgE-mediated reactions are typically delayed many hours to several days after ingesting the triggering foods (3). The pathogenic processes underlying non-IgE-mediated allergic reactions are poorly understood, but most are predominantly mediated by T cells and involve delayed type hypersensitivity (1). Non-IgE-mediated allergic conditions predominantly present with gastrointestinal (GI) manifestations and often overlap with many GI conditions, such as gastroesophageal reflux disease (GERD), functional dyspepsia, and lactose intolerance. Unlike IgE-mediated conditions, the definitive prevalence of non-IgE-mediated diseases is elusive due to the lack of clear diagnostic criteria and confirmatory tests.

Most non-IgE-mediated food allergies occur at a young age (e.g., infancy and toddlerhood) and milk is the most prevalent food allergen. The majority of these clinical syndromes resolve after 1–5 years. The most common clinical non-IgE-mediated allergies include food protein-induced allergic enterocolitis syndrome (FPIES), food protein enteropathy, and food protein-induced allergic proctocolitis (FPIAP) (2). Conditions such as eosinophilic esophagitis (EoE), other eosinophilic gastrointestinal diseases (EGID), and atopic dermatitis are mediated by both IgE- and non-IgE-mediated pathways (4).

 DOI: 10.1201/9780429322570-13

13.2 NON-IgE-MEDIATED FOOD ALLERGIES

13.2.1 FOOD PROTEIN-INDUCED ALLERGIC ENTEROCOLITIS SYNDROME

FPIES can be acute or chronic and the usual age of onset of symptoms is around 1–3 months of age or a few weeks later, when infants are exposed to the triggering foods such as rice and oats as cereals (5, 6). The incidence varies between 0.15–8 per 1,000 in children aged less than 3 years (7, 8). In most cases, patients present with repetitive emesis within 4 hours after intake of the triggering food. Symptoms can be severe with repeated episodes of projectile emesis with or without accompanying diarrhea. Patients can be pale, lethargic, dehydrated, and hypotensive. The chronic presentation is rare and includes persistent emesis, poor weight gain, and bloody stools. The diagnosis is often delayed due to the lack of specificity of these symptoms and the lack of familiarity with this condition among many primary care and emergency department clinicians. The most common triggers for FPIES include milk, soy, rice, and oats (9). FPIES typically resolve by 3–5 years of age (10). Adult-onset FPIES is rare and in most cases is secondary to seafood exposure such as fish, shellfish, and mollusks (5, 6).

The pathogenesis of FPIES is not clear. However, robust actuation of innate immune mechanisms after food ingestion has been implicated (10). T cell stimulation and activation of monocytes, neutrophils, and eosinophils have been reported in patients with active FPIES but not in those who had already outgrown their FPIES. T cells have also been implicated in the production of inflammatory cytokines, such as tumor necrosis factor-alpha (TNF-α), resulting in an increase in intestinal permeability and dysmotility (6).

FPIES is diagnosed based on clinical manifestations (high index of suspicion) and subsequent improvement with elimination of the food trigger (5, 11). There are no laboratory tests specific for FPIES, but abnormalities may include elevated white cell count with increased absolute neutrophil count, increased platelet count, metabolic acidosis, and methemoglobinemia. Abnormalities in stool may include increased leukocyte or eosinophil count (11). Families of children with FPIES should be well educated regarding this condition and carry a written action plan (explicitly explaining the management of FPIES) since many emergency department staff may not be familiar with FPIES (11). Ondansetron and intravenous corticosteroids should be considered to treat more severe reactions (5, 11). A supervised oral food challenge can be performed in a controlled setting, when it is anticipated that the patient may have outgrown their FPIES (usually 1–2 years after the most recent reaction).

13.2.2 FOOD PROTEIN-INDUCED ALLERGIC PROCTOCOLITIS

FPIAP occurs early in life and the prevalence is roughly 0.16% among healthy infants (12). In infants with rectal bleeding, the prevalence ranges between 18% and 64% (13). The presentation is mostly subacute and occurs between 2 and 8 weeks of life. Often, thriving infants present with stools mixed with mucus or blood (14). The pathogenesis involves T cells, but the exact mechanisms have not been elucidated. Cow milk proteins and, less commonly, soy protein are the common offending allergens (15). Breastfed infants can be affected due to the presence of small amounts of these proteins absorbed intact and excreted into the breast milk (14). Elimination of cow's milk protein or soy protein from the infant's diet is achieved by eliminating these proteins from the mother's diet in breastfed infants or in formula-fed babies by switching to an extensively hydrolyzed formula. Unlike FPIES, this condition lacks systemic manifestations (hypotension, shock), vomiting, diarrhea, and growth failure.

13.2.3 FOOD PROTEIN-INDUCED ENTEROPATHY

The prevalence of food protein-induced enteropathy is unknown but generally considered rare and most often noted in infants and young children (16). It presents with chronic intractable diarrhea, fat malabsorption (steatorrhea), and poor weight gain (14). Cow's milk is the most common trigger that causes immune-mediated damage to the intestinal mucosa. Other noted food allergens include soy, poultry, rice, and fish. Severe malabsorption could also lead to anemia, hypoalbuminemia, and vitamin K deficiency. Treatment involves strict avoidance of the allergen and most patients will outgrow this condition by 2–3 years of age. A food challenge can be planned after this age to evaluate whether the condition is outgrown.

13.3 MIXED IgE- AND NON-IgE-MEDIATED ALLERGIC FOOD REACTIONS

13.3.1 ATOPIC DERMATITIS

Atopic dermatitis affects approximately 10% of children (17) and is likely due to complex interactions between a defective cutaneous barrier, immune dysregulation, and environmental triggers (e.g., food allergens, infections, irritants) in genetically susceptible individuals (17, 18). The exact role of food allergies in causing atopic dermatitis is not clearly known. However, in a subset of young children, food allergies can either induce or worsen eczematous lesions. Infants with atopic dermatitis have an increased chance of developing IgE-mediated food allergic reactions and, later in life, asthma and allergic rhinitis. This concept is popularly referred to as the "atopic march" (17, 19).

Milk, egg, wheat, soy, and peanut are the most common food allergens accounting for the majority (up to 90%) of food-induced atopic dermatitis in young children (17, 18). Various forms of cutaneous reactions have been noted in children with atopic dermatitis after intake of the triggering food. Immediate IgE-mediated cutaneous reactions, such as urticaria and angioedema, may occur within 1–2 hours of ingestion. Late IgE-mediated reactions involving a transient morbilliform rash can manifest in 6–10 hours. Isolated eczematous type delayed reactions can often be noted in 6–48 hours with flares of eczema at the expected sites of the exanthem (18). These delayed-onset (6–48 hours after exposure) cutaneous symptoms are mediated by T helper 2 (T_H2) cells (2). Caution must be exerted before empirically eliminating foods to assure the nutritional adequacy of the diet (17). Apart from eliminating the triggering food antigen, the focus of management should be aimed at other contributors, such as barrier dysfunction, and treating or preventing coexisting infections.

13.3.2 Cow Milk Protein Allergy

Cow milk protein allergy is discussed separately because it has protean presenting manifestations. Symptoms of cow milk protein allergy are usually difficult to recognize due to the lack of a clear time-related association between exposure and onset of symptoms (1). The prevalence of cow milk protein allergy during infancy is 2–3% and the most common food allergen in this age group (20). The exact mechanisms of these disorders are still poorly understood, but both IgE- and non-IgE-mediated pathways could be involved. Early manifestations may be due to IgE-mediated immediate-type reactions, such as urticaria and angioedema. Late onset non-IgE-mediated presentations include intractable GERD, refractory eczema, bloody stools (infantile proctocolitis), persistent crying, and altered bowel habits (either excessively loose stools or constipation) (1). Clinicians often have difficulty in diagnosing this entity due to similarities between cow milk protein allergy and many common conditions of infancy, such as GERD, infantile colic, and dyschezia. Cow milk protein allergy should be in the differential diagnosis of GERD in infants and a 2–4-week trial of a hypoallergenic formula is recommended (21). Rarely, cow milk protein has been implicated in pulmonary hemosiderosis (Heiner's syndrome), which manifests as recurrent lung infiltrates, GI bleeding, iron-deficiency anemia, and poor growth. This has been associated with non-IgE-mediated hypersensitivity to cow's milk where peripheral eosinophilia and cow's milk precipitins may be noted.

13.3.3 Eosinophilic Esophagitis

EoE is a chronic, immunologic, antigen-mediated, clinicopathological condition with varied clinical manifestations and disease severity that affects both children and adults (22). It is characterized by infiltration of the esophageal mucosa predominantly by eosinophils leading to esophageal dysfunction. It is one of the leading causes of dysphagia and food impaction. After the initial recognition of EoE as a new entity in the early 1990s, the definition of EoE has undergone several changes. Based on the most recent consensus statement, EoE is diagnosed in the presence of symptoms of esophageal dysfunction and esophageal biopsy showing at least 15 eosinophils per high-power field (eos/hpf) or approximately 60 eosinophils per mm^2 after a thorough evaluation and exclusion of other conditions contributing to esophageal eosinophilic infiltrations (23, 24) (Table 13.1).

Although EoE is a global disease, the incidence widely varies across geographic regions. Both the incidence and prevalence of EoE have been increasing (25). The estimated incidence of EoE in North America and Europe is 4/100,000 person-years and the estimated prevalence is 23–90/100,000 (25–27). For patients who underwent an esophagogastroduodenoscopy (EGD) for diverse GI symptoms, the prevalence of EoE was 2–7% (25). The same study also reported a prevalence as high as 12–23%

TABLE 13.1

Causes of Esophageal Eosinophilia

- Eosinophilic esophagitis
- Gastroesophageal reflux disease
- Eosinophilic gastroenteritis
- Achalasia
- Vasculitis/Connective tissue disorder
- Hypereosinophilic syndrome
- Viral and fungal infections
- Inflammatory bowel disease – Crohn's disease
- Drug hypersensitivity response
- Celiac disease
- Pill esophagitis
- Graft vs. host disease
- Pemphigus

---

in patients for whom the endoscopy was done for dysphagia and 46–63% in patients who presented for food impaction. Most patients present between late childhood and mid adulthood (<50 years of age), although the disease can occur at all ages (infancy through late adulthood) (27). Males are more commonly affected than females (nearly 70% male) (24, 28). Although EoE has been reported across all races and ethnicities, there is a slight predominance in Caucasians (27).

The pathogenic mechanism of EoE remains elusive but involves a complex interaction between various factors, including genetic, environmental, and host immune response to ingested food allergens leading to the development of mucosal infiltration by eosinophils (22). All of these factors ultimately elicit a T_H2 response mediated predominantly by interleukins (IL)-4, 5, and 13 (29, 30). Food allergens have been strongly implicated in the pathogenesis of EoE. Seasonal variation in the diagnosis of EoE with increasing clusters during pollen seasons makes an argument for its association with aeroallergens (31, 32). EoE is also more prevalent in cold and arid climate zones and rural communities with low population density (33–35).

Although food triggers have a crucial role in the pathogenesis of EoE, only 15–43% of the patients have documented IgE-mediated food hypersensitivity (36, 37). Emerging evidence suggests that IgE might not have a critical role in the pathogenesis of EoE, although EoE patients have mildly increased IgE levels. This is further supported by clinical trials in which the anti-IgE antibody, omalizumab, failed to demonstrate a decrease in esophageal eosinophilia or an improvement in clinical manifestations (38, 39). Studies have shown that IgG_4 reactive to specific foods are elevated in the serum and esophageal tissue of patients with EoE and may be involved in disease pathogenesis (40). Similar to various other atopic conditions, several factors associated with eliciting a T_H2 response have been associated with the development of EoE in children, including early exposure to antibiotics, Cesarean section, preterm birth, formula feeding, and use of acid-suppressive medications during infancy (41–43).

Patients with EoE will frequently have a history of environmental allergies and also a family member with atopy (44–46). The presence of a comorbid atopic condition in patients with EoE is associated with severe symptoms and poor response to treatment with steroids. Due to this strong association of atopy with EoE, all patients with EoE should be evaluated for comorbid allergic disorders.

Symptoms of EoE are the manifestations of esophageal dysfunction. The presenting symptoms vary widely with the age of the patients. Infants and toddlers typically present with feeding issues (gagging, choking on feeds, refusal to feed), non-specific GI symptoms (vomiting, frequent spit-ups), or poor weight gain (24, 47, 48). School-age children usually present with reflux symptoms, abdominal pain, and heartburn. Adolescents may present with dysphagia, heartburn, and epigastric pain. Most common manifestations in adults include dysphagia followed by food impaction and, less commonly, reflux, heartburn, and abdominal pain. Food impaction may occur due to esophageal dysmotility or stricture.

Stricture is a late complication, especially in those with a prolonged duration of untreated EoE. The uncontrolled inflammatory cascade promotes subepithelial fibrosis leading to esophageal remodeling and stricture formation (48). Many patients describe recurrent episodes of food impaction that is relieved by drinking fluids or forcibly vomiting. In developed nations, EoE is now the leading cause of dysphagia and food impaction in children, adolescents, and young adults (26). Many patients might have subconsciously developed compensatory maneuvers to overcome dysphagia, such as eating slowly and meticulously, drinking copious quantities of liquids while eating, and breaking food into small pieces. In patients who present with symptoms suggestive of EoE, clinicians should specifically inquire about the aforementioned maneuvers to assess the severity of the condition.

Common endoscopic findings seen in EoE are longitudinal furrows, mucosal edema, white plaques or exudates, esophageal rings (also called feline rings, felinization, or trachealization), strictures, and mucosal fragility or crêpe paper appearance (24) (Figure 13.1).

Similar to the clinical presentation, the endoscopic findings differ between children and adults. Commonly in children, pallor or decreased vasculature (58%) and white plaques (38%) are seen, while in adults, esophageal rings (57%) and strictures (25%) are more frequent (49). The common occurrence of strictures and rings in adults is believed to be related to the chronicity of the inflammation leading to fibrosis and stricture formation. Biopsies of the gastric and duodenal mucosa are also needed to exclude other causes of esophageal eosinophilia such as EGIDs, celiac disease, and Crohn's disease.

Multiple esophageal biopsies from different regions of the esophagus are recommended to increase the diagnostic yield (50, 51). One study demonstrated that a single biopsy showed a sensitivity of 55% in diagnosing EoE, which increased to 100% with five biopsy specimens (51). Another study examined 1,342 biopsies and found that the probability of finding ≥15 eos/hpf in one, four, five, and six biopsies as 63%, 98%, 99%, and > 99% respectively (50). Because inflammatory changes in EoE often have a patchy distribution, experts recommend biopsies from different levels (mid and distal) of the esophagus and in areas with abnormal findings, such as plaques, furrows, and rings (51–53).

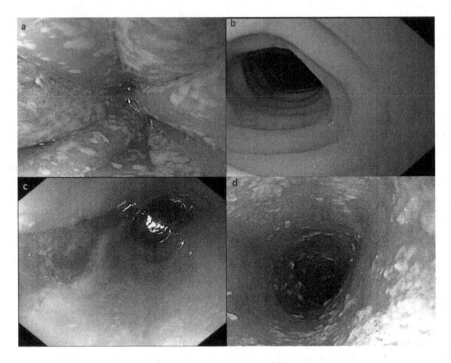

FIGURE 13.1 Endoscopic pictures of patients with eosinophilic esophagitis demonstrating (a) mucosal edema with longitudinal furrows and white plaques, (b) trachealization of the esophagus, (c) mucosal tear of the esophagus, and (d) white plaques due to eosinophilic infiltration.

Source: **Figure 13.1b courtesy of Jonathan Moses, MD.**

GERD is the most common differential diagnosis for EoE with overlapping clinical manifestations and histopathological findings (52, 54). Both disorders may even coexist and contribute to each other (55). EoE can lead to secondary GERD due to dysmotility or reduced esophageal compliance. Alternatively, GERD can disrupt or reduce the esophageal epithelial barrier and lead to antigen exposure and increased eosinophilic activity. The histologic criteria of ≥15 eos/hpf has a sensitivity of 100% and a specificity of 96% for diagnosing EoE (56). On the contrary, in GERD, the increased eosinophils are mostly noted in distal esophageal biopsies and usually <5 eos/hpf (53, 57).

Radiological investigations have a very limited role in the diagnosis of EoE. Contrast studies have poor sensitivity for the diagnosing the mucosal changes of EoE (58). However, an esophagram can be valuable in evaluating for a small-caliber esophagus and strictures (24, 59, 60). Several biomarkers have been evaluated for either enhancing the diagnostic accuracy of biopsies or reducing the need for frequent endoscopic disease monitoring, although a limitation in the majority of these biomarkers is the lack of clear-cut differentiation between EoE and other atopic conditions (61). In preliminary studies, esophageal sampling utilizing either cytosponge or string was found to be useful in monitoring EoE activity and further studies are needed to explore their role.

The main goals of EoE treatment are to improve symptoms and resolve esophageal inflammation to avoid long-term complications. Treatment strategies involve three main approaches: (i) pharmacological therapy; (ii) dietary modifications; and (iii) treatment of complications (Figure 13.2). The mode of therapy depends on many patient factors (choice of therapy, affordability, feasibility, and understanding about therapies) and stage of EoE. Many experts consider histologic remission as <5 eos/hpf and a response to treatment as 5–14 eos/hpf (62).

Currently, proton pump inhibitor (PPI) therapy is considered the first line of treatment prior to dietary therapy or steroids (62, 63). Previously, PPI-responders were termed as having PPI-responsive esophageal eosinophilia and prior guidelines recommended an 8-week trial with PPI to diagnose this condition (52). However, current evidence shows that PPI-responsive esophageal eosinophilia has all clinical features similar to EoE and is essentially indistinguishable from EoE. Hence, response to PPI is no longer a criterion to diagnose or rule out EoE (23, 63). Histologic remission with PPI therapy is reported to occur in between 23–83% of patients (64, 65). The long-term effectiveness of PPIs on EoE has not yet been elucidated.

Corticosteroids are the mainstay of pharmacological treatment in those who do not respond to PPI therapy. Fluticasone metered-dose inhaler or oral viscous budesonide have been used as topical corticosteroids in EoE. Topical corticosteroids are not approved for treating EoE by the United States Food and Drug Administration (FDA) and are utilized as off-label therapy. Histologic remission occurs in approximately three quarters of patients when topical corticosteroids are used as first- or second-line therapy (62). Almost 10% of the population have EoE

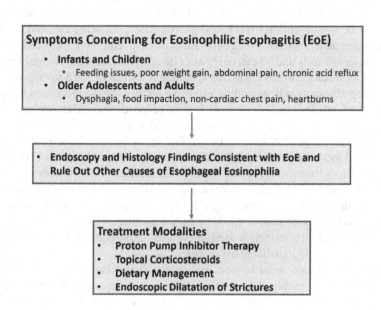

FIGURE 13.2 Overview of management of eosinophilic esophagitis.

refractory to topical steroid treatment. Discontinuation of topical steroids may result in disease recurrence. Approximately 10–15% of patients on topical corticosteroids may develop asymptomatic esophageal candidiasis and about 2–3% may develop oral candidiasis, which could be prevented by rinsing the mouth with water after administration of medications (66–68). Adrenal suppression occurs in a small number of children with EoE who receive topical corticosteroids (69). Topical corticosteroid usage in pediatric populations is also associated with a reduction of growth velocity (70). Systemic corticosteroids are no longer recommended due to associated side effects, rapid recurrence of EoE with discontinuation, and evidence that topical steroids are as effective but also with significantly lesser adverse effects (22, 53, 64, 67).

For patients who do not want or respond to pharmacological interventions, dietary therapy is advocated. Dietary modifications include three types: (i) elemental; (ii) specific-food elimination; and (iii) targeted-food elimination. The elemental diet, which involves a diet comprising exclusively elemental amino acid-based formulas, has the highest remission rate close to 90% but is difficult to maintain due to poor palatability and may result in frequent relapses due to poor adherence (48, 71).

The most popular elimination diet is the six-food elimination diet (6FED), which includes elimination of dairy, wheat, eggs, soy, nuts (peanut and tree nuts), and fish (including shellfish) (71). In this diet, all types of fruits, vegetables, rice, beans, non-wheat grains, poultry, and red meat are allowed without restriction. The 6FED has a remission rate of 70% in both adults and children (48, 71, 72). A repeat EGD is recommended to evaluate for histological response 6–8 weeks after the introduction of the 6FED. If the biopsies show remission, eliminated diet groups are systematically introduced in succession followed by a repeat biopsy.

The four-food elimination diet (4FED) does not restrict nuts and fish. In a prospective study involving 78 children with EoE, the most common allergens identified were cow's milk (85%), egg (35%), wheat (33%), and soy (19%) (73). After 8 weeks on the 4FED, 64% of children had histologic remission. Allowing nuts and fish in the diet increases adherence but with a decrease in disease remission. Elimination of just two foods (cow's milk and wheat) has lower efficacy but has the advantage of patients having more dietary choices (74). This approach is termed the step-up approach.

Targeted elimination is guided by extensive allergy testing to various foods and eliminating foods to which the patient is most reactive. Skin prick testing alone or in combination with atopic patch testing are utilized for choosing the diets to be eliminated. Atopic patch testing lacks validity and is not standardized in EoE (22). The targeted food elimination diet has a response rate of less than 50% (71). Patients may have difficulty adhering to the dietary modifications or have poor response to it. Patients should be thoroughly informed about the pros and cons of different treatment modalities, and management by a multidisciplinary team (gastroenterologist, allergist, dietitian) is preferred. Working with a dietitian is critical to educate families in understanding elimination diets, preventing cross-contamination of food, and preventing or treating nutritional deficiencies.

Esophageal dilation helps to treat esophageal narrowing. Esophageal strictures and narrow caliber esophagus are most often seen in late adolescents and adults. Esophageal dilation in EoE patients is relatively safe with <1% risk of perforation (75). Esophageal dilations do not treat inflammation related to EoE. Serial dilations are usually necessary to alleviate symptoms of esophageal narrowing.

Dupilumab (a fully human monoclonal antibody, blocks interleukin-4 and interleukin-13 signaling) has been shown to be very effective in the management of EoE and currently approved for adults and children ≥ 12 years of age (76). Other monoclonal antibodies targeting the T_H2 inflammatory cascade have been evaluated in the treatment of EoE (77–80). Even though these biologics improved histologic findings of EoE, they failed to show substantial clinical improvement.

13.3.4 OTHER EOSINOPHILIC GASTROINTESTINAL DISEASES

The true incidence of EGID is unknown (81). In one study, the estimated prevalence of eosinophilic gastritis, eosinophilic gastroenteritis, and eosinophilic colitis were 6.3, 8.4, and 3.3 per 100,000, respectively (82). Eosinophilic gastroenteritis was more prevalent in children <5 years, eosinophilic gastritis was more prevalent in older population, and no specific age groups were noted in eosinophilic colitis. The etiopathogenesis of EGID is not precisely known, but affected patients have a significant history of food allergy and other atopic conditions suggesting a possible allergic response to ingested foods (82, 83).

EGID can also involve different layers of the GI tract and presenting symptoms vary based on the involved layer (81). Symptoms with mucosal involvement may include nausea, recurrent emesis, abdominal pain, diarrhea, hematochezia, and weight loss (81, 84, 85). Severe mucosal involvement may lead to protein-losing enteropathy, resulting in malnutrition. Muscular involvement may cause obstruction (e.g., gastric outlet obstruction if antrum or pylorus is involved). Serosal and subserosal involvement may result in ascites. Patients may have peripheral eosinophilia and elevated IgE. Endoscopic testing with demonstration of eosinophilic infiltration on biopsy is the gold standard for diagnosis. Oral corticosteroids are the mainstay of therapy. The goal of corticosteroid therapy is to control severe GI symptoms, followed by a quick taper to low-dose maintenance therapy. There are limited data on the use of dietary therapy in these disorders. In one study among children with eosinophilic gastritis, dietary restriction resulted in 82% clinical response and 78% histological response (86). However, similar studies in both adult and pediatric patients with eosinophilic gastroenteritis did not show significant improvement with dietary modifications (87, 88). Other treatment options in EGID with limited efficacy include mast cell stabilizers, leukotriene antagonists, anti-IL-5 antibodies, and anti-IgE antibodies (81, 85).

13.4 NOVEL APPROACHES

Endoluminal functional luminal imaging (EndoFLIP®) is a minimally invasive medical device that helps measure the distensibility (stiffness) of the esophagus and is useful in diagnosing early fibrostenotic complications of EoE (89). Newer topical corticosteroid formulations, such as premixed oral budesonide suspension or oral dispersible budesonide or fluticasone tablets, are being investigated, aimed at enhanced and reliable drug delivery (90, 91). Many newer biologics targeting IL-13, IL-4, and IL-5 are being investigated for their efficacy and safety in EGIDs (92). Sialic acid-binding immunoglobulin-like lectin 8 (Siglec-8) is a surface receptor found in eosinophils and mast cells; and antolimab, a monoclonal antibody against Siglec-8, selectively binds to this receptor and induces apoptosis (93). This mechanism of action is being explored for its therapeutic efficacy in both EoE and other EGIDs (93, 94).

13.5   INCORRECT/OUTDATED PRACTICES

Until recently, patients with esophageal eosinophilia who had a favorable response to PPIs were considered to have PPI-responsive esophageal eosinophilia and prior guidelines recommended an 8-week trial with PPIs to diagnose this condition. However, current evidence shows that PPI-responsive esophageal eosinophilia has all manifestations similar to EoE and is essentially indistinguishable from EoE. Hence, response to PPIs is no longer a criterion to diagnose or rule out EoE. Alternatively, PPI is now considered a treatment for EoE. Use of systemic corticosteroids in EoE is not recommended and has significant side effects. Omalizumab (anti-IgE) and infliximab (anti-TNF-α) were noted to be ineffective for EoE (92, 95, 96). Similarly, sodium cromoglycate and antihistamines have no role in the management of EoE (53).

PRACTICE PEARLS

- Because EoE is a patchy disease, multiple biopsies (2–4) from both proximal and distal parts of the esophagus are recommended for diagnosis.
- Efforts should be made to rule out other causes of esophageal eosinophilia before a diagnosis of EoE is made.
- PPI should not be used to diagnose PPI-responsive esophageal eosinophilia or exclude EoE but rather used as first-line treatment for EoE.
- Patients who do not respond to PPI should be offered topical corticosteroids or dietary therapy (elimination diets vs. elemental diet).
- Systemic steroids are not recommended in the treatment of EoE.
- A multidisciplinary team with expertise in EoE involving a gastroenterologist, an allergist, and a dietitian is necessary to provide a holistic care for patients with EoE.

REFERENCES

1. Davis CM, Kelso JM. Food allergy management. Immunol Allergy Clin North Am. 2018;38(1):53–64.
2. Yu W, Freeland DMH, Nadeau KC. Food allergy: Immune mechanisms, diagnosis and immunotherapy. Nat Rev Immunol. 2016;16(12):751–65.
3. D'Auria E, Abrahams M, Zuccotti GV, Venter C. Personalized nutrition approach in food allergy: Is it prime time yet? Nutrients. 2019;11(2).
4. Muraro A, Werfel T, Hoffmann-Sommergruber K, Roberts G, Beyer K, Bindslev-Jensen C, et al. EAACI food allergy and anaphylaxis guidelines: Diagnosis and management of food allergy. Allergy. 2014;69(8):1008–25.
5. Bingemann TA, Sood P, Jarvinen KM. Food protein-induced enterocolitis syndrome. Immunol Allergy Clin North Am. 2018;38(1):141–52.

6. Tan JA, Smith WB. Non-IgE-mediated gastrointestinal food hypersensitivity syndrome in adults. J Allergy Clin Immunol Pract. 2014;2(3):355–7 e1.
7. Mehr S, Frith K, Barnes EH, Campbell DE, Allen K, Barnes E, et al. Food protein-induced enterocolitis syndrome in Australia: A population-based study, 2012–2014. J Allergy Clin Immunol. 2017;140(5):1323–30.
8. Kuan-Wen S, Martin V, Seay HL, Shreffler WG, Yuan Q. Incidence and clinical presentation of food protein-induced enterocolitis syndrome in a prospective healthy infant cohort. J Allergy Clin Immunol. 2019;143(2):AB157.
9. Caubet JC, Ford LS, Sickles L, Jarvinen KM, Sicherer SH, Sampson HA, et al. Clinical features and resolution of food protein-induced enterocolitis syndrome: 10-year experience. J Allergy Clin Immunol. 2014;134(2):382–9.
10. Goswami R, Blazquez AB, Kosoy R, Rahman A, Nowak-Wegrzyn A, Berin MC. Systemic innate immune activation in food protein-induced enterocolitis syndrome. J Allergy Clin Immunol. 2017;139(6):1885–96 e9.
11. Nowak-Wegrzyn A, Chehade M, Groetch ME, Spergel JM, Wood RA, Allen K, et al. International consensus guidelines for the diagnosis and management of food protein-induced enterocolitis syndrome: Executive summary—workgroup report of the adverse reactions to foods committee, American Academy of Allergy, Asthma & Immunology. J Allergy Clin Immunol. 2017;139(4):1111–26 e4.
12. Elizur A, Cohen M, Goldberg MR, Rajuan N, Cohen A, Leshno M, et al. Cow's milk associated rectal bleeding: A population based prospective study. Pediatr Allergy Immunol. 2012;23(8):765–9.
13. Nowak-Węgrzyn A, editor. Food protein-induced enterocolitis syndrome and allergic proctocolitis. Allergy and asthma proceedings: OceanSide Publications, 2015.
14. Panel NI-SE, Boyce JA, Assa'ad A, Burks AW, Jones SM, Sampson HA, et al. Guidelines for the diagnosis and management of food allergy in the United States: report of the NIAID-sponsored expert panel. J Allergy Clin Immunol. 2010;126(6 Suppl):S1–58.
15. Chafen JJS, Newberry S, Riedl M, Bravata DM, Maglione MA, Booth M, et al. Prevalence, natural history, diagnosis, and treatment of food allergy: A systematic review of the evidence: Santa Monica, CA: RAND Corporation, WR-757-1, 2010.
16. Nowak-Węgrzyn A, Katz Y, Mehr SS, Koletzko S. Non – IgE-mediated gastrointestinal food allergy. J Allergy Clin Immunol. 2015;135(5):1114–24.
17. Greenhawt M. The role of food allergy in atopic dermatitis. Allergy Asthma Proc. 2010;31(5):392–7.
18. Bergmann MM, Caubet J-C, Boguniewicz M, Eigenmann PA. Evaluation of food allergy in patients with atopic dermatitis. J Allergy Clin Immunol Pract. 2013;1(1):22–8.
19. Hill DA, Spergel JM. The atopic march: Critical evidence and clinical relevance. Ann Allergy Asthma Immunol. 2018;120(2):131–7.
20. Wood RA, Sicherer SH, Vickery BP, Jones SM, Liu AH, Fleischer DM, et al. The natural history of milk allergy in an observational cohort. J Allergy Clin Immunol. 2013;131(3):805–12.
21. Rosen R, Vandenplas Y, Singendonk M, Cabana M, DiLorenzo C, Gottrand F, et al. Pediatric gastroesophageal reflux clinical practice guidelines: Joint recommendations of the North American Society for Pediatric Gastroenterology, Hepatology, and Nutrition and the European Society for Pediatric Gastroenterology, Hepatology, and Nutrition. J Pediatr Gastroenterol Nutr. 2018;66(3):516–54.
22. Liacouras CA, Furuta GT, Hirano I, Atkins D, Attwood SE, Bonis PA, et al. Eosinophilic esophagitis: updated consensus recommendations for children and adults. J Allergy Clin Immunol. 2011;128(1):3–20 e6; quiz 1–2.
23. Dellon ES, Liacouras CA, Molina-Infante J, Furuta GT, Spergel JM, Zevit N, et al. Updated international consensus diagnostic criteria for eosinophilic esophagitis: Proceedings of the AGREE conference. Gastroenterol. 2018;155(4):1022–33. E10.

24. Furuta GT, Liacouras CA, Collins MH, Gupta SK, Justinich C, Putnam PE, et al. Eosin-ophilic esophagitis in children and adults: A systematic review and consensus recom-mendations for diagnosis and treatment. Gastroenterol. 2007;133(4):1342–63.

25. Dellon ES. Epidemiology of eosinophilic esophagitis. Gastroenterol Clin North Am. 2014;43(2):201–18.

26. Arias A, Perez-Martinez I, Tenias JM, Lucendo AJ. Systematic review with meta-analy-sis: The incidence and prevalence of eosinophilic oesophagitis in children and adults in population-based studies. Aliment Pharmacol Ther. 2016;43(1):3–15.

27. Dellon ES, Jensen ET, Martin CF, Shaheen NJ, Kappelman MD. Prevalence of eosino-philic esophagitis in the United States. Clin Gastroenterol Hepatol. 2014;12(4):589–96 e1.

28. Liacouras CA, Spergel JM, Ruchelli E, Verma R, Mascarenhas M, Semeao E, et al. Eosinophilic esophagitis: A 10-year experience in 381 children. Clin Gastroenterol Hepatol. 2005;3(12):1198–206.

29. Mishra A, Hogan SP, Lee JJ, Foster PS, Rothenberg ME. Fundamental signals that regu-late eosinophil homing to the gastrointestinal tract. J Clin Invest. 1999;103(12):1719–27.

30. Hogan SP, Mishra A, Brandt EB, Foster PS, Rothenberg ME. A critical role for eotaxin in experimental oral antigen-induced eosinophilic gastrointestinal allergy. Proc Natl Acad Sci U S A. 2000;97(12):6681–6.

31. Wolf WA, Jerath MR, Dellon ES. De-novo onset of eosinophilic esophagitis after large volume allergen exposures. J Gastrointestin Liver Dis. 2013;22(2):205–8.

32. Fahey L, Robinson G, Weinberger K, Giambrone AE, Solomon AB. Correlation between aeroallergen levels and new diagnosis of eosinophilic esophagitis in New York City. J Pediatr Gastroenterol Nutr. 2017;64(1):22–5.

33. Hurrell JM, Genta RM, Dellon ES. Prevalence of esophageal eosinophilia varies by cli-mate zone in the United States. Am J Gastroenterol. 2012;107(5):698–706.

34. Jensen ET, Hoffman K, Shaheen NJ, Genta RM, Dellon ES. Esophageal eosinophilia is increased in rural areas with low population density: Results from a national pathology database. Am J Gastroenterol. 2014;109(5):668–75.

35. Elitsur Y, Aswani R, Lund V, Dementieva Y. Seasonal distribution and eosinophilic eso-phagitis: The experience in children living in rural communities. J Clin Gastroenterol. 2013;47(3):287–8.

36. Prasad GA, Alexander JA, Schleck CD, Zinsmeister AR, Smyrk TC, Elias RM, et al. Epidemiology of eosinophilic esophagitis over three decades in Olmsted county, Minne-sota. Clin Gastroenterol Hepatol. 2009;7(10):1055–61.

37. Almansa C, Krishna M, Buchner AM, Ghabril MS, Talley N, DeVault KR, et al. Sea-sonal distribution in newly diagnosed cases of eosinophilic esophagitis in adults. Am J Gastroenterol. 2009;104(4):828–33.

38. Erwin EA, Tripathi A, Ogbogu PU, Commins SP, Slack MA, Cho CB, et al. IgE antibody detection and component analysis in patients with eosinophilic esophagitis. J Allergy Clin Immunol Pract. 2015;3(6):896–904 e3.

39. Clayton F, Fang JC, Gleich GJ, Lucendo AJ, Olalla JM, Vinson LA, et al. Eosinophilic esophagitis in adults is associated with IgG4 and not mediated by IgE. Gastroenterol. 2014;147(3):602–9.

40. Wright BL, Kulis M, Guo R, Orgel KA, Wolf WA, Burks AW, et al. Food-specific IgG4 is associated with eosinophilic esophagitis. J Allergy Clin Immunol. 2016;138(4):1190–2 e3.

41. Radano MC, Yuan Q, Katz A, Fleming JT, Kubala S, Shreffler W, et al. Cesarean section and antibiotic use found to be associated with eosinophilic esophagitis. J Allergy Clin Immunol Pract. 2014;2(4):475–7 e1.

42. Jensen ET, Kappelman MD, Kim HP, Ringel-Kulka T, Dellon ES. Early life expo-sures as risk factors for pediatric eosinophilic esophagitis. J Pediatr Gastroenterol Nutr. 2013;57(1):67–71.

43. Jensen ET, Kuhl JT, Martin LJ, Rothenberg ME, Dellon ES. Prenatal, intrapartum, and postnatal factors are associated with pediatric eosinophilic esophagitis. J Allergy Clin Immunol. 2018;141(1):214–22.

44. Assa'ad AH, Putnam PE, Collins MH, Akers RM, Jameson SC, Kirby CL, et al. Pediatric patients with eosinophilic esophagitis: An 8-year follow-up. J Allergy Clin Immunol. 2007;119(3):731–8.

45. Simon D, Marti H, Heer P, Simon HU, Braathen LR, Straumann A. Eosinophilic esophagitis is frequently associated with IgE-mediated allergic airway diseases. J Allergy Clin Immunol. 2005;115(5):1090–2.

46. Assa'ad A. Eosinophilic esophagitis: Association with allergic disorders. Gastrointest Endosc Clin N Am. 2008;18(1):119–32; x.

47. Dellon ES, Liacouras CA. Advances in clinical management of eosinophilic esophagitis. Gastroenterol. 2014;147(6):1238–54.

48. Munoz-Persy M, Lucendo AJ. Treatment of eosinophilic esophagitis in the pediatric patient: An evidence-based approach. Eur J Pediatr. 2018;177(5):649–63.

49. Kim HP, Vance RB, Shaheen NJ, Dellon ES. The prevalence and diagnostic utility of endoscopic features of eosinophilic esophagitis: A meta-analysis. Clin Gastroenterol Hepatol. 2012;10(9):988–96 e5.

50. Nielsen JA, Lager DJ, Lewin M, Rendon G, Roberts CA. The optimal number of biopsy fragments to establish a morphologic diagnosis of eosinophilic esophagitis. Am J Gastroenterol. 2014;109(4):515–20.

51. Gonsalves N, Policarpio-Nicolas M, Zhang Q, Rao MS, Hirano I. Histopathologic variability and endoscopic correlates in adults with eosinophilic esophagitis. Gastrointest Endosc. 2006;64(3):313–19.

52. Dellon ES, Gonsalves N, Hirano I, Furuta GT, Liacouras CA, Katzka DA. ACG clinical guideline: Evidenced based approach to the diagnosis and management of esophageal eosinophilia and eosinophilic esophagitis (EoE). Am J Gastroenterol. 2013;108(5):679–92.

53. Lucendo AJ, Molina-Infante J, Arias Á, von Arnim U, Bredenoord AJ, Bussmann C, et al. Guidelines on eosinophilic esophagitis: Evidence-based statements and recommendations for diagnosis and management in children and adults. United Eu Gastroenterol J. 2017;5(3):335–58.

54. Spechler SJ, Genta RM, Souza RF. Thoughts on the complex relationship between gastroesophageal reflux disease and eosinophilic esophagitis. Am J Gastroenterol. 2007;102(6):1301–6.

55. Kia L, Hirano I. Distinguishing GERD from eosinophilic oesophagitis: Concepts and controversies. Nat Rev Gastroenterol Hepatol. 2015;12(7):379.

56. Dellon ES, Speck O, Woodward K, Covey S, Rusin S, Shaheen NJ, et al. Distribution and variability of esophageal eosinophilia in patients undergoing upper endoscopy. Mod Pathol. 2015;28(3):383–90.

57. Dellon ES, Gibbs WB, Fritchie KJ, Rubinas TC, Wilson LA, Woosley JT, et al. Clinical, endoscopic, and histologic findings distinguish eosinophilic esophagitis from gastroesophageal reflux disease. Clin Gastroenterol Hepatol. 2009;7(12):1305–13.

58. Binkovitz LA, Lorenz EA, Di Lorenzo C, Kahwash S. Pediatric eosinophilic esophagitis: Radiologic findings with pathologic correlation. Pediatr Radiol. 2010;40(5):714–19.

59. Menard-Katcher C, Swerdlow MP, Mehta P, Furuta GT, Fenton LZ. Contribution of esophagrám to the evaluation of complicated pediatric eosinophilic esophagitis. J Pediatr Gastroenterol Nutr. 2015;61(5):541–6.

60. Gentile N, Katzka D, Ravi K, Trenkner S, Enders F, Killian J, et al. Oesophageal narrowing is common and frequently under-appreciated at endoscopy in patients with oesophageal eosinophilia. Aliment Pharmacol Ther. 2014;40(11–12):1333–40.

61. Hines BT, Rank MA, Wright BL, Marks LA, Hagan JB, Straumann A, et al. Minimally invasive biomarker studies in eosinophilic esophagitis: A systematic review. Ann Allergy Asthma Immunol. 2018;121(2):218–28.

62. Laserna-Mendieta EJ, Casabona S, Savarino E, Perello A, Perez-Martinez I, Guagnozzi D, et al. Efficacy of therapy for eosinophilic esophagitis in real-world practice. Clin Gastroenterol Hepatol. 2020;18(13):2903–2911.e4.

63. Molina-Infante J, Bredenoord AJ, Cheng E, Dellon ES, Furuta GT, Gupta SK, et al. Proton pump inhibitor-responsive oesophageal eosinophilia: An entity challenging current diagnostic criteria for eosinophilic oesophagitis. Gut. 2016;65(3):524–31.

64. Dellon ES, Liacouras CA, Molina-Infante J, Furuta GT, Spergel JM, Zevit N, et al. Updated international consensus diagnostic criteria for eosinophilic esophagitis: Proceedings of the AGREE conference. Gastroenterol. 2018;155(4):1022–33 e10.

65. Lucendo AJ, Arias A, Molina-Infante J. Efficacy of proton pump inhibitor drugs for inducing clinical and histologic remission in patients with symptomatic esophageal eosinophilia: A systematic review and meta-analysis. Clin Gastroenterol Hepatol. 2016;14(1):13–22 e1.

66. Chuang MY, Chinnaratha MA, Hancock DG, Woodman R, Wong GR, Cock C, et al. Topical steroid therapy for the treatment of eosinophilic esophagitis (EoE): A systematic review and meta-analysis. Clin Transl Gastroenterol. 2015;6:e82.

67. Schaefer ET, Fitzgerald JF, Molleston JP, Croffie JM, Pfefferkorn MD, Corkins MR, et al. Comparison of oral prednisone and topical fluticasone in the treatment of eosinophilic esophagitis: A randomized trial in children. Clin Gastroenterol Hepatol. 2008;6(2):165–73.

68. Dellon ES, Woosley JT, Arrington A, McGee SJ, Covington J, Moist SE, et al. Efficacy of budesonide vs fluticasone for initial treatment of eosinophilic esophagitis in a randomized controlled trial. Gastroenterol. 2019;157(1):65–73 e5.

69. Philpott H, Dougherty MK, Reed CC, Caldwell M, Kirk D, Torpy DJ, et al. Systematic review: Adrenal insufficiency secondary to swallowed topical corticosteroids in eosinophilic oesophagitis. Aliment Pharmacol Ther. 2018;47(8):1071–8.

70. Kumar S, Choi SS, Gupta SK. Eosinophilic esophagitis: Current status and future directions. Pediatr Res. 2020;88(3):345–347.

71. Arias A, Gonzalez-Cervera J, Tenias JM, Lucendo AJ. Efficacy of dietary interventions for inducing histologic remission in patients with eosinophilic esophagitis: A systematic review and meta-analysis. Gastroenterol. 2014;146(7):1639–48.

72. Kagalwalla AF, Sentongo TA, Ritz S, Hess T, Nelson SP, Emerick KM, et al. Effect of six-food elimination diet on clinical and histologic outcomes in eosinophilic esophagitis. Clin Gastroenterol Hepatol. 2006;4(9):1097–102.

73. Kagalwalla AF, Wechsler JB, Amsden K, Schwartz S, Makhija M, Olive A, et al. Efficacy of a 4-food elimination diet for children with eosinophilic esophagitis. Clin Gastroenterol Hepatol. 2017;15(11):1698–707 e7.

74. Molina-Infante J, Arias Á, Alcedo J, Garcia-Romero R, Casabona-Frances S, Prieto-Garcia A, et al. Step-up empiric elimination diet for pediatric and adult eosinophilic esophagitis: The 2–4–6 study. J Allergy Clin Immunol. 2018;141(4):1365–72.

75. Moawad F, Cheatham J, DeZee K. Meta-analysis: The safety and efficacy of dilation in eosinophilic oesophagitis. Aliment Pharmacol Ther. 2013;38(7):713–20.

76. Dellon ES, Rothenberg ME, Collins MH, Hirano I, Chehade M, Bredenoord AJ, Lucendo AJ, Spergel JM, Aceves S, Sun X, Kosloski MP, Kamal MA, Hamilton JD, Beazley B, McCann E, Patel K, Mannent LP, Laws E, Akinlade B, Amin N, Lim WK, Wipperman MF, Ruddy M, Patel N, Weinreich DR, Yancopoulos GD, Shumel B, Maloney J, Giannelou A, Shabbir A. Dupilumab in Adults and Adolescents with Eosinophilic Esophagitis. N Engl J Med. 2022;387(25):2317–2330. doi: 10.1056/NEJMoa2205982. PMID: 36546624.

77. Spergel JM, Rothenberg ME, Collins MH, Furuta GT, Markowitz JE, Fuchs G, 3rd, et al. Reslizumab in children and adolescents with eosinophilic esophagitis: Results of a double-blind, randomized, placebo-controlled trial. J Allergy Clin Immunol. 2012;129(2):456–63, 63 e1–3.

78. Straumann A, Conus S, Grzonka P, Kita H, Kephart G, Bussmann C, et al. Anti-inter-leukin-5 antibody treatment (mepolizumab) in active eosinophilic oesophagitis: A ran-domised, placebo-controlled, double-blind trial. Gut. 2010;59(01):21–30.

79. Assa'ad AH, Gupta SK, Collins MH, Thomson M, Heath AT, Smith DA, et al. An anti-body against IL-5 reduces numbers of esophageal intraepithelial eosinophils in children with eosinophilic esophagitis. Gastroenterology. 2011;141(5):1593–604.

80. Rothenberg ME, Wen T, Greenberg A, Alpan O, Enav B, Hirano I, et al. Intravenous anti – IL-13 mAb QAX576 for the treatment of eosinophilic esophagitis. J Allergy Clin Immunol. 2015;135(2):500–7.

81. Licari A, Votto M, D'Auria E, Castagnoli R, Caimmi SME, Marseglia GL. Eosin-ophilic gastrointestinal diseases in children: A practical review. Curr Pediatr Rev. 2020;16(2):106–14.

82. Jensen ET, Martin CF, Kappelman MD, Dellon ES. Prevalence of eosinophilic gastritis, gastroenteritis, and colitis: Estimates from a national administrative database. J Pediatr Gastroenterol Nutr. 2016;62(1):36–42.

83. Bischoff SC. Food allergy and eosinophilic gastroenteritis and colitis. Curr Opin Allergy Clin Immunol. 2010;10(3):238–45.

84. Ingle SB, Hinge Ingle CR. Eosinophilic gastroenteritis: An unusual type of gastroenteri-tis. World J Gastroenterol. 2013;19(31):5061–6.

85. Uppal V, Kreiger P, Kutsch E. Eosinophilic gastroenteritis and colitis: A comprehensive review. Clin Rev Allergy Immunol. 2016;50(2):175–88.

86. Ko HM, Morotti RA, Yershov O, Chehade M. Eosinophilic gastritis in children: Clinico-pathological correlation, disease course, and response to therapy. Am J Gastroenterol. 2014;109(8):1277–85.

87. Grandinetti T, Biedermann L, Bussmann C, Straumann A, Hruz P. Eosinophilic gastro-enteritis: Clinical manifestation, natural course, and evaluation of treatment with corti-costeroids and vedolizumab. Dig Dis Sci. 2019;64(8):2231–41.

88. Reed C, Woosley JT, Dellon ES. Clinical characteristics, treatment outcomes, and resource utilization in children and adults with eosinophilic gastroenteritis. Dig Liver Dis. 2015;47(3):197–201.

89. Menard-Katcher C, Benitez AJ, Pan Z, Ahmed FN, Wilkins BJ, Capocelli KE, et al. Influence of age and eosinophilic esophagitis on esophageal distensibility in a pediatric cohort. Am J Gastroenterol. 2017;112(9):1466.

90. Comer GM, Bush MA, Dellon ES, Marino MT. Effect of food intake and body position on the pharmacokinetics of swallowed APT-1011, a fluticasone orally disintegrating tab-let, in healthy adult volunteers. J Clin Pharmacol. 2020;60(6):734–43.

91. Lucendo AJ, Miehlke S, Schlag C, Vieth M, von Arnim U, Molina-Infante J, et al. Effi-cacy of budesonide orodispersible tablets as induction therapy for eosinophilic esophagi-tis in a randomized placebo-controlled trial. Gastroenterol. 2019;157(1):74–86. E15.

92. Choudhury S, Baker S. Eosinophilic esophagitis: The potential role of biologics in its treatment. Clin Rev Allergy Immunol. 2019:1–10.

93. Beveridge C, Falk GW. Novel therapeutic approaches to eosinophilic esophagitis. Gas-troenterol Hepatol. 2020;16(6):295.

94. Dellon E, Peterson K, Murray J. Efficacy and safety of AK002 in adult patients with active eosinophilic gastritis and/or eosinophilic gastroenteritis: Primary results from a randomized, double-blind, placebo-controlled phase 2 trial (ENIGMA study). Am J Gastroenterol. 2019;114:S36.

95. Rocha R, Vitor AB, Trindade E, Lima R, Tavares M, Lopes J, et al. Omalizumab in the treatment of eosinophilic esophagitis and food allergy. Eur J Pediatr. 2011;170(11):1471.

96. Straumann A, Bussmann C, Conus S, Beglinger C, Simon H-U. Anti-TNF-[alpha] (infliximab) therapy for severe adult eosinophilic esophagitis. J Allergy Clin Immunol. 2008;122(2):425.

14 Nonalcoholic Fatty Liver Disease

Arunkumar Krishnan and Tinsay Woreta

14.1 INTRODUCTION

Nonalcoholic fatty liver disease (NAFLD) is the most common cause of liver disease worldwide. It affects approximately 25%–30% of the adult population worldwide and one-third of the population in the United States (1). It is present in 15% of non-obese patients (body mass index [BMI] <30), 65% of obese patients (BMI 30–39), and 85% of extremely obese patients (BMI ≥40)(2). It ranges from isolated excessive accumulation of triglyceride in hepatocytes (nonalcoholic fatty liver [NAFL]) to hepatic triglyceride accumulation associated with inflammation and hepatocyte injury (nonalcoholic steatohepatitis [NASH]), which can lead to hepatic fibrosis and cirrhosis (Figure 14.1) (3). It is a growing cause of the end-stage liver disease (ESLD) globally and is recognized as an etiology of hepatocellular cancer (HCC), even in the absence of underlying cirrhosis (4). Besides the strong correlation for liver-related morbidity and mortality, NAFLD is also associated with an increased risk for cardiovascular disease and solid neoplasms (2, 5). NAFLD is a multifactorial, complex disease with multiple factors, including genetics, dietary habits, and physical activity, interacting to form the NAFLD phenotype (6). In addition, nutrition and diet play important roles in the gut microbiome that may contribute to the development and progression of NAFLD (7). At present, there is no approved pharmacological or surgical therapy for the management of NAFLD. The current therapeutic approaches focus on lifestyle modification with dietary intervention and regular cardiovascular exercise to achieve weight loss. Studies have shown that a healthy diet and weight loss in the early stages of NAFLD could be sufficient to prevent disease progression (8).

14.2 IMPACT OF NUTRIENTS ON THE DEVELOPMENT OF NAFLD

The mechanisms in NAFLD development and progression are complex, since many factors contribute to fat deposition within the liver. The "multiple hit" hypothesis suggests a complex interaction among genetic, epigenetic, and environmental (mostly unhealthy dietary patterns and unbalanced nutrient) factors, resulting in dysregulated lipid metabolism and excessive intrahepatic lipid deposition. Many factors, including insulin resistance, lipotoxicity, adipocytokines, and disruption in the intestinal microbiota, can act in parallel or synergistically in a genetically susceptible host and lead to the development of NAFLD (9).

DOI: 10.1201/9780429322570-14

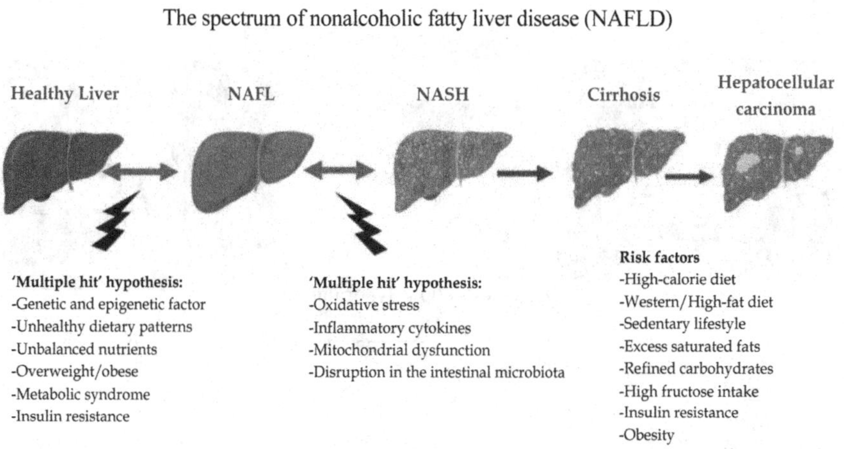

The spectrum of nonalcoholic fatty liver disease (NAFLD)

'Multiple hit' hypothesis:
-Genetic and epigenetic factor
-Unhealthy dietary patterns
-Unbalanced nutrients
-Overweight/obese
-Metabolic syndrome
-Insulin resistance

'Multiple hit' hypothesis:
-Oxidative stress
-Inflammatory cytokines
-Mitochondrial dysfunction
-Disruption in the intestinal microbiota

Risk factors
-High-calorie diet
-Western/High-fat diet
-Sedentary lifestyle
-Excess saturated fats
-Refined carbohydrates
-High fructose intake
-Insulin resistance
-Obesity

FIGURE 14.1 The spectrum of nonalcoholic fatty liver disease (NAFLD): NAFLD includes a spectrum of disease severity ranging from nonalcoholic fatty liver (NAFL; simple steatosis without evidence of hepatocellular injury) to nonalcoholic steatohepatitis (NASH; hepatic steatosis and inflammation with hepatocyte injury [ballooning] with or without fibrosis). NASH may further progress to advanced fibrosis and cirrhosis, which is the strongest independent risk factor for the development of hepatocellular carcinoma (HCC).

14.3 INFLUENCE OF MACRONUTRIENTS ON NAFLD

Excessive consumption of calories leading to obesity and its related comorbidities is a leading risk factor for NAFLD (8). Interestingly, the distribution of macronutrient composition also affects liver fat accumulation. Hepatic steatosis is associated with a constellation of adverse alterations in glucose, fatty acid, and lipoprotein metabolism. Abnormalities in fatty acid metabolism, in conjunction with adipose tissue, hepatic, and systemic inflammation, are critical factors involved in developing dyslipidemia, insulin resistance, and other cardiometabolic risk factors associated with NAFLD (10). Diets high in fructose, saturated fats, and cholesterol, and lower in polyunsaturated fatty acids (PUFAs) and fiber, are associated with the development of NAFLD (Figure 14.2) (11). These are often linked to lifestyle risk factors, such as excessive caloric intake and reduced physical activity.

14.3.1 DIETARY CARBOHYDRATES

High carbohydrate consumption contributes to insulin resistance and hepatic steatosis by activating the carbohydrate response element-binding protein (ChREBP). Postprandial hyperglycemia raises hepatic concentrations of phosphorylated intermediates, causing activation of ChREBP and induction of its target genes (12). Both enzymes of lipogenesis and glycolysis pathways and glucose 6-phosphatase are involved, which may result in insulin resistance. High carbohydrate intake leads

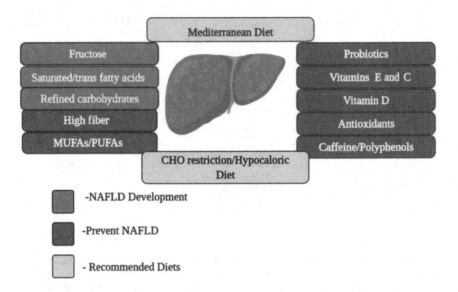

FIGURE 14.2 Contribution of macro- and micronutrients to NAFLD pathogenesis. Depiction of nutritional elements involved in the prevention or development of NAFLD and NAFLD-related metabolic complications. MUFAs: monounsaturated fatty acids; PUFAs; polyunsaturated fatty acids; CHO: carbohydrates.

to increased circulating insulin concentrations, which contribute to elevated fasting triglyceride concentrations even under isocaloric conditions (13). In addition, carbohydrate consumption can stimulate hepatic lipogenesis by converting excess glucose to fatty acids, which, combined with a low-fat meal, promotes the development of a NAFLD through increased de novo fatty acid and triglyceride synthesis (14).

Several studies suggest that low carbohydrate diets can improve insulin resistance by reducing glycemic load and β-cell insulin secretion (15). It can also reduce serum triglycerides, insulin, and glucose; increase high-density lipoprotein (HDL); promote weight loss; decrease intrahepatic triglyceride content; and improve the metabolic parameters of patients with obesity (16). We recommend that patients with NAFLD consume a low-carbohydrate and low saturated-fat diet and increase their consumption of fruits and vegetables.

14.3.2 Fructose

A diet with high fructose content stimulates de novo lipogenesis and increases the hepatic synthesis of triglyceride (17). Moreover, high intake of fructose also inhibits leptin secretion and satiety cannot be achieved (18). Similarly, a high-fructose diet reduces peroxisome proliferator-activated receptor alpha (PPARα) activity and hepatic lipid oxidation and stimulates nuclear factor kappa-light-chain-enhancer of activated B cells (NF-κB) expression; these lead to oxidative stress, hepatic steatosis, and fibrosis (19, 20).

Fructose intake is also associated with alterations in intestinal microflora, increased gut permeability, and bacterial overgrowth in the small intestine, which increases the endotoxin levels in the portal vein and may contribute to inflammation in NASH (21, 22). Fructose additionally stimulates the production of uric acid, which may cause insulin resistance and oxidative stress. Serum uric acid has been shown to be associated with the development of NAFLD and a positive dose-response association with a raised serum alanine aminotransferase (ALT) irrespective of BMI (23, 24).

14.3.3 Dietary Protein

The role of protein intake in the development and treatment of NAFLD is still unclear. However, an increment in dietary protein content has been shown to reduce the risk of hepatic steatosis during a high-fat diet both in rodents and humans (25, 26), whereas protein malnutrition leads to steatosis (27). A high-protein diet has favorable effects on treating NAFLD by increasing hepatic lipid oxidation (23). Recent evidence shows that a low-calorie high-protein diet leads to improvement of glucose homeostasis, lipid profile, and liver enzymes in patients with NAFLD (26).

14.3.4 Dietary Fats

Western diets and increased intake of saturated fat have been linked to impaired postprandial lipid metabolism and insulin resistance. Western diets contain more saturated fatty acids (SFAs), trans-fatty acids, and vegetable oil rich in omega-6 (n-6) PUFA and less omega-3 (n-3) PUFA (28). The proatherogenic effect of trans-fatty acids is in part attributed to increased triglyceride, low-density lipoprotein (LDL), cholesterol, and lipoprotein, and reduced plasma high-density lipoprotein (HDL) (27). However, little is known about the influence of trans-fatty acids on hepatic lipid metabolism. Nevertheless, studies have shown that an increased intake of trans- and saturated fatty acids and also a high ratio of n-6 to n-3 PUFAs are linked with NAFLD (29, 30). We can categorize fats into three types: saturated, mono-, and polyunsaturated fats.

14.3.4.1 Saturated Fatty Acids

Diets rich in SFA induce endoplasmic reticulum stress in the liver and contribute to the damage of hepatocytes in animal models (31). SFA intake is also correlated with impaired glutathione metabolism, which can lead to oxidative stress. They also promote apoptosis of hepatocytes, possibly leading to the progression of NAFL to NASH (32, 33). Restriction of SFA intake to <7% of total energy does not lead to any further improvements in blood lipids in patients with insulin resistance and may even be detrimental for patients. Recommended daily intake of fat should compose ≤30% of total calories (SFA >7% and <10% of total calories) for patients with NAFLD (20).

14.3.4.2 Monounsaturated Fatty Acids

Monounsaturated fatty acids (MUFAs) induce a more favorable plasma lipid profile, with reduced oxidized LDL, triglyceride, cholesterol, and a lower total cholesterol/HDL ratio. MUFA decreases the serum level of triglyceride by activation of PPARα (34). An increase in MUFA intake decreases the accumulation of triglyceride in the liver and improves postprandial triglyceride level and glucose response in patients with insulin resistance. In addition, it may offset the proinflammatory effects of SFAs and decrease insulin resistance and hepatic steatosis (37). Incorporating MUFA into the diet, especially as a replacement for SFA, may reduce the risk of metabolic syndrome and NAFLD.

14.3.4.3 Polyunsaturated Fatty Acids

A diet rich in n-3 PUFA protects against fatty liver because it prevents hepatic fat accumulation and reduces hepatic steatosis (32). PUFAs might influence NAFLD by inhibiting transcription factor sterol regulatory element-binding protein-1 (SREBP-1) and activating PPARα (23). PUFA concentrations are lower in patients with NAFLD and low levels of circulating n-3 PUFAs are associated with increased intrahepatic saturated fat content (i.e., higher de novo lipogenesis), increased hepatic uptake of circulating free fatty acids, and decreased fatty acid oxidation. The n-3 PUFAs eicosapentaenoic acid (EPA) and docosahexaenoic acid (DHA) are essential modulators of the inflammatory pathway and, therefore, may inhibit proinflammatory eicosanoid production by inflammatory cells related to hepatic injury in NAFLD (35). Supplementation with 1 g/day of n-3 PUFA could decrease hepatic fat infiltration; 2 g/day reduces triglyceride, serum fasting glucose, and hepatic enzyme levels, as well as hepatic steatosis, inflammation, and fibrosis (36).

14.3.5 Dietary Fiber

Dietary fibers help in the reduction of caloric intake by increasing satiety and contributing to intestinal regulation. Daily recommended fiber intake varies from 20–40 g/day (5–15 g/day from soluble fibers) (37). Soluble fibers slow gastric emptying and glucose and cholesterol absorption, whereas insoluble fibers modulate gut microbiota composition and activity. In patients with NAFLD, reduced fiber intake may contribute to disease progression by promoting microbiome depletion and increased gut permeability, inducing insulin resistance, inflammation, and oxidative stress (38). Clinical studies suggest that an increased intake of fiber is inversely correlated with insulin resistance, LDL, cholesterol, and hepatic lipid accumulation (39). Patients with NAFLD on high-fiber diets had lower serum aminotransferase and cholesterol levels, less hepatic steatosis, and lower NAFLD fibrosis scores (40). Dietary fibers that are derived from whole grains demonstrated the benefits of their consumption and the reduction of comorbidities associated with NAFLD and metabolic syndrome.

14.3.6 Dietary Patterns

Dietary patterns as a whole, rather than individual constituents of food, may have a significant influence on NAFLD development, since dietary patterns also take into account interactions between various nutrients. Ideally, lifestyle modifications with dietary interventions should promote the maintenance of weight loss. Given the strong relationship between dietary patterns and NAFLD, nutritional intervention is currently the backbone of patients' management strategy with NAFLD.

14.3.6.1 Mediterranean Diet

The Mediterranean diet has benefits in cardiovascular risk reduction, improvements in insulin sensitivity, and prevention of hypertension, hypercholesterolemia, and obesity (41, 42). The Mediterranean diet is characterized by a high intake of fruits, vegetables, nuts, cereals, whole grains, and olive oil, as well as moderate consumption of fish, poultry, and dairy products (mostly yogurt and cheese) and a low intake of red meat and red wine (Figure 14.3) (43).

The Mediterranean diet has compounds, such as polyphenols, vitamins, and other biomolecules, that have anti-inflammatory effects. Foods rich in polyphenols include fruits, vegetables, red wine, wild herbs, spices, nuts, and olives, especially extra virgin olive oil. Additionally, the Mediterranean diet is rich in MUFA and low in SFA, and it provides glutathione, antioxidants, and a balanced ratio of n-6/n-3 PUFA. The intake of MUFA has been demonstrated to reduce postprandial adiponectin expression and improve plasma lipid levels (44). High n-3 PUFA intake increases insulin sensitivity, reduces intrahepatic triglyceride content, and ameliorates NASH (45–47). Foods composing the Mediterranean diet, mainly rich in protein, insoluble fibers, and unsaturated fatty acids, also have significant effects on the gut microbiome and its secretion of metabolites that modulate immune function and various inflammatory

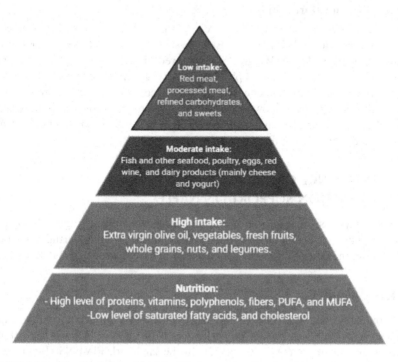

FIGURE 14.3 The food pyramid of the Mediterranean diet. MUFA: monounsaturated fatty acid; PUFA: polyunsaturated fatty acid.

and metabolic pathways (48). Although clinical studies evaluating the efficacy of the Mediterranean diet for NAFLD are still limited, joint clinical practice guidelines from the European Association for the Study of the Liver (EASL), the European Association for the Study of Diabetes (EASD), and the European Association for the Study of Obesity (EASO) recommend the Mediterranean diet as the best dietary pattern for patients with NAFLD (49). Although the Mediterranean diet advocates consumption of wine in moderation, there is no safe threshold of alcohol established for patients with NAFLD, so regular alcohol use should be avoided.

14.3.6.2   Low-Carbohydrate Diet

A low-carbohydrate diet (LCD) is defined as having <40% of the total daily energy intake provided by carbohydrates (50). LCD has gained popularity as a means of rapid weight loss and improvement in insulin resistance, along with other parameters of metabolic syndrome, potentially offering a treatment option for NAFLD. It has been shown to decrease intrahepatic triglycerides and improve metabolic parameters of patients with obesity (51). A recent meta-analysis suggests that both LCD and low/moderate fat (≤30% of daily calories) intake have similar effects on reducing liver transaminases (52). LCD, especially foods rich in fiber, can decrease glucose absorption, reducing the hepatic influx of glucose and de novo lipogenesis. Additionally, the fiber content of LCD can positively act on the gut microbiome (53, 54). However, long-term studies are required to assess liver-related outcomes in patients with NAFLD.

14.3.6.3   Hypocaloric Diet

The American Association for the Study of Liver Diseases (AASLD) guidelines suggest a hypocaloric diet and increased physical activity with weight loss to help patients with NAFLD (3). Weight loss, achieved either by hypocaloric diet alone or in combination with increased physical activity, generally reduces liver steatosis. Weight loss achieved by a hypocaloric diet also reduces hepatic inflammation and fibrosis (55). Studies have shown that 7%–10% weight loss results in improvements in NAFLD, and among patients with ≥10% weight loss, 90% had resolution of NASH and 45% had regression of fibrosis (55).

14.4   INFLUENCE OF MICRONUTRIENTS AND NUTRITION SUPPORT ON NAFLD

The liver plays a significant role in micronutrient metabolism (Figure 14.1). Thus, micronutrients have been studied as possible coadjuvant therapies during a nutritional intervention. In addition, NAFLD patients tend to have micronutrient deficiencies.

14.4.1   Vitamin E

Since oxidative stress is one of the key mechanisms of hepatocellular injury, micronutrients with antioxidant properties, such as vitamin E, have been studied in the treatment of patients with NASH. In the landmark PIVENS (Pioglitazone, Vitamin E, or Placebo for the Treatment of Nondiabetic Patients with Nonalcoholic Steatohepatitis) trial, vitamin E 800 IU/day reduced hepatic necroinflammation and facilitated resolution of NASH in non-diabetic patients with biopsy-proven NASH when compared with placebo. However, there was no improvement in fibrosis scores (56). The AASLD guidelines recommend consideration of vitamin E 800 IU/day for non-diabetic patients with biopsy-proven NASH to improve liver histology patterns; however, its use is not recommended in diabetic patients with NASH in cryptogenic or NASH-related cirrhosis, or NAFLD without a liver biopsy (3). Clinicians must discuss the risks and benefits with patients prior to initiating this therapy due to the concern of an increase in all-cause mortality and association with an increased risk of hemorrhagic stroke and prostate cancer (57).

14.4.2 PROBIOTICS

Gut dysbiosis could promote de novo hepatic lipogenesis by stimulating expression of lipogenic enzymes (58). Disruptions in this microbiome have been associated with different disorders, including metabolic diseases and obesity-related NAFLD (59). Metabolism of bile acids can be altered by microbiota and a high-fat diet, contributing to NAFLD. Gut-derived lipopolysaccharide may cross intestine tight junctions inducing liver injury through the activation of Kupffer cells, thus contributing to the onset of liver fibrosis (60). However, the specific microbes involved in the pathogenesis of NAFLD have yet to be elucidated (61). Despite the promising role of probiotics in animal models, evidence for the use of probiotics for the treatment of NAFLD in human subjects is still lacking (62).

14.4.3 CHOLINE

Choline is an essential nutrient found in animal protein and egg yolks. It is a phospholipid component of cell membranes and metabolized mainly in the liver into phosphatidylcholine and a precursor of phosphatidylcholine, a critical component of very low-density lipoprotein (VLDL). The lack of choline causes hepatocytes to be unable to secrete triglycerides in the form of VLDL and triglycerides accumulate in the hepatocytes (63). In addition, choline deficiency may induce NAFLD by inducing irregular phospholipid synthesis, lipoprotein secretion flaws, and oxidative damage due to mitochondrial dysfunction (64). Choline deficiency is significantly associated with increased fibrosis in postmenopausal women with NAFLD (65). Although associations between dietary choline and NAFLD exist, no controlled interventional studies are currently available. Further studies are needed to investigate whether there is a therapeutic benefit of choline supplementation for NAFLD.

14.4.4 VITAMIN D

In the liver, vitamin D receptors are broadly expressed and vitamin D may down-regulate the expression of the NF-κB and improve expression of PPARα. Moreover, vitamin D decreases lipolysis in adipose tissue and increases adiponectin secretion, stimulates insulin secretion, and improves the expression of GLUT-4 receptors in skeletal muscle (66). Epidemiological studies have, however, shown conflicting results on the correlation of vitamin D deficiency and NAFLD (67, 68). Short-term vitamin

D supplementation did not consistently improve dyslipidemia or NAFLD histological features (72), while longer-term supplementation was associated with reduced inflammation and lipid peroxidation (69). High-dose vitamin D did not improve insulin resistance, liver enzymes, or hepatic steatosis (70, 71). Further studies are necessary to better understand the role of vitamin D in NAFLD pathogenesis and treatment.

14.4.5   VITAMIN C

Vitamin C is a potent antioxidant that balances the effects of reactive oxygen species (ROS) in cells by scavenging free radicals (72). Vitamin C could play a beneficial role in NAFLD by acting as a free radical scavenger. In in vitro models, vitamin C can reduce the formation of ROS and increase the activity of superoxide dismutase and glutathione peroxidase (73). In NAFLD, this scavenging mechanism may protect cells from lipotoxicity-induced cellular oxidative stress. In addition, vitamin C can promote the production of adiponectin and decrease insulin resistance and inflammation (74). There are no clinical trials on the effect of vitamin C supplementation alone on NAFLD. However, the combination of vitamins C and E (1000 IU and 1000 mg, respectively) was found to reduce hepatic fibrosis in diabetic patients with NASH, however without improvement in inflammation or ALT levels (75).

14.4.6   COPPER

In the liver, copper is a co-factor for several antioxidant enzymes (76). Low levels of hepatic copper are linked with diabetes, systemic metabolic disease, and liver diseases, such as alcoholic liver disease and NAFLD, whereas low ceruloplasmin levels are associated with NAFLD in children and adults (77, 78). Copper deficiency in NAFLD patients may exacerbate lipotoxicity and oxidative stress from the upregulation of triglyceride synthesis and impairment of the mitochondria. Moreover, dietary copper deficiency and high fructose consumption synergistically worsen liver damage and accelerate hepatic steatosis, inflammation, and fibrogenesis. Fructose also acts as an inhibitor of duodenal copper absorption and thus increases the impairment of oxidant defense and lipid peroxidation (79). Similarly, a deficiency of copper is observed in patients with NAFLD and is associated with insulin resistance, steatosis, and an accelerated progression of NASH (80).

14.4.7   COFFEE

Coffee consumption has been associated with several health benefits, such as a reduction in mortality and a lower risk of cardiovascular disease, Parkinson's disease, and cancer (81). Coffee has a hepatoprotective effect; drinking coffee ≥2 cups/day is independently associated with a lower risk for NAFLD and a significant reduction in the risk of fibrosis among NASH patients (82). Fibrosis improvement is due to polyphenols in the coffee that contribute to this antifibrotic effect rather than caffeine. (83) Coffee consumption has also been demonstrated to have an inverse association with cirrhosis and hepatocellular carcinoma (84, 85).

14.5   NOVEL APPROACHES

The approach for treating patients with NAFLD is weight loss, attainable through lifestyle modification, gradual weight reduction, and increased physical activity. Unfortunately, weight loss sustainability is poor and recidivism is frequently encountered. Any form of healthful eating habits (Mediterranean diet, low-fat, or low-carbohydrate), which will lead to calorie reduction and long-term adherence, should be encouraged. The most effective form of long-term therapy for NAFLD and NASH remains diet therapy with lifestyle modification.

14.6   INCORRECT/OUTDATED PRACTICES

Abnormal levels of hepatic aminotransaminases are among the most frequent reasons for a patient to be referred to hepatology. Hepatic ALT and aspartate aminotransaminase (AST) are markers for hepatocellular injury, although ALT is more specific. However, ALT levels can be normal across the disease spectrum in up to 30% of patients. Therefore, the presence of a fatty liver in a radiological study requires further investigation and management, even in the presence of a normal ALT level. Assuming that patients with normal ALT have no chance of progression to NASH is incorrect.

Currently, no pharmacological treatment has been approved for NAFLD/NASH; that does not mean there is no treatment for patients who have NAFLD. Poor dietary composition is an important factor in the progression of NAFLD. The majority of NAFLD cases arise due to excess intake of simple carbohydrates and total SFA with reduced intake of dietary fiber and n-3 PUFA-rich foods. Lifestyle modifications, including dietary changes and exercise that ultimately lead to a weight loss of 7%–10% total body weight, remain the keystone of NAFLD management.

PRACTICE PEARLS

- Lifestyle interventions consisting of diet, exercise, and weight loss are the mainstay of treatment for patients with NAFLD.
- To manage this growing health problem, clinicians need to advise patients with NAFLD to achieve a minimum of 7%–10% weight reduction through lifestyle modifications.
- NAFLD patients, whether normal weight or obese, should be informed that a healthy diet has benefits beyond weight reduction.
- Dietary recommendations to manage NAFLD include a diet that is focused on the following principles:
  - Calorie restriction
  - Avoidance of consumption of processed food and products with added fructose

- Avoidance of consumption of refined carbohydrates, saturated and trans fats, and replacement of saturated/trans fats with MUFA or n-3 PUFA
- Consumption of low-to-moderate carbohydrate diet with adequate protein intake to regulate and prevent the overconsumption of fats and carbohydrates
- Increasing intake of dietary fibers, vegetables, and fruits rich in antioxidants, vitamins, and minerals
- Consumption of coffee which lowers the risk of metabolic syndrome and improves liver fibrosis
- Consideration of daily supplementation of vitamin E 800 IU/day, which has been shown to reduce hepatic inflammation in non-diabetic adults with biopsy-proven NASH

REFERENCES

1. Younossi ZM, et al. Global epidemiology of nonalcoholic fatty liver disease meta-analytic assessment of prevalence, incidence, and outcomes. Hepatol 2016;64:73–84.
2. Schugar RC, Crawford PA. Low-carbohydrate ketogenic diets, glucose homeostasis, and nonalcoholic fatty liver disease. Curr Opin Clin Nutr Metab Care 2012;15:374–380.
3. Chalasani N, et al. The diagnosis and management of non-alcoholic fatty liver disease: Practice guideline by the American Association for the Study of Liver Diseases, American College of Gastroenterology, and the American Gastroenterological Association. Hepatol 2012;55:2005–2023.
4. Estes C, Razavi H, Loomba R, Younossi Z, Sanyal AJ. Modeling the epidemic of non-alcoholic fatty liver disease demonstrates an exponential increase in burden of disease. Hepatol 2018;67:123–133.
5. European Association for the Study of the Liver (EASL). European Association for the Study of Diabetes (EASD) & European Association for the Study of Obesity (EASO) clinical practice guidelines for the management of non-alcoholic fatty liver disease. J Hepatol 2016;64:1388–1402.
6. Gaemers IC, Groen AK. New insights in the pathogenesis of nonalcoholic fatty liver disease. Curr Opin Lipidol 2006;17:268–273.
7. Mokhtari Z, Gibson DL, Hekmatdoost A. Nonalcoholic fatty liver disease, the gut microbiome, and diet. Adv Nutr 2017;8:240–252.
8. Perdomo CM, Frühbeck G, Escalada J. Impact of nutritional changes on nonalcoholic fatty liver disease. Nutr. 2019;11:677.
9. Buzzetti E, Pinzani M, Tsochatzis EA. The multiple-hit pathogenesis of non-alcoholic fatty liver disease (NAFLD). Metab 2016;65:1038–1048.
10. Koteish A, Diehl AM. Animal models of steatosis. Semin Liver Dis 2001;21:89–104.
11. Ouyang X, Cirillo P, Sautin Y, et al. Fructose consumption as a risk factor for nonalcoholic fatty liver disease. J Hepatol 2008;48:993–999.
12. Agius L. High-carbohydrate diets induce hepatic insulin resistance to protect the liver from substrate overload. Biochem Pharmacol 2013;85:306–312.
13. York LW, Puthalapattu S, Wu GY. Nonalcoholic fatty liver disease and low-carbohydrate diets. Annu Rev Nutr 2009;29:365–379.

14. McLaughlin T, Abbasi F, Lamendola C, Yeni-Komshian H, Reaven G. Carbohydrate-induced hypertriglyceridemia: An insight into the link between plasma insulin and triglyceride concentrations. J Clin Endocrinol Metab 2000;85:3085–3088.

15. Ebbeling CB, Swain JF, Feldman HA, Wong WW, Hachey DL, Garcia-Lago E, et al. Effects of dietary composition on energy expenditure during weight-loss maintenance. JAMA 2012;307:2627–2634.

16. Santos FL, Esteves SS, da Costa Pereira A, Yancy Jr WS, Nunes JP. Systematic review and meta-analysis of clinical trials of the effects of low carbohydrate diets on cardiovascular risk factors. Obes Rev 2012;13:1048–1066.

17. Poulsom R. Morphological changes of organs after sucrose or fructose feeding. Prog Biochem Pharmacol 1986;21:104–134.

18. Zivkovic AM, German JB, Sanyal AJ. Comparative review of diets for the metabolic syndrome: Implications for nonalcoholic fatty liver disease. Am J Clin Nutr 2007;86:285–300.

19. Roglans N, Vila L, Farre M, et al. Impairment of hepatic STAT-3 activation and reduction of PPARα activity in fructose-fed rats. Hepatol 2007;45:778–788.

20. Wei Y, Wang D, Topczewski F, et al. Fructose-mediated stress signaling in the liver: Implications for hepatic insulin resistance. J Nutr Biochem 2007;18:1–9.

21. Vos MB, McClain CJ. Fructose takes a toll. Hepatol 2009;50:1004–1006.

22. Wit NJW, Afman LA, Mensink M, Müller M. Clinical application of basic science phenotyping the effect of diet on non-alcoholic fatty liver disease. J Hepatol 2012;57:1370–1373.

23. Xu C, Yu C, Xu L, Miao M, Li Y. High serum uric acid increases the risk for nonalcoholic Fatty liver disease: A prospective observational study. PloS One 2010;5:e11578.

24. Zelber-Sagi S, Ben-Assuli O, Rabinowich L, Goldstein A, Magid A, Shalev V, et al. The association between the serum levels of uric acid and alanine aminotransferase in a population-based cohort. Liver Int 2015;59:109–116.

25. Shertzer HG, Woods SE, Krishan M, Genter MB, Pearson KJ. Dietary whey protein lowers the risk for metabolic disease in mice fed a high-fat diet. J Nutr 2011;141:582–587.

26. Schwarz J, Tome D, Baars A, Hooiveld GJ, Muller M. Dietary protein affects gene expression and prevents lipid accumulation in the liver in mice. PloS One 2012;7:ee47303.

27. Zivkovic AM, German JB, Sanyal AJ. Comparative review of diets for the metabolic syndrome: Implications for nonalcoholic fatty liver disease. Am J Clin Nutr 2007;86:285–300.

28. Bedogni G, Bellentani S. Fatty liver: How frequent is it and why? Ann Hepatol 2004;3:63–65.

29. Tanaka N, Sano K, Horiuchi A, Tanaka E, Kiyosawa K, Aoyama T. Highly purified eicosapentaenoic acid treatment improves nonalcoholic steatohepatitis. J Clin Gastroenterol 2008;42:413–418.

30. Kien CL. Dietary interventions for metabolic syndrome: Role of modifying dietary fats. Curr Diabetes Rep. 2009;9:43–50.

31. Zivkovic AM, German JB, Sanyal AJ. Comparative review of diets for the metabolic syndrome: Implications for nonalcoholic fatty liver disease. Am J Clin Nutr 2007;86:285–300.

32. Cao J, Dai DL, Yao L, Yu HH, Ning B, Zhang Q, Cheng WH, Shen W, Yang ZX. Saturated fatty acid induction of endoplasmic reticulum stress and apoptosis in human liver cells via the PERK/ATF4/CHOP signaling pathway. Mol Cell Biochem 2012;364:115–129.

33. Leamy AK, Egnatchik RA, Young JD. Molecular mechanisms and the role of saturated fatty acids in the progression of non-alcoholic fatty liver disease. Prog Lipid Res 2013;52:165–174.

34. Assy N, Nassar F, Nasser G, Grosovski M. Olive oil consumption and nonalcoholic fatty liver disease. World J Gastroenterol 2009;15:1809–1815.

35. Nobili V, Alisi A, Musso G, Scoreltti E, Calder PC, Byrne CD. Omega-3 fatty acids: Mechanisms of benefit and therapeutic effects in pediatric and adult NAFLD. Crit Rev Clin Lab Sci 2016;53:106–120.
36. Capanni M, Calella F, Biagini MR, et al. Prolonged n-3 polyunsaturated fatty acid supplementation ameliorates hepatic steatosis in patientswith non-alcoholic fatty liver disease: A pilot study. Aliment Pharmacol Ther 2006;23:1143–1151.
37. European Association for Cardiovascular Prevention & Rehabilitation, Reiner Z, Catapano AL, et al. ESC/EAS guidelines for the management of dyslipidaemias: The task force for the management of dyslipidaemias of the European Society of Cardiology (ESC) and the European Atherosclerosis Society (EAS). Eur Heart J 2011;32:1769–1818.
38. Makki K, et al. The impact of dietary fiber on gut microbiota in host health and disease. Cell Host Microbe 2018;23:705–715.
39. Chen JP, et al. Dietary fiber and metabolic syndrome: A meta-analysis and review of related mechanisms. Nutrients 2017;10:24.
40. Krawczyk M, et al. Gut permeability might be improved by dietary fiber in individuals with nonalcoholic fatty liver disease (NAFLD) undergoing weight reduction. Nutrients 2018;10:E1793.
41. Romagnolo DF, Selmin OI. Mediterranean diet and prevention of chronic diseases. Nutr Today 2017;52:208–222.
42. Estruch R, Ros E, Salas-Salvado J, et al. Primary prevention of cardiovascular disease with a Mediterranean diet. N Engl J Med 2013;368:1279–1290.
43. Bach-Faig A, Berry EM, Lairon D, Reguant J, Trichopoulou A, Dernini S, Medina FX, Battino M, Belahsen R, Miranda G, et al. Mediterranean diet foundation expert group. Mediterranean diet pyramid today. Science and cultural updates. Public Health Nutr 2011;14:2274–2284.
44. Godos J, Federico A, Dallio M, Scazzina F. Mediterranean diet and nonalcoholic fatty liver disease: Molecular mechanisms of protection. Int J Food Sci Nutr 2017;68:18–27.
45. Argo CK, Patrie JT, Lackner C, Henry TD, de Lange EE, Weltman AL, et al. Effects of n-3 fish oil on metabolic and histological parameters in NASH: A double-blind, randomized, placebo-controlled trial. J Hepatol 2015;62:190–197.
46. Storlien LH, Kraegen EW, Chisholm DJ, Ford GL, Bruce DG, Pascoe WS. Fish oil prevents insulin resistance induced by high-fat feeding in rats. Sci 1987;237:885–888.
47. Levy JR, Clore JN, Stevens W. Dietary n-3 polyunsaturated fatty acids decrease hepatic triglycerides in Fischer 344 rats. Hepatol 2004;39:608–616.
48. Richards JL, Yap YA, McLeod KH, Mackay CR, Mariño E. Dietary metabolites and the gut microbiota: An alternative approach to control inflammatory and autoimmune diseases. Clin Transl Immunology 2016;5:e82.
49. Diabetes Obesity. EASL-EASD-EASO clinical practice guidelines for the management of non-alcoholic fatty liver disease. J Hepatol 2016;64:1388–1402.
50. Crowe TC. Safety of low-carbohydrate diets. Obes Rev 2005;6:235–245.
51. Hu T, Mills KT, Yao L, et al. Effects of low-carbohydrate diets versus low-fat diets on metabolic risk factors: A meta-analysis of randomized controlled clinical trials. Am J Epidemiol 2012;176:S44–S54.
52. Katsagoni CN, Georgoulis M, Papatheodoridis GV, Panagiotakos DB, Kontogianni MD. Effects of lifestyle interventions on clinical characteristics of patients with non-alcoholic fatty liver disease: A meta-analysis. Metab 2017;68:119–132.
53. Rusul E, Dragomir A, Posea M. Metabolic effects of low glycaemic index diets. Nutr J 2009;8:5.
54. Parnell JA, Reimer AR. Prebiotic fiber modulation of the gut microbiota improves risk factors for obesity and the metabolic syndrome. Gut Microbes 2012;3:29–34.

55. Vilar-Gomez E, Martinez-Perez Y, Calzadilla-Bertot L, Torres- Gonzalez A, Gra-Ora-mas B, Gonzalez-Fabian L, et al. Weight loss through lifestyle modification significantly reduces features of nonalcoholic steatohepatitis. Gastroenterol 2015;149:367–378.

56. Sanyal AJ, Chalasani N, Kowdley KV, McCullough A, Diehl AM, Bass NM, et al. Pioglitazone, vitamin E, or placebo for nonalcoholic steatohepatitis. N Engl J Med 2010;362:1675–1685.

57. Albanes D, Till C, Klein EA, Goodman PJ, Mondul AM, Weinstein SJ, et al. Plasma tocopherols and risk of prostate cancer in the selenium and vitamin E cancer prevention trial (SELECT). Cancer Prev Res (Phila) 2014;7:886–895.

58. Parnell JA, Raman M, Rioux KP, Reimer RA. The potential role of prebiotic fibre for treatment and management of non-alcoholic fatty liver disease and associated obesity and insulin resistance. Liver Int 2012;32:701–711.

59. Mokhtari Z, Gibson DL, Hekmatdoost A. Nonalcoholic fatty liver disease, the gut micro-biome, and diet. Adv Nutr (Bethesda Md) March 2017;8:240–252.

60. Duseja A, Chawla YK. Obesity and NAFLD: The role of bacteria and microbiota. Clin Liver Dis 2014;18:59–71.

61. Aqel B, DiBaise JK. Role of the gut microbiome in nonalcoholic fatty liver disease. Nutr Clin Pract 2015;30:780–786.

62. Tarantino G, Finelli C. Systematic review on intervention with prebiotics/probiot-ics in patients with obesity-related nonalcoholic fatty liver disease. Future Microbiol 2015;10:889–902.

63. Maher JJ. New insights from rodent models of fatty liver disease. Antioxid Redox Signal 2011;15:535–550.

64. Wit NJW, Afman LA, Mensink M, Müller M. Clinical application of basic sci-ence phenotyping the effect of diet on non-alcoholic fatty liver disease. J Hepatol 2012;57:1370–1373.

65. Guerrerio AL, Colvin RM, Schwartz AK, Molleston JP, Murray KF, Diehl A, et al. Cho-line intake in a large cohort of patients with nonalcoholic fatty liver disease. Am J Clin Nutr 2012;95:892–900.

66. Shi H, Norman AW, Okamura WH, Sen A, Zemel MB. 1alpha,25-Dihydroxyvita-min D3 modulates human adipocyte metabolism via nongenomic action. FASEB J 2011;15:2751–2753.

67. Eliades M, Spyrou E, Agrawal N, et al. Meta-analysis: Vitamin D and non-alcoholic fatty liver disease. Aliment Pharmacol Ther August 2013;38:246–254.

68. Wang X, Li W, Zhang Y, Yang Y, Qin G. Association between vitamin D and non-alco-holic fatty liver disease/non-alcoholic steatohepatitis: Results from a meta-analysis. Int J Clin Exp Med 2015;8:17221–17234.

69. Sharifi N, Amani R, Hajiani E, Cheraghian B. Does vitamin D improve liver enzymes, oxidative stress, and inflammatory biomarkers in adults with nonalcoholic fatty liver disease? A randomized clinical trial. Endocrine 2014;47:70–80.

70. Barchetta I, Del Ben M, Angelico F, et al. No effects of oral vitamin D supplementation on non-alcoholic fatty liver disease in patients with type 2 diabetes: A randomized, dou-ble-blind, placebo-controlled trial. BMC Med June 29, 2016;14:92.

71. Kitson MT, Pham A, Gordon A, Kemp W, Roberts SK. High-dose vitamin D supplemen-tation and liver histology in NASH. Gut April 2016;65:717–718.

72. Naidu KA. Vitamin C in human health and disease is still a mystery? Nutr J 2003;2:7.

73. Valdecantos MP, Perez-Matute P, Quintero P, Martinez JA. Vitamin C, resveratrol and lipoic acid actions on isolated rat liver mitochondria: All antioxidants but different. Redox Rep 2010;15:207–216.

74. Rose FJ, Webster J, Barry JB, Phillips LK, Richards AA, Whitehead JP. Synergistic effects of ascorbic acid and thiazolidinedione on secretion of high molecular weight adiponectin from human adipocytes. Diabetes Obes Metab 2010;12:1084–1089.

75. Harrison SA, Torgerson S, Hayashi P, Ward J, Schenker S. Vitamin E and vitamin C treatment improves fibrosis in patients with nonalcoholic steatohepatitis. Am J Gastroenterol 2003;98:2485–2490.
76. Lai CC, Huang WH, Klevay LM, Gunning WT 3rd, Chiu TH. Antioxidant enzyme gene transcription in copper-deficient rat liver. Free Radic Biol Med 1996; 21:233–240.
77. Nobili V, Siotto M, Bedogni G, Rava L, Pietrobattista A, Panera N, Alisi A, Squitti R. Levels of serum ceruloplasmin associate with pediatric nonalcoholic fatty liver disease. J Pediatr Gastroenterol Nutr 2013;56:370–375.
78. Aigner E, Strasser M, Haufe H, Sonnweber T, Hohla F, Stadlmayr A, Solioz M, Tilg H, Patsch W, Weiss G, Stickel F, Datz C. A role for low hepatic copper concentrations in nonalcoholic fatty liver disease. Am J Gastroenterol 2010;105:1978–1985.
79. Dongiovanni P, Lanti C, Riso P, Valenti L. Nutritional therapy for nonalcoholic fatty liver disease. J Nutr Biochem 2016;29:1–11.
80. Aigner E, Strasser M, Haufe H, et al. A role for low hepatic copper concentrations in nonalcoholic Fatty liver disease. Am J Gastroenterol 2010;105:1978–1985.
81. Poole R, Kennedy OJ, Roderick P, Fallowfield JA, Hayes PC, Parkes J. Coffee consumption and health: Umbrella review of meta-analyses of multiple health outcomes. BMJ 2017;359:5024.
82. Shen H, Rodriguez AC, Shiani A, et al. Association between caffeine consumption and nonalcoholic fatty liver disease: A systemic review and meta-analysis. Ther Adv Gastroenterol January 2016;9:113–120.
83. Chen S, Teoh NC, Chitturi S, Farrell GC. Coffee and non-alcoholic fatty liver disease: Brewing evidence for hepatoprotection? J Gastroenterol Hepatol March 2014;29:435–441.
84. Liu C, Li J, Xiang X, et al. PDGF receptor-alpha promotes TGF-beta signaling in hepatic stellate cells via transcriptional and posttranscriptional regulation of TGF-beta receptors. Am J Physiol Gastrointest Liver Physiol October 1, 2014;307:G749–G759.
85. Paradis V, Perlemuter G, Bonvoust F, et al. High glucose and hyperinsulinemia stimulate connective tissue growth factor expression: A potential mechanism involved in progression to fibrosis in nonalcoholic steatohepatitis. Hepatol October 2001;34:738–744.

15 Hepatic Cirrhosis and Acute Liver Failure

Sriya Muralidharan, Nikhil Kapila, and Matthew Kappus

15.1 INTRODUCTION

Hepatic dysfunction presents a constellation of challenges in nutritional management (Figure 15.1). Patients with cirrhosis often experience anorexia as with other chronic illnesses associated with malnutrition.[1] Not only does the compressive effect of ascites contribute to early satiety and appetite loss, but patients with cirrhosis have twice the fasting levels of leptin compared with healthy controls. The increased serum leptin contributes to appetite loss.[2] Additionally, the inflammatory state of cirrhosis leads to the upregulation of markers of catabolism of healthy body mass. This combination of effects leads to protein-calorie malnutrition (PCM) and a variable use of energy substrates in patients with liver disease.

15.2 SARCOPENIA AND PROTEIN-ENERGY MALNUTRITION

Sarcopenia is positively correlated with higher Child-Pugh scores, and interventions aimed at protein-energy malnutrition (PEM) treatment must consider the variable resting energy expenditure (REE) in patients with cirrhosis. Diagnosis of PEM typically includes assessment of functional capacity, degree of weight loss, nutritional intake, evidence of muscle wasting, and subcutaneous fat loss. PEM is noted in over 20% of patients with compensated cirrhosis and between 50% and 100% of patients with decompensated cirrhosis.[3] This increased REE may contribute to PEM. Hypermetabolism is defined as a REE >120% of the predicted value and is identified in acute liver failure (ALF) and patients with cirrhosis.[4] This increase in REE is thought to stem from higher circulating levels of catecholamines, which may be precipitated by gastrointestinal bacterial translocation, the stress state of cirrhosis, or possibly neural dysregulation secondary to overall sympathetic overstimulation.[4]

15.3 HEPATIC ENCEPHALOPATHY AND PEM

When patients with cirrhosis develop decompensation with hepatic encephalopathy, the presence of PEM and sarcopenia is a poor prognostic indicator. PEM in patients with cirrhosis is defined as a state of critically decreased protein and fat stores that is exacerbated by poor functional status and nutrition in an already hypermetabolic state. Understanding the pathogenesis of hyperammonemia is important in understanding the role it plays in progressive muscle loss and PEM. Ammonia metabolism

DOI: 10.1201/9780429322570-15

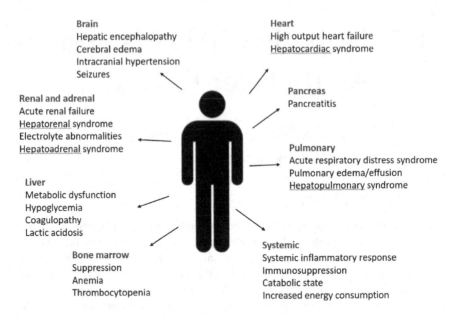

Brain
Hepatic encephalopathy
Cerebral edema
Intracranial hypertension
Seizures

Heart
High output heart failure
Hepatocardiac syndrome

Renal and adrenal
Acute renal failure
Hepatorenal syndrome
Electrolyte abnormalities
Hepatoadrenal syndrome

Pancreas
Pancreatitis

Pulmonary
Acute respiratory distress syndrome
Pulmonary edema/effusion
Hepatopulmonary syndrome

Liver
Metabolic dysfunction
Hypoglycemia
Coagulopathy
Lactic acidosis

Bone marrow
Suppression
Anemia
Thrombocytopenia

Systemic
Systemic inflammatory response
Immunosuppression
Catabolic state
Increased energy consumption

FIGURE 15.1 Complications of liver disease create a complex set of nutritional barriers for patients.

begins with enterocyte and colonic flora ammonia production from ingested nitrogenous substrates. Once ammonia is produced, its metabolism is dependent on a balance of the peri-portal hepatocyte urea cycle and skeletal muscle glutaminase, with renal excretion of the glutamine product. Renal glutamine may recirculate and reach the enterocytes where it is re-metabolized into ammonia[5] (Figure 15.2). Patients with cirrhosis lose the function of ammonia metabolism in the hepatocyte, implicating skeletal muscle to assume a greater share of ammonia breakdown. This increase in skeletal muscle ammonia content stimulates myostatin, promoting myocyte autophagy leading to sarcopenia and resultant PEM.[6]

15.4 MACRONUTRIENT DEFICIENCY IN CIRRHOSIS

In addition to PEM, cirrhosis begets altered macronutrient and micronutrient metabolism in an attempt to meet altered energy demands. The absence of functional hepatocytes in patients with cirrhosis leads to impaired non-oxidative glucose metabolism (Table 15.1).

During episodes of fasting (e.g., between meals or overnight), energy metabolism must rely instead on fatty acid oxidation, leading to a starvation state and reliance on breakdown of skeletal muscle. Impaired gluconeogenesis between meals and overnight causes accelerated breakdown of skeletal muscle and lean body mass. This starvation state promotes insulin resistance and the development of type 2 diabetes mellitus. This dysregulation of glucose is a poor prognosticator. It is important to note that patients with cirrhosis may have normal fasting plasma

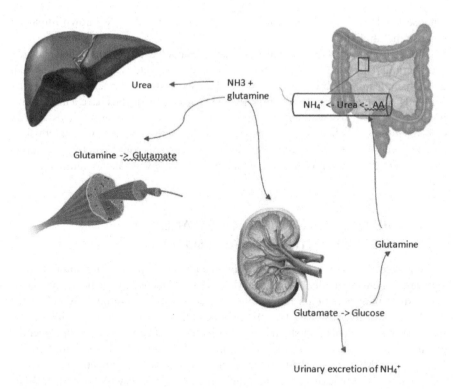

FIGURE 15.2 In vivo ammonia metabolism. Ammonia metabolism begins with enterocyte and colonic flora ammonia production from ingested nitrogenous substrates/amino acids (AA). Renal glutamine re-circulates and reaches the enterocytes where it is re-metabolized into ammonia.[5] Patients with cirrhosis lose the function of ammonia metabolism in the hepatocyte, implicating skeletal muscle to assume a greater share of ammonia breakdown. This increase in skeletal muscle ammonia content stimulates myostatin, promoting myocyte autophagy leading to sarcopenia and resultant protein-energy malnutrition.

TABLE 15.1

Normal Fasting State versus Fasting State in Setting of Cirrhosis

	Normal Metabolic Fasting	Fasting with Cirrhosis
Fatty acid oxidation	Increased	Increased
Gluconeogenesis	Increased	Decreased
Glycogenesis	Decreased	Decreased
Glycolysis	Decreased	Decreased
Skeletal muscle catabolism	Low	Increased

glucose levels or lower hemoglobin A1c measurements despite known impaired glucose metabolism.[7]

In patients with cirrhosis, globulin production is decreased due to synthetic hepatic dysfunction. Therefore, patients with cirrhosis compensate with increased protein catabolism, leading to breakdown of skeletal muscle utilizing branched-chain amino acids (BCAAs) for energy production. Patients with cirrhosis thus have a faster elimination rate of BCAAs with a lower ratio of BCAAs to aromatic amino acids. BCAA supplementation has been shown to have survival benefit in patients with sarcopenia, but not in those with normal muscle mass.[8] For this reason, long-term BCAA supplementation (0.25 g/kg/day) is recommended regardless of vegetable or animal protein source.[9]

15.5   MICRONUTRIENT METABOLISM AND FAT-SOLUBLE VITAMIN MALABSORPTION

The etiology of cirrhosis may be important in addressing specific micronutrient deficiencies. Patients with alcohol use disorder and subsequent development of cirrhosis suffer from poor nutritional intake and deficiencies in B vitamins long before the development of liver disease. Thiamine (B1) deficiency is important to address routinely in these patients and should be coordinated while addressing hypoglycemia, given the risk of Wernicke-Korsakoff syndrome. The European Society for Clinical Nutrition and Metabolism (ESPEN) recommends empiric supplementation of B vitamins, vitamin D, manganese, magnesium, and zinc in patients with cirrhosis.[10] When considering diseases which can result in pancreatic insufficiency concomitant with liver disease, fat-soluble vitamins A, D, E, and K should be supplemented.

15.6   NUTRITIONAL ASSESSMENT OF PATIENTS WITH CIRRHOSIS

Cirrhosis presents several challenges not only in optimization, but in nutritional assessment. Extravascular volume and deficiencies in protein metabolism are key confounders of traditional markers of nutritional assessment. Consequently, percent ideal body weight or serum albumin measurements do not accurately reflect nutritional status in patients with cirrhosis. Existing methods for quantifying skeletal muscle include focusing on muscle volume, the quality of the skeletal muscle, muscle function, or the fiber type (type I vs. II). Some common objective assessments (DEXA, anthropometry) intrinsically utilize the fat and fat-free mass (FFM) of body composition, which in turn is determined by hydration and density fractions that are not accurate in patients with cirrhosis due to imbalance in intra- and extravascular volume. Anthropometric indices such as mid-arm muscle circumference are affected by edema and anasarca. Hand-grip strength utilizing dynamometry has been shown to be a sensitive and specific marker of body mass depletion in patients with cirrhosis and is positively correlated to total protein stores in the body.[4] While hand-grip strength as a correlate for nutritional status was shown to be a valid measurement in men (with loss of strength having a negative correlation to survival), a similar correlation was not demonstrated in women.[4]

Other studies in patients awaiting hepatic transplantation have trialed cross-sectional computed tomography (CT) or magnetic resonance imaging (MRI) to assess degree of core muscle sarcopenia. Skeletal muscle cross-sectional area on a single CT image at the level of the third lumbar vertebra (L3) has been used as a surrogate for whole body muscle mass since cross-sectional imaging is already being obtained for patients undergoing screening for hepatocellular carcinoma.[11-14] The cross-sectional area is then normalized to height, creating the Skeletal Muscle Index (SMI), which can be used as a marker for sarcopenia-related mortality. Notably, it has been hypothesized that female patients will preferentially utilize fat stores prior to the usage of muscle stores, such that when they do present with sarcopenia, they are at a more severe level of PEM compared with their male counterparts. Existing studies have been underpowered in answering this question.[15] In 2012, Carey et al. conducted a multi-center retrospective study to assess the parameters for diagnosis of sarcopenia in patients with end-stage liver disease using SMI as determined on MRI or CT followed by body segmentation analysis.[16] They determined the appropriate diagnostic cutoffs for SMI (cm^2/m^2) to be 50 cm^2/m^2 in males and 39 cm^2/m^2 in females. Patients with SMI less than those cutoffs were defined as having sarcopenia; a correlation between sarcopenia and higher waitlist mortality was established with these cutoffs. While the use of CT or MR imaging remains costly and cumbersome for clinical work, the accurate identification of sarcopenia via cross-sectional imaging is useful in assessing the risk of sepsis, length of hospital stay, and post-transplant mortality as a prognostic tool.

There are screening tools developed in patients with cirrhosis for identifying patients at risk for malnutrition. One such tool is the Royal Free Hospital-Nutritional Prioritizing Tool (RFH-NPT), which uses the patient's nutritional history and complications of their liver disease from acute hepatitis to cirrhosis in an effort to stratify patients into low risk (0 points), moderate risk (1 point), and high risk (2–7 points) categories for malnutrition[17] (Figure 15.3). The RFH-NPT starts with identifying high-risk patients who present with acute hepatitis. Risk is further stratified based on the presence of ascites or edema (moderate risk). This simple-to-use and short tool allows clinicians to readily identify nutritionally at-risk patients and reassess risk. The dynamic change in the RFH-NPT score uniquely indicates improving or increased risk of clinical worsening.[17]

15.7 OPTIMIZING NUTRITION IN CIRRHOSIS

15.7.1 PROTEIN AND CALORIE REQUIREMENTS

The increased REE in patients with cirrhosis must be met by increased energy and protein intake. A total energy intake of 30–35 kcal/kg/day and a protein intake of 1.2–1.5 g/kg/day are recommended for patients with malnutrition or patients requiring maintenance of normal body mass index status. In patients with obesity, the ESPEN guidelines note that enteral nutrition (EN) can be given as long as the target intake for ideal body weight is 25 kcal/kg/day with an increased protein intake of 2.0–2.5 g/kg/day.[9] Table 15.2 demonstrates the nutritional recommendations necessary for patients with chronic liver disease.

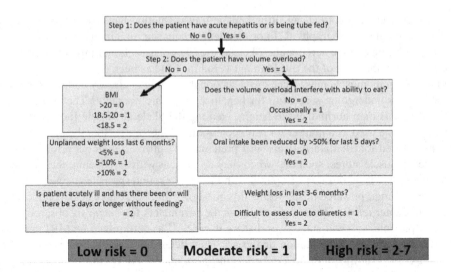

FIGURE 15.3 Royal Free Hospital Nutritional Prioritizing Tool.

TABLE 15.2

Nutritional Recommendations for Patients with Chronic Liver Disease

	Summary of Recommendations		
Macronutrient	BMI <40	BMI >40	Nocturnal Supplementation
Total caloric intake	30–35 kcal/kg/day	25 kcal/kg/day	700 calories
Carbohydrate	45–75% of caloric intake		30–50%
Protein	1.2–1.5 g/kg/day	2.0–2.5 g/kg/day	15–25%
BCAA	0.25 g/kg/day		
Fat	20–30% of caloric intake		30–40%
Fluid restriction	1–1.5 L/day		
Micronutrients	B complex and fat-soluble vitamins (A, D, E, K), manganese, zinc		
Probiotic supplementation	Consideration, with *Lactobacillus*		

Fluid management in patients with cirrhosis is essential. Hyponatremia (sodium <130 mEq/L) is an important prognostic indicator of changes in circulatory volume in the setting of ascites and reflects renal dysfunction and increased renal response to antidiuretic hormone.[18] Free water restriction and diuresis can assist in management of hyponatremia in cirrhosis, but the primary etiology is mediated by neurohormonal mechanisms and splanchnic vasodilation, so these interventions alone are frequently insufficient. Consequently, ESPEN guidelines recommend the use of enteral supplements with high caloric density, while limiting additional fluids to less than 1–1.5 L/day.

Regarding protein intake, achieving a positive nitrogen balance is imperative in optimizing nutritional status in patients with cirrhosis.[19] The nitrogenous source – vegetable or animal protein – does not seem to have significant clinical impact; however, a vegetable source may also provide fiber that has prebiotic function that can prevent negative gut flora alterations and decrease gut transit time to increase ammonia excretion, resulting in improvements in hepatic encephalopathy. Vegetable protein intake may assist patients attempting to lower their body mass index (BMI) as well.[4]

In a randomized controlled trial (RCT) that addressed the practice of restricting protein intake to limit nitrogenous load in patients with decompensated cirrhosis and hepatic encephalopathy, 30 patients were randomized to either a low-protein diet or a normal protein diet; at day 2 and day 14, protein synthesis and breakdown were evaluated by assessing urinary excretion of stable (15)N-glycine isotope, a marker of protein turnover. The study demonstrated that patients with acute hepatic encephalopathy receiving the recommended increased protein diet did not have any worsening of encephalopathy. Those patients receiving a low-protein diet experienced increased protein breakdown and muscle wasting. This higher protein breakdown is attributed to the acute stress of cirrhosis decompensation, poor voluntary enteral intake given acute encephalopathy, and the need for protein metabolism to provide sufficient energy.[20] While most prior studies of BCAA efficacy had evaluated encephalopathy as the primary outcome, Marchesini et al. found that BCAA supplementation over the course of 1 year significantly lowered the rates of hospital admission and the durations of hospital stays with improvement of their secondary outcomes including a decrease in Child-Pugh score, anorexia, and improvement in health-related quality of life.[21] Furthermore, Muto et al. found that daily administration of oral BCAA at 12 g/day over 2 years provided event-free survival benefit while generally increasing serum albumin concentrations and overall quality of life in the patient population.[22] In all randomized trials studying BCAA supplementation, long-term compliance is a challenge but, given the benefits, can be encouraged in patients with advanced cirrhosis.

15.7.2 Nocturnal Supplementation

Patients with cirrhosis exhibit a predisposition to fasting state metabolism, leading to increased lean body weight catabolism. Normal controls who undergo starvation for 2–3 days rely on fat oxidation and gluconeogenesis to maintain adequate cell function. However, in patients with cirrhosis, a single evening of fasting resulted in decreased glycogenolysis due to reduced glycogen storage capacity, leading to increased fat oxidation and gluconeogenesis.[23] The primary substrate for gluconeogenesis in patients with cirrhosis becomes skeletal muscle protein. Due to the replacement of the hepatic parenchyma with fibrosis, glycogenesis and the ability to store glycogen are reduced. Without these stores, patients with advanced liver disease utilize lean muscle mass as a primary energy substrate. In patients with chronic liver disease, nocturnal feeding is utilized to reduce the effect of the "starvation state," which results in protein catabolism from the skeletal muscle. These studies, which evaluated both short- and long-term assessment of total body protein stores, recommended a bedtime oral nutritional supplement to meet approximately 700 calories with 15–25% protein, 30–50% carbohydrate, and 30–40% fat (typically 2 cans of oral nutrition supplement depending on the patient's glycemic control) to interrupt the overnight fast and progression of nocturnal gluconeogenesis. In an RCT conducted by Plank et al., total body protein stores improved significantly in patients using nocturnal supplementation with a total body protein gain of 2 kg over the year, while those only receiving daytime supplementation did not experience this same benefit. The ideal composition of the evening supplementation includes BCAA as well.[24] In patients with liver disease, the provision of small meals more frequently than traditional mealtimes allows for better glycemic load and utilization of oral macronutrients instead of body store breakdown during fasting states. For this reason, patients should limit fasting periods to no longer than 3–6 hours.[4] Per the ESPEN guidelines, 3–5 meals/day and a late evening snack are recommended.

15.7.3 GUT FLORA MODIFICATION

It is unclear why patients with cirrhosis have variable rates of progression. One theory suggests that changes to the gut microbiome, dependent on the etiology of cirrhosis, may contribute to the variability in decompensation. In cirrhosis, the "metabolic neural pathway" (gut–liver–brain) has an evident role in the management of hepatic encephalopathy. The portal vein is a main conduit for transfer of lipopolysaccharide and other bacterial products from the intestines to the liver. In a study of 219 patients with cirrhosis and 25 age-matched controls who underwent stool microbiota pyrosequencing,[25] the microbiota and the Cirrhosis Dysbiosis Ratio (CDR) remained unchanged in stable outpatients with cirrhosis, but there was a significant dysbiosis with a drop in CDR after onset of decompensation (specifically hepatic encephalopathy). The lower the CDR, the more endotoxemia and more decompensated the cirrhosis. Additionally, in patients with decompensated cirrhosis (hepatic encephalopathy, spontaneous bacterial peritonitis), a high Model for End Stage Liver Disease (MELD) score correlated with lower levels of native bacteria. In patients with cirrhosis, RCTs have shown probiotics with *Firmicutes* and *Actinobacteria* phyla to be potentially beneficial. In patients with hepatic encephalopathy, those patients receiving *Lactobacillus* probiotic demonstrated reduced dysbiosis through an increased level of native bacteria relative to *Bacteroidetes* phylum.[26] There is more to learn about the potential benefits of nutritional intervention of both pre- and probiotics.

15.7.4 PARENTERAL NUTRITION IN HEPATIC DYSFUNCTION

Parenteral nutrition (PN) should be utilized in patients with cirrhosis only when oral or enteral feeding is not feasible. PN is indicated in such patients particularly if they are fasting for over 72 hours or if there is concomitant compromise of the patient's airway due to impaired swallow or cough reflex.[27] Complications of PN are primarily infectious, but also related to the potential for worsened cholestasis. In both pediatric and adult populations, PN can cause a range of clinical and pathologic changes from transient but benign elevation in transaminases to steatosis and intrahepatic cholestasis. Fibrogenesis of cirrhosis is exacerbated in patients who are on PN for prolonged periods or if patients with cirrhosis have comorbidities that predispose them to cholestasis, including short bowel syndrome, prior surgeries and infections, or Crohn's disease.[28] Furthermore, prolonged PN promotes intestinal dysbiosis that affects important intestinal functions, including immunoprotection, gut motility, and nutrient absorption. The provision of small amounts of enteral food with BCAAs and prokinetic medications (cholecystokinin or erythromycin) may address some of these intestinal complications of PN use. Purposeful limitation of micronutrients like copper and manganese or drugs with biliary excretion is also a key component of managing PN-related complications in patients with cirrhosis.[28]

15.8 REFEEDING SYNDROME

In patients with cirrhosis and PEM, it is important to consider the risk of refeeding syndrome. One tactic to consider is introducing nutrition at a minimal 10 kcal/kg/day building up to maintenance levels and close monitoring of electrolytes.[9]

15.9 ACUTE LIVER FAILURE

ALF is different from chronic liver disease with a different range of nutritional implications (Table 15.3). ALF is a clinical syndrome characterized by the development of acute, severe liver injury associated with abnormal liver chemistries, coagulopathy, and hepatic encephalopathy in a patient with no prior history of liver disease.[29] Acetaminophen toxicity is the leading cause of ALF in the United States and Europe,

TABLE 15.3
Acute versus Chronic Liver Disease

	Acute Liver Failure	Cirrhosis (Chronic Liver Disease)
Resting Energy Expenditure	High	Low/normal/high
Protein-Energy Malnutrition	High	High
Body Composition	Normal Sarcopenia Obese	Sarcopenic, low muscle mass Sarcopenic obesity
Branched-Chain Amino Acid Use	High	High
Protein Use	High	High
Energy Use	High	High

while viral hepatitis is the most frequent cause in Africa and Asia.[30] The United States ALF Study Group studied 1,147 patients enrolled at 23 sites from 1998 to 2007 and observed that nearly two-thirds of patients were women with an average age of 38 years.[31]

Malnutrition in patients with ALF differs from those with chronic liver disease or cirrhosis because patients tend to be younger and lack associated comorbidities that are observed in patients with chronic liver disease. ALF, however, is associated with rapid loss of hepatocellular function resulting in severe metabolic derangements due to alterations in protein, carbohydrate, and lipid metabolism.[9]

15.10   NUTRITIONAL ASSESSMENT IN ALF

Nutritional status prior to the development of ALF has prognostic and clinical significance. The ALF Study group prospectively enrolled 782 adults with ALF during a 6-year span and found that obese (BMI >30 kg/m^2) and severely obese patients (BMI >35 kg/m^2) were significantly more likely to undergo liver transplantation or die compared with non-obese patients.[32] Anorexia nervosa has also been identified as a cause of ALF. In a series of 12 patients with a mean BMI of 11.3 kg/m^2, the authors suggested that an alternative pathway to ALF may involve nutritional deprivation leading to autophagy-associated hepatocyte dysfunction.[33]

Traditional scoring systems such as the Mini Nutritional Assessment and the Malnutrition Screening Tool are commonly used to assess nutritional status in patients admitted to the hospital.[34] These scoring systems, however, have not been validated in the critical care setting and should not be routinely used to assess the nutritional status of patients with ALF. The Nutrition Risk in Critically Ill (NUTRIC) score and Nutrition Risk Screening (NRS) 2002 have been studied in critically ill patients and are able to stratify both nutrition status and disease severity.[35]

Guidelines from the American Association for the Study of Liver Diseases (AASLD)[36] and the European Association for the Study of the Liver (EASL)[29] do not make any recommendations regarding routine estimation of energy expenditure in patients with ALF. However, ESPEN advocates for routine assessment of energy expenditure due to significant variability in an individual's predicted energy expenditure.[9] Assessing energy expenditure with direct calorimetry is cumbersome and impractical. Hand-held devices calculate only the mean volume of oxygen consumed and assume the respiratory quotient is 0.85. The devices are portable and simple to use, and require the patient to breathe into a mask. These hand-held devices are more accurate than predictive models and therefore may help guide clinical decision making in the critically ill ALF patient.

15.11   CARBOHYDRATE METABOLISM AND MANAGEMENT IN ALF

In ALF, hypoglycemia is believed to result from depletion of glycogen stores, insulin resistance, deranged gluconeogenesis, and failure of compensatory renal gluconeogenesis. Alterations in splanchnic circulation result in markedly impaired glucose tolerance, increased levels of glucagon, and markedly reduced sensitivity to insulin.[9]

The development of hypoglycemia is an ominous development in ALF and is associated with increased mortality. Altered mentation in hypoglycemia may be mistaken for hepatic encephalopathy and can be identified by frequent monitoring of blood sugar. Monitoring of blood sugars should take place every 1–2 hours and can be readily performed with bedside, point-of-care devices. Ultimately, the goal is to maintain normoglycemia with blood sugars between 150–180 mg/dL. This goal can be achieved with intravenous glucose infusion; boluses of concentrated glucose should be avoided since they may precipitate large osmotic fluid shifts. On the contrary, hyperglycemia (>300 mg/dL) may further increase cerebral intracranial pressure and therefore should be avoided and managed with insulin.

15.12 METABOLIC DERANGEMENTS IN ALF

Electrolyte and metabolic derangements in patients with ALF are multifactorial in etiology, but often due to increased systemic production and decreased hepatic clearance associated with the rapid loss of liver function. Elevated lactate levels occur due to increased systemic production of lactic acid and decreased hepatic clearance. Indeed, both elevated levels of lactic acid and acidosis are independent risk factors for mortality in patients with ALF due to acetaminophen toxicity and are included in scoring systems that assess risk of mortality in these patients. In patients with sub-acute liver failure, the acidifying effect of lactic acid may be balanced by the alkalinizing effect of hypoalbuminemia that is observed in patients with ALF not induced by acetaminophen.

Hyponatremia is common in patients with ALF with up to one-third of patients with acetaminophen-induced ALF.[29] Murphy et al. demonstrated that using hypertonic saline infusion to maintain serum sodium between 145–155 mEq/L was associated with reduced incidence and severity of intracranial hypertension.[37] Serum sodium >150 mEq/L may be associated with cell damage and therefore serum sodium should be closely monitored and maintained between 140–145 mEq/L. As with other critically ill patients, rapid shifts in serum sodium should be avoided when using hypertonic saline to prevent the development of central pontine myelinolysis.

Derangements of other electrolytes, including phosphate, magnesium, potassium, and calcium, may be observed due to respiratory failure, tissue ischemia/infarction, and renal impairment. Hyperphosphatemia may serve as an independent predictor of poor prognosis in patients with acetaminophen-induced ALF. Patients with a serum phosphate >1.2 mEq/L at 48 to 96 hours after ingestion of acetaminophen have a low chance of spontaneous survival. Electrolytes must be closely monitored and repletion protocols should be implemented when necessary. In instances with progressive kidney injury, anuria, or severe metabolic derangements that are not amenable to medical therapy, renal replacement therapy may be required.

15.13 AMINO ACID METABOLISM AND MANAGEMENT IN ALF

In ALF, a three- to four-fold increase in amino acids has been observed with a relative increase in tryptophan, aromatic, and sulfur-containing amino acids, and a corresponding decrease in BCAA. Due to loss of significant hepatocyte function in ALF, there is decreased uptake of amino acids in the splanchnic circulation and this disturbed milieu may contribute to increased production of ammonia. Elevated arterial ammonia is associated with increased risk of cerebral edema and intracranial hypertension, and therefore regular monitoring of arterial ammonia with the introduction of EN is recommended.

Though studies have observed no adverse impact on the administration of amino acids in patients with chronic liver disease, the rapid loss of hepatocyte function and the disturbed pathways of amino acid metabolism in patients with ALF put them at increased risk for complications. In patients with hyper-acute ALF, deferring protein administration for 24–48 hours may allow liver function to improve and prevent further ammonia production.[9] Although in patients with chronic liver disease serial monitoring of ammonia is of little clinical value, in patients with ALF, arterial ammonia should be monitored at regular intervals with the initiation of EN or PN. Although venous ammonia samples are often obtained, societal guidelines recommend monitoring arterial instead of venous ammonia.[9, 29] Ammonia levels can be falsely elevated if a tourniquet is applied for a prolonged period of time or if the serum sample is not kept on ice and tested within 15 minutes of obtaining the specimen.

15.14 WHEN AND HOW TO FEED IN ALF

Due to the rapid presentation and relative infrequency of ALF, there are limited clinical trials that assess nutritional intervention in these patients. Many of the recommendations for management of nutrition are extrapolated from the critical care literature and based on expert opinion. Due to the dramatic onset of ALF, many patients will not be malnourished at initial presentation. In patients with ALF and no evidence of malnutrition, EN or PN should be started in whom it is unlikely that normal oral intake would be resumed within 5 days. If patients have evidence of malnutrition, EN or PN should be instituted immediately.

Patients with minimal hepatic encephalopathy can safely tolerate an oral diet as long as there is an intact cough and gag reflex. All patients should undergo nutritional assessment as outlined earlier. There should be a low threshold for oral nutritional supplements if patients are unable to maintain adequate oral nutrition. If unable to meet caloric needs, a nasogastric tube may be inserted to facilitate enteral feeding. The risks of nasogastric tube placement need to be considered on a case-by-case basis, including bleeding during placement as well as the risk of micro-aspiration in the setting of large gastric residual.

The selection of enteral formula should be similar to that for other critically ill patients. According to the American Society for Parenteral and Enteral Nutrition (ASPEN),[35] patients should receive standard polymeric formula that is isotonic or near isotonic. There is no evidence that enteral feeding reinforced with BCAA improves outcomes when compared to standard, whole-protein formulations. As mentioned earlier, arterial ammonia should be monitored at regular intervals with initiation of EN in patients with ALF.

Nearly 75% of European centers surveyed use PN in patients with ALF.[38] PN should be initiated in patients who are unable to tolerate oral or enteral nutrition and should be considered if enteral feeding is unable to meet more than 60% of a patient's nutritional requirement. Initiation and monitoring of PN should be undertaken with the guidance of a multidisciplinary team[39] that includes a registered dietitian and a pharmacist. Prior to initiating PN, complications that need to be considered include the development of bacterial and fungal infections, liver injury, hyperglycemia, electrolyte imbalances, and complications associated with long-term central venous access including venous thromboembolism.

The most commonly used lipid emulsions include medium- and long-chain triglycerides and appear to be relatively well tolerated in patients with ALF.[38] Contrary to other critical illnesses, ALF is characterized by the release of fatty acids from the splanchnic circulation as opposed to other conditions, such as sepsis, in which fatty acids are absorbed. Additionally, ALF may be associated with profound mitochondrial dysfunction and impaired lipid metabolism. Therefore, serum triglyceride levels should be routinely monitored with a goal serum triglyceride level of less than 3 mmol/L.[29]

15.15 NOVEL APPROACHES

Standard of care for outpatients with cirrhosis includes achieving a protein intake of 1.2–1.5 g/kg/day and a total energy intake of 30–35 kcal/kg/day.[9] Nutritional education should be provided to all patients and their caregivers. Information including protein and caloric intake should be shared, as well as an emphasis on reducing periods of fasting, with the inclusion of a complex carbohydrate evening snack. In cirrhosis, there is a significant burden of patient and caregiver fatigue. Therefore, information about nutritional intake can be easily lost or prioritized lower. It is crucial that the healthcare team help in making patients and their caregivers aware of these important points. Patient-created informational guides, such as from https://wellnesstoolbox.ca/cirrhosis/, can be helpful for patients. It is also recommended that if a patient screens positive for malnutrition, they be referred to a dietitian.

Inpatients admitted with cirrhosis or ALF should universally be evaluated by a dietitian.[9] There is a move towards standardizing this practice, since this has not always been a readily available resource. Early consideration for nasogastric or nasojejunal feeding should be considered.[29] Further work is being explored on the role of BCAA supplementation for the reversal or improvement of frailty and malnutrition.

15.16 INCORRECT/OUTDATED PRACTICES

Use of serum albumin alone is no longer recommended as adequate for evaluation of nutritional status in patients with liver disease. Albumin is a byproduct of hepatic metabolism and will be impacted by the reduced metabolic capacity of the liver. Albumin is also affected by the administration of intravenous albumin and intra/extracellular fluid shifts, further complicating the reliability of this serum marker as a measurement for malnutrition.

Serum ammonia is another biomarker that has little utility in the care of patients with cirrhosis and is limited by both time from initial sampling and storage temperature. Serum ammonia is unable to adequately diagnose hepatic encephalopathy or assess the response to treatment of hepatic encephalopathy.

PRACTICE PEARLS

- Patients with cirrhosis lose the function of ammonia metabolism in the hepatocyte, implicating skeletal muscle to assume a greater share of ammonia breakdown.
- Impaired gluconeogenesis between meals and overnight causes accelerated breakdown of skeletal muscle and lean body mass.
- Patients with chronic liver failure should have a protein intake of 1.2–1.5 g/kg/day; higher if the patient also has obesity.
- BCAA supplementation of 12 g/day over 2 years is recommended for patients with advanced cirrhosis.
- Nocturnal supplementation with a mixed nutritional supplement reduces the downstream effects of the nighttime starvation state in patients with cirrhosis.
- For patients with ALF, consider EN or PN if normal oral intake does not return after 5 days or sooner if already malnourished.

REFERENCES

1. Cheung K, Lee SS, Raman M. Prevalence and mechanisms of malnutrition in patients with advanced liver disease, and nutrition management strategies. *Clin Gastroenterol Hepatol*. Feb 2012;10(2):117–25. Doi:10.1016/j.cgh.2011.08.016.
2. Kalaitzakis EBI, Ohman L, et al. Altered postprandial glucose, insulin, leptin, and ghrelin in liver cirrhosis: Correlations with energy intake and resting energy expenditure. *Am J Clin Nutr*. 2007;85:808–15.
3. Juakiem W, Torres DM, Harrison SA. Nutrition in cirrhosis and chronic liver disease. *Clin Liver Dis*. Feb 2014;18(1):179–90. Doi:10.1016/j.cld.2013.09.004.
4. Amodio P, Bemeur C, Butterworth R, et al. The nutritional management of hepatic encephalopathy in patients with cirrhosis: International Society for Hepatic Encephalopathy and Nitrogen Metabolism consensus. *Hepatol*. Jul 2013;58(1):325–36. Doi:10.1002/hep.26370.
5. Dasarathy S, Merli M. Sarcopenia from mechanism to diagnosis and treatment in liver disease. *J Hepatol*. Dec 2016;65(6):1232–44. Doi:10.1016/j.jhep.2016.07.040.
6. Jindal A, Jagdish RK. Sarcopenia: Ammonia metabolism and hepatic encephalopathy. *Clin Mol Hepatol*. 9, 2019;25(3):270–9. Doi:10.3350/cmh.2019.0015.
7. Nishida T. Diagnosis and clinical implications of diabetes in liver cirrhosis: A focus on the oral glucose tolerance test. *J Endocr Soc*. 2017;1(7):886–96. Doi:10.1210/js.2017-00183.
8. Hanai T, Shiraki M, Nishimura K, et al. Sarcopenia impairs prognosis of patients with liver cirrhosis. *Nutrition*. Jan 2015;31(1):193–9. Doi:10.1016/j.nut.2014.07.005.
9. Plauth M, Bernal W, Dasarathy S, et al. ESPEN guideline on clinical nutrition in liver disease. *Clin Nutr*. Apr 2019;38(2):485–521. Doi:10.1016/j.clnu.2018.12.022.
10. Cruz-Jentoft AJ, Baeyens JP, Bauer JM, et al. Sarcopenia: European consensus on definition and diagnosis: Report of the European working group on sarcopenia in older people. *Age Ageing*. Jul 2010;39(4):412–23. Doi:10.1093/ageing/afq034.

11. Carey EJ, Lai JC, Wang CW, et al. A multicenter study to define sarcopenia in patients with end-stage liver disease. *Liver Transpl.* May 2017;23(5):625–33. Doi:10.1002/lt.24750.

12. Montano-Loza AJ. Skeletal muscle abnormalities and outcomes after liver transplantation. *Liver Transpl.* Nov 2014;20(11):1293–5. Doi:10.1002/lt.23995.

13. Montano-Loza AJ. Muscle wasting: A nutritional criterion to prioritize patients for liver transplantation. *Curr Opin Clin Nutr Metab Care.* May 2014;17(3):219–25. Doi:10.1097/MCO.0000000000000046.

14. Montano-Loza AJ, Duarte-Rojo A, Meza-Junco J, et al. Inclusion of sarcopenia within MELD (MELD-Sarcopenia) and the prediction of mortality in patients with cirrhosis. *Clin Transl Gastroenterol.* Jul 16 2015;6:e102. Doi:10.1038/ctg.2015.31.

15. Tandon P, Ney M, Irwin I, et al. Severe muscle depletion in patients on the liver transplant wait list: Its prevalence and independent prognostic value. *Liver Transpl.* Oct 2012;18(10):1209–16. Doi:10.1002/lt.23495.

16. Carey EJ, Lai JC, Wang CW, et al. A multicenter study to define sarcopenia in patients with end-stage liver disease. *Liver Transplant Offic Pub Am Assoc Stud Liver Dis Int Liver Transplant Soc.* 2017;23(5):625–33. Doi:10.1002/lt.24750.

17. Borhofen SM, Gerner C, Lehmann J, et al. The royal free hospital-nutritional prioritizing tool is an independent predictor of deterioration of liver function and survival in cirrhosis. *Dig Dis Sci.* Jun 2016;61(6):1735–43. Doi:10.1007/s10620-015-4015-z.

18. John S, Thuluvath PJ. Hyponatremia in cirrhosis: Pathophysiology and management. *World J Gastroenterol.* 2015;21(11):3197–3205. Doi:10.3748/wjg.v21.i11.3197.

19. Nielsen K, Kondrup J, Martinsen L, Stilling B, Wikman B. Nutritional assessment and adequacy of dietary intake in hospitalized patients with alcoholic liver cirrhosis. *Br J Nutr.* May 1993;69(3):665–79. Doi:10.1079/bjn19930068.

20. Cordoba J, Lopez-Hellin J, Planas M, et al. Normal protein diet for episodic hepatic encephalopathy: Results of a randomized study. *J Hepatol.* Jul 2004;41(1):38–43. Doi:10.1016/j.jhep.2004.03.023.

21. Marchesini G, Bianchi G, Merli M, et al. Nutritional supplementation with branched-chain amino acids in advanced cirrhosis: A double-blind, randomized trial. *Gastroenterol.* Jun 2003;124(7):1792–801. Doi:10.1016/s0016-5085(03)00323-8.

22. Muto Y, Sato S, Watanabe A, et al. Effects of oral branched-chain amino acid granules on event-free survival in patients with liver cirrhosis. *Clin Gastroenterol Hepatol.* Jul 2005;3(7):705–13. Doi:10.1016/s1542-3565(05)00017-0.

23. Plank LD, Gane EJ, Peng S, et al. Nocturnal nutritional supplementation improves total body protein status of patients with liver cirrhosis: A randomized 12-month trial. *Hepatol.* Aug 2008;48(2):557–66. Doi:10.1002/hep.22367.

24. Tsien CD, McCullough AJ, Dasarathy S. Late evening snack: Exploiting a period of anabolic opportunity in cirrhosis. *J Gastroenterol Hepatol.* Mar 2012;27(3):430–41. Doi:10.1111/j.1440-1746.2011.06951.x.

25. Bajaj JS, Heuman DM, Hylemon PB, et al. Altered profile of human gut microbiome is associated with cirrhosis and its complications. *J Hepatol.* May 2014;60(5):940–7. Doi:10.1016/j.jhep.2013.12.019.

26. Acharya C, Bajaj JS. Gut microbiota and complications of liver disease. *Gastroenterol Clin North Am.* Mar 2017;46(1):155–69. Doi:10.1016/j.gtc.2016.09.013.

27. Plauth M, Schuetz T, Working group for developing the guidelines for parenteral nutrition of the German association for nutritional M. hepatology – guidelines on parenteral nutrition, Chapter 16. *Ger Med Sci.* 2009;7:Doc12-Doc12. Doi:10.3205/000071.

28. Guglielmi FW, Boggio-Bertinet D, Federico A, et al. Total parenteral nutrition-related gastroenterological complications. *Dig Liver Dis.* Sep 2006;38(9):623–42. Doi:10.1016/j.dld.2006.04.002.

29. Wendon J, Cordoba J, Dhawan A, et al. EASL clinical practical guidelines on the management of acute (fulminant) liver failure. *J Hepatol.* May 2017;66(5):1047–81. Doi:10.1016/j.jhep.2016.12.003.

30. Bernal W, Wendon J. Acute liver failure. *N Engl J Med.* Dec 26, 2013;369(26):2525–34. Doi:10.1056/NEJMra1208937.

31. Lee WM, Squires RH, Jr., Nyberg SL, Doo E, Hoofnagle JH. Acute liver failure: Summary of a workshop. *Hepatol.* Apr 2008;47(4):1401–15. Doi:10.1002/hep.22177.

32. Rutherford A, Davern T, Hay JE, et al. Influence of high body mass index on outcome in acute liver failure. *Clin Gastroenterol Hepatol.* Dec 2006;4(12):1544–9. Doi:10.1016/j.cgh.2006.07.014.

33. Rautou PE, Cazals – Hatem D, Moreau R, et al. Acute liver cell damage in patients with anorexia nervosa: A possible role of starvation-induced hepatocyte autophagy. *Gastroenterol.* 2008;135(3):840–48.e3. doi:10.1053/j.gastro.2008.05.055.

34. Anthony PS. Nutrition screening tools for hospitalized patients. *Nutr Clin Pract.* Aug–Sep 2008;23(4):373–82. Doi:10.1177/0884533608321130.

35. McClave SA, Taylor BE, Martindale RG, et al. Guidelines for the provision and assessment of nutrition support therapy in the adult critically ill patient: Society of critical care medicine (SCCM) and American society for parenteral and enteral nutrition (A.S.P.E.N.). *JPEN J Parenter Enteral Nutr.* Feb 2016;40(2):159–211. Doi:10.1177/0148607115621863.

36. Lee WM, Stravitz RT, Larson AM. Introduction to the revised American association for the study of liver diseases position paper on acute liver failure 2011. *Hepatol.* Mar 2012;55(3):965–7. Doi:10.1002/hep.25551.

37. Murphy N, Auzinger G, Bernel W, Wendon J. The effect of hypertonic sodium chloride on intracranial pressure in patients with acute liver failure. *Hepatol.* Feb 2004;39(2):464–70. Doi:10.1002/hep.20056.

38. Schutz T, Bechstein WO, Neuhaus P, Lochs H, Plauth M. Clinical practice of nutrition in acute liver failure – a European survey. *Clin Nutr.* Oct 2004;23(5):975–82. Doi:10.1016/j.clnu.2004.03.005.

39. Dalton MJ, Schepers G, Gee JP, Alberts CC, Eckhauser FE, Kirking DM. Consultative total parenteral nutrition teams: The effect on the incidence of total parenteral nutrition-related complications. *JPEN J Parenter Enteral Nutr.* Mar–Apr 1984;8(2):146–52. Doi:10.1177/0148607184008002146.

16 Liver Transplantation

Sherifatu Abu, Peng-sheng Ting,
and Po-Hung (Victor) Chen

16.1 INTRODUCTION

The liver is a major metabolic organ that integrates various biochemical pathways to process carbohydrates, lipids, proteins, and vitamins to maintain a well-nourished state. As a result, individuals with end-stage liver disease (ESLD) develop protein-energy malnutrition (PEM) that, if uncorrected, influences the progression of hepatic disease. For instance, hypoalbuminemia potentiates hydroelectric imbalance that can result in complications such as variceal bleeding, ascites, hydrothorax, hepatic encephalopathy (HE), and hepatorenal syndrome and, therefore, worsen one's morbidity and mortality.[1] Fortunately, liver transplantation corrects metabolic derangements due to ESLD, but it requires patients to improve their nutritional status to promote healing, especially in the acute period.[2] There is growing consensus that a greater focus on the nutritional status of ESLD patients is needed to reduce the short- and long-term mortality in patients undergoing liver transplantation and improve graft survival after transplantation.

16.2 NUTRITIONAL ASSESSMENT OF PRE-TRANSPLANT PATIENT

The initial assessment of patients undergoing liver transplantation (LT) includes a history and physical examination.[6] The history should contain documentation of weight loss, anorexia, nausea, diets, and supplements. The physical examination should include monitoring changes in oral mucosa, skin, and hair, as well as any evidence of muscle and subcutaneous fat loss.[3] Several nutritional screening questionnaires have been validated in ESLD populations. They include questionnaires not specific to any particular disease – such as the Nutritional Risk Screening (NRS-2002), Malnutrition Universal Screening Tool (MUST), Nutritional Risk Index (NRI), Birmingham Nutritional Risk Score (BNR), Short Nutritional Assessment Questionnaire (SNAQ), and the Subjective Global Assessment (SGA) – and liver disease-specific nutritional assessments such as the Royal Free Hospital Nutritional Prioritizing Tool (RFH-NPT) and Liver Disease Undernutrition Screening Tool (LDUST). Only SGA provides an independent prognosticator of 1-year mortality after adjusting for sex, age, disease etiology, and Model for End Stage Liver Disease (MELD) score.[5–8] With SGA as the reference standard, RFH-NPT and LDUST are the most accurate in detecting malnutrition in advanced liver disease (area under the curve 0.885 and 0.892; sensitivity 97.4% and 94.9%; and specificity 73.3% and 58%, respectively).[7] Ultimately, SGA remains a popular nutritional assessment tool in liver disease and is endorsed by both the European Society for Clinical Nutrition and Metabolism (ESPEN) and the European Association for the Study of the Liver

DOI: 10.1201/9780429322570-16

(EASL) (Table 16.1).[9] It predicts post-transplantation outcome, demonstrates a strong association with postoperative anthropometric indices,[10–12] and is more sensitive in detecting malnutrition than other bedside tools (sensitivity is 92.0% for SGA vs. 87.1% for NRS-2002 vs. 82.0% for MUST).[12]

Biochemical tests have intrinsic limitations. For example, serum transferrin levels correlate with inflammation and severity of liver damage and thus can be falsely low in individuals with concurrent severe liver disease. Similarly, serum albumin does not sensitively and dynamically reflect hepatic function in ESLD since its synthesis is markedly reduced in this population;[13] thus, it correlates more with the severity of liver disease than with malnutrition.[14] Prealbumin (transthyretin) is a better marker of nutritional status because of its shorter half-life (2–3 days). Other markers such as CD8 cell counts, low total lymphocyte counts, abnormal skin anergy tests, and immune complexes levels are also currently being evaluated as potential markers for nutritional status in this population, although levels may be affected by concurrent illnesses (e.g., alcohol abuse, infections) and hypersplenism.[3]

Anthropometric measurements such as BMI, skin fold thickness (biceps, triceps, or subscapular), and mid upper-arm muscle circumference are less expensive and quicker alternatives for nutritional assessment. The classical anthropometric measurements such as weight and BMI are often overestimated by ascites and peripheral edema due to the difficulty of accurately deducting areas of fluid collection from the calculation.[6] Skinfold thickness and mid-upper arm circumference are less sensitive to edema and are shown to detect malnutrition in ESLD patients despite high interobserver variability.[6, 15–17]

Hand-grip/strength dynamometry is another technique used to assess and monitor nutritional status and the effects of interventions. It reflects upper extremity strength and can be used in conjunction with bioelectrical impedance analysis (BIA) to assess the effects of adopted nutritional therapy regimens.[18] The hand grip strength test is easy to perform and non-invasive. When compared with the SGA and nutritional prognostic index (NPI) in 50 outpatient, compensated, cirrhotic patients, the hand grip strength test (68% vs. 28% by SGA and 19% by NPI) was best at predicting poor clinical outcomes in malnourished individuals,[14, 19] ESLD complications, and PEM.[6, 20, 21] ESPEN recommends using the hand grip test to assess mortality risk;[22] grip strength is a good predictor of complication rates within the next year regardless of sex.[17] In general, grip strength seems better preserved in patients with viral cirrhosis vs. alcohol-related liver disease, cholestatic liver disease, or other liver etiologies.[22]

Sarcopenia or loss of muscle is a key feature of malnutrition and can be diagnosed using radiographic techniques, such as dual-energy X-ray absorptiometry (DEXA), computed tomography (CT), and BIA.[5] BIA measures body cell mass or metabolically active components of a cell including fat, bone, muscle, and intra- and extracellular water. It determines the body's resistance or impedance to flow across various points of contact using water as a conductor. As a result, its accuracy is limited in patients with fluid retention; however, it is a great modality for determining mortality in patients with liver cirrhosis. Similarly, CT imaging of skeletal muscle in the L3 region correlates with whole body muscle mass and is associated with

TABLE 16.1

Elements of Subjective Global Assessment

	Well-Nourished	Mild Malnutrition	Moderate Malnutrition	Severe Malnutrition
Muscle wasting	None	Mild	Moderate	Severe
Subcutaneous fat loss	None	Mild	Moderate	Severe
Duration of inadequate dietary intake	<2 weeks	2–3 weeks	3–5 weeks	>5 weeks
Functional capacity	Full	Suboptimal	Requires assistance with activities of daily living	Minimally ambulatory or bedridden

Source: Adapted from Detsky, AS, McLaughlin, JR, et al. *J Parenter Enteral Nutr* 1987.

mortality in ESLD, obese liver cirrhosis, patients waiting for LT, and orthotopic LT recipients.[23–26]

Currently, there is no consensus on the best method to quantify and classify malnutrition. However, given the range of techniques available, ESPEN recommends using SGA, anthropometry, or hand grip strength as bedside screening tools to identify individuals at risk of malnutrition and selecting patients in need of nutrition therapy.[17] Other nutrition scoring techniques such as DEXA and CT/magnetic resonance imaging (MRI) can be used to diagnose sarcopenia (a strong predictor of morbidity and mortality) in patients with non alcoholic steatohepatitis (NASH), cirrhosis, and LT;[17] however, it does not add prognostic information to the bedside screening tools.[14, 18]

16.3 NUTRITIONAL THERAPY BEFORE LIVER TRANSPLANTATION

The main goal of pre-LT nutritional therapy is to prevent further nutrient and muscle deterioration. Nutritional therapy can be enteral or parenteral, but the former is generally preferred.[5, 17] Individuals receiving a living donor transplant should start an early and planned nutritional intervention several months before transplantation.[5, 14] LT patients with the highest MELD score or those who cannot maintain oral intake above 60% of the recommended nutritional intervention for more than 10 days should receive additional nutrition support to increase skeletal muscle mass.[17] ESPEN guidelines also recommend delaying surgery so patients with severe nutritional risk can receive nutrition support for at least 10–14 days prior to major surgery since underfeeding is a risk factor for postoperative complications.[27]

Enteral nutrition via an endoscopically placed large-bore gastrostomy or jejunostomy feeding tube helps patients who cannot consume food orally, achieve adequate nutritional intake, and maintain the integrity of the gastric mucosa and gut
barrier. The gut barrier guards against bacterial translocation by providing antigenic
stimulation of the gut lymphoid tissue and facilitating release of biliary secretions
containing immunoglobulin A (IgA).[28] Complications associated with enteral feeding are usually secondary to excessive feeding (resulting in food intolerances such as
diarrhea, bloating, or vomiting) and less likely due to infection. However, the presence
of ascites is a relative contraindication to placing gastrostomy or jejunostomy feeding tubes.[17, 29] Ascites increases the difficulty of properly and securely inserting the
feeding tube. The open communication between the skin, subcutaneous tissue, and
ascitic fluid – in combination with hypocomplementemia and decreased opsoniza-
tion in cirrhotic ascites – increases the risk of bacterial peritonitis. Puncturing of
variceal vessels or small collateral subcutaneous vessels in patients with portal
hypertension during tube placement can also occur.[17] Alternatively, ESPEN recommends that patients with fulminant hepatic failure, coma, and moderate-to-severe
malnutrition who cannot achieve adequate intake orally or via enteral access (due
to bowel obstruction, ileus, or esophageal bleeding) should receive parenteral nutrition.[17] Unfortunately, the parenteral route carries risks of infection, fluid overload,
and electrolyte imbalance.[17]

16.3.1 MACRONUTRIENT SUPPLEMENTATION PRE-TRANSPLANT

For stable patients without fluid overload or other signs of liver decompensation,
standardized nutritional formulas can include maintenance fluids, glucose infusions
(in patients fasting or unable to receive enteral nutrition for more than 12 hours),
vitamins, or liver-adapted solutions containing high levels of branched-chain amino
acids (BCAA) and low levels of aromatic amino acids (AAA). Regardless of the formulation, for patients with liver failure, the nutritional goal is to provide adequate
protein and energy equivalent to patients' daily energy expenditure to encourage
mobilization of native fat stores and prevent muscle breakdown.[3, 5, 13]

Carbohydrate intake should exclusively be provided by glucose and cover
50–60% of non-protein energy requirements. However, patients with liver failure have alterations in glucose homeostasis and are at risk of hypoglycemia but
can also develop hyperglycemia secondary to impaired glucose tolerance, insulin resistance, hyperinsulinemia, and hyperglucagonemia,[3, 17, 30] while concurrently
having depleted hepatic glycogen stores. As a result, ESLD patients undergo accelerated starvation or increased gluconeogenesis, lipid oxidation, and protein catabolism resulting in subcutaneous fat tissue and muscle wasting during prolonged
periods of fasting (usually at night).[3, 31] This is prevented with continuous monitoring
of blood glucose levels, the use of glucose infusions to maintain 2–3 g/kg of body
weight per day of glucose and the use of appropriate amount of insulin to help maintain euglycemia.[17]

Lipids consumption should cover 40–50% of non-protein energy requirements. Patients with cirrhosis typically have decreased plasma levels of essential fatty acids and their polyunsaturated derivates.[3, 32] As a result, enteral and

parenteral nutrition provide various sources of fatty acids. Omega-3 fatty acid lipid emulsions can reduce the occurrence of diet-induced and parenteral nutrition-induced hepatic steatosis, improve cholestasis, and reduce inflammation.[32, 33] Fat restriction is not advisable unless the patient has fat malabsorption. For such individuals, medium-chain triglycerides can help, since they do not require bile salts for absorption.[34] Medium-chain triglycerides are available via enteral and parenteral routes of nutrition administration.

Protein replenishment, however, is more challenging. It requires balancing the need for hypercaloric diets and the risks of hyperammonemia and HE. Nonetheless, protein intake should not be restricted since it can aggravate protein deficiency especially in patients with sarcopenia.[4, 17] Typically, whole-protein formulations containing adequate proportions of the nine essential amino acids are used in the clinical setting, but BCAA-enriched formulas (i.e., leucine, isoleucine, valine) are preferred in patients with cirrhosis and HE.[4, 5, 13] BCAAs are metabolized extrahepatically, making them suitable for patients with liver failure. BCAAs can lower ammonia, improve albumin/prealbumin levels, promote liver regeneration, stimulate the maturation of dendritic cells, and boost immune system function.[18] In contrast, AAA (i.e., phenylephrine, tryptophan, and tyrosine) are not effectively metabolized in liver failure and thus accumulate.[3] As a result, patients with liver failure often do not meet the expected 3.5:1 Fischer's ratio (BCAA: AAA) but instead have a 1:1 ratio.[3] The resulting transport of AAA across the blood–brain barrier can contribute to HE.[3] The metabolism of AAA creates weak neurotransmitters that compete with endogenous neurotransmitters and inhibit excitatory stimulation of the brain.[3, 14] In addition, tryptophan is metabolized to 5-hydroxytryptophan (serotonin), which can also exacerbate lethargy.[3] Despite the purported physiologic benefits of a BCAA-rich diet, ESPEN guidelines do not recommend specialized formulas, since there is no evidence that they are superior to standard whole-protein formulas for improving patient outcomes.[17] Nonetheless, initial protein intake should be at least 1 g/kg/day then gradually titrated up to 1.8–2.0 g/kg/day.[1, 3, 5]

Overall, patients with ESLD should maintain a total energy intake of at least 1.3 times the resting energy expenditure (24 kcal/kg/day), preferably as measured by indirect calorimetry.[17, 35] Complex and simple carbohydrates should compose 50–60% of the total non-protein energy requirements and lipids should contribute the remaining 40–50%. Patients should avoid excess calories, but frequent meals can minimize periods of fasting and catabolic state. A small bedtime snack and nocturnal glucose supplementation allow an increase in carbohydrate, but a decrease in lipid and protein oxidation rates by the next morning, which prevents undernutrition, significant basal energy expenditure changes, and total body protein losses; it also improves nitrogen balance.[36, 37]

16.3.2 Micronutrient Supplementation Pre-Transplant

Additionally, patients with ESLD are susceptible to severe micronutrient deficiencies. Thiamine, folate, vitamin B6, vitamin B12, anti-oxidant micronutrients (i.e., selenium, vitamin E, vitamin C), and vitamin K are typically depleted in this population,[17] resulting in higher risks of oxidative stress, elevated brain ammonia concentrations, and coagulopathy.[38] Magnesium and zinc deficiencies are also common in patients with decompensated cirrhosis due to diuretic-induced urinary excretion and decreased absorption. Clinically, zinc deficiency presents as anosmia and dysgeusia, deranged protein metabolism, and HE. Vitamin D and calcium deficiencies are also prevalent among LT candidates and have been associated with acute cellular rejection and liver osteodystrophy.[39] Liver osteodystrophy or abnormal bone morphology in liver disease is secondary to several physiologic changes that promote bone loss, including parathyroid and calcitonin hormone imbalances, cholestasis-associated malabsorption, increased circulating cytokines, poor diet, physical inactivity, and alcohol ingestion. Diets or supplementation rich in calcium and vitamin D are encouraged to prevent osteoporosis and osteopenia and improve immune tolerance of liver allograft.[39]

In addition to the aforementioned micronutrients, patients with alcohol-associated or cholestatic liver disease can have reduced vitamin A stores, resulting in blindness and infertility.[40] Standard replacement dosing is often appropriate. However, casual vitamin A supplementation in patients with ongoing hazardous alcohol consumption can further aggravate liver injury and is not recommended. High levels of ethanol appear to potentiate the hepatotoxicity of retinol and beta-carotene, which results in a narrow therapeutic window.[41]

16.3.3 USE OF SYNBIOTICS TO IMPROVE GUT MICROBIOTA

Collectively, probiotics can alter the gut microbiota, reduce endotoxin production, and prevent bacterial translocation across the gut mucosa.[14] Prebiotics are non-digestible dietary fiber that pass through the upper gastrointestinal (GI) tract unchanged to nourish the gut microbiota. Synbiotics are foods that combine both probiotics and prebiotics to provide a health benefit to the consumer. The addition of synbiotics to ESLD patients' diets in the preoperative setting may attenuate the postoperative systemic inflammatory response, decrease post-LT infections, and shorten the length of antibiotics.[42] These favorable outcomes are specifically attributed to the beneficial effects of *Lactobacillus*, which include facilitating immunoglobulin production, modulating lymphocyte and macrophage activities, eliminating toxins, and strengthening the gut mucosal barrier.[43, 44]

16.4 NUTRITIONAL CONSIDERATIONS AFTER LIVER TRANSPLANTATION

Many of the nutritional abnormalities associated with chronic liver disease correct with a new functioning liver. However, sarcopenia and other alterations in body composition can persist for at least 12 months after LT.[45] This is partly due to the hypercatabolic state that endures up to 4 weeks post-transplantation. As a result, nutritional therapy that meets the patient's energy and protein requirements is needed early. Unfortunately, LT can also interrupt the vagal innervation and cause a loss of autonomic regulatory control on nutrient absorption, metabolism, glucose and lipid homeostasis, and appetite signaling.[46] Chronic immunosuppressive therapy addition-ally predisposes post-LT patients to weight gain, obesity, diabetes, and multiple vita-min deficiencies. Nuanced nutritional prescriptions also attempt to minimize these effects by ensuring a patient's protein and non-protein requirements do not exceed their caloric needs.

16.4.1 Metabolic Complications Following Liver Transplantation

In the first hours following transplantation, glucose utilization falls substantially due to the newly transplanted liver's impaired glycolytic and aerobic respiration path-ways.[5] Energy generation predominately comes from fatty acid oxidation for the first 6 hours post-LT before shifting to glucose utilization in functioning allografts. It is advisable to administer a small amount of glucose (without insulin) immedi-ately after transplantation to minimize peripheral fat mobilization and breakdown.[18] However, patients with a history of diabetes prior to transplantation may require sliding-scale insulin in response to episodes of hyperglycemia.[47]

The eventual restoration of Insulin sensitivity in the functioning liver allows energy expenditure to normalize. The expenditure is highest during the early weeks after LT and can persist for up to 4 weeks postoperatively. Generally, the post-LT diet should contain adequate calories comprising low-fat, lean-protein foods. Patients will require 1.5–2.0 g/kg/day of protein immediately after transplantation, given the marked increase in protein consumption during wound healing and liver recovery.[4, 17] Non-protein energy needs can vary according to the patient's metabolic and inflam-matory status but estimates commonly range between 25–30 kcal/kg/day.[4, 5, 17] Clinicians should strive to avoid excessive or reductive caloric intake during the early phase post-LT. Chronically exceeding the caloric need can cause weight gain, hyperlipidemia, hyperglycemia, insulin resistance, hypertension, and hepatic steato-sis, whereas withholding nutritional support and inducing a cumulative net caloric deficit of >10,000 kcal can impair survival.[48]

Clinicians should also monitor for potential electrolyte abnormalities, particularly potassium, phosphorous, and magnesium, during the initial post-LT period due to the risk of refeeding syndrome in malnourished patients. Additionally, con-tinued diuretic use in volume-overloaded individuals and immunosuppressant-induced nephrotoxicity can both lead to electrolyte derangements.[49] It is standard to recommend a salt-restrictive diet (3 g sodium/day) after LT to reduce steroid-associated water retention.[50] Pre-transplant vitamin A and zinc deficiencies typically normalize immediately after LT, but they can persist (as can other pre-transplant micronutrient derangements) if the allograft function is poor.[51] Finally, clinicians should consider vitamin D and calcium supplementation, particularly for patients with pre-LT osteopenia/osteoporosis, malnutrition, or muscle wasting, since bone loss can occur within the first 3–6 months after LT.[52] In more severe cases, bisphos-phonates can help to prevent further bone loss.

Overall, the goals of post-LT nutritional support are (1) to provide enough pro-tein and energy intake to minimize soft tissue breakdown and (2) to replenish appropriate electrolytes and vitamins when deficient. A common strategy is to resume enteral nutrition within 12 hours of LT then slowly transitioning to small, frequent oral meals based on the patient's tolerance and ability to meet their nutritional requirements consistently.[53]

16.4.2 LONG-TERM NUTRITIONAL SUPPORT AFTER LIVER TRANSPLANTATION

After LT, most patients will require immunosuppressive therapy indefinitely. Despite the advancement of medical therapy and reduced side effects, increased survival rates have highlighted the unwelcome metabolic implications of calcineurin inhibitors (i.e., tacrolimus, cyclosporine), mTOR inhibitors (i.e., rapamycin, everolimus), and corticosteroids (Table 16.2).[5, 54]

New-onset diabetes or glucose intolerance is a common complication of tacrolimus use. Oral hypoglycemics, insulin, and dietary diabetic restrictions are often needed to prevent hyperglycemia. However, simply maintaining tacrolimus at an even trough level of 3–8 ng/mL can also reduce its diabetogenic potential without increasing the risk of acute rejection.[55, 56] Additionally, tacrolimus and cyclosporine affect energy metabolism and restrict muscle mass growth by inhibiting calcineurin, a promoter of skeletal muscle differentiation and hypertrophy.[57] Similarly, corticosteroids increase proteolysis, appetite, and fat deposition; impair protein synthesis, and decrease fat oxidation,[58] which effectively worsen sarcopenia, muscle wasting, and osteoporosis. Close monitoring of these medication effects allows for timely dietary adjustments.

Another long-term complication of LT is weight gain, which is exacerbated by the appetite stimulation of immunosuppressive therapy, insulin resistance, and post-operative cytokine release.[59] The most rapid weight gain typically occurs during the first 6–12 postoperative months and favors fat over muscle mass recovery.[5] However, the poorly balanced weight gain often continues beyond the first year, resulting in frequent overweight, obesity, and relative sarcopenia among LT recipients.[49] Excessive weight gain can be especially notable in patients who had severe dietary restrictions or GI symptoms before transplantation.[60] Metabolic syndrome, diabetes mellitus, and cardiovascular events are some of the unfortunate, long-term adverse outcomes in this population.[61, 62] Regular consultation with an experienced transplant dietitian can help calibrate the day-to-day dietary recommendations as the LT recipient's nutritional needs evolve after the transplantation.

16.5 NOVEL APPROACHES

PEM, frailty, and sarcopenia are three interrelated risk factors of adverse clinical outcomes in cirrhosis. Dynamic protein-calorie repletion and micronutrient supplementation are critical to the proper clinical management of patients with ESLD. Several diagnostic methods currently exist to quantify malnutrition, frailty, or sarcopenia. These include the SGA, anthropometry, and computed tomography-assisted assessment of skeletal muscle composition. There is currently no unifying consensus on the "best method" in patients with cirrhosis, with some older studies showing that imaging tools do not provide additional prognostic information to the bedside screening tools (e.g., SGA, anthropometry, etc.).[14, 18] Nonetheless, recent research continues to demonstrate the benefit of imaging. For instance, a 2018 study

TABLE 16.2

Severity of Adverse Metabolic Effects from Common Immunosuppression Medications for Liver Transplantation

	Tacrolimus	Cyclosporine	Sirolimus (Rapamycin)	Corticosteroids	Mycophenolate Mofetil
Hypertension	Moderate	Moderate	Mild	Mild	None
Diabetes	Moderate	Mild	None	Severe	None
Dyslipidemia	Mild	Mild	Severe	Mild	None
Abdominal obesity	None	None	None	Mild	None
Osteopenia/ Osteoporosis	None	None	None	Severe	None
Gastrointestinal	None	None	None	Mild (stress ulcer)	Mild (diarrhea)

Source: Adapted from Lucey MR, Terrault N, et al. *Liver Transpl.* 2013.

demonstrated substantial nutritional deficits in ESLD patients are seen on CT when not adequately measured by laboratory testing.[63] Thus, with continued research, the use of imaging modalities to test for malnutrition may yet become the standard of care.

16.6 INCORRECT/OUTDATED PRACTICES

Reductive caloric intake for patients with liver disease is an outdated practice that can lead to undesirable outcomes, such as reduced graft or patient survival. Instead, it is recommended that patients achieve a caloric goal of 30 kcal/kg/day and 1.5 g/kg/day of protein during the perioperative period. Postoperative goals are similar: 1.5–2.0 g/kg/day of protein and 25–30 kcal/kg/day of non-protein energy, with variations in specific caloric goals depending on the clinical scenario.[4, 5, 17] Other than limited clinical scenarios (e.g., bowel obstruction), parenteral nutrition is generally not preferred given risks of infection and fluid overload. Instead, oral or enteral nutrition is ideal when the use of flavoring agents, such as herbs and spices, may improve taste and stimulate appetite.

PRACTICE PEARLS

- Aggressive nutritional repletion is essential in maintaining adequate hepatic function and improving outcomes after LT.
- There are no gold standard nutritional assessment techniques available. However, conducting a bedside physical examination and using nutritional assessment tools, anthropometric measurements, or hand-grip strength testing are paramount to assessing PEM during the pre- and post-LT periods.
- Radiographic tools have not consistently demonstrated additional prognostic information when compared with bedside screening tools.

- Oral or enteral nutrition is preferred, but parenteral nutrition can be considered in patients who cannot maintain enteral feeding above 60% of the recommended nutritional intervention for more than 10 days.
- Nutritional therapy *before* LT: maintain a total energy intake of at least 1.3 times the resting energy expenditure (24 kcal/kg/day). Carbohydrates and lipids should provide 50–60% and 40–50%, respectively, of non-protein energy requirements. Protein intake should not be restricted. Use whole-protein formulations to maintain an initial intake of 1 g/kg/day.
- Nutritional therapy *after* LT should consist of low-fat, lean-protein meals for up to 4 weeks post-LT. Target 25–30 kcal/kg/day of non-protein energy and 1.5–2.0 g/kg/day of protein energy immediately after LT. Consider limiting salt intake (3 g sodium/day) to reduce steroid-associated water retention.
- Avoid excessive or reductive caloric intake during the early post-LT phase to minimize adverse events.
- LT corrects many cirrhosis-related nutritional abnormalities (e.g., electrolyte derangements, micronutrient deficiencies), but sarcopenia can persist up to 12 months post-LT.
- Use the lowest level of immunosuppression needed to prevent allograft rejection and minimize adverse metabolic effects. Regularly monitor adverse effects and make timely dietary adjustments when indicated.

REFERENCES

1. Kondrup J. Nutrition in end stage liver disease. *Best Pract Res Clin Gastroenterol.* 2006;20(3):547–60. doi:10.1016/j.bpg.2006.02.001.
2. Merli M, Giusto M, Gentili F, et al. Nutritional status: Its influence on the outcome of patients undergoing liver transplantation. *Liver Int.* Feb 2010;30(2):208–14. doi:10.1111/j.1478-3231.2009.02135.x.
3. Aranda-Michel J. Nutrition in hepatic failure and liver transplantation. *Curr Gastroenterol Rep.* Aug 2001;3(4):362–70. doi:10.1007/s11894-001-0061-0.
4. Yao CK, Fung J, Chu NHS, Tan VPY. Dietary interventions in liver cirrhosis. *J Clin Gastroenterol.* 9, 2018;52(8):663–73. doi:10.1097/MCG.0000000000001071.
5. Anastácio LR, Davisson Correia MI. Nutrition therapy: Integral part of liver transplant care. *World J Gastroenterol.* Jan 2016;22(4):1513–22. doi:10.3748/wjg.v22.i4.1513.
6. Nunes G, Santos CA, Barosa R, Fonseca C, Barata AT, Fonseca J. Outcome and nutritional assessment of chronic liver disease patients using anthropometry and subjective global assessment. *Arq Gastroenterol.* Jul–Sept 2017;54(3):225–31. doi:10.1590/S0004-2803.201700000-28.
7. Georgiou A, Papatheodoridis GV, Alexopoulou A, et al. Evaluation of the effectiveness of eight screening tools in detecting risk of malnutrition in cirrhotic patients: The KIRRHOS study. *Br J Nutr.* 12 2019;122(12):1368–1376. doi:10.1017/S0007114519002277.
8. Ferreira LG, Anastácio LR, Lima AS, Correia MI. Assessment of nutritional status of patients waiting for liver transplantation. *Clin Transplant.* Mar–Apr 2011;25(2):248–54. doi:10.1111/j.1399-0012.2010.01228.x.

9. Detsky AS, McLaughlin JR, Baker JP, et al. What is subjective global assessment of nutritional status? *JPEN J Parenter Enteral Nutr.* Jan–Feb 1987;11(1):8–13. doi:10.1177/014860718701100108.

10. Stephenson GR, Moretti EW, El-Moalem H, Clavien PA, Tuttle-Newhall JE. Malnutrition in liver transplant patients: Preoperative subjective global assessment is predictive of outcome after liver transplantation. *Transplant.* Aug 2001;72(4):666–70. doi:10.1097/00007890-200108270-00018.

11. Kyle UG, Kossovsky MP, Karsegard VL, Pichard C. Comparison of tools for nutritional assessment and screening at hospital admission: A population study. *Clin Nutr.* Jun 2006;25(3):409–17. doi:10.1016/j.clnu.2005.11.001.

12. Lim HS, Kim HC, Park YH, Kim SK. Evaluation of malnutrition risk after liver transplantation using the nutritional screening tools. *Clin Nutr Res.* Oct 2015;4(4):242–9. doi:10.7762/cnr.2015.4.4.242.

13. Campos AC, Matias JE, Coelho JC. Nutritional aspects of liver transplantation. *Curr Opin Clin Nutr Metab Care.* May 2002;5(3):297–307. doi:10.1097/00075197-200205000-00010.

14. O'Brien A, Williams R. Nutrition in end-stage liver disease: Principles and practice. *Gastroenterol.* May 2008;134(6):1729–40. doi:10.1053/j.gastro.2008.02.001.

15. Thuluvath PJ, Triger DR. Evaluation of nutritional status by using anthropometry in adults with alcoholic and nonalcoholic liver disease. *Am J Clin Nutr.* Aug 1994;60(2):269–73. doi:10.1093/ajcn/60.2.269.

16. Romeiro FG, Augusti L. Nutritional assessment in cirrhotic patients with hepatic encephalopathy. *World J Hepatol.* Dec 2015;7(30):2940–54. doi:10.4254/wjh.v7.i30.2940.

17. Plauth M, Bernal W, Dasarathy S, et al. ESPEN guideline on clinical nutrition in liver disease. *Clin Nutr.* 4, 2019;38(2):485–521. doi:10.1016/j.clnu.2018.12.022.

18. Hammad A, Kaido T, Aliyev V, Mandato C, Uemoto S. Nutritional therapy in liver transplantation. *Nutr.* Oct 2017;9(10). doi:10.3390/nu9101126.

19. Alvares-da-Silva MR, Reverbel da Silveira T. Comparison between handgrip strength, subjective global assessment, and prognostic nutritional index in assessing malnutrition and predicting clinical outcome in cirrhotic outpatients. *Nutr.* Feb 2005;21(2):113–17. doi:10.1016/j.nut.2004.02.002.

20. Augusti L, Franzoni LC, Santos LA, et al. Lower values of handgrip strength and adductor pollicis muscle thickness are associated with hepatic encephalopathy manifestations in cirrhotic patients. *Metab Brain Dis.* 8, 2016;31(4):909–15. doi:10.1007/s11011-016-9828-8.

21. de Lima DC, Ribeiro HS, Cristina R, et al. Functional status and heart rate variability in end-stage liver disease patients: Association with nutritional status. *Nutr.* Jul–Aug 2015;31(7–8):971–4. doi:10.1016/j.nut.2015.01.014.

22. Peng S, Plank LD, McCall JL, Gillanders LK, McIlroy K, Gane EJ. Body composition, muscle function, and energy expenditure in patients with liver cirrhosis: A comprehensive study. *Am J Clin Nutr.* May 2007;85(5):1257–66. doi:10.1093/ajcn/85.5.1257.

23. Carey EJ, Lai JC, Wang CW, et al. A multicenter study to define sarcopenia in patients with end-stage liver disease. *Liver Transpl.* 5, 2017;23(5):625–33. doi:10.1002/lt.24750.

24. Durand F, Buyse S, Francoz C, et al. Prognostic value of muscle atrophy in cirrhosis using psoas muscle thickness on computed tomography. *J Hepatol.* Jun 2014;60(6):1151–7. doi:10.1016/j.jhep.2014.02.026.

25. Montano-Loza AJ, Meza-Junco J, Prado CM, et al. Muscle wasting is associated with mortality in patients with cirrhosis. *Clin Gastroenterol Hepatol.* Feb 2012;10(2):166–73, 173.e1. doi:10.1016/j.cgh.2011.08.028.

26. Hanai T, Shiraki M, Nishimura K, et al. Sarcopenia impairs prognosis of patients with liver cirrhosis. *Nutr.* Jan 2015;31(1):193–9. doi:10.1016/j.nut.2014.07.005.

27. Weimann A, Braga M, Carli F, et al. ESPEN guideline: Clinical nutrition in surgery. *Clin Nutr.* 6, 2017;36(3):623–50. doi:10.1016/j.clnu.2017.02.013.

28. Nagpal R, Yadav H. Bacterial translocation from the gut to the distant organs: An overview. *Ann Nutr Metab.* 2017;71 Suppl 1:11–16. doi:10.1159/000479918.

29. Baltz JG, Argo CK, Al-Osaimi AM, Northup PG. Mortality after percutaneous endoscopic gastrostomy in patients with cirrhosis: A case series. *Gastrointest Endosc.* Nov 2010;72(5):1072–5. doi:10.1016/j.gie.2010.06.043.

30. Müller MJ, Pirlich M, Balks HJ, Selberg O. Glucose intolerance in liver cirrhosis: Role of hepatic and non-hepatic influences. *Eur J Clin Chem Clin Biochem.* Oct 1994;32(10):749–58. doi:10.1515/cclm.1994.32.10.749.

31. McCullough AJ, Tavill AS. Disordered energy and protein metabolism in liver disease. *Semin Liver Dis.* Nov 1991;11(4):265–77. doi:10.1055/s-2008-1040445.

32. Yang J, Fernández-Galilea M, Martínez-Fernández L, et al. Oxidative stress and non-alcoholic fatty liver disease: Effects of omega-3 fatty acid supplementation. *Nutr.* Apr 2019;11(4). doi:10.3390/nu11040872.

33. Jump DB, Lytle KA, Depner CM, Tripathy S. Omega-3 polyunsaturated fatty acids as a treatment strategy for nonalcoholic fatty liver disease. *Pharmacol Ther.* 1, 2018;181:108–125. doi:10.1016/j.pharmthera.2017.07.007.

34. Juárez-Hernández E, Chávez-Tapia NC, Uribe M, Barbero-Becerra VJ. Role of bioactive fatty acids in nonalcoholic fatty liver disease. *Nutr J.* 08 2016;15(1):72. doi:10.1186/s12937-016-0191-8.

35. Nielsen K, Kondrup J, Martinsen L, et al. Long-term oral refeeding of patients with cirrhosis of the liver. *Br J Nutr.* Oct 1995;74(4):557–67. doi:10.1079/bjn19950158.

36. Tsien CD, McCullough AJ, Dasarathy S. Late evening snack: Exploiting a period of anabolic opportunity in cirrhosis. *J Gastroenterol Hepatol.* Mar 2012;27(3):430–41. doi:10.1111/j.1440-1746.2011.06951.x.

37. Verboeket-van de Venne WP, Westerterp KR, van Hoek B, Swart GR. Energy expenditure and substrate metabolism in patients with cirrhosis of the liver: Effects of the pattern of food intake. *Gut.* Jan 1995;36(1):110–6. doi:10.1136/gut.36.1.110.

38. Butterworth RF. Thiamine deficiency-related brain dysfunction in chronic liver failure. *Metab Brain Dis.* Mar 2009;24(1):189–96. doi:10.1007/s11011-008-9129-y.

39. Bitetto D, Fabris C, Falleti E, et al. Vitamin D and the risk of acute allograft rejection following human liver transplantation. *Liver Int.* Mar 2010;30(3):417–44. doi:10.1111/j.1478-3231.2009.02154.x.

40. McClain CJ, Van Thiel DH, Parker S, Badzin LK, Gilbert H. Alterations in zinc, vitamin A, and retinol-binding protein in chronic alcoholics: A possible mechanism for night blindness and hypogonadism. *Alcohol Clin Exp Res.* Apr 1979;3(2):135–41. doi:10.1111/j.1530-0277.1979.tb05287.x.

41. Leo MA, Lieber CS. Alcohol, vitamin A, and beta-carotene: Adverse interactions, including hepatotoxicity and carcinogenicity. *Am J Clin Nutr.* Jun 1999;69(6):1071–85. doi:10.1093/ajcn/69.6.1071.

42. Sugawara G, Nagino M, Nishio H, et al. Perioperative synbiotic treatment to prevent postoperative infectious complications in biliary cancer surgery: A randomized controlled trial. *Ann Surg.* Nov 2006;244(5):706–14. doi:10.1097/01.sla.0000219039.20924.88.

43. Mou H, Yang F, Zhou J, Bao C. Correlation of liver function with intestinal flora, vitamin deficiency and IL-17A in patients with liver cirrhosis. *Exp Ther Med.* Nov 2018;16(5):4082–8. doi:10.3892/etm.2018.6663.

44. Rayes N, Seehofer D, Hansen S, et al. Early enteral supply of lactobacillus and fiber versus selective bowel decontamination: A controlled trial in liver transplant recipients. *Transplant.* Jul 2002;74(1):123–7. doi:10.1097/00007890-200207150-00021.

45. Giusto M, Lattanzi B, Di Gregorio V, Giannelli V, Lucidi C, Merli M. Changes in nutritional status after liver transplantation. *World J Gastroenterol*. Aug 2014;20(31):10682–90. doi:10.3748/wjg.v20.i31.10682.

46. Yi CX, la Fleur SE, Fliers E, Kalsbeek A. The role of the autonomic nervous liver innervation in the control of energy metabolism. *Biochim Biophys Acta*. Apr 2010;1802(4):416–31. doi:10.1016/j.bbadis.2010.01.006.

47. Peláez-Jaramillo MJ, Cárdenas-Mojica AA, Gaete PV, Mendivil CO. Post-liver transplantation diabetes mellitus: A review of relevance and approach to treatment. *Diabetes Ther*. Apr 2018;9(2):521–43. doi:10.1007/s13300-018-0374-8.

48. Driscoll DF, Blackburn GL. Total parenteral nutrition 1990. A review of its current status in hospitalised patients, and the need for patient-specific feeding. *Drugs*. Sep 1990;40(3):346–63. doi:10.2165/00003495-199040030-00003.

49. Anastácio LR, Ferreira LG, Ribeiro HS, et al. Sarcopenia, obesity and sarcopenic obesity in liver transplantation: A body composition prospective study. *Arq Bras Cir Dig*. 2019;32(2):e1434. doi:10.1590/0102-672020190001e1434.

50. Dougkas A, Vannereux M, Giboreau A. The impact of herbs and spices on increasing the appreciation and intake of low-salt legume-based meals. *Nutr*. Dec 2019;11(12). doi:10.3390/nu11122901.

51. Pescovitz MD, Mehta PL, Jindal RM, Milgrom ML, Leapman SB, Filo RS. Zinc deficiency and its repletion following liver transplantation in humans. *Clin Transplant*. Jun 1996;10(3):256–60.

52. Giannini S, Nobile M, Ciuffreda M, et al. Long-term persistence of low bone density in orthotopic liver transplantation. *Osteoporos Int*. 2000;11(5):417–24. doi:10.1007/s001980070109.

53. Amodio P, Bemeur C, Butterworth R, et al. The nutritional management of hepatic encephalopathy in patients with cirrhosis: International society for hepatic encephalopathy and nitrogen metabolism consensus. *Hepatol*. Jul 2013;58(1):325–36. doi:10.1002/hep.26370.

54. Lucey MR, Terrault N, Ojo L, et al. Long-term management of the successful adult liver transplant: 2012 practice guideline by the American Association for the Study of Liver Diseases and the American Society of Transplantation. *Liver Transpl*. Jan 2013;19(1):3–26. doi:10.1002/lt.23566.

55. Song JL, Gao W, Zhong Y, et al. Minimizing tacrolimus decreases the risk of new-onset diabetes mellitus after liver transplantation. *World J Gastroenterol*. Feb 2016;22(6):2133–41. doi:10.3748/wjg.v22.i6.2133.

56. Shivaswamy V, Boerner B, Larsen J. Post-transplant diabetes mellitus: Causes, treatment, and impact on outcomes. *Endocr Rev*. Feb 2016;37(1):37–61. doi:10.1210/er.2015-1084.

57. Hudson MB, Price SR. Calcineurin: A poorly understood regulator of muscle mass. *Int J Biochem Cell Biol*. Oct 2013;45(10):2173–8. doi:10.1016/j.biocel.2013.06.029.

58. Peckett AJ, Wright DC, Riddell MC. The effects of glucocorticoids on adipose tissue lipid metabolism. *Metab*. Nov 2011;60(11):1500–10. doi:10.1016/j.metabol.2011.06.012.

59. Richards J, Gunson B, Johnson J, Neuberger J. Weight gain and obesity after liver transplantation. *Transpl Int*. Apr 2005;18(4):461–6. doi:10.1111/j.1432-2277.2004.00067.x.

60. Richardson RA, Garden OJ, Davidson HI. Reduction in energy expenditure after liver transplantation. *Nutrition*. 2001 Jul–Aug 2001;17(7–8):585–9. doi:10.1016/s0899-9007(01)00571-8.

61. Kallwitz ER. Metabolic syndrome after liver transplantation: Preventable illness or common consequence? *World J Gastroenterol*. Jul 2012;18(28):3627–34. doi:10.3748/wjg.v18.i28.3627.

62. Laish I, Braun M, Mor E, Sulkes J, Harif Y, Ben Ari Z. Metabolic syndrome in liver transplant recipients: Prevalence, risk factors, and association with cardiovascular events. *Liver Transpl.* Jan 2011;17(1):15–22. doi:10.1002/lt.22198.

63. Bush WJ, Davis JP, Maluccio MA, Kubal CA, Salisbury JB, Mangus RS. Computed tomography measures of nutrition in patients with end-stage liver disease provide a novel approach to characterize deficits. *Transplant Proc.* Dec 2018;50(10):3501–7. doi:10.1016/j.transproceed.2018.06.006.

17 Nutrition Management in Oncology

Gastroenterology, Breast, Esophageal, Head and Neck, Gynecologic, Lung, Prostate Cancers, and Palliative Care

Pankaj Vashi, Julia Fechtner, and Kristen Trukova

17.1 INTRODUCTION

The prevalence of malnutrition in people with cancer has been estimated to be up to 85%, particularly in cancers that affect the gastrointestinal (GI) tract. According to the National Cancer Institute (NCI), 20%–40% of people with cancer die from malnutrition, cachexia, or complications attributed to these conditions. Therefore, any unintended weight loss should be evaluated during cancer treatment. It has been reported that as little as a 5% weight loss can reduce tolerance to chemotherapy, increase side effects, and decrease quality of life. Weight loss can also interfere with patients' ability to complete or stay on track with their prescribed cancer therapy.

Cancer and cancer treatments can impact patients' ability to ingest, digest, absorb, and metabolize nutrients, making the management of nutritional status challenging in this population. Over the last decade, many new therapeutic modalities like immunotherapies and precision medicine focused targeted drugs have created new nutritional challenges with unique side effect profiles. For this reason, most evidence-based guidelines for oncology nutrition recommend that all patients being treated for cancer be screened for malnutrition and rescreened throughout treatment. Some of the main goals of nutrition therapy for those at risk are as follows:

- Prevent or treat nutrition deficiency and problems, including preventing muscle and bone loss
- Decrease or manage symptoms that impact nutrition
- Maintain the immune system to help fight infection
- Aid recovery and healing from surgery, chemotherapy, and/or radiation therapy
- Maintain or improve the patient's strength, energy, and quality of life

DOI: 10.1201/9780429322570-17

Also, for patients who are well nourished, good nutrition and physical activity behaviors are important during and after treatment. All patients, especially those with excess body weight, should be counseled on eating and activity behaviors to help them achieve and maintain a healthy body weight, since obesity has been associated with poorer outcomes during treatment, as well as an increase in risk of recurrence in some cancers.

This chapter outlines approaches to nutrition screening, assessment, interventions, and monitoring in the oncology population. The chapter begins with a review of screening tools that have been validated for use in this population. After that, a review of many of the most common cancers will include a brief overview of the cancer, risk factors, and common treatments, including some nutrition interventions. Finally, the appendices in this chapter can serve as a reference to help the provider anticipate side effects of common treatments as well as offer suggestions for nutritional management of those symptoms.

17.2 NUTRITION SCREENING AND ASSESSMENT

17.2.1 SCREENING

Nutrition screening in the oncology population is used for the early identification of patients who are malnourished or at nutritional risk. A nutrition screen can be completed by any qualified healthcare professional, including those other than the registered dietitian (RD). Screening for malnutrition enables a timely referral for nutrition assessment and intervention. Owing to the duration of cancer treatments, adjustments in regimens and modalities, and changes in an individual's tolerance to treatment over time, it is imperative that patients are screened at initial presentation and regularly rescreened at each clinic visit thereafter.[1] There should be a process in place whereby a positive screening alerts the RD for referral. Once a patient is referred, nutrition interventions and education require continuous modification to meet the patient's dynamic needs.

A screening tool provides a valid, standardized, and efficient method to identify nutrition impact symptoms and clinical signs of malnutrition (see Chapter 1). Based on the Academy of Nutrition and Dietetics Evidence Analysis Library (EAL), there are four nutrition screening tools that have proven to be valid and reliable in the inpatient setting, two of which are appropriate in the outpatient setting (Table 17.1).

17.2.2 ASSESSMENT

The purpose of the oncology nutrition assessment is to perform a comprehensive evaluation of the patient's nutritional status, nutrition impact symptoms, and nutritional requirements. Furthermore, the assessment is utilized by the RD to form individualized interventions, monitoring, and continued evaluation as appropriate. As stated by the EAL Oncology Work Group, "An adult oncology nutrition assessment should characterize and document the presence of (or expected potential for) altered nutrition status and nutrition impact symptoms that may result in a measurable adverse

TABLE 17.1
Nutrition Screening Tools Validated in the Oncology Population

Screening Tool	Components Assessed	Inpatient	Outpatient
Patient-Generated–Subjective Global Assessment (PG–SGA)	Weight, nutrition impact symptoms, intake, and functional status	×	×
Malnutrition Screening Tool (MST)	Weight and appetite	×	×
Malnutrition Screening Tool for Cancer Patients (MSTC)	Intake, weight, ECOG, and BMI	×	
Malnutrition Universal Screening Tool (MUST)	BMI, weight, acute illness, and intake	×	
Weight Loss	Percentage of lean body weight		

Source: Onc: Nutrition screening tools. 2012. Academy of Nutrition and Dietetics Evidence Analysis Library. www.andeal.org/topic.cfm?cat=5452&conclusion_statement_id=251796&highlight=oncology%20assessment&home=1. Updated 2012. Accessed March 2015. Nutrition Management in Oncology 67.

effect on body composition, function, quality of life (QOL) or clinical outcome, and may include indicators of malnutrition."[2]

The Subjective Global Assessment (SGA) and Patient-Generated Subjective Global Assessment (PG–SGA) nutrition assessment tools have been validated by the EAL for use among adult oncology patients in acute care and ambulatory settings.[3] Both tools include assessment of intake, weight, GI symptoms, and functional status. However, the SGA incorporates a physical examination, while the PG–SGA covers a more comprehensive review of nutrition impact symptoms.

Malnutrition is extremely prevalent in the oncology population, with incidence rates estimated to be between 40% and 80%.[4,5] Malnutrition is defined as "a state of nutrition in which a deficiency, excess or imbalance of energy, protein, and other nutrients causes adverse effects on body form, function and clinical outcome."[4] Complications of malnutrition include increased therapy-related toxicity, poor performance status, lower quality of life, reduced survival, increased number of hospitalizations and length of stay, and increased healthcare costs.[5–8] PG–SGA remains the most used screening tool in oncology due to its simplicity and objective validated interventions.

The oncology nutrition assessmInt is a multifactorial approach that should be completed at every clinic visit for patients who are at risk for malnutrition or are already malnourished. Evaluation of nutrition impact symptoms that the patient is already experiencing, or is at risk for developing, is critical in helping to maintain or improve their nutritional status. Nutrition impact symptoms are defined as side effects from treatment or the cancer itself that impair intake, digestion, or absorption.

Examples commonly seen in the oncology setting include nausea, vomiting, diarrhea, constipation, dysphagia, odynophagia, anorexia, mucositis, early satiety, and alterations in taste and smell.

The careful monitoring of weight status and implementation of nutritional interventions to support a healthy body weight is a key component of the nutrition assessment. Cancer-induced weight loss and more recently, lean body mass, have both been used as primary outcomes in clinical trials.

Patients with significant weight loss and/or sarcopenia have been associated with greater treatment toxicity and shorter survival. Significant weight loss is defined as 1%–2% in 1 week, 5% in 1 month, 7.5% in 3 months, and 10% in 6 months. Computerized tomography (CT) images, bioelectrical impedance analysis (BIA), dual-energy X-ray absorptiometry (DXA), and anthropometry are used to assess changes in lean body mass. A recent study found that the presence of sarcopenia surpasses the presence of malnutrition as a predictor of survival in colorectal cancer. When sarcopenia and malnutrition are present, survival is worse in colorectal cancer compared to just one of those conditions being present.[9, 10]

In addition to using a validated assessment tool, the oncology nutrition assessment should encompass each component of the nutrition care process, including an in-depth diet history, medication list review, anthropometric measurements, biochemical data, nutrition-focused physical exam, and psychosocial factors. Recently, sarcopenia determined by skeletal muscle mass index using a validated software at the third lumber vertebra on a routine CT scan has been shown to be a very sensitive tool to determine muscle mass loss in cancer patients. In fact, sarcopenia supersedes PG–SGA in certain cancer types.[10] Early nutritional interventions can improve outcomes in these oncology patients.

17.3 GASTROENTEROLOGY

17.3.1 INTRODUCTION

The gastrointestinal (GI) tract refers to the route from the mouth to the anus that is responsible for digestion, absorption, and elimination. The GI tract is also host to a plethora of microorganisms that are responsible for 70% of the body's immune function, making it the largest immune tissue in the body.

The GI tract is a very complex and dynamic system that is impacted by what we eat and by exposure to toxins. Chronic inflammation is linked to breakdown in this complex immune system, which triggers the formation of cancerous growth. GI cancers include organs in the upper and lower GI tract, namely, the esophagus, stomach, pancreas, liver, gallbladder, colon/rectum, and anus. These cancers can cause alterations in anatomy and function that can affect nutritional status, quality of life, and treatment outcomes. Aberrations commonly experienced with GI cancers that make nutritional management challenging will be covered. Cancers of the head and neck and esophagus are discussed in their own section.

17.3.1.1 Statistics/Survival

Cancers of the GI tract are collectively some of the most lethal cancers worldwide. Lifetime risk of developing a cancer in the GI tract ranges from 0.2% to 5%, depending on location and tumor type, with anal cancer being the least common and colorectal being the most common. Survival rates depend on stage at diagnosis and tumor type, with advanced stages having much less favorable prognoses.[11]

17.3.1.2   Risk Factors

Common risk factors for GI cancers include tobacco use; alcohol consumption; history of infection, such as *Helicobacter pylori*, chronic hepatitis, Epstein–Barr virus, and human papilloma virus; and genetics and chronic inflammation.[12] Obesity affects 2/3 of US population and has now become an independent risk factor for many cancers including colon cancer.[13] Diet plays a key role in the development of several GI cancers.

For example, high saturated fat and low-fiber intake has been linked to colorectal cancers, and intake of smoked, salted, cured, and pickled foods are known risk factors for stomach cancer.[12, 14] Furthermore, it is estimated that 15%–50% of GI cancers are preventable by diet, activity, weight management, and screening.[12]

17.3.1.2.1   Symptoms

Recognizing symptoms that are considered "red flags" for GI cancers is important for early detection.

These include:

- Unexplained weight loss
- Abdominal pain that lasts longer than 4 weeks
- Unexplained loss of appetite
- Change in bowel habits
- Nausea and vomiting lasting for more than a week
- Symptoms related to anemia (fatigue, shortness of breath, and weakness)
- New onset of unexplained back pain
- Gastrointestinal bleeding

Early detection of GI cancers is difficult due to latent signs and symptoms and lack of routine screening tests. It is very important to recognize these warning signs so that timely referral to a gastroenterologist can be made.

Nutrition assessment should include a determination of energy and protein needs. Although predictive equations have been proposed for the outpatient and home care population, specific recommendations related to the type of cancer may lead to more accurate provision of nutrients (see Table 17.2).

17.3.2   Treatment Options

17.3.2.1   Enteral Feeding

In patients with esophageal and proximal gastric cancer, dysphagia is the most predominant symptom that impacts nutrition. Dysphagia can get worse with radiation treatment and thus early placement of enteral tube (either percutaneous endoscopic gastrostomy [PEG] or surgical jejunostomy [J-tube]) is crucial to prevent worsening nutritional status. Another new modality of treatment is liquid nitrogen spray cryotherapy for metastatic esophageal cancer. This can help patients continue to eat and has been shown to help maintain good nutrition and improve survival.[14]

TABLE 17.2
Estimating Energy and Protein Requirements

Cancer Type	Energy (kcal/kg/day Actual Weight)	Protein (g/kg/day Actual Weight)	Fluid
Stomach, pancreas, gallbladder, colon, rectum, anus	30–35: Repletion, weight gain 25–30: Inactive, nonstressed 35: Hypermetabolic 25–30: Sepsis	1.0–1.5: Cancer 1.5–2.5: Cancer cachexia 1.0–1.5: Inflammatory bowel disease 1.5–2.0: Short bowel syndrome	20–40 mL/kg/day or 1 mL/kcal
Liver	25–40: Based on dry weight 35–40: Stable cirrhosis 25–35: Without encephalopathy 35: Acute encephalopathy 30–40: Stable, malnourished	1.0–1.5: All except those with encephalopathy 0.6–0.8: Acute encephalopathy	

Source: Adapted from Huhmann M. *Oncology Nutrition for Clinical Practice*. 3rd ed. Chicago, IL: Oncology Nutrition Dietetic Practice Group of the Academy of Nutrition and Dietetics; 2013:14.

17.3.2.2   Surgical Management

The presence of cancer in the GI tract predisposes one to malnutrition. Patients who are malnourished preoperatively are significantly more likely to have longer lengths of hospital stay and postoperative morbidity and mortality.[16–19] Nutrition screening is essential for identifying patients at increased risk for perioperative morbidity, and early intervention is critical to improving outcomes.

Optimization of nutritional status preoperatively is imperative. In patients who are at severe nutritional risk, nutrition support should be implemented for 10–14 days preoperatively, and surgery should be postponed until this is achieved. Severe nutritional risk is defined as one of the following:[18]

- Weight loss of 10%–15% within 6 months
- Body mass index (BMI) <18.5 kg/m^2
- Subjective Global Assessment Grade C

In oncology patients unable to consume above 60% of estimated intake for more than 10 days or in whom inadequate intake is anticipated for more than 7 days perioperatively, regardless of nutritional status, it is recommended that nutrition support via the enteral route (oral or tube feeding) be implemented without delay.[18] Preoperative parenteral nutrition (PN) for 7–15 days has been shown to reduce postoperative morbidity and should be considered in severely malnourished patients in whom oral or enteral nutrition (EN) is contraindicated or insufficient.[20–22]

Postoperatively, the traditional practice of holding oral or enteral feeds until return of bowel sounds is without evidence, yet pervasive as a standard of care.[23] Early feeding should be initiated to promote bowel hypertrophy and anastomotic healing.[24] Feeding proximal to an anastomosis may prevent disruption or leak.[25] If feeding is started within 24 hours, dysmotility can be attenuated, even in the absence of peristalsis.[26] In patients undergoing gastrectomy, rectal and pelvic surgery, pancreaticoduodenectomy, and colon resection, a normal diet should be offered on postoperative day one without restrictions, and patients should be advised caution in increasing intake according to tolerance. Early feeding reduces the risk of infection and length of hospital stay.[27-30]

Immunonutrition or pharmaconutrition refers to immune-modulating formulas containing supraphysiological doses of arginine, with or without glutamine, omega-3 fatty acids, and nucleotides, which are recommended for their effect on reducing postoperative infectious complications and hospital length of stay.[28] Results from a systematic review and meta-analysis of randomized controlled trials evaluating the effect of pharmaconutrition on postoperative clinical outcomes compared with standard nutritional provision highlight the importance of timing in the provision of immunonutrition.[28] Preoperative provision, as defined by 5–7 days prior to surgery, shows no advantage on outcomes over standard nutrition. However, perioperative and postoperative administration are associated with significantly reduced infectious complications and length of stay.

Additionally, perioperative administration was associated with significant reduction in anastomotic dehiscence and postoperative administration was associated with reduction in noninfectious complications. Perioperative nutrition was defined as 5–7 days before surgery plus postoperative day (POD) commencement via jejunal tube on POD 1–2 until POD 7 or until oral intake was established.

Postoperative nutrition was defined as pharmaconutrition commencement via jejunal tube on POD 1–2 until POD 7 or until oral intake was established.

17.3.2.3 ERAS Protocol (Enhanced Recovery after Surgery)

The ERAS program is an evidence-based, multimodal, and patient-centered approach to optimizing patient care and experience during perioperative care. This particular guideline consists of 23 items including preoperative counseling, preoperative carbohydrate loading, perioperative nutrition, avoidance of bowel preparation, no routine use of surgical drain, thromboembolism prophylaxis, antibiotic prophylaxis, minimally invasive approach, intraoperative fluid restriction, multimodal analgesia, prevention of hypothermia, early oral fluid and normal diet intake, glycemic control, prevention of delayed gastric emptying, stimulation of bowel movement, early mobilization, prevention of postoperative nausea and vomiting, fluid management, and systematic audit. Majority of the recommendations were based on evidence from colorectal surgery but has been found to be effective in many other surgeries.[27]

17.3.2.4 Dumping Syndrome

Partial or total gastrectomy and pancreaticoduodenectomy may disrupt gastric motility, resulting in delayed emptying or rapid transit of stomach contents into the small intestine, known as dumping syndrome. Removal or manipulation of the pyloric valve during surgery predisposes one to dumping syndrome. Early symptoms manifest as cramping, bloating, nausea, and diarrhea within 10–15 minutes of eating due to the influx of fluid into the small intestine in response to concentrated simple carbohydrates. Hypotension, weakness, and faintness may follow. Late symptoms of dumping syndrome occur 2–3 hours after eating when the sugar from the intestines is absorbed and the body's response to hyperglycemia is accelerated. Elevated insulin levels cause hypoglycemia. Symptoms include high heart rate, dizziness, shakiness, sweating, fainting, and confusion.[31, 32]

To prevent or manage the occurrence of postoperative dumping syndrome, follow these guidelines for 6–8 weeks:

- Eat slowly and chew foods thoroughly to liquefy the bolus since the digestive capability of the stomach is decreased or naught.
- Eat 6–8 small meals per day.
- Consume fluids 45 minutes before eating or 1 hour after eating, not with meals.
- Avoid raw fruits and vegetables and other fibrous foods, including whole grains, nuts, seeds, peas, and beans.
- Limit frui½o 1/2 cup cooked or canned at a time.
- Limit or avoid milk or milk products if unable to tolerate.
- Consume protein foods with each meal and snack.
- Avoid high-sugar foods such as fruit juice, sugar-sweetened beverages, honey, jam, jelly, molasses, ice cream, pudding, pastries, pies, cake, fruit ice, sherbet, and gelatin.
- Avoid foods that contain sugar, honey, corn syrup, fructose, lactose, dextrose, maltose, sorbitol, xylitol, or mannitol in the first 3 ingredients.[31]

17.3.2.5 Delayed Gastric Emptying

The presence of gastric and pancreatic tumors, duodenal ulcers, subtotal gastrectomy, Whipple procedure, and narcotic use are common etiologies for gastroparesis in the oncology setting. Symptoms include protracted nausea and vomiting, decreased appetite, bloating, fullness, early satiety, and alteration in glucose control. Oral diet manipulation includes small frequent meals, use of liquid calories, and avoidance of high-fiber and high-fat foods. Prokinetic and antiemetic agents should accompany diet modification. In cases of severe gastroparesis or when symptom management is unsuccessful, jejunal feeding should be considered to prevent malnutrition. When delayed emptying occurs as a result of gastrectomy, supplementation with vitamin B12, vitamin D, calcium, and a multivitamin with minerals should be considered.[33, 34]

Removing segments of the small intestine can alter digestion and absorption. Symptoms may include nausea, abdominal cramping, and diarrhea. Functional adaptation can occur; however, significant loss of small bowel may require PN support to maintain fluid and electrolyte balance. Diet guidelines for the first 4–6 weeks after small bowel surgery include the following:

- Eat small, frequent meals.
- Chew foods thoroughly.
- Consume protein with each meal or snack.
- Avoid high-fiber foods; limit total fiber to <20 g per day.

After 4–6 weeks, add new foods back to the diet one at a time and assess for tolerance prior to continuing transition to regular diet.[35] If short bowel syndrome (SBS) is severe, more extensive nutrition support may be required.

17.3.2.6 Ostomy Placement

Diversion of fecal transit may be required temporarily or permanently for management of bowel obstruction or removal of GI malignancy. A colostomy is performed when it is necessary to bypass or remove the distal colon, rectum, or anus. Removal of the colon typically requires minimal diet modification (except for ascending colostomy, covered below). Sufficient fiber and fluid can prevent constipation. In cases of loose stool, thickening foods may be beneficial. Similarly, reducing gaseous and odorous foods may be advised.[36]

Removal or bypass of the entire colon and rectum requires an ileostomy. High fluid output can cause dehydration and electrolyte imbalance for patients with ileostomies and ascending colostomies.

Also, risk of stoma blockage exists because the ileal lumen is <1 inch in diameter. Large amounts of insoluble fibers should be avoided. Follow these guidelines for nutritional management status post-ileostomy placement[36]:

- Eat small frequent meals.
- Chew foods well to prevent foods from causing a blockage or obstruction as stool exits the ileostomy.
- Stay hydrated. Do not attempt to control diarrhea by restricting fluids. Monitor ostomy output and consume 1 L fluid in addition to output volume.
- Avoid fiber. Avoid stringy vegetables, foods with skins, and dried fruits. Limit foods to those with 2 g or less of fiber per serving.
- Choose low-fat foods. Avoid meats with casings.
- Avoid simple sugars (sweetened beverages and sugary foods).

After 6–8 weeks, add new foods back to the diet one at a time and assess for tolerance prior to continuing transition to regular diet.

17.3.2.7 Fat Maldigestion

Fat maldigestion can occur following GI surgeries and in the presence of GI malignancies. Following gastrectomy, accelerated transit of food into the small intestine can prevent adequate mixing of food contents with bile salts and digestive enzymes. Additionally, large food particles entering the small intestine may impair adequate degradation by enzymes. Alternatively, pancreatic exocrine insufficiency (PEI) may accompany a diagnosis of pancreatic cancer or bile duct blockage or may occur during nonsurgical treatment and/or following Whipple surgery. PEI can be ruled in by measuring pancreatic elastase. In cases of PEI, pancreatic enzyme replacement and fat-soluble vitamin supplementation may be warranted.[31]

17.3.2.8 Short Bowel Syndrome

Surgical resection of the small bowel leaving <200 cm is termed short bowel syndrome. Initially, PN and or EN will be necessary to achieve adequate nutritional provision, but over approximately 2 years, the remaining gut adapts, whereby the surface area and absorptive capacity of the small bowel increases. Loss of the terminal ileum and the ileal break mechanism results in gastric hypersecretion and accelerated transit. Without the terminal ileum, the site for bile salt reabsorption, bile salts enter the colon and cause choleric diarrhea. Cholestyramine can be helpful if <100 cm of distal ileum is resected, and the colon is intact, but should be avoided if >100 cm of terminal ileum is resected. Antimotility agents such as loperamide, diphenoxylate, and opiates can be used to slow transit and should be administered 30 minutes before meals.[35]

Patients with SBS are at risk for deficiency of fat-soluble vitamins, vitamin B12, and magnesium.

Supplementation with a liquid or chewable vitamin/mineral supplement should be considered.

Bowel adaptation occurs with macronutrient exposure. Whole food and/or use of a polymeric formula maximizes intestinal stimulation. Semi elemental EN formulas can be considered if needed, but elemental formulas should be avoided because they are hypertonic. PN may be required to maintain electrolyte and fluid balance. Oral diet guidelines for patients with SBS include the following[32]:

- Macronutrient composition should be 20%–30% carbohydrate, 20%–30% protein, and 50%–60% fat for patients with jejunostomies/ileostomies.
- Macronutrient composition should be 50%–60% carbohydrate, 20%–30% protein, and 20%–30% fat for patients with intact colon.
- Avoid concentrated sweets/fluids.
- Chew foods well.
- Limit fluids with meals and drink isotonic beverages.

Recently, development of a unique intestinal growth hormone, teduglutide, has helped many patients get off PN dependency.[36]

17.3.2.9 Obstruction

Mechanical obstruction of the small bowel can occur from adhesions from previous abdominal GI surgeries or from the presence of gastrointestinal tumors. Colonic pseudo-obstruction can develop from narcotic use and lead to significant constipation. Symptoms of obstruction include nausea, vomiting, abdominal pain, abdominal distention, and inability to pass flatus or stool.[33] Nutritional management for partial small bowel obstruction includes liquid oral nutrition drink supplements and foods that are moist and soft. For partial colonic obstruction, a very low-fiber diet and stool softeners are recommended. Complete bowel obstruction warrants nil per os (NPO) to limit bowel distension. In the presence of weight loss and/or malnutrition, or anticipation of prolonged NPO, PN should be initiated. In some patients with chronic obstruction, PN is required long term. For patients in whom surgical intervention is appropriate, refer to the "Surgical Management" section of this chapter. A venting gastrostomy tube is found to be effective in reducing obstructive symptoms and helps palliation in terminally ill patients.

17.3.2.10 Small Intestinal Bacterial Overgrowth

Small intestinal bacterial overgrowth (SIBO) is a condition in which mostly anaerobic bacteria colonize the small intestine in larger than normal quantities, causing symptoms of gas, bloating, abdominal distention, diarrhea, and weight loss. SIBO should be suspected in GI cancer patients with gastroparesis, impaired peristalsis, removal of the ileocecal valve, PEI, stricture/obstruction/adhesion of the GI tract, gastrocolic fistula, surgical blind loops, intestinal pseudo-obstruction, and/or hypochlorhydria/achlorhydria.[34, 37] SIBO is diagnosed by an ileal aspirate and culture; however, the practice of empirically treating patients for SIBO without diagnostic confirmation is not uncommon.[34]

Treatment includes antibiotic therapy and dietary manipulation. Since carbohydrates are fermented by bacteria and fermentation in the small bowel can contribute to symptoms, the diet should be modified to reduced carbohydrate and fiber. Fat should be substituted for carbohydrates to supply adequate calories and reduce the production of gas and bloating.[37] Nutrients of concern requiring monitoring include calcium, magnesium, iron, vitamin B12, and fat-soluble vitamins.[34]

17.3.2.11 Fistulas

A fistula is an abnormal passageway or connection between two organs or structures. Enteric fistulas are connections of the small intestine/bowel with other abdominal organs or with the chest or skin.

They are named by the originating segment of bowel (gastro-, duodeno-, entero-, jejuno-, ileo-, colo-, recto-) and the point of termination (-cutaneous, -enteric, -colonic, -rectal, -vesical, -vaginal, -aortic).

Etiologies include distal obstruction, radiation, and infection and can occur from the presence of tumors and from injury during surgery.[35] Malnutrition preoperatively increases the risk of fistula development.

Fistulas requiring nutritional management include those that have a high output of fluid and nutrients (a high-output fistula drains more than 500 mL/day) or increased output stimulated by PO intake that prevents the fistula from closing. In either case, NPO may be indicated and PN will be necessary. Patients with high-output fistulas who are not on PN may require extra vitamin/mineral supplementation.[35] When output is <500 mL/day, enteral feeding may be possible; feeding proximal to the fistula enhances absorptive area. Fiber-free formulas or diets should be used when the fistula is distal and fiber-containing products or diets can be used when the fistula is proximal to the site of feeding entry.[35]

17.3.2.12 Summary

GI cancers pose nutritional challenges that require a knowledgeable dietitian and team of providers.

The functions of digestion and absorption may be altered or severely compromised; in many cases, multimodal treatment requires medical therapy and dietary modification or nutrition support to prevent or reverse malnutrition. Nutrition support or supplemental nutrition individualized by a dietitian is necessary for optimal management of GI cancer patients.

17.4 BREAST CANCER

17.4.1 INTRODUCTION

17.4.1.1 Statistics/Survival

Breast cancer remains the most diagnosed cancer in women, and the second leading cause of cancer death in women in the United States. Between 2010 and 2019, breast cancer occurrence rates increased for all ethnic groups. Asian and Pacific Islanders had the largest increase at 2.1%, with Caucasian women experiencing an 0.5% increase and a 0.7% increase among African American women. Death rates from breast cancer decreased by 43% from 1989 to 2020 related to advances in early diagnosis and treatment. For all women, 5-year survival is 99% for women with local disease (stages 0 and I, some stage II), 87% for regional disease (stage II and some stage III), and 30% for advanced disease (stage IIIc and stage IV).[36]

17.4.1.2 Subtypes

Subtypes of breast cancer are determined by the presence of biological markers or receptors present on tumor cells. Pathologists classify a breast tumor as estrogen receptor (ER) positive or negative, progesterone receptor (PR) positive or negative, as well as human epidermal growth factor 2 (HER2neu) positive or negative through the examination of tissue biopsied or excised.

Tumors identified as ER positive and/or PR positive are generally less aggressive and less responsive to chemotherapy. Typically, these tumors respond to hormonal therapies. HER2 positive tumors are often more aggressive than HER2 negative tumors. Women diagnosed with triple negative tumors (no ER, PR, or HER2 receptors on the tumor cell) unfortunately have a poorer short-term prognosis, in part related to the lack of specific therapies toward this tumor type.[36] Triple negative cancers are in general more responsive to chemotherapy.

17.4.1.3 Lifestyle Risk Factors

Lifestyle factors that increase the risk of breast cancer include weight gain after age 18, excess body fat (related to postmenopausal breast cancer), and alcohol. Physical activity and breastfeeding have been shown to reduce risk.[38]

17.4.1.3.1 Weight

Obesity has also been strongly correlated with the risk of postmenopausal breast cancer. In addition, overweight and obesity status at diagnosis increases the risk of recurrence and adversely impacts breast cancer and all-cause mortality. Data have shown this obesity effect regardless of stage, treatment, and menopausal status. Molecular studies have shown that adipocytes interact with cancer cells to impair ability to mitigate insulin resistance as well as upregulate estrogen production.[39] Further, weight gain through breast cancer treatment is correlated with poor prognosis. In one study, a >10% weight gain after diagnosis was associated with increased mortality.[37]

Unfortunately, a breast cancer event increases a woman's risk of weight gain. Recent studies have shown an average weight gain of 5–14 pounds.[40] In the HEAL study of breast cancer survivors, 68% of women gained weight, and 74% gained body fat and maintained that gain at 3 years from diagnosis.[41]

Weight gain after diagnosis is most related to chemotherapy, compared to radiation and hormonal therapy. Premenopausal status and decreased physical activity levels appear to be the most impactful variables contributing to weight gain after breast cancer.[42]

Research has suggested that it may be beneficial for women to focus on healthy weight loss during treatment, which is much different from other cancer types.[40, 43] Clinicians are encouraged to guide women toward appropriate dietary and physical activity goals.

17.4.1.3.2 Physical Activity

The benefits of adequate physical activity for health cannot be understated. The Nurse's Health

Study documented in a cohort of 2,987 women diagnosed with breast cancer stages I–III who achieved 3–5 hours of walking per week (>3 metabolic equivalent task-hours per week, MET-h/week) reduced their risk of dying from breast cancer by half. The Collaborative Women's Longevity Study (CWLS) followed 4,400 American women ages 20–79 beginning at breast cancer diagnosis for 6 years and noted that women with >2.9 MET-h/week had a reduced risk of breast cancer and all-cause mortality. Results showed that increased physical activity consistently provided a survival benefit regardless of age, stage of breast cancer, and BMI.[42]

17.4.1.3.3 Diet

The World Cancer Research Foundation and the American Institute for Cancer Research (WCRF/AICR) have published comprehensive reports on the evidence linking diet and lifestyle to cancer.

Their general cancer recommendations are to follow a plant-based diet rich in vegetables, fruits, whole grains, beans, and limited in red and processed meats, high-calorie and high-sugar foods, and alcohol.

While no specific nutrients or foods (other than alcohol) are consistently linked to breast cancer risk, two large-scale trials reviewed diet changes and risk of breast cancer recurrence. Specifically, the Women's Healthy Eating and Living (WHEL) trial implemented a low-fat (goal 15%–20% dietary fat) and increased fruit and vegetable regimen (3 fruit and 5 vegetable servings daily).

Women in the intervention group were successful in increasing produce intake to goal and reducing dietary fat from 28% to 21% on average (did not meet target).

No significant benefit of this intervention was found in relation to breast cancer recurrence after 7 years.[44]

The Women's Intervention Nutrition Study (WINS) focused specifically on reducing fat intake to 15%–20% of diet to decrease risk of breast cancer recurrence. Women were able to meet the goal of 20% dietary fat or less. This trial of nearly 2,500 women, begun in 1987, did find a significant reduction in recurrent breast cancer.[43] However, a large percentage of women also experienced weight loss. Therefore, it is not possible to determine if diet change or weight loss or the combination most impacted the risk reduction noted in this study. However, both diet and maintaining a healthy weight are advantageous for breast cancer survivors, who are also at risk for cardiovascular disease.

17.4.1.3.4 Alcohol

The AICR found convincing dose–response evidence that alcohol intake is a risk factor for cancer. One standard drink per day increased breast cancer risk by 10%.[38] There are several specific mechanisms by which alcohol causes cell damage. Firstly, alcohol influences estrogen breakdown and effects, and persons who heavily consume alcohol may have nutrient-poor diets. Secondly, the detoxification of alcohol produces carcinogens and free radicals, and alcohol enhances the absorption of free radicals into cells. Finally, increased folate intake may partially reduce the risk of alcohol damage.

17.4.1.3.5 Omega-3 Fatty Acids

In vitro and animal studies elucidated several mechanisms by which eicosapentanoic acid and docosahexanoic acid may inhibit breast cancer by reducing inflammation.[45] Research in humans has been inconsistent but promising; more large-scale studies are needed. One report from the WHEL study noted that food intake of 73 mg EPA daily provided a 25% reduced risk of breast cancer recurrence, but this has not been replicated.[46] A recent meta-analysis showed that only 3 of 14 studies showed statistically significant reduction in breast cancer risk.[47] It is appropriate to recommend two to three servings of oily fish per week. It is important to note that flax seed oil primarily contains alpha-linolenic acid (ALA), and only 5%–10% of ALA is converted to EPA and DHA by the liver, therefore limiting effective vegan options to increase intake of EPA/DHA.

17.4.1.3.6 Phytoestrogens

Soy foods contain phytoestrogens from isoflavone components. In the past, there was concern about phytoestrogen intake promoting ER+ breast tumor growth. Soy foods are recommended for children and adolescents to reduce breast cancer risk.[48] Further studies have shown no detriment to the intake of soy food up to three servings daily for breast cancer survivors, and potential benefit on the effectiveness of tamoxifen.[49, 50]

It is prudent to recommend whole food sources of soy such as tofu, soy milk, soy nuts, tempeh, or miso because one serving provides 30 mg isoflavones. The isoflavone content of processed soy protein powders or soy isoflavone supplements may exceed the daily recommended limit of 100 mg. Soy foods that do not contain soy protein, such as soybean oils or soy sauce, do not contain isoflavones.

Other foods such as legumes, nuts, and some fruits do contain minute amounts of isoflavones.

However, the quantity is measured in micrograms (mcg), making it unlikely to approach the daily limit of 100 mg with diet alone.

17.4.1.3.7 Cruciferous Vegetables

Vegetables from the Brassica family have been investigated for their content of glucosinolates, including indole-3-carbinol. This phytochemical participates in liver detoxification and is involved in the breakdown of estrogen. In vitro studies have shown antiapoptotic and antiangiogenetic effects.[51] Large-scale human studies have not been carried out to review the effects of increased consumption of cruciferous vegetables on breast cancer risk. However, increasing consumption is obviously part of a plant-based diet.

17.4.1.3.8 Lignans

Lignans are present in nearly all plant foods such as grains, vegetables, seeds, tea, and coffee, but flax seeds are the most significant source. Lignans are phytoestrogens, which have been proposed to have protective effects for breast cancer. These compounds have been investigated for anticancer effects, and benefit has been seen in vitro and in rodent studies. Human data have been mixed, with one study of over 1,200 women showing lower risk of aggressive breast tumors, and another of nearly 335,000 women not showing any relationship between dietary lignans and breast cancer risk over 11.5 years.[52, 53]

17.4.1.3.9 Green Tea

While all tea is a source of antioxidants, green tea is specifically noted for its catechin content, specifically epigallocatechin-3-gallate (EGCG). It is known that tea catechins have antioxidant, antiangiogenic, anti-inflammatory, and antiproliferative actions in the body. As yet, data relating green tea to breast cancer are limited to in vitro and epidemiological evidence only. Some observational studies have linked a higher intake of green tea to a reduced risk of breast cancer while others have shown no effect. A cohort from the Sister Study looked at over 45,000 siblings of women with breast cancer. This study found it beneficial to drink 5 cups of black or green tea weekly to reduce risk of breast cancer.[44]

17.4.1.4 Energy and Protein Requirements

Typical energy requirements are between 25 and 30 kcal/kg actual weight and protein requirements vary 1–1.5 g/kg for normal women.[54]

17.4.1.4.1 Survivorship Considerations

The cardiotoxicity of breast cancer therapies is well established, and is a concern in patients who now survive decades after completing treatment. Patnaik et al. found that in older breast cancer survivors, cardiovascular disease surpassed breast cancer recurrence as cause of mortality.[55] It remains the number one cause of death for US women. This highlights the value of a plant-based, low-fat diet and physical activity for breast cancer survivors, in addition to reducing use of tobacco and alcohol.

Bone health is an important focus for this population due to the adverse effects on bone related to chemotherapy and aromatase inhibitor therapies.[46] Women should consume adequate calcium and vitamin D from food or supplements as indicated by the Dietary Reference Intakes (DRI).

Although a 25-hydroxyvitamin D (25(OH)D) level of >20 ng/mL is appropriate for bone health, some researchers have suggested that the most beneficial level of 25(OH)D for breast cancer risk is between 40 and 60 ng/dL.[46, 48] This topic remains controversial, but it is valuable to assess serum vitamin D status in this population to assure adequate levels, minimally for bone health.

Dietary Reference Intakes for Bone Health			
Age	**Calcium**	**Age**	**Vitamin D**
19–50 years	1000 mg/day	19–70 years	600 IU[a]/day
51+ years	1200 mg/day	71+ years	800 IU/day

Source: Institute of Medicine (US) Committee to Review Dietary Reference Intakes for Vitamin D and Calcium; In: Ross AC et al. eds. *Dietary Reference Intakes for Calcium and Vitamin D.* Washington (DC): National Academies Press (US); 2011.

[a] International units.[56]

Vitamin D has been investigated in the last few decades for anticancer benefits. While research is ongoing, potential mechanisms include induction of cell differentiation and apoptosis, inhibition of abnormal cell proliferation, and tumor angiogenesis.

17.4.2 Treatment Options

17.4.2.1 Surgery

The most common surgical interventions are lumpectomy, mastectomy, and breast reconstruction.

While there are no nutrition-related side effects, it is recommended to ensure that the daily protein needs of 1–1.2 g/kg are met.

17.4.2.2 Chemotherapy

Chemotherapy was traditionally given in the breast cancer population as an adjuvant treatment, that is, after a surgical procedure to remove the tumor. However, it is increasingly employed as a neoadjuvant therapy to assess the tumor's response to the treatment, reduce the quantity of tissue resected, and target any cells outside the immediate breast region.

Side effects of chemotherapy vary based on type of drug, dose, and single- versus multiple-agent therapy; frequency of treatment; and individual differences. See Appendices 1 and 2 for specific interventions related to each drug or symptom.

Common therapeutic drugs used for breast cancer:

- Capecitabine (Xeloda)
- Carboplatin (Paraplatin)

- Cyclophosphamide (Cytoxan)
- Docetaxel (Taxotere)
- Doxorubicin (Adriamycin)
- Epirubicin (Ellence)
- Eribulin (Halaven)
- Fluorouracil (5-FU)
- Gemcitabine (Gemzar)
- Ixabepilone (Ixempra)
- Methotrexate (MTX)
- Paclitaxel (Taxol)
- Paclitaxel albumin-stabilized nanoparticle formulation (Abraxane)
- Vinorelbine (Navelbine)

Common multiple-agent chemotherapy regimen acronyms used in breast cancer:

- TAC (Taxotere/Adriamycin/Cytoxan)
- A/C, then T (Adriamycin/Cytoxan, usually followed by Taxol)
- THP (Taxotere/Herceptin/Perjeta)
- TCHP (Taxotere/Cytoxan/Herceptin/Perjeta)[57]

17.4.2.3 Endocrine Therapy

Common Side Effects of Common Endocrine Therapies		
Treatment	Nutrition-Related Side Effect	Nutrition Recommendations
Tamoxifen (Nolvadex)	Mild nausea	Take with a glass of water
Anastrozole (Arimidex)	Mild nausea	
Exemestane (Aromasin)	Mild nausea, abdominal pain	Take with food
Letrozole (Femara)	Nausea, weight gain	May elevate cholesterol levels
Fulvestrant (Faslodex)	Nausea, vomiting, diarrhea, constipation	
Leuprolide (Lupron)	None	
Goserelin (Zoladex)	None	

17.4.2.4 Monoclonal Antibodies

Common Side Effects of Biologic Agents		
Agent	Nutrition-Related Side Effect	Nutrition Recommendations
Pertuzumab (Perjeta)	Nausea, diarrhea, mucositis	
Lapatinib (Tykerb)	Nausea, vomiting, diarrhea	Take 1 hour before, or 1 hour after eating; no grapefruit juice
Everolimus (Afinitor)	Mucositis, diarrhea	Take with water, with or without food; monitor serum lipids
Trastuzumab (Herceptin)	Diarrhea	
Pembrolizumab (Keytruda)	Nausea, vomiting, diarrhea (colitis), anorexia	
Fam-trastuzumab deruxtecan-nxki (Enhertu)	Diarrhea[58]	

17.4.2.5 Radiation Therapy

Common Radiation Treatment Areas in Breast Cancer

Area of Body	Nutrition-Related Side Effect	Nutrition Recommendations
Breast/chest wall	Minimal	Protein intake 1–1.2 g/kg daily
Intraoperative radiation	None	None therapy (IORT)
Brain	Potential nausea/vomiting, hyperglycemia	Monitor blood glucose levels
Hip/spine	Minimal	None

17.4.3 NUTRITION INTERVENTION SUMMARY

Dietitians are most frequently called upon in this population to manage nutrition impact symptoms during chemotherapy, provide counseling and support, and guide food choices. In the survivorship phase, dietitians remain indispensable to help patients implement a plant-based, heart-healthy diet and work toward weight loss, if indicated. Finally, dietitians can encourage weight-bearing exercise and assure adequate calcium and vitamin D intake to reduce the risk of osteoporosis.

17.5 ESOPHAGEAL, HEAD, AND NECK CANCERS

17.5.1 INTRODUCTION

Cancers of the esophagus (EC) or head and neck are often very distressing due to the potential impairment of speech, swallowing, and breathing, and frequent effects on the patient's physical appearance and social functioning.[57] Patients with these cancers have one of the highest rates of malnutrition, with 25%–50% of these patients identified as nutritionally compromised prior to diagnosis or treatment, and nutrition status is likely to worsen with treatment initiation. [57, 59] Significant weight loss and malnutrition are indicative of poor prognosis and are associated with decreased physical functioning and quality of life, and may reduce response to treatment or cause treatment delay, which may result in shorter periods of remission and increase mortality.[60, 61] Early assessment and management by an RD and speech and language pathologist (SLP) along with effective symptom management are imperative to achieve best nutrition and quality of life outcomes.[62] EC is the eighth most common cancer in the world and its prevalence continues to rise in the United States. EC is commonly classified into two types: squamous cell carcinomas (SCC), and adenocarcinomas of the esophagus (AE).[60] In 2022, approximately 19,000 new cases of EC were diagnosed and deaths reported. Early diagnosis, localized stage, and early treatment intervention can improve outcome and more than double survival. The 5-year survival for all cases of EC is 19%.[61] Head and neck cancers (HNCs) account for 3% of all cancer cases in the United States. In 2022, there were 48,000 new cases of HNC diagnosed in US.[59] Five main types of HNC exist in the United States, including oral and oropharyngeal cancer, salivary gland cancer, laryngeal and hypopharyngeal cancer, nasopharyngeal cancer, and nasal cavity and paranasal sinus cancer.

Early detection increases the chance of survival. Five-year survival rates for HNC are approximately 90% when detected and treated while in early stages 1 and 2, but are much lower in advanced-stage disease.[60]

17.5.2 RISK FACTORS

Both EC and HNC are most diagnosed in males. EC cases are three to four times more common in men than women, and the median age of diagnosis is 67 years.[61] The most notable and modifiable risk factors for EC, and HNC (oral cavity, oropharynx, hypopharynx, and larynx) are smoking and alcohol consumption. It has been reported that at least 75% of HNCs are caused by human papilloma virus (HPV) or tobacco and alcohol use and that most cases of EC are preventable by appropriate diet and avoidance of the associated risk factors. HPV vaccination has been shown to help prevent HNC.[58, 63] Salivary cancer is an exception: older age and exposure to radiation and toxins, particularly asbestos, in the workplace are common risk factors. Infection from *Helicobacter pylori* is also a risk factor for SCC of the esophagus.[64] The Centers for Disease Control (CDC) reported that more than 2,370 cases of HPV-associated oropharyngeal cancers are diagnosed in women and nearly 9,360 cases in men each year in the United States.[64] Esophageal achalasia, an esophageal motility disorder, also increases risk of EC. Infection with Epstein–Barr virus has also been identified as a risk factor for nasopharynx and salivary gland cancer.[38]

Gastroesophageal reflux disease (GERD) is a primary risk factor for AE due to the damage that occurs to the esophageal tissue from the gastric acids. GERD also increases the risk of developing Barrett's esophagus, which is associated with a 30–60-fold increase in the risk of AE.[58] Recent studies have identified that obesity (classified as BMI >40 kg/m^2) elevates the risk of esophageal adenocarcinoma independent of other risk factors, especially in males, and even more prevalent when BMI >40 and GERD exist together.[65]

As mentioned, alcohol intake and tobacco usage are the greatest risk factors, although there is some evidence to support that consumption of processed meats, red meats, and certain preserved or salted foods may increase risk of HNCs and ECs.[38]

17.5.3 SYMPTOMS AND SUPPORT

The most common symptoms of HNCs are a nonhealing lump or sore, a sore throat that does not go away, swallowing difficulty (dysphagia), and a change or hoarseness of the voice.[66] Unfortunately, symptoms of EC do not usually occur until the disease is developing into a more advanced stage.

When symptoms do occur, patients often experience dysphagia, heartburn-like symptoms, pain, hoarseness, coughing, anorexia, and unintentional weight loss.[67, 68]

17.5.3.1 AICR Guidelines and Diet Recommendations for Prevention

There are a few studies that show that regular consumption of non-starchy vegetables, fruits, and carotenoid-rich foods may have the potential to protect against HNC and EC. Foods containing vitamin C, fiber, folate, pyridoxine, and vitamin E may also provide protection.[68]

17.5.3.2 Estimated Energy and Nutrient Requirements

It is generally acknowledged that the energy expenditure (EE) for most cancer patients is increased, although some recent studies demonstrate that EE may vary between various cancer diagnoses.

A small study estimated energy requirements of EC patients between 30 and 35 kcal/kg, which is consistent with the usual recommendations for nutrition repletion for oncology patients.[69]

Energy needs for obese patients are recommended at 21–25 kcal/kg actual body weight.[70] Protein requirements, assuming normal renal function, range between 1 and 1.5 g/kg for stable, non-stressed patients, and 1.5 and 2.0 g/kg for stressed or nutritionally compromised patients.[71] Fluid needs are typical of other patients without heart failure or renal impairment at 30–35 mL/kg, although may be higher in patients experiencing GI losses or drains. It is recommended that HNC and EC patients take a vitamin and mineral supplement to meet 100% of the DRI, particularly being mindful that many of these patients' oral intakes may have been inadequate for some time related to symptoms or lifestyle that may have included excessive alcohol consumption prior to diagnosis.[72, 73]

17.5.3.3 Nutrition Support

Dysphagia and weight loss are the most common nutrition impact symptoms in EC and are present in over 70% of patients diagnosed worldwide.[74] Despite aggressive nutrition interventions, including diet modifications, oral nutrition supplementation, symptom management, and medication management, oral intakes may not sustain nutritional status throughout aggressive chemotherapy and/or radiation therapy, and may require EN via a percutaneous endoscopic gastrostomy (PEG) tube or jejunostomy tube (J-tube). Temporary feeding tubes will also be placed after surgical resections from glossectomy, esophagectomy, base of tongue or pharynx tumor excisions, and tracheostomy.

Prophylactic feeding tubes remain controversial but have resulted in fewer hospital admissions for dehydration and malnutrition, fewer treatment interruptions, and/or delays, and maintain a higher quality of life during treatment when compared to patients solely relying on oral intakes.[75] Nutrition assessment is recommended for patients prior to treatment and frequent reassessments throughout treatment to ensure appropriate nutrition intervention are in place to prevent further nutrition decline or treatment delay. Modifications to enteral feeding formulas, schedules, water flushes, or addition of motility agents may be needed as treatment continues and requires frequent monitoring.

Close follow-up after completion of therapy is essential to help avoid long-term dependence on enteral feedings and to support the transition back to an oral diet.[76]

17.5.4 Treatment Options

Treatment for EC and HNC often include esophageal dilation, chemotherapy, radiation therapy, chemoradiation (CRT), cryotherapy, targeted therapy, and surgery.[66, 77, 78, 79] Treatment options will be determined by the patient and physician and often depends on tumor stage, size and location, primary subtype, metastasis of tumor (if present), and patient's overall health and other comorbidities.

17.5.4.1 Chemotherapy and Nutrition

Chemotherapy may be used alone or as either neoadjuvant (before) or adjuvant (after) therapy in combination with radiation or surgery. Advances in chemoradiation have led to increased survival and local and regional tumor control for patients with EC and HNC, but often cause significant toxicity to the patient.[80] The following is a list of common chemotherapeutic drugs commonly used to treat EC and HNC. See Appendix 1 for specific interventions related to each drug or symptom.

Common chemotherapeutic drugs used in EC and HNC:

- Bevacizumab (Avastin®)
- Cetuximab (Erbitux®)
- Cisplatin (as single-agent or combined modality) with 5-Fluorouracil (5-FU®) or capecitabine (Xeloda®) • Capecitabine (Xeloda)
- Oxaliplatin and either 5-FU or capecitabine
- ECF: Epirubicin (Ellence®), cisplatin, and 5-FU
- DCF: Docetaxel (Taxotere®), cisplatin, and 5-FU
- Carboplatin and paclitaxel (Taxol®)

Other chemotherapy or targeted therapy drugs that have been used in these cancers:

- Doxorubicin (Adriamycin®)
- Bleomycin
- Mitomycin
- Vinorelbine (Navelbine®)
- Topotecan
- Ifosafamide
- Irinotecan (Camptosar®)
- Trastuzumab (Herceptin®)

17.5.4.2 Radiation Therapy and Nutrition

Radiation therapy acts by directing X-rays to cancerous cells or regions to cause DNA damage, inhibiting the cells' ability to replicate. Rapidly dividing cells are the most susceptible to radiation damage, such as the lining of the oral and gut mucosa and blood and hair cells.[78] Radiation may be used alone or combined with chemotherapy. It may also be given preoperatively in an attempt to shrink tumors or postoperatively to help ensure that tumor bed and surrounding margins or lymph nodes are clear of disease. The goal of therapy is to eradicate tumor cells while minimizing damage to healthy tissues. The amount of radiation a patient receives is measured in gray (Gy) and the number of treatments a person receives is referenced in fractions (fx). Radiation has a cumulative effect which means that side effects continue to worsen with each additional fraction received, with most side effects starting between 10 and 15 fractions (after 2–3 weeks of treatment) and intensifying throughout the remainder of therapy. A common treatment for EC and HNC may include CRT, 2.0 per fraction to 70 Gy in 7 weeks with single-agent cisplatin given every 1–3 weeks.[81] The following section is a list of potential side effects from radiation therapy and nutrition management. Radiation may also exacerbate tooth decay and patients may be required to have previously damaged teeth removed prior to therapy. Late side effects may occur months or even years after completion of therapy.

Owing to the rapid decline in nutritional status that can occur during radiation to the head and neck or esophagus and the potential need for alternative nutrition, close monitoring throughout the entire course of therapy and recovery is strongly recommended.

Common Side Effects of Common Radiation Treatments

Nutrition-Related Side Effect	Nutrition Recommendations
Xerostomia/thick saliva	Eat small frequent meals.
	Alternate bites and sips at meals.
	Add extra sauces, gravy, and broths to foods.
	Maintain adequate hydration, sip throughout the day. Suck on hard candies, frozen fruits. Chew sugar-free gum.
	Avoid alcohol, caffeine, acidic, or spicy foods.
	Use a humidifier at home to help moisten the air.
Trismus	Eat slowly with small bites of food.
	Modify food textures to optimize intake.
	Use oral nutrition supplements.
	Follow aspiration precautions.
	SLP consult
Oral candidiasis	Practice good oral hygiene.
	Choose soft-textured, low-acid foods.
	Avoid sugar or yeast-derived foods. May try 1 tbsp yogurt held in mouth, 5 minutes daily.

17.5.4.3 Surgery and Nutrition

The goal of surgery is to remove the tumor with a margin of healthy tissue. If the cancer has spread, some surrounding lymph nodes may also need to be removed. Surgeries to treat EC or HNC will commonly result in swallowing difficulties, dependent on the degree and site of the resection. Side effects of surgery may also include pain, swelling, structural deformities such as tooth loss or hemiglossectomy (partial removal of the tongue), or tracheostomy, which may make it difficult to chew or swallow after surgery and potentially limit oral intakes.[72] EC patients eligible for surgery commonly undergo either esophagectomy or esophagogastrectomy with jejunostomy tube placement.

Data show that intensive nutrition support provided by an RD is associated with weight maintenance and fewer postoperative complications in these patients.[70, 82] Frequent monitoring by an SLP is also recommended to assist in preservation and/ or regaining of muscle function to the affected areas. Potential side effects of these surgeries are listed in Table 17.3.

TABLE 17.3

Common Side Effects to Common Surgical Procedures

Treatment	Nutrition-Related Side Effect	Enteral Nutrition	Oral Nutrition Recommendations
Esophagectomy or Esophagogastrectomy	Dumping syndrome (early or late)	Temporary jejunostomy tube *See feeding recommendations.	**Anti-Dumping Diet** • Limit foods in concentrated sugars. • Limit fats and fried, greasy foods. • Increase soluble fiber foods. • Drink liquids 30 minutes before/after meals. • Eat 5–6 small frequent meals • Eat slowly.
	Reflux		Eat small frequent meals. Anti-reflux diet.
	Esophagus or gastric dysmotility		Low-fat, low-fiber diet is recommended for dysmotility, and possible initiation of motility agents.
	Early satiety		Eat 5–6 small frequent meals. Choose carbohydrate- and protein-dense foods. Use oral supplements between meals to help meet needs and prevent weight loss.
Tracheostomy		Gastrostomy tube (PEG tube) with or without ability to take oral intakes. *See feeding recommendations.	**SLP therapy** When determined to have safe swallowing function, often patients will be able to tolerate liquids and soft foods, and occasionally solids. Monitor for ability to wean EN.
Glossectomy – full or partial		Temporary nasogastric tube or PEG tube *See feeding recommendations.	**SLP therapy** Once safe swallow function established, diet will start with variety of viscous liquids, then slowly advance to soft/semi-solid foods as tolerated.

*Recommended enteral jejunostomy feedings post-esophagectomy/esophagogastrectomy:

Early initiation of feedings with a full-strength isotonic polymeric formula is recommended, 1 vs. 1.5 kcal/mL based on patient needs. Typically, feedings start at 24 hours continuously, then transition to nocturnal feedings to help optimize oral feedings, once diet is advanced. If a standard formula is not tolerated, then transition to semi-elemental or elemental formula is recommended. These formulas are typically reserved for patients with small bowel dysfunction or malabsorption.

*Recommended enteral feedings for gastrostomy tubes post-tracheostomy, glossectomy, or chemotherapy and radiation:

Use full-strength standard formula, typically 1.5–2.0 kcal/mL, but individually selected based on patient's energy needs. Bolus feeding, typically 3–4 times per day, is preferred to help simulate regular mealtimes and is usually well tolerated. If a patient is unable to tolerate bolus feedings, then transitioning to gravity feeding bags or even a feeding pump is indicated. Regardless of tube type, it is important to provide adequate hydration via water flushes to meet hydration needs, because many of these patients are temporarily unable to take oral intake. Use of modulars such as protein or fiber powders may be indicated to meet nutrient needs or aid in symptom management.

17.5.4.3.1   Diet

Patients with EC and HNC are at increased risk for malnutrition and cachexia requiring a high-calorie, high-protein diet and frequent supplementation with oral nutrition beverages. Diet modifications are often required to help support patients throughout chemotherapy and radiation therapy due to multiple nutrition impact symptoms or alterations to the GI tract as a result of surgical alteration or tumor obstruction. The RD will help direct patients toward appropriate texture modifications, nutrient-dense food and liquids, and adequate hydration, and adjust timing of meals and snacks to maximize intake.

17.5.4.3.2   Medications and Supplements Commonly Used

Patients may require a variety of medications to achieve optimal symptom management throughout therapy, including antiemetics, acid reflux and pain medications, stool softeners, antimotility agents, and soothing mouth rinses. Ensuring appropriate medication administration and tolerance is imperative in this population because many of these patients suffer from dysphagia and may need medications modified to liquid or patch forms when available, or even administered through feeding tubes. It is important to review medications carefully because some drugs are not safe to crush and alternatives may need to be prescribed.

Glutamine is an amino acid that is used by rapidly dividing cells and has been shown to help protect the upper and lower GI tract mucosa from harmful effects of chemotherapy and radiation therapy. Multiple studies have proven the benefit in reduction of severity and duration of oral mucositis and esophagitis.[74] There are some concerns that glutamine might stimulate tumor growth, and therefore, negatively impact the outcomes of anticancer treatment, although studies showing this are very limited (in vitro) and further evaluation is needed.[75] Typical dosing for glutamine during radiation therapy provides 10 g three times daily, mixed into 3–4 ounces of a liquid, usually juice or water, or even applesauce or yogurt.

Oral nutrition supplement packets containing β-hydroxy-β-methylbutyrate (HMB), and essential amino acids glutamine and arginine, may also be recommended during radiation and recovery. A preliminary study showed HMB's potential for increase in weight and fat-free mass and that it may potentially inhibit cachexia.[75, 83] Additional studies demonstrated HMB's potential to lessen radiation-induced inflammation and mucosal atrophy and prevention of radiation dermatitis.[83, 84] Consumption of one packet mixed into 8 ounces of water or juice twice daily orally or via PEG tube is recommended to try to achieve these results.

Medi-honey is a medical-grade honey that has the potential to accelerate wound healing and is more commonly used topically on open wounds or burns, but can be safely consumed orally to treat mucositis and esophagitis. Recommended dosing is 1 tbsp taken orally 15 minutes prior to radiation therapy, 15 minutes after radiation therapy, and one additional dose 6 hours later.

17.5.5   Nutrition Intervention Summary

EC and HNC patients are a complex population with a wide range of nutritional challenges. Early nutrition intervention by an RD prior to treatment initiation and ongoing throughout treatment and recovery are crucial. Preventing decline in the patient's nutritional status by limiting weight loss and preserving lean body mass, in addition to effective symptom management, improves treatment outcomes by preventing treatment delays and unplanned hospitalizations, while also improving patients' performance status and quality of life.

17.6 GYNECOLOGIC CANCERS

Gynecologic cancers are those involving female reproductive organs found in the pelvic region of the body, including endometrial/uterine, cervical, and ovarian. Treatment options depend on cancer type and stage, and include surgery, radiation, and chemotherapy either alone or in combination.

The endometrium is the lining of the uterus, with tissue that is regenerated regularly during the menstrual cycle. Symptoms of this cancer type are often exhibited early, allowing diagnosis to be made in early stages.[85] Endometrial cancer is considered the most common of the gynecologic cancers and the fifteenth most common cancer overall with an estimated 66,200 new cases in the United States in 2023.[86] Most of these new cases were diagnosed in women over the age of 60. Eighty-two percent of women with this cancer type survive up to 5 years. Endometrial cancer is twice as common in overweight women (BMI 25 to 29.9), and more than 3 times as common in obese women (BMI > 30).[86] Research shows that increase in overall body adipose tissue, particularly in the abdominal region, increases the risk of developing endometrial cancer.[87] A high-fat diet can increase the risk of many cancers, including endometrial cancer due to increased risk of obesity. Endometrial cancer is twice as common in women with type 2 diabetes, and diets that are high in refined carbohydrates and sugary beverages are also believed to increase risk.[88] Regular physical activity is considered protective against developing this disease.

Medications that affect hormone levels such as estrogen, birth control pills, and Tamoxifen can increase risk of endometrial cancer. Risk also increases with history of breast or ovarian cancer, or polycystic ovarian syndrome (PCOS) and number of pregnancies.[88]

The ovaries are organs responsible for the production of oocytes, in addition to hormones such as estrogen and progesterone, in the female body. Ovarian cancer afflicts about 20,000 women and is the eighth most common cancer among women in the United States, but it is considered the deadliest of the female cancers.[86] The 5-year survival rate of is currently at 50%.[89] Overweight and obesity, tall stature, and smoking can increase the risk of ovarian cancer.[87] Family history inherited risk through BRCA 1 and BRCA 2 genes, Lynch syndrome, and endometriosis increase risk of ovarian cancer.

Hereditary ovarian cancer accounts for almost 20% of all ovarian cancer cases.[86] Tests are available to help detect gene mutations for individuals determined to be at risk for hereditary disease. Age of 55 and older and use of hormone replacement therapy are independent risk factors for developing this disease.[87] Unfortunately, ovarian cancer may not cause early signs or symptoms, often leading to these cancers being diagnosed at advanced stages. Signs or symptoms may include:

- Pain, swelling, or feeling of pressure in the abdomen or pelvis
- Sudden or frequent urge to urinate

- Trouble eating or feeling full
- Gastrointestinal problems, such as gas, bloating, or constipation[87]

Advanced metastatic ovarian cancer can often be complicated by recurrent ascites and bowel obstruction which can cause maintaining adequate nutrition to be very challenging, often requiring the need for parenteral nutrition.

The cervix is found at the base of the uterus, being the portion of tissue connecting to the vagina. Cervical cancer is the least common of the gynecologic cancers, with an estimated 13,960 new cases diagnosed in 2023 in the United States.[85, 90] It is the fourth most common cancer in women worldwide and seventh overall.[85]

It is most diagnosed in women ages 35–44.[91] Sixty-seven percent of women survive 5 years with this disease. Human papilloma virus (HPV), smoking, and overweight and obesity are considered risk factors.[85] At this time, there is no strong evidence connecting diet, amount of physical activity, or weight to increased risk. HPV vaccination and regular cervical cancer screenings help with cervical cancer prevention.[87]

17.6.1 TREATMENT OPTIONS

Treatments include surgery, chemotherapy, or surgery/chemotherapy, radiation, hormone therapy, targeted therapy, and brachytherapy. Patients with advanced gynecological cancers that require major tumor debulking surgeries may require the placement of an ostomy or occasionally a venting gastrostomy tube. Radiation treatments for cervical cancer and endometrial cancer may include external beam radiation therapy (EBRT) and intensity-modulated radiation therapy (IMRT). Brachytherapy or internal radiation therapy may be used for cervical cancer. Intraperitoneal radiation therapy is currently being studied as an option to treat some cases of advanced ovarian cancer.[70]

Common Chemotherapy Regimens by Tumor Site

Uterine/Endometrial	Ovarian	Cervical
Combination regimens:	• Taxanes (Paclitaxel, Docetaxel)	• Cisplatin
• Docetaxel/carboplatin	• Platinum (Cisplatin, Carboplatin)	• Paclitaxel
• Carboplatin/paclitaxel	• Altretamine	• Bevacizumab
• Doxorubicin/cisplatin/ifosfamide	• Capecitabine	• Carboplatin
• Carboplatin/paclitaxel/doxorubicin	• Cyclophosphamide	• Topotecan
Single-agent options:	• Etoposide	• Gemcitabine
• Paclitaxel	• Gemcitabine	• 5-FU (5-fluorouracil)
• Doxorubicin/liposomal	• Ifosfamide	• Irinotecan
doxorubicin	• Irinotecan	• Mitomycin
• Carboplatin	• Liposomal doxorubicin	• Vinorelbine
• Cisplatin	• Melphalan	• Docetaxel
• Ifosfamide	• Pemetrexed	• Ifosfamide
• Docetaxel	• Topotecan	
	• Vinorelbine	

Note: See Appendices 1 and 2 for common side effects and nutritional management.

17.6.2 Nutrition Intervention Summary

Patients may initially present in good health status with no or few nutritional impact symptoms.

Maintaining nutritional status is important to help patients tolerate treatment and prevent treatment delay. With initiation of treatment, nutrition-related side effect management becomes paramount. Pre- and postsurgical health complications that may hinder surgical outcomes, such as uncontrolled blood sugar levels or excessive body fatness, must be addressed. Since patients may undergo chemotherapy and/ or radiation treatments, managing nutrition-related side effects should be mitigated with attempts to improve the patient's quality of life. Nutrition support may or may not be warranted; the goal of patient care should be the context of intervention within the interdisciplinary team.

17.7 LUNG CANCER

17.7.1 Introduction

Lung cancer remains the leading cause of cancer-related death and is the second most common cancer in men and women.[91] Two main types of lung cancer compose 95% of cases: non-small cell lung cancer (85%) and small cell lung cancer (10%–15%).[92] Lung cancer is often diagnosed at advanced stages, and 45%–69% of patients exhibit signs of cachexia at diagnosis.[92] Various treatments for lung cancer can pose many nutrition challenges. Patients often experience side effects that include esophagitis, dysphagia, anorexia, nausea and vomiting, taste changes, and fatigue. Continued weight loss after diagnosis contributes to poorer treatment response and increased mortality.[93]

17.7.2 Treatment Options

The primary treatments for lung cancer include chemotherapy and immunotherapy, radiation therapy, and surgery. Depending on the stage of the disease, two or more modalities may be recommended.

17.7.2.1 Surgery

Surgery is an ideal way to address lung cancer if patients can tolerate it. Many patients are not surgical candidates at diagnosis due to current lung function, malnutrition or performance status, or comorbid conditions. Surgical options include lobectomy (removal of an entire lobe), pneumonectomy (removal of the entire lung), and wedge resection (removal of a section of the lung).[94, 95] Depending on the histology, cytology, and stage of the lung tumor, surgery can be a successful option for patients with a curative intent. The type of operation recommended depends on how well a patient will tolerate the procedure, size of the tumor, and location and extent of the disease.

As with most major surgeries, adequate calorie and protein intake is essential for healing and to decrease nutrition-related complications. A low BMI prior to surgery has been linked to increased mortality.[96] In one study, patients with normal nutritional status had a median survival of 58 months compared to 36 months in patients with impaired nutritional status.[89, 97]

17.7.2.2 Radiation

Radiation therapy uses beams of high energy to injure and kill cancer cells, shrink tumors, and stop the growth of cancer cells.[98] The most common types of radiation therapy delivery methods are external beam radiation and internal radiation. External beam radiation involves focusing radiation from outside the body onto the cancerous cells within the body. Radiation oncologists can use sophisticated software and imaging techniques to adjust the size and shape of the beam while maximizing the dose of radiation to the tumor. This helps to minimize the impact on healthy surrounding tissue and organs and lessen side effects from treatment. The number of external beam radiation treatments can vary from days to weeks depending on the physician's plan of care for the patient. External beam radiation is more likely to cause side effects that impact ability to eat, especially if the esophagus is near the targeted treatment area.

Internal radiation therapy, also known as high dose rate (HDR) brachytherapy, involves placing radioactive material into the tumor itself or near the cancer cells. Brachytherapy is especially helpful to shrink tumors of the bronchi, thereby relieving symptoms of breathing difficulty, and is less likely to cause nutrition impact symptoms.[95]

Radiation can be used at different times during treatment. Radiation can be used as the main treatment for lung cancer with or without chemotherapy, particularly if the tumor cannot be removed by surgery or the patient is not an ideal surgical candidate. It can also be used after surgery to kill any residual cancer cells that are still present. The physician may also recommend radiation before surgery in conjunction with chemotherapy to help shrink the lung tumor to make future surgery less extensive.

Due to the nature of radiation therapy and the area of treatment, patients most commonly experience painful swallowing, dysphagia, mucus, and fatigue.

The tissues of the esophagus can become irritated and sore, and patients often complain of painful swallowing or having a "lump" in the throat. Symptoms of esophagitis may not become apparent until the second or third week of radiation and can subside two to three weeks after completion of treatment. Dietary modifications include chopping foods into small pieces, avoiding acidic or spicy foods, drinking oral nutritional supplements, and eating soft or moistened foods. Another side effect of radiation can be thick mucus buildup in the esophagus. Patients often complain of thick ropey mucus that can cause them to gag or have reflux. Encouraging patients to drink at least 6–8 cups of water per day and drinking lemon or lime beverages can help reduce mucus.

Swallowing function can also become compromised during radiation therapy to the lung. Consultation with a speech and language pathologist (SLP) is essential before and during radiation. An SLP can provide appropriate exercises and techniques to maintain muscle integrity and swallowing to help reduce long-term complications. In addition, the SLP may recommend diet texture changes or thickened liquids and may refer patients back to the dietitian for guidance. Depending on the severity of the radiation esophagitis, the physician may prescribe pain medication or swish-and-swallow numbing agents to reduce painful swallowing. Some patients may often require PEG placement to provide nutrition while bypassing the esophagus.

Fatigue during radiation is one of the most common side effects, which is exacerbated by inadequate nutrition. Radiation fatigue can often lead to decreased physical activity and loss of lean muscle mass.

Patients with weight loss greater than 5% and fatigue correlated with a low Karnofsky performance score and quality of life.[99] Adequate calorie/protein intake and increasing physical activity as tolerated has been shown to improve visceral protein stores. Patients may benefit from regular physical therapy sessions.

17.7.2.3 Chemotherapy and Targeted Therapy

Chemotherapy is a drug used to destroy cancer cells. Targeted therapies are drugs that can block the growth and spread of cancer. Depending on the agent, dose, and frequency of chemotherapy and targeted therapy, the nutritional implications vary. Appendix 1 is a chart that includes therapies commonly associated with lung cancer treatment and the nutritional side effects.

17.7.2.4 Lung Cancer and Lifestyle Interventions

Lung cancer risk is convincingly increased with high beta-carotene supplement intake as well as drinking water with high arsenic intake (mainly in unregulated water supplies). There is limited/suggestive evidence from AICR that increased intake of red meats, processed meats, and alcohol may increase the risk of lung cancer.[38]

17.7.3 Nutrition Intervention Summary

Patients undergoing treatment for lung cancer will most likely have significant nutritional challenges related to malnutrition. All patients should undergo nutrition assessment prior to treatment. Based on the patient's plan of care, continued surveillance during treatment is warranted to help patients manage treatment-related side effects, prevent weight loss, and improve outcomes.

17.8 PROSTATE CANCER

17.8.1 Introduction

Prostate cancer is the second most frequent cancer diagnosis made in men and the fifth leading cause of death worldwide.[100] In 2023, it is estimated that 288,300 new cases of prostate cancer diagnosed in the United States, representing 7.1% of all cancers in men.[99] Incidence and mortality rates are strongly related to age with the highest incidence, nearly 60%, in elderly men (>65 years of age) and highest incidence in African American men worldwide.[90] Prostate cancer treatment depends on the stage of the cancer. In early stages, it can be asymptomatic and can often only require active surveillance. In advanced prostate cancer, hormone therapy (or androgen deprivation therapy), chemotherapy, radiation, and/or a combination may be used for treatment.

The 5-year survival rate is around 98%, with a median survival rate of 1–2 years for metastatic prostate cancer.[91] All treatments for prostate cancer have potential side effects. Side effects and nutrition recommendations to aid with side effects are listed in this chapter for chemotherapy, radiation therapy, and surgery.

Nutrition, including diet and lifestyle, play a role in prostate cancer risk worldwide.[102] A low-fat, plant-based diet including a variety of fruits and vegetables along with increased physical activity may help prevent prostate cancer.[102] Obesity is a key factor linked to increased risk for advanced prostate cancer. Maintaining a healthy weight and regular physical activity is protective against not only prostate cancer, but many other cancers as well.

17.8.2 NUTRITION RECOMMENDATIONS

- Achieve and maintain a healthy weight. Increase physical activity.
- Decrease intake of high animal fat foods. High-calorie intake of saturated animal fat has shown to increase the growth of prostate cancer cells by increasing the circulating levels of androgens.[102]
- Studies show high intake of dairy (>4 servings per week), particularly full-fat dairy, is linked to prostate cancer and recurrence of prostate cancer.[99] Recurrence risk increases three-fold if overweight (BMI >27). Eat or drink low-fat dairy in moderation. Substitute soymilk for extra health benefits.

The following nutrition recommendations have shown benefit in early studies, although more recent studies have not provided the same results and was not always statistically significant. Incorporating these foods may still provide cancer-fighting benefits along with other health benefits.

- Lycopene is a phytochemical found in red fruits and vegetables, such as tomatoes, watermelon, and grapefruit. High-lycopene foods may help promote cancer cell death in prostate cancer.[98] Strive to get at least one lycopene-rich food daily.
- Adding whole soy products into the diet may have potential for reducing prostate cancer risk. Substituting soymilk for cow's milk, snacking on soy nuts, and cooking with tofu are ways to increase soy consumption.[103]
- Studies have shown that 1 cup or 8 fl oz of 100% pomegranate juice daily may slow the progression of localized cancer and potentially lengthen the time in which it takes the prostate specific antigen (PSA) score to double. [104]
- Ground flaxseed may help decrease prostate cancer proliferation. The goal is to incorporate three tablespoons daily into foods, drinks, and smoothies. [105]
- Green tea consumption of 6–7 cups per day may reduce prostate cancer risk, help increase prostate cancer cell death, and prevent progression by inhibiting cell growth.[106, 107]
- Some studies have shown that turmeric, a spice with strong anti-inflammatory properties, may help increase prostate cancer cell death, reduce progression, and may aid in stopping the formation of metastases in prostate cancer.[108]

17.8.3 TREATMENT OPTIONS

17.8.3.1 Chemotherapy, Hormone Therapy, and Immunotherapy

Chemotherapy	Hormone Therapy	Immunotherapy
Doxetaxol (Taxotere)	Lupron (Eligard)	Sipuleucel-T (Provenge)
Cabazitaxel (Jevtana)	Degarelix (Firmagon)	Pembrolizumab (Keytruda)
Mitoxantrone (Novantrone)	Zoladex (Goserelin)	
Estramustine (Emcyt)	Bicalutamide (Casodex)	
Carboplatin (Paraplatin)	Abiraterone (Zytiga)	
Oxaliplatin (Eloxatin)	Enzalutamide (Xtandi)	
Cisplatin (Platinol)	Flutamide (Eulexin)	
	Triptorelin Pamoate (Trelstar)	

17.8.3.2 Radiation Therapy

Radiation therapy (also called radiotherapy) is a prostate cancer treatment that uses targeted energy to kill cancer cells and stop them from spreading. At low doses, radiation is used as an X-ray to see inside your body and take pictures, such as X-rays of your teeth and bones. Radiation used in prostate cancer treatment works in much the same way, except that it is given in higher doses. Radiation therapy can be external beam (when a machine outside the body aims radiation at prostate cancer cells) or via brachytherapy, which is seed implantation or interstitial radiation therapy (when radiation is temporarily or permanently put inside the body, in or near the prostate cancer cells). Sometimes people get both forms of radiation therapy at different intervals. Radiation therapy is a commonly used cancer treatment option. It may be given as a single therapy, along with chemotherapy and/or hormone therapy, or postsurgery. For some early-stage cancer diagnoses, radiation therapy can be effective and used as a single treatment option for cure.

Common Side Effects to Common Radiation Treatments

Treatment	Nutrition-Related Side Effect
Stereotactic Body Radiation Therapy (SBRT) or Cyberknife (typically 1–5 treatments)	Diarrhea
External Beam Radiation Therapies (EBRT) Intensity Modulated Radiation Therapy (IMRT), Three-Dimensional Conformal Radiation Therapy (3D-CRT)	Diarrhea, inflammation in GI tract, lactose intolerance, nausea/vomiting, fatigue
Brachytherapy	Fatigue, diarrhea
Radiopharmaceuticals given IV (Xofigo, Pluvicto) indicated for metastatic prostate cancer	Diarrhea, fatigue, nausea, loss of appetite, constipation, dry mouth
Proton Beam Radiation Therapy – uses protons instead of X-rays	Urinary incontinence, diarrhea
Deep Tissue Hyperthermia (typically given in combination with chemotherapy and/or radiation therapy)	Fatigue

17.8.3.3 Surgery

Surgery is the most common treatment option to try to cure prostate cancer if it is not thought to have spread outside the gland (stage 1 or 2 cancers). The main type of surgery for prostate cancer is known as a radical prostatectomy. Nutrition-related side effects are not common, but may include loss of lean body mass, nausea/vomiting, and fatigue. Deep tissue hyperthermia (DTH) and brachytherapy may also be treatment options to treat prostate cancer. Fatigue is the most common side effect of these deep tissue hyperthermia (DTH) and brachytherapy; fatigue is the most common side effect of these. Prostate surgery can be a very effective treatment option for prostate cancer and can be used as a single treatment option or along with chemotherapy and/or hormone therapy.

17.8.4 NUTRITION INTERVENTION SUMMARY

Nutrition is an integral part of prostate cancer throughout all stages of treatment. Chemotherapy, radiation therapy, and surgery are all options that may cause symptoms for patients with prostate cancer. Once prostate cancer is in remission, it is recommended to follow the American Institute of Cancer Research guidelines. These guidelines encourage a diet high in plant-based proteins, fruits, vegetables, and omega-three fatty acids, and limited in saturated fat, simple sugars, and salt. Achieving and maintaining a healthy body weight is important for prostate cancer.[101, 109]

17.9 PALLIATIVE CARE

17.9.1 OVERVIEW

What is palliative care?

> Palliative care is an exercise in forward planning and prevention rather than a model of crisis intervention.
>
> Dr. Ronald S. Schonwetter

> Palliative care is an approach that improves the quality of life of patients and their families facing the problems associated with life-threatening illness, through the prevention and relief of suffering by means of early identification and impeccable assessment and treatment of pain and other problems, physical, psychosocial, and spiritual.
>
> World Health Organization

Palliative care:

- Provides relief from pain and other distressing symptoms
- Affirms life and regards dying as a normal process
- Intends neither to hasten nor postpone death
- Integrates the psychological and spiritual aspects of patient care
- Offers a support system to help patients live as actively as possible until death

- Offers a support system to help the family cope during the patient's illness and in their own bereavement
- Uses a team approach to address the needs of patients and their families, including bereavement counseling, if indicated
- Will enhance quality of life, and may also positively influence the course of illness
- Is applicable early in the course of illness, in conjunction with other therapies that are intended to prolong life, such as chemotherapy or radiation therapy, and includes those investigations needed to better understand and manage distressing clinical complications

17.9.1.1 Comparison of Palliative Care versus Hospice Care

Palliative Care	Hospice Care
Provide QOL throughout treatment	Provides QOL toward end of life
Provides care for caregivers + patient	Provides care for caregivers + patient
Prevents/treats symptoms of diagnosis	Provides medications, supplies, equipment, and hospital services relate to the terminal illness
Begins at time of initial diagnosis	Begins with less than 6 months left to live
Billed through insurance as a typical treatment	Reimbursed to hospice company at a daily rate for all services

17.9.1.2 Model of Palliative Care for Oncology

Palliative care is specialized medical care for people with serious illnesses. It focuses on providing patients with relief from the symptoms and stress of a serious illness. The goal is to improve quality of life for both the patient and the family.[110] Palliative care is provided by a specially trained team of doctors, nurses, dietitians, and other specialists who work together with a patient's other doctors to provide an extra layer of support. It is appropriate at any age and at any stage in a serious illness and can be provided along with curative treatment.[111–114]

17.9.1.3 Challenges That Occur with Oncology Patients

What role does nutrition play in oncologic palliative care?

In palliative care, nutrition has a major impact on oncology patients' quality of life. Symptoms can not only adversely affect food and fluid intake, but a patient's nutritional intake can also influence their symptoms and overall well-being.

Although not typically painful, anorexia and cachexia in oncology patients are unmistakable indications that the underlying disease is not under control and that death is approaching. Food and eating are some of the highest pleasures in life and often fade away in affected patients and can often lead to a condition called cachexia-related suffering (CRS). CRS is defined as negative emotions associated with reduced nutritional intake and weight loss. CRS affects both patients and caregivers. Patients may be embarrassed about the visibility of loss of weight or feel harassed by their caregivers. Caregivers may feel personally rejected.

Oncology patients often experience a series of losses: loss of weight and the desire to eat; loss of the ability to smell, taste, chew, and swallow food; loss of the ability to digest and absorb nutrients, and loss of the ability to eliminate waste products independently.[115, 116]

17.9.1.4 Multistep Approach to Nutritional Care of Palliative Care Patients

Step 1: Nutrition screening and assessment
Step 2: Developing a care plan
Step 3: Recognizing changes in nutritional needs
Step 4: Education: patient, family, multidisciplinary team

17.9.2 PALLIATIVE CARE FOR ONCOLOGY PATIENTS

Cancer is known to be among a long list of chronically progressive diseases that unfortunately may lose their therapeutic options. When in conjunction with other comorbidities/diseases such as HIV infection, COPD, CHF, or neurologic disorders, the challenges can be even greater. Anorexia and cachexia can cause negative emotions and may be unmistakable indications that the underlying disease is not under control and that death is approaching.

Psychosocial issues related to sustaining life with food are often known as CRS. CRS is explored in advanced cancer diseases and may manifest into what is known as cancer cachexia syndrome (CCS).

CRS and its relationship to CCS include aspects of distress suffered by patients, caregivers, partners, and a patient's healthcare professionals. CRS is more prevalent in caregivers than in patients. Emotions may be but are not limited to anxiety, anger, feeling upset, bother, concern, frustration, and guilt.

Patients may even be embarrassed by their change in appearance or feel harassed by their caregivers.

Conversely, caregivers may feel rejected or incompetent if they are declined by the patient.

There are constructive and adverse reactions to CRS. Recognizing the terminal nature of the disease and acceptance is the key to relief of CRS. Instead of solely focusing on food, caregivers may find other ways to care for the patient versus pressuring about food. Adverse reactions can occur if CCS is not recognized or accepted. Adversely, encouraging more food intake may put more pressure on the patient verbally and nonverbally. Pushing patients may cause pain, nausea, anticipatory nausea, and even vomiting.

17.9.2.1 Palliative Care and Nutrition: Artificial Nutrition and Hydration

Artificial hydration is the provision of water or electrolyte solutions through any nonoral route.

Artificial nutrition includes PN and EN by nasogastric tube (NGT), percutaneous endoscopic gastrostomy (PEG) tube, percutaneous endoscopic gastrostomy jejunostomy (PEG-J) tube, gastrostomy tube, or gastrojejunostomy tube.[115]

There is limited evidence showing increased survival and quality of life in patients receiving artificial nutrition. Current literature lacks high-quality randomized trials that might yield clear indications and guide practice. The American Gastroenterological Association (AGA) endorses PEG tube placement for prolonged tube feeding (defined as greater than 30 days) and NGT feedings when feeding is required for shorter periods. The American College of Physicians advises that the routine use of PN should be discouraged in patients undergoing chemotherapy, and that, when it is used in patients with cancer with malnutrition, physicians should consider the possibility of increased risk.

In other countries, PN continues to be used regularly for patients with advanced cancer.[114]

In hospice settings, parenteral hydration is not routine, but may be considered in instances in which the patient is experiencing neuropsychiatric symptoms such as delirium, myoclonus, and agitation,[115] although these symptoms are also related to the dying process and parenteral hydration may not add comfort. It is important to consider the positive and negative when considering appropriate route of artificial nutrition and hydration (ANH) for each individual patient. Consider the following table when considering EN ANH. Per the AGA, EN is appropriate to consider when the patient cannot or will not eat, the gut is functional, and the patient can tolerate the placement of the device.[115]

Positive Considerations	Negative Considerations
Duration of survival	Pharyngeal/esophageal/bowel perforation
Improved comfort	Accidental bronchial insertion of NG/OG tube
Reduction or healing of pressure ulcer	NGTs fall out about 25% of the time or accidental removal occurs
Reduction in aspiration	Infection at insertion site
Prevents hunger and thirst	Peristomal leaks
	Sepsis
	Necrotizing fasciitis
	Fluid overload
	Pain
	Possibility of restraints

Current Levels of Evidence for Artificial Nutrition in the Oncology Population

Type of Artificial Nutrition	Outcome	*Classification	*Level of Evidence
PN	During chemotherapy	III	B1
Prophylactic EN before treatment in head and neck cancer	Weight stabilization	IIa	B2
EN before surgery	Gastrointestinal cancer	IIa	A

* Description of classification based on levels of evidence:
IIa – Weight of evidence/opinion is in favor of usefulness/efficacy
III – Intervention is not useful/effective and may be harmful
B1 – Limited evidence from single, randomized trial
B2 – Limited evidence from other nonrandomized studies
 A – Sufficient evidence from multiple randomized trials

Inconsistent results have been generated from randomized studies in patients with a variety of tumors and therapies. Because no statistical benefit from PN has been demonstrated in survival, treatment tolerance, treatment toxicity, or tumor response in patients receiving PN during chemotherapy or radiotherapy, PN has not been consistently used in advanced cancer care in the United States. Subsequent studies evaluating PN and EN remain mixed.[115]

PN and EN have been able to improve some nutritional indices, such as body weight, fat mass, nitrogen balance, and whole-body potassium. Prealbumin and retinol-binding protein levels increase only with PN. Immune indices such as complement factors and lymphocyte number improve only with EN. PN and EN both appear to prevent further deterioration of the nutritional state and may even show some improvement which will allow for cancer treatment to continue.[115]

It is important to reinforce that current data regarding ANH have significant methodological weaknesses and limited evidence for current practice as described in these sections. Providers should critically consider the patient, their wishes, and the overall potential benefits and risks before making a decision in regard to providing or not providing ANH.

17.9.2.2   Assessment

Nutrition needs will change as the patient transitions through the palliative care spectrum. In the early phase of palliative care, the goal of nutrition treatment is to manage malnutrition risk and mitigate symptoms. Early identification and management of malnutrition risk improves and protects nutrition status and quality of life (QOL) throughout the stages of treatment and disease.

Rescreening should be repeated routinely. Through the patient's cancer journey, the nutrition status will change as well as the goals. The presence of cancer cachexia does not always indicate end of life or need for hospice. In the later stages of palliative care, the goal of nutrition therapy should transition to QoL including comfort, symptom relief, and food enjoyment if able. Toward the last days of life, the aim of care should provide comfort for the patient and caregiver.

The assessment should include biochemical data, medical tests, procedures, nutrition-focused physical findings, and client-reported history. In the assessment, the RDN should consider the stage of the cancer cachexia.

17.9.3   End of Life

Nutrition care at the end of life requires a sensible, informed, and personalized approach. Helping make the right food choices and removing any anxieties about food and fluid intake often gives valuable relief and comfort to both patients and caregivers and may also provide some precious time.

Both religion and culture play an important role when end-of-life issues are at stake; therefore, it is paramount to explore and understand a patient's religious and cultural background in order to reach a consensus regarding nutrition support.

Checklist to establish religious beliefs, cultural affiliation, and family background when end-of-life decisions are necessary:

- What do they think of the sanctity of life?
- What is their definition of death?

- What is their religious background and how active are they presently?
- What do they believe are causal agents in illness and how do these relate to the dying process?
- What is the patient's social support system?
- Who makes decisions about matters of importance in the family?

When nutrition support is withdrawn, it is important for the clinician to discuss with family/caregivers' key points regarding end of life.

The consideration to withdraw nutrition is often not well received; therefore, factual information is necessary.

- Neither thirst nor hunger is experienced at the end of life.
- Lack of fluid and food allows for ketosis and a release of opioids in the brain, which may, in fact, produce a sense of euphoria.
- Physiological adaptation to lack of nourishment prevents discomfort.
- Dehydration results in azotemia, hypernatremia, and hypercalcemia, which are all assumed to produce a calming effect prior to death.
- Curtailing food and fluid can decrease oral and bronchial secretion, reduce the need to urinate, and ease coughing from pulmonary congestion.
- Withholding artificial nutrition/hydration is not painful and dehydration may actually enhance comfort during the dying process.

17.9.3.1 Ethical Considerations

- Advanced directives, living wills, and durable powers of attorney are legal documents that allow individuals to express their decision about end-of-life care to family, friends, and healthcare providers.
- Often, living wills or advanced directives do not stipulate whether nutrition interventions, such as ANH, are desired.

Though a patient and family may request artificial nutrition be continued once hospice is established, most insurance companies dictate whether PN is a covered benefit and most hospice facilities decide if they will accept the patient even if artificial nutrition and hydration is a known covered benefit.

17.9.3.2 Professional Consensus Statement on Nutritional Care in Palliative Care Patients

- Nutritional care:

  - Is an essential aspect of palliative care
  - Is individualized
  - Is fluid through life

    – Nutrition needs are fluid through life and from person to person. Respect this fluidity and be ready to educate. You are the nutrition expert, and you will be educating the patient/care giver/interdisciplinary team.

  - Must be delivered safely and with compassion and dignity
  - Must encompass physical/social/cultural/emotional aspects
  - Matters for all palliative care professionals

- Staff and volunteers should receive regular training on nutrition in palliative care
- Healthcare organizations are responsible for delivering nutritional care

It is important to consider end of life not only in oncology but throughout all stages of life to improve quality for both the patient and the patient's family. Utilization of a specialized team of clinicians to help patients and caregivers understand the difference between palliative care and hospice care is vital for a successful transition. It can be overwhelming for everyone involved but it does not have to be with the right team by one's side.

REFERENCES

1. Onc: Nutrition Screening Tools. 2012. *Academy of Nutrition and Dietetics Evidence Analysis Library*. http://www.andeal.org/topic.cfm?cat=5452&conclusion_statement_id=251796&highlight=oncology%20 assessment&home=1. Updated 2012. Accessed March 2015.
2. Onc: Nutrition Assessment for Adult Oncology Patients. 2013. *Academy of Nutrition and Dietetics Evidence Analysis Library*. www.andeal.org/topic.cfm?format_tables=0&-cat=5164. Updated 2013. Accessed March 2015.
3. Onc: Nutrition Assessment Tools. 2012. *Academy of Nutrition and Dietetics Evidence Analysis Library*. www.andeal.org/topic.cfm?cat=5453&conclusion_statement_id=251792&highlight=nutrition%20assessment%20for%20adult%20oncology%20 patients&home=1. Updated 2012. Accessed March 2015.
4. Harris D, Haboubi N. Malnutrition screening in the elderly population. *J R Soc Med*. 2005 Sep;98(9):411–14.
5. Nutrition in Cancer Care (PDQ®): Nutrition Screening and Assessment. *National Cancer Institute Website*. www.cancer.gov/cancertopics/pdq/supportivecare/nutrition/HealthProfessional/page4#_50_toc. Updated September 3, 2014. Accessed March 2015.
6. Nutrition and the Adult Oncology Patient. *Academy of Nutrition and Dietetics Evidence Analysis Library*. www.andeal.org/files/Docs/Nutrition%20and%20the%20Adult%20Oncology%20Patient_09262013FINAL. Updated 2013. Accessed March 2015.
7. Grant M, Rivera LM. Impact of dietary counseling on quality of life in head and neck patients undergoing radiation therapy. *Qual Life Res*. 1994;3:77–8.
8. Nitenberg G, Raynard B. Nutritional support of the cancer patient: Issues and dilemmas. *Crit Rev Oncol Hematol*. 2000 Jun;34(3):137–68.
9. Vashi P, Gorsuch K, Wan L et al. Sarcopenia supersedes subjective global assessment as a predictor of survival in colorectal cancer. PLoS One;14(6):e0218761. https://doi.org/10.1371/journal.
10. De Pergola G, Silvestris F. Obesity as a major risk factor for cancer. J Obes. 2013:291546. https://doi.org/10.1155/2013/291546.
11. Cancer Types. *American Cancer Society Website*. www.cancer.org/cancer/showallcancertypes/index. Accessed March 28, 2015.
12. Mehta M, Shike M. Diet and physical activity in the prevention of colorectal cancer. *J Natl Compr Canc Netw*. 2014 Dec;12(12):1721–6.
13. Cancer Prevention: By the numbers. *American Institute for Cancer Research Website*. www.aicr. org/reduce-your-cancer-risk/cancer-prevention/reduce_cancer_by_numbers. html. Accessed March 28, 2015.
14. Kachaamy T, Prakash R, Kundranda M, Batish R, Weber J et al. Liquid nitrogen spray cryotherapy for dysphagia palliation in patients with inoperable esophageal cancer. *GIE*, Sept 2018. doi:10.1016/j.gie.2018.04.2362.

15. Morgan TM, Tang D, Stratton KL et al. Preoperative nutritional status is an important predictor of survival in patients undergoing surgery for renal cell carcinoma. *Eur Urol.* 2011 Jun;59(6):923–8.
16. Garth AK, Newsome CM, Simmance N, Crowe TC. Nutritional status, nutrition practices and postoperative complications in patients with gastrointestinal cancer. *J Hum Nutr Diet.* 2010 Aug;23(4):393–401.
17. Perioperative total parenteral nutrition in surgical patients. The veterans' affairs total parenteral nutrition cooperative study group. Gordon P. Buzby, Gordon P, M.D., et. al. *N Engl J Med.* 1991 Aug 22;325(8):525–32.
18. Weimann A, Braga M, Harsanyi L et al. ESPEN guidelines on enteral nutrition: Surgery including organ transplantation. *Clin Nutr.* 2006 Apr;25(2):224–44.
19. Braga M, Ljungqvist O, Soeters P, Fearon K, Weimann A, Bozzetti F, ESPEN. ESPEN guidelines on parenteral nutrition: Surgery. *Clin Nutr.* 2009 Aug;28(4):378–86.
20. Martindale RG, McClave SA, Taylor B, Lawson CM. Perioperative nutrition: What is the current landscape? *J Parenter Enteral Nutr.* 2013 Sep;37(5 Suppl):5S–20S.
21. Gabor S, Renner H, Matzi V et al. Early enteral feeding compared with parenteral nutrition after oesophageal or oesophagogastric resection and reconstruction. *Br J Nutr.* 2005 Apr;93(4):509–13.
22. Osland E, Yunus RM, Khan S, Memon MA. Early versus traditional postoperative feeding in patients undergoing resectional gastrointestinal surgery: A meta-analysis. *J Parenter Enteral Nutr.* 2011 Jul;35(4):473–87.
23. Kalff JC, Türler A, Schwarz NT et al. Intra-abdominal activation of a local inflammatory response within the human muscularis externa during laparotomy. *Ann Surg.* 2003 Mar;237(3):301–15.
24. Mortensen K, Nilsson M, Slim K et al. Consensus guidelines for enhanced recovery after gastrectomy: Enhanced Recovery After Surgery (ERAS®) Society recommendations. *Br J Surg.* 2014 Sep;101(10):1209–29.
25. Gustafsson UO, Scott MJ, Schwenk W et al. Guidelines for perioperative care in elective colonic surgery: Enhanced recovery after surgery (ERAS®) society recommendations. *Clin Nutr.* 2012 Dec;31(6):783–800.
26. Lassen K, Coolsen MM, Slim K et al. Guidelines for perioperative care for pancreaticoduodenectomy: Enhanced recovery after surgery (ERAS®) society recommendations. *Clin Nutr.* 2012 Dec;31(6):817–30.
27. Nygren J, Thacker J, Carli F et al. Guidelines for perioperative care in elective rectal/pelvic surgery: Enhanced recovery after surgery (ERAS®) Society recommendations. *Clin Nutr.* 2012 Dec;31(6):801–16.
28. Osland E, Hossain MB, Khan S, Memon MA. Effect of timing of pharmaconutrition (immunonutrition) administration on outcomes of elective surgery for gastrointestinal malignancies: A systematic review and meta-analysis. *JPEN J Parenter Enteral Nutr.* 2014 Jan;38(1):53–69.
29. Frantz D, Munroe C et al. Gastrointestinal disease. In: Mueller, C et al. eds. *ASPEN Adult Nutrition Support Core Curriculum*. 2nd ed. Silver Spring, MD: A.S.P.E.N.; 2012:426–53.
30. Huhmann M. Nutrition management of the surgical oncology patient. In: Leser, M, Ledesma, N, Bergerson, S, Trujillo, E eds. *Oncology Nutrition for Clinical Practice*. 3rd ed. Chicago, IL: Oncology Nutrition Dietetic Practice Group of the Academy of Nutrition and Dietetics; 2013:14.
31. Gill C. Nutrition management for cancers of the gastrointestinal tract. In: Leser, M, Ledesma, N, Bergerson, S, Trujillo, E eds. *Oncology Nutrition for Clinical Practice*. 3rd ed. Chicago, IL: Oncology Nutrition Dietetic Practice Group of the Academy of Nutrition and Dietetics; 2013:20.
32. Massironi S, Cavalcoli F, Rausa E, Invernizzi P, Braga M et al. Understanding short bowel syndrome: Current status and future perspectives. *Dig Liver Dis.* 2020;52(3):253–61.

33. Bordeianou L, Yeh DD. *Overview of Management of Small Bowel Obstruction in Adults.* UpToDate.com website. www.uptodate.com/contents/overview-of-management-of-mechanical-small-bowelobstruction-in-adults?source=related_link. Accessed April 10, 2015.

34. Vanderhoof JA, Pauley-Hunter RJ. *Treatment of Small Intestinal Bacterial Overgrowth.* UpTo-Date.com website. www.uptodate.com/contents/treatment-of-small-intestinal-bacterial-overgrowth?source=search_result&search=small+bowel+bacterial+overgrowth&select edTitle=1%7E121. Accessed April 9, 2015.

35. Stein SL. *Overview of Enteric Fistulas.* UpToDate.com website. www.uptodate.com/contents/overview-of-enteric-_stulas?source=search_result&search=_stula&selected Title=1%7E150. Accessed April 9, 2015.

36. Breast Cancer Facts and Figures 2022–2024. Pages 6, 11. *The American Cancer Society Website.* www.cancer.org. Accessed December 10, 2022.

37. Irwin ML, McTiernan A, Baumgartner RN et al. Changes in body fat and weight after a breast cancer diagnosis: Influence of demographic, prognostic, and lifestyle factors. *J Clin Oncol.* 2005 Feb 1;23(4):774–82.

38. World Cancer Research Fund/American Institute for Cancer Research Continuous Update Project Expert Report 2018. Diet, nutrition, physical activity and breast cancer. dietandcancerreport.com.

39. Picon-Ruiz M, Morata-Tarifa C, Valle-Goffin J, Friedman E, Slingerland J. Obesity and adverse breast cancer risk and outcome: Mechanistic insights and strategies for intervention. *CA Cancer J Clin.* 2017 Sep–Oct; 67(5): 378–97.

40. Pierce JP, Faerber S, Wright F et al. A randomized trial of the effect of a plant-based dietary pattern on additional breast cancer events and survival: The women's healthy eating and living (WHEL) study. *Control Clin Trials.* 2002 Dec;23(6):728–56.

41. Majed B, Moreau T, Asselain B, Curie Institute Breast Cancer Group. Overweight, obesity and breast cancer prognosis: Optimal body size indicator cut-points. *Breast Cancer Res Treat.* 2009 May;115(1):193–203.

42. Holick CN, Newcomb PA, Trentham-Dietz A et al. Physical activity and survival after diagnosis of invasive breast cancer. *Cancer Epidemiol Biomarkers Prev.* 2008 Feb;17(2):379–86.

43. Blackburn GL, Wang KA. Dietary fat reduction and breast cancer outcome: Results from the women's intervention and nutrition study (WINS). *Am J Clin Nutr.* 2007 Sep;86(3):s878–81.

44. Zhang D, Nichols HB, Troester M, Cai J, Bensen JT et al. Tea consumption and breast cancer risk in a cohort of women with a family history of breast cancer. *Int J Cancer.* 2020 Aug 1;147(3):876–886.

45. Patterson RE, Flatt SW, Newman VA et al. Marine fatty acid intake is associated with breast cancer prognosis. *J Nutr.* 2011 Feb;141(2):201–6.

46. Hadji P, Body JJ, Aapro MS et al. Practical guidance for the management of aromatase inhibitor associated bone loss. *Ann Oncol.* 2008 Aug;19(8):1407–16.

47. Lee KH, Seong HJ, Kim G, Jeong GH, Kim JY et al. Consumption of fish and omega-3 fatty acids and cancer risk: An umbrella review of meta-analyses of observational studies. *Adv Nutr.* 2020 Sep;11 (5): 1134–49.

48. Ross AC, Manson JE, Abrams SA et al. The 2011 report on dietary reference intakes for calcium and vitamin D from the institute of medicine: What clinicians need to know. *J Clin Endocrinol Metab.* 2011 Jan;96(1):53–8.

49. Mahabir S. Association between diet during preadolescence and adolescence and the risk for breast cancer during adulthood. *J Adolesc Health.* 2013 May;52(5Suppl):S30–5.

50. Caan BJ, Natarajan L, Parker B et al. Soy food consumption and breast cancer prognosis. *Cancer Epidemiol Biomarkers Prev.* 2011 May;20(5):854–8.

51. Liu X, Lv K. Cruciferous vegetables intake is inversely associated with risk of breast cancer: A meta-analyis. *Breast.* 2013 Jun;22(3):309–13.

52. McCann SE, Hootman KC, Weaver AM et al. Dietary intakes of total and specific lignans are associated with clinical breast tumor characteristics. *J Nutr.* 2012 Jan;142(1):91–8.

53. Zamora-Ros R, Ferrari P, Gonzalez CA et al. Dietary flavonoid and lignin intake and breast cancer risk according to menopause and hormone receptor status in the European perspective investigation into cancer and nutrition (EPIC) study. *Breast Cancer Res Treat.* 2013 May;139(1):163–76.

54. Newman V. Medical nutrition therapy for breast cancer. In: Marian, M, Roberts, S eds. *Clinical Nutrition in Oncology Patients.* Sadbury, MA: Jones and Barlett; 2010;7:176.

55. Mehta L, Watson K, Barac A, Beckie TM, Bittner V. Cardiovascular disease and breast cancer: Where these entities intersect. *Circulation.* 2018 Feb 20;137(8):e30–e66.

56. Institute of medicine (US) committee to review dietary reference intakes for vitamin D and calcium. In: Ross, AC, Taylor, CL, Yaktine, AL, Del Valle, HB. eds. *Dietary Reference Intakes for Calcium and Vitamin D.* Washington, DC: National Academies Press (US); 2011.

57. Polovich M, Olsen M, LeFebvre K eds. *Chemotherapy and Biotherapy Guidelines for Treatment and Recommendations for Practi*[ce]. 4th ed. Pittsburgh, PA: Oncology Nursing Society; 2014:27–47.

58. American Cancer Society: Cancer Facts and Figures 2013. *American Cancer Society Website*. http://www.cancer.org/research/cancerfacts_gures/cancerfacts_gures/cancer-facts-_gures-2013. Accessed March 4, 2015.

59. Terrell JE. Quality of life assessment in head and neck cancer patients. *Hematol Oncol Clin North Am.* 1999 Aug;13(4):849–65.

60. Isenring E. Esophageal and head and neck cancer. In: Marian, M, Roberts, S eds. *Clinical Nutrition in Oncology Patients.* Sadbury, MA: Jones and Barlett; 2010;7:165–85.

61. Lesser, M. Medical nutrition therapy for esophageal cancer. In: Leser, M, Ledesma, N, Bergerson, S, Trujillo, E eds. *Oncology Nutrition for Clinical Practice.* Chicago, IL: Oncology Nutrition Dietetic Practice Group of the Academy of Nutrition and Dietetics; 2013;19:181–6.

62. Santarpia L, Contaldo F, Pasanisi F. Nutrition screening and early treatment of malnutrition in cancer patients. *J Cachexia Sarcopenia Muscle.* 2011 Mar;2(1):27–35.

63. Riddle B, Davidson W, Elliot R, Basillie F, Porceddu S. Collaborative management of acute side effects for head and neck cancer patients receiving radiotherapy. *Asia Pac J Clin Oncol.* 2005;1(Suppl):A18.

64. Melhado RE, Alderson D, Tucker O. The changing face of esophageal cancer. *Cancers (Basel).* 2010 Jun 28;2(3):1379–404.

65. What You Need to Know About Cancer of the Esophagus. *National Cancer Institute Website.* Www. cancer.gov/cancertopics/wyntk/esophagus. Revised April 2013. Accessed June 4, 2013.

66. Chemotherapy for Cancer of the Esophagus. *American Cancer Society Website.* www.cancer.org/cancer/esophaguscancer/detailedguide/esophagus-cacner-treating-chemotherapy. Accessed March 13, 2015.

67. Surveillance Epidemiology and End Results. *SEER Stat Fact Sheets: Esophagus Cancer. National Cancer Institute Website.* http://seer.cancer.gov/statfacts/html/esoph.html. Accessed March 5, 2012.

68. Esophagus Cancer. *American Cancer Society Website.* www.cancer.org/Cancer/Esophagus Cancer/Detailed Guide. Revised January 18, 2013. Accessed March 1, 2015.

69. Nguyen A, Nadler E. Medical nutrition therapy for head and neck cancer. In: Leser, M, Ledesma, N, Bergerson, S, Trujillo, E eds. *Oncology Nutrition for Clinical Practice.* Chicago, IL: Oncology Nutrition Dietetic Practice Group of the Academy of Nutrition and Dietetics; 2013;21:201–8.

70. Ligthart-Melis GC, Weijs PJ, Te Boveldt ND et al. Dietitian-delivered intensive nutritional support is associated with a decrease in severe postoperative complications after surgery in patients with esophageal cancer. *Dis Esophagus*. 2013;26(6):587–93.

71. Festi D, Scaioli E, Baldi F et al. Body weight, lifestyle, dietary habits and gastroesophageal re_\flux disease. *World J Gastroenterol*. 2009;15(14):1690–701.

72. Nguyen A, Nadler E. Head and neck cancer: Defining effective medical nutrition therapy for nutritional phases observed during chemoradiation. *Oncol Nutr Connect*. 2012;20(1):3–21.

73. Hurst JD, Gallagher AL. Energy, macronutrient, micronutrient, and fluid requirements. In: Elliott, L, Molseed, LL, McCallum, PD eds. *The Clinical Guide to Oncology Nutriti*^{on}. 2nd ed. Chicago, IL: American Dietetic Association; 2006:54–71.

74. Topkan E, Parlak C, Topuk S, Pehlivan B. Influence of oral glutamine supplementation on of survival outcomes patients treated with concurrent chemoradiotherapy for locally advanced non-small cell lung cancer. *BMC Cancer*. 2012 Oct 31;12:502.

75. Berk L, James J, Schwartz A et al. A randomized, double-blind, placebo-controlled trial of betahydroxyl beta-methly butyrate, glutamine, and arginine mixture for the treatment of cancer cachexia. *Support Cancer Care*. 2008;16(10):1179–88.

76. Lopes AB, Fagundes RB. Esophageal squamous cell carcinoma-precursor lesions and early diagnosis. *World J Gastrointest Endosc*. 2012;16;4(1):9–16.

77. Fietkau R. Principles of feeding cancer patients via enteral or parenteral nutrition during radiotherapy. *Strahlenther Onkol*. 1998;174(suppl III):47–51.

78. Esophageal Cancer Treatment; Treatment Option Overview (PDQ®). *National Cancer Institute Website*. www.cancer.gov/cancertopics/pdq/treatment/esophageal/HealthProfessional/page4. Accessed November 5, 2012.

79. Forastiere A, Trotti A, Pfister D, Grandis J. Head and neck cancer: Recent advances and new standards of care. *J Clin Oncol*. 2006;24:2603–5.

80. Chemotherapy Drugs and Often Used During Chemotherapy. *Chemocare Website*. http://chemocare.com/chemotherapy/drug-info/default.aspx. Accessed March 13, 2015.

81. NCCN Guidelines for treatment of cancer by site. *National Comprehensive Cancer Network (NCCN) Website*. www.nccn.org/professionals/physician_gls/pdf/head-and-neck.pdf. Accessed November 16, 2012.

82. Gaurav K, Goel RK, Shukla M, Pandey M. Glutamine: An approach to novel chemotherapy-induced toxicity. *Indian J Med Paediatr Oncol*. 2012 Jan;33(1):13–20.

83. Imai T, Matsuura K, Asada Y et al. Effect of HMB/Arg/Gln on the prevention of radiation dermatitis in head and neck cancer patients treated with concurrent chemoradiotherapy. *Jpn J Clin Oncol*. 2014;44(5):422–7.

84. Yavas C, Yavas G, Acar H et al. Amelioration of radiation-induced acute inflammation and mucosal atrophy by beta-hydroxy-beta-methylbutyrate, L-glutamine, and L-arginine: Results of an experimental study. *Support Cancer Care*. 2013;21(3):883–8.

85. National Cancer Institute. *Surveillance, Epidemiology, and End Results Program (SEER) Stat Fact Sheets*. www.cancer.gov/types/ovarian/patient/ovarian-epithelial-treatment-pdq. https://seer.cancer.gov/statfacts/html/corp.html. Accessed October 9, 2022.

86. National Cancer Institute. *Surveillance, Epidemiology, and End Results Program (SEER) Stat Fact Sheets: Cervix Uteri Cancer*. http://seer.cancer.gov/statfacts/html/cervix.html. Accessed October 9, 2022.

87. American Cancer Society. www.cancer.org/cancer/endometrial-cancer/about/key-statistics.html, www.cancer.org/cancer/cervical-cancer/treating/chemotherapy.html. Accessed October 9, 2022.

88. World Cancer Research Fund International. www.wcrf.org/cancer-trends/cervical-cancer-statistics/. Accessed October 9, 2022. National Cancer Institute. Surveillance, epidemiology, and end results program (SEER) stat fact sheets: Ovary cancer. http://seer.cancer.gov/statfacts/html/ovary.html. Accessed March 13, 2015.

89. Cranganu A, Camporeale J. Nutrition aspects of lung cancer. *Nutr Clin Pract.* 2009 Dec;24(6):688–700.

90. Rawla P. Epidemiology of prostate cancer. World J Oncol. 2019 Apr;10(2):63–89. doi: 10.14740/wjon1191. Epub 2019 Apr 20. PMID: 31068988; PMCID: PMC6497009.

91. Bray F, Ferlay J, Soerjomataram I, Siegel RL, Torre LA, Jemal A. Global cancer statistics 2018: GLOBOCAN estimates of incidence and mortality worldwide for 36 cancers in 185 countries. CA Cancer J Clin. 2018;68(6):394–424. doi: 10.3322/caac.21492.

92. What Are the Key Statistics about Lung Cancer? *American Cancer Society Website.* www.cancer.org/cancer/lungcancer-non-smallcell/detailedguide/non-small-cell-lung-cancer-key-statistics. Accessed March 19, 2015.

93. Martin-Ucar AE, Nicum R, Oey I, Edwards JG, Waller DA. En-bloc chest wall and lung resection for non-small cell lung cancer. Predictors of 60-day non-cancer related mortality. *Eur J Cardiothorac Surg.* 2003 Jun;23(6):859–64.

94. Lung Cancer. *American Cancer Society Website.* www.cancer.org/cancer/lungcancer/index. Accessed March 16, 2015.

95. Non-Small Cell Lung Cancer Treatment (PDQ®). *National Cancer Institute.* www.cancer.gov/cancertopics/pdq/treatment/non-small-cell-lung/Patient/page4. Accessed March 16, 2015.

96. Trestini I, Sperduti I, Sposito M, Kadrija D, Drudi A. Evaluation of nutrition status in non-small-cell lung cancer: Screening, assessment and correlation with treatment outcome. *ESMO Open.* 2020;5(3).

97. Tewari N., Martin-Ucar AE, Black E et al. Nutritional status affects long term survival after lobectomy for lung cancer. *Lung Cancer.* 2007 Sep;57(3):389–94.

98. Soares NDCP, Elias MB, Lima Machado C, Trindade BB, Borojevic R, Teodoro AJ. Comparative analysis of lycopene content from different tomato-based food products on the cellular activity of prostate cancer cell lines. Foods. 2019 Jun 10;8(6):201. doi: 10.3390/foods8060201. PMID: 31185698; PMCID: PMC6617171.

99. American Institute of Cancer Research (AICR). *Prostate Cancer,* last updated September 1, 2020. www.aicr.org/research/the-continuous-update-project/prostate-cancer/. Accessed October 9, 2022.

100. Scott H, McMillan DC, Brown DJ, Forrest LM, McArdle CS, Milroy R. A prospective study of the impact of weight loss and the systemic inflammatory response on quality of life in patients with inoperable non-small cell lung cancer. *Lung Cancer.* 2003 Jun;49(3):295–9.

101. Wilson KM, Shui IM, Mucci LA, Giovannucci E. Calcium and phosphorus intake and prostate cancer risk: A 24-y follow-up study. Am J Clin Nutr. 2015 Jan;101(1):173–83. doi: 10.3945/ajcn.114.088716. Epub 2014 Nov 19. PMID: 25527761; PMCID: PMC4266887.

102. National Cancer Institute (NCI). www.cancer.gov/types/prostate/patient/prostate-prevention-pdq#_12, www.cancer.org/cancer/prostate-cancer/treating/radiation-therapy.html, www.cancer.org/cancer/prostate-cancer/treating/vaccine-treatment.html, www.cancer.org/cancer/prostate-cancer/treating/chemotherapy.html, www.cancer.gov/about-cancer/treatment/cam/patient/prostate-supplements-pdq#_446. Accessed October 9, 2022.

103. Tat D, Kenfield SA, Cowan JE, Broering JM, Carroll PR, Van Blarigan EL, Chan JM. Milk and other dairy foods in relation to prostate cancer recurrence: Data from the cancer of the prostate strategic urologic research endeavor (CaPSURE™). Prostate. 2018 Jan;78(1):32–9. doi: 10.1002/pros.23441. Epub 2017 Nov 6. PMID: 29105845; PMCID: PMC5716878.

104. Applegate CC, Rowles JL, Ranard KM, Jeon S, Erdman JW. Soy consumption and the risk of prostate cancer: An updated systematic review and meta-analysis. Nutr. 2018 Jan 4;10(1):40. doi: 10.3390/nu10010040. PMID: 29300347; PMCID: PMC5793268.

105. Naiko A, Chewonarin T, Tang M et al. Ellagic acid, a component of pomegranate fruit juice, suppresses androgen-dependent prostate carcinogenesis via induction of apoptosis. Prostate. 2015 Feb;75(2):151–60.

106. Azrad M, Vollmer RT, Madden J, Dewhirst M, Polascik TJ, Snyder DC, Ruffin MT, Moul JW, Brenner DE, Demark-Wahnefried W. Flaxseed-derived enterolactone is inversely associated with tumor cell proliferation in men with localized prostate cancer. J Med Food. 2013 Apr;16(4):357–60. doi: 10.1089/jmf.2012.0159. PMID: 23566060; PMCID: PMC3624628.

107. Kumar NB, Hogue S, Pow-Sang J, Poch M, Manley BJ, Li R, Dhillon J, Yu A, Byrd DA. Effects of green tea catechins on prostate cancer chemoprevention: The role of the gut microbiome. Cancers (Basel). 2022 Aug 18;14(16):3988. doi: 10.3390/cancers14163988. PMID: 36010981; PMCID: PMC9406482.

108. Guo Y, Zhi F, Chen P, Zhao K, Xiang H, Mao Q, Wang X, Zhang X. Green tea and the risk of prostate cancer: A systematic review and meta-analysis. Medicine (Baltimore). 2017 Mar;96(13):e6426. doi: 10.1097/MD.0000000000006426. PMID: 28353571; PMCID: PMC5380255.

109. Katta S, Srivastava A, Thangapazham RL, Rosner IL, Cullen J, Li H, Sharad S. Curcumin-gene expression response in hormone dependent and independent metastatic prostate cancer cells. Int J Mol Sci. 2019 Oct 2;20(19):4891. doi: 10.3390/ijms20194891. PMID: 31581661; PMCID: PMC6801832.

110. Eliassen AH, Colditz GA, Rosner B, Willett WC, Hankinson SE. Adult weight change and risk of postmenopausal breast cancer. *JAMA*. 2006;296(2):193–201.

111. Hossain S, Beydoun MA, Beydoun HA, Chen X, Zonderman AB et al. Vitamin D and breast cancer: A systematic review and meta-analysis of observational studies. Clin Nutr ESPEN. 2019 Apr;30:170–84.

112. Aune D, Navarro Rosenblatt DA, Chan DS, Vieira AR, Vieira R, Greenwood DC et al. Dairy products, calcium, and prostate cancer risk: A systematic review and meta-analysis of cohort studies. Am J Clin Nutr. 2015;101:87–117.

113. Parikh RB. Early specialty palliative care – Translating data in oncology into practice [Sounding Board]; *N Engl J Med*. 2013;369(24):2347–51.

114. Palliative Care in Cancer. *National Cancer Institute Website*. www.cancer.gov/cancer-topics/factsheet/Support/palliative-care. Published 2010. Accessed January 25, 2015.

115. Oberholzer R. The concept of cachexia-related suffering (CRS) in palliative care. In: Preedy, VR ed. *Diet and Nutrition in Palliative Care*. Boca Raton, FL: Taylor & Francis Group, LLC; 2011:3–16.

116. Hospice and End of Life Care. *National Resource Center on Nutrition, Physical Activity & Aging Website*. http://nutritionandaging._u.edu/creative_solutions/hospice.asp. Published June 2005. Accessed January 27, 2015.

117. Berger AM, Shuster JL, Von Roenn JH. *Principles and Practice of Palliative Care and Supportive Oncology*. 4th ed. Philadelphia, PA: Lippincott Williams & Wilkins; 2013:779–89.

Recognition is given to the authors of this chapter in the first edition:

Rachel Winston, MS, RDN, CSO; Stephanie Paver, RDN, CSO, CNSC; Kamorin Samson, RDN, CSO, LDN; Renee Pieroth, RDN, CSO, LDN; Crystal Langlois, RDN, CSO, LD; Nathan Schober, MS, RDN, CNSC; Maureen Geboy, RDN, LD; Andrea Swartz, RDN, LD; Roberta Scheuer, RDN, LD; Matt Rinehart, MS, RDN, CSO, LD; Jessica Smith, MS, RDN, CSO, LD; Gabrielle Taylor, MS, RDN, LD; Kalli Castille, MS, RDN, LD, FAND; Jessica Engelbrecht, MS, RDN, CSR, LD, CNSC; Brooke McIntyre, RDN, CSO, LD, CNSC; and Jasmyn Walker, MS, RDN, LD, CSO, CNSC.

Appendix 1

Chemotherapeutic Agent	Common Nutritional Side Effects	Notes
Abraxane	Low white blood cell and red blood counts, nausea, weakness/fatigue	
Afatinib (Gilotrif®)	Diarrhea, mouth sores, dry mouth	Taken on empty stomach a few hours before a meal with 8 oz of water
Bevacizumab (Avastin®)	Anorexia, abdominal pain, upper respiratory infection, constipation, low white blood cell count, proteinuria, diarrhea, mouth sores, generalized weakness	Of note: Patient has to be off Avastin for 4 weeks prior to surgery related to wound healing issues. If needing nutrition support consider the timeline/delays encountered.
Bleomycin (Blenoxane®)	Nausea, vomiting, mucositis, weight loss, anorexia	
Carboplatin (Paraplatin®)	Low white/red/platelet counts, nausea, vomiting, taste changes, low magnesium levels	Adequate hydration is a concern with all the platinum-based therapies.
Casodex	Rapid weight gain	
Cisplatin (Platinol®)	Nausea, vomiting, kidney toxicity, low magnesium/calcium/potassium, low white/red/platelet counts	Watch for refractory low potassium related to low magnesium.
Capecitabine (Xeloda®)	Nausea, vomiting, diarrhea	
Cetuximab (Erbitux)	Nausea, vomiting, diarrhea, constipation, low magnesium	
Crizotinib (Xalkori®)	Nausea, vomiting, diarrhea, taste changes, edema	TKI mechanism; avoid grapefruit/St. John's Wort
Cyclophosphamide (Cytoxan®)	Nausea, vomiting	
Dacarbazine		
Docetaxel (Taxotere®)	Low red/white blood cell counts, fluid retention, nausea, diarrhea, peripheral neuropathy, mouth sores	
Doxorubicin (Adriamycin®) (Rubex®)	Nausea, vomiting, low white/red/platelet counts, mouth sores	
Epirubicin (Ellence®)	Nausea, vomiting, diarrhea, mucositis	

(Continued)

(*Continued*)

Chemotherapeutic Agent	Common Nutritional Side Effects	Notes
Erlotinib (Tarceva®)	Diarrhea, anorexia, nausea, vomiting	Taken by mouth on empty stomach a few hours before a meal with full glass of water at the same time every day. Avoid grapefruit/St. John's Wort.
Etoposide (VP-16, Toposar®)	Low red/white/platelet counts, nausea, vomiting, mouth sores, anorexia, metallic taste, peripheral neuropathy	
Firmagon	Peripheral edema, fatigue, osteoporosis, decrease in lean body mass, elevated lipids, hot flashes	
Fluraeal 5-FU	Increased triamine, stomatitis, nausea, vomiting, diarrhea	
Gefitinib	HTN, dry skin, anorexia, nausea, vomiting, mucositis	
Gemcitabine (Gemzar®)	Flu symptoms, fever, nausea, vomiting, anorexia, low red/white/platelet counts	
Ifosfamide (Ifex®)	Low red/white/platelet counts, nausea, vomiting, anorexia, blood in urine	Hydration is important with this medication to help clear bladder.
Irinotecan (Camptosar®)	Diarrhea, nausea, vomiting, weakness, anorexia, fever, weight loss, low red/white/platelet counts	St. John's Wort is contraindicated.
Ixabepilone (Ixempra®)	Diarrhea, constipation, mucositis	
Lupron	Peripheral edema, fatigue, osteoporosis, decrease in lean body mass, elevated lipids, hot flashes	
Methotrexate (MTX®)	Mucositis, nausea	
Mitomycin (Mutamycin)	Low red/white/platelet count, mouth sores, anorexia, fatigue	
Paclitaxel (Taxol®)	Low red/white/platelets, peripheral neuropathy, nausea, vomiting, diarrhea, mouth sores	
Pazopanib		Take one hour before eating or two hours after. Avoid grapefruit and grapefruit juice.

(*Continued*)

Chemotherapeutic Agent	Common Nutritional Side Effects	Notes
Pemetrexed (Alimta®)	Low red/white/platelet counts, nausea, vomiting, constipation, anorexia, diarrhea, stomatitis, esophagitis, taste change, difficulty swallowing	Typical supplementation with Alimta to prevent severe anemia: Folic acid (350–1000 Mcg) by mouth 1 week prior to first treatment and to continue daily. B12 (1000 Mcg) injections given 1 week prior to first treatment then every 3 cycles.
Ramucirumab (Cyramza®)	Rare	
Sunitinib	HTN, diarrhea, stomatitis, dysgeusia, neutropenia, abdominal pain	
Topotecan	Nausea, vomiting, diarrhea, mucositis	
Trastuzumab (Herceptin®)	Nausea, vomiting, diarrhea	
Trelstar	Peripheral edema, fatigue, osteoporosis, decrease in lean body mass, elevated lipids, hot flashes	
Vinblastine (Velban®)	Low red/white/platelets, nausea, vomiting, constipation	Avoid St. John's Wort/ grapefruit. Constipation prevention is helpful because severe constipation can occur with medication.
Vincristine	Neuropathy, mucositis, diarrhea	
Vinorelbine (Navelbine®)	Low red/white/platelet counts, nausea, vomiting, muscle weakness, constipation	
Xtandi (Enzulatamide)	Diarrhea, fatigue, hot flashes	
Zoladex	Peripheral edema, fatigue, osteoporosis, decrease in lean body mass, elevated lipids, hot flashes	
Zytiga (Abiraterone)	Fatigue, diarrhea, hot flashes, upset stomach, HTN, hypokalemia, edema	

Appendix 2

Chemotherapy-Related Side Effects	Management of Nutrition Impact Symptoms
Low red blood cell counts	Ensure adequate calories, protein, iron, copper, B12, and folic acid intake and adequate physical activity.
	Iron food examples are beef, pork, turkey, chicken, fish, enriched grains, nuts, dried beans, etc. An iron supplement may also be needed if iron saturation is low. Add vitamin C-rich foods with non-heme sources.
	Copper food examples are nuts, seeds, and lentils.
	Folic acid food examples are dark leafy greens, asparagus, broccoli, beans/lentils, and enriched grains.
	B-12 food examples are animal protein and enriched grains.
	Avoid caffeine with meals, which can decrease iron absorption.
	Physical activity: minimum of 30 minutes of moderate physical activity most days of the week.
	Medications that may be added could include but are not limited to Procrit and Aranesp.
Low white blood cell counts	Ensure adequate calories/protein/vitamin/minerals for recovery.
	If white blood cell counts are below 2.5 mcL or ANC < 1.0 mcL then special care and diet restrictions should be heeded to prevent unwanted infection.
	See United States Department of Agriculture and Food and Drug Administration report on "Food Safety For People with Cancer." (www.fda.gov/downloads/Food/FoodborneIllnessContaminants/UCM312761.pdf)
	A low microbial diet may also be recommended. Usually what is recommended is avoiding undercooked foods and choosing cooked foods instead. Examples include cooked fruits/vegetables, cooked meat, pasteurized milks, etc. Avoid yogurt and other probiotic foods until white counts have recovered. Avoid buffets, and ensure leftovers are only kept a few days and then reheated to at least 165 degrees F.
	Medications that may be added could include but are not limited to Neulasta and Neupogen.
Low platelet counts	No direct causal link to help with recovery but a naturopathic doctor may have suggestions of certain supplements that may help to recover these counts.
	Take extra care when preparing foods not to cut yourself, since the bleeding may be more difficult to stop.
	Interventions that may be added could include but are not limited to corticosteroids, platelet transfusion, and splenectomy.

(*Continued*)

Chemotherapy-Related Side Effects	Management of Nutrition Impact Symptoms
Nausea/vomiting	Prevent dehydration by drinking plenty of fluids (ginger tea, water, sports drinks, watered-down juice, broths, popsicles, clear sodas, slushies, ice chips, etc.). Foods well tolerated include crackers, canned fruit, mashed potatoes, oatmeal, dry toast, pretzels, rice, and small frequent meals. Drink fluids between meals instead of with meals. Avoid strong smells (cold/room temp foods help with this), greasy foods, acidic foods, spicy foods, and caffeine. High-protein foods combined with ginger may be helpful. Ginger is a well-known anti-nausea tool and can be consumed as ginger ale (if actually formulated with ginger), ginger tea, ginger chew candies, etc. Try wearing sea bands. Medications that may be added could include but are not limited to Zofran, Kytril, Compazine, Ativan, Sancuso patch, scopolamine patch, and many more.
Constipation	Ensure adequate hydration (At least 64 oz fluid daily unless specified by healthcare provider) and adequate fiber intake (25–35 g fiber per day) along with 30–60 minutes of moderate physical activity most days of the week if medically feasible. High-fiber foods/Supplements include wheat bran cereal, whole grain bread/products, brown rice, raw vegetables, fruits, ground flax seed, chia seeds, and Metamucil. Try 4–8 oz warm prune juice or black cherry juice. Also, probiotic foods can help promote intestinal health and include yogurt, kefir, and miso. Medications that may be added could include but are not limited to stool softeners, laxatives, enemas, etc. Items such as vitamin C and magnesium may be added at the right dose to help with bowel movements as well.
Diarrhea	Prevention of dehydration and electrolyte disturbances is key. An easy rule of thumb is to weigh at start of day and end of day: every pound lost is close to 16 oz of fluid along with the minimum of 64 oz water. Example of oral rehydration solution from *Oley.org*: 3/8 tsp salt, ¼ tsp salt substitute (potassium chloride), ½ tsp baking soda, 2 tbsp + 2 tsp table sugar, add tap water to make 1 Liter (can add NutraSweet/Splenda for better taste). Other hydration options: water is good but alternate with other options, such as sports drinks, juice, Pedialyte, etc. to maximize absorption and prevent electrolyte issues. Foods recommended: BRATY diet (bananas, white rice, applesauce, white toast, and yogurt), oatmeal, barley, citrus, etc. Can add pectin powder or similar product to smoothies to help slow diarrhea. Drink/eat cold/room temperature foods. Milk alternatives or Lactaid milk. Try Banatrol 1–3 packets a day or other soluble fiber supplement.

(*Continued*)

Chemotherapy-Related Side Effects	Management of Nutrition Impact Symptoms
	Avoid lactose (regular cow milk/goat milk, cheese, etc.), hot foods, caffeine, drinking and eating at same time, insoluble fiber (uncooked fruits/vegetables, whole grains, particularly whole-wheat products), vitamin C supplements, etc.
	Consider sources of probiotics – yogurt, kefir, and/or supplements.
	Medications that may be added could include but are not limited to Imodium, Lomotil, Questran, and many more.
Anorexia	Small frequent meals with protein at all meals and snacks. Aim to eat every 2–3 hours.
	Add in high-calorie/high-protein foods such as avocado dips, hummus, hard-boiled eggs, cottage cheese, smoothies with whey protein powder, milk/soy milk, nuts/seeds/nut butters, etc.
	Supplements may include Boost, Ensure, Orgain, Boost Very High Calorie, whey protein powder, ENU, etc.
	In severe cases nutrition support may be indicated if anorexia is causing significant weight loss and poor intake is expected to be for an extended period of time.
	Consider food and/or supplement sources of EPA.
	Medications that may be added could include but are not limited to corticosteroids, Marinol, Megace, Remeron, and many more.
Mouth sores	Can be painful to chew and certain foods like those high in acid may be painful. Keep mouth clean by brushing and using a healthcare-approved mouthwash that is alcohol free.
	Try to avoid foods high in acid such as tomatoes, oranges, lemons, etc. Also avoid spices, alcohol/alcohol-based mouth rinses, sharp foods like chips, buffalo sauce, etc.
	Try soft, moist, bland foods such as smoothies, mashed potatoes, Boost/Ensure/Orgain/ENU supplements, puddings, room temperature soup, eggs, and soft fruit.
	Suck on hard candy, chew gum.
	Medications that may be added could include but are not limited to Episil® oral gel, magic mouth wash, baking soda/salt/water mouth rinse used multiple times per day.
Taste changes	Can be bitter, metallic, salty, sweet, or just "wrong."
	Zinc supplements have been shown to help with taste changes; typical dose is usually 30 mg or more per day in split doses.
	If metallic taste, avoid red meats, switch to plastic utensils for eating, and try cooking in ceramic/glass instead of metal dishes.
	If lack of taste, ensure rinsing mouth several times per day with healthcare-approved mouth wash that is alcohol free, use "extra" spices (typically not salt) to flavor foods, and try more gravy/sauce with foods.
	Medications that may be added could include but are not limited to zinc supplementation and alcohol-free mouth washes multiple times per day.

(Continued)

Chemotherapy-Related Side Effects	Management of Nutrition Impact Symptoms
Edema	Ensuring adequate protein and calories, avoiding excess salt (typically more than 2 g/day), and ensuring adequate thiamine level are first steps to nutritionally help with edema.
	If malnourished, low albumin can cause edema or cause it to become worse. Try small frequent meals and add nutritional supplements to try to increase calories/protein; consider nutrition support if unable to increase intake to a sufficient amount.
	Excess salt can cause fluid to leak into areas of the body; avoid processed foods (frozen/canned) and eat more fresh foods, watch meat for saline additives, use other spices instead of salt when cooking, read all labels for sodium content.
	Poor intake and weight loss can also cause vitamin deficiencies; edema can be caused by a thiamine deficiency that is unrelated to cancer treatment. If poor intake is suspected, then along with increasing calories and protein, add a thiamine supplement that meets at a minimum 100% of the RDA.
	Medications that may be added could include but are not limited to diuretics and albumin.
Hot flashes	Foods that may trigger hot flashes include caffeine, alcohol, sugar/refined sugar, and spicy foods.

18 Home Enteral Nutrition

Michelle Romano, Elizabeth Bobo,
and Angela Matthewson

18.1 HOME ENTERAL NUTRITION

18.1.1 INTRODUCTION/OVERVIEW

Enteral nutrition is defined as a "system of providing nutrition directly into the gastrointestinal tract via a tube, catheter, or stoma that bypasses the oral cavity" (Robinson et al. 2018). This therapy is used in individuals who are malnourished or at risk for malnutrition because they are unable to consume adequate nutrients by mouth. An early report using representative sampling and the Centers for Medicare and Medicaid Services (CMS) data estimate the home enteral nutrition (HEN) population to be increasing yearly and was approximately 148,000 in 1991 (Oley Foundation 1993). More recent estimates place the HEN population at 437,882 patients; including 248,846 adults and 189,036 pediatric patients (Mundi et al. 2017, 799). The American Society for Parenteral and Enteral Nutrition (ASPEN) developed Home and Alternate Site Care Standards for clinicians caring for patients requiring home nutrition support, and described this group as "a multi-disciplinary team with expertise in nutrition support [which] should be involved in the planning, education, implementation, and monitoring of HEN patients" (Durfee et al. 2014). Studies reporting on the team approach have noted reduced hospitalization rates (Klek et al. 2011, 383; Hall et al. 2014). Successful HEN therapy requires the expertise of multiple clinicians in order to achieve the best possible outcome. The following chapter outlines the steps that are needed to achieve clinical and patient goals.

18.1.2 ASSESSMENT

There are several criteria that make up an adult home enteral nutrition candidate. Ultimately this individual is one who cannot meet their nutrient requirements orally, who has sufficient bowel length for absorption of nutrients, and who is able to conduct therapy at home (ASPEN 2002). Reduced oral intake can be a result of impaired swallowing, motility disorder, or obstruction. Small bowel length greater than 100 cm is needed for adequate absorption of nutrients. Table 18.1 outlines common diagnoses for patients on HEN. Frequently, HEN is initiated in patients with swallow dysfunction related to stroke or neoplasm of the head and neck, or dysmotility or obstruction of the upper gastrointestinal tract. Contraindications for enteral nutrition include patients with obstruction, refractory nausea and vomiting, high-output fistulas, and severe malabsorption.

DOI: 10.1201/9780429322570-18

TABLE 18.1
Common Diagnoses for Home Enteral Nutrition

Neoplasm
Crohn's disease (adult and pediatric)
Neurologic swallow dysfunction
Motility disorder (gastroparesis)
Chronic obstruction
Congenital bowel dysfunction (chronic pseudo-obstruction)
Prematurity
Cystic fibrosis
Inborn errors of metabolism
Eosinophilic esophagitis

TABLE 18.2
Home Enteral Nutrition Care Plan

Nutrition goals; short term and long term, anticipated duration of therapy
Patient/caregiver education
Feeding route
Nutrition prescription
Infusion schedule
Drug-nutrient interactions
Care of access device
Infusion equipment
Monitoring frequency
Planned re-evaluation of care plan at least every three months or as needed based on patient status

Once the patient undergoes a full nutrition assessment, a plan of care will be developed taking into account the patient's therapy goals. See Table 18.2 for components of a full nutrition care plan.

Assessment of the patient should also include past medical history, available laboratory data, swallowing ability, and bowel habits. The patient may have additional medical conditions that will impact the decision of enteral formula and enteral feeding route choices. For example, a patient that also has heart failure would need a fluid restriction, and a concentrated formula might be used with reduced water flushes. A nutrition-focused physical examination should be undertaken to determine muscle or fat wasting, dehydration, or evident vitamin or mineral deficiency. Medications should be reviewed with special consideration of medication that can or should be crushed, food-nutrient interaction, and dosing schedule (i.e., insulin, medications that need to be taken with or without food). A pharmacist should review each medication to determine whether the enterally administered medication will be safe, stable, and compatible as ordered (Boullata 2017, 79). See Table 18.3 for potential enteral nutrition-drug interactions (Verdell and Rollins 2017, 373–374).

The patient and/or caregiver and the home environment need to be considered during the planning of HEN. The patient/caregiver should be assessed for the ability to conduct safe home therapy, including willingness, cognitive ability, and physical ability. The home should have adequate water supply, electricity,

---

TABLE 18.3

Specific Drug-Enteral Nutrition Interactions

Phenytoin
- Absorption may be reduced due to binding to enteral nutrition components or enteral tubing.
- Generally recommended to hold enteral nutrition for at least one hour and possibly 2 hours pre- and post-dose.
- Monitor serum phenytoin concentration.
- Consistence of administration is important.
- Dilute phenytoin suspension when administered through a feeding tube.

Carbamazepine
- Enteral nutrition can reduce bioavailability, more so for post-pyloric feeding than gastric feeding, since it is acid stable.
- Adequate dilution of the suspension (or slurry from crushed tablet) at least 1:1 (or up to 3:1) with water prior to administration via feeding tube may help reduce drug loss.
- If dilution and flushing fail in patients with post-pyloric administration, it would be reasonable to hold feedings before and after administration.

Fluoroquinolones
- Bioavailability appears to be reduced by enteral nutrition formulas.
- Data are limited for each of the fluoroquinolones' interaction with enteral feedings. It is currently recommended to hold enteral feedings for 1 hour pre- and 2 hours post-dose. This practice is supported with ciprofloxacin and norfloxacin; however, holding feedings with other fluoroquinolones should not be done routinely.

Warfarin
- Two proposed mechanisms of reduced warfarin absorption are binding with an enteral nutrition component (likely protein) or to polyurethane tubing; however, the interactions have not been clearly delineated.
- Potential methods of reducing the warfarin-enteral nutrition interaction include:
  - Using concentrated drug administered rapidly to minimize contact with the feeding tube
  - Separating warfarin administration from enteral nutrition administration
  - Increasing the warfarin dose until a therapeutic PT/INR is achieved
  - Changing to an alternate anticoagulation therapy that does not interact with enteral nutrition
  - Holding enteral nutrition for at least 1 hour before and after dose
  - Routine monitoring of PT/INR, especially with changes to enteral nutrition regimen so as not to place the patient at risk for bleeding

Source: Verdrell and Rollins (2017).

telephone, and adequate storage area for formula and enteral equipment (Boullata 2017, 17).

18.2 PEDIATRIC INDICATIONS

As practiced in adult care, enteral nutrition is the preferred route of nutrition support for pediatric patients since it has fewer deleterious effects than parenteral support, and is more physiologic. The primary indications for HEN of a pediatric patient are insufficient oral intake to promote growth and development, oral motor dysfunction, gastrointestinal abnormality that prohibits sufficient oral nutrient intake, and as primary therapy, such as for metabolic disorders (Braegger et al. 2010, 112; Vermilyea and Goh 2016, 59–60).

18.2.1 INSUFFICIENT ORAL INTAKE

Insufficient oral intake to meet nutrient needs is a common indicator for HEN in the pediatric population. It may manifest as either a reduction in appetite, such as seen in children undergoing oncologic treatment, or as an inability to meet nutrient needs when needs are elevated above that seen in the general population. For example, children with cystic fibrosis, burns, and congenital heart defects have increased energy requirements and may be unable to meet their needs via an oral diet alone (Hannah and John 2013, 568; Braegger et al. 2010, 122). Insufficient oral intake may also present secondary to a developed food aversion, such as is seen in some infants with severe gastroesophageal reflux disease, or in children with sensory integration problems, such as avoidant restrictive food intake disorder or autism. Criteria for insufficient oral intake includes an inability to consume >60%–80% of nutrient needs for >5 days in children greater than 1 year of age and >3 days in children less than 1 year of age (Vermilyea and Goh 2016, 59; Boullata et al. 2017, 37). HEN provides the child with additional nutrition so that their needs in relation to their energy expenditure are met.

18.2.2 ORAL MOTOR DYSFUNCTION

Oral motor dysfunction is a common issue in infants born prematurely because the suck–swallow–breathe reflex is not developed until 34 weeks gestation. Plus, after birth these infants are often intubated for ventilatory support, which inhibits the development of feeding skills and leads to oral motor dysfunction. These infants also tend to have elevated energy requirements. Thus, it is not uncommon for a premature infant to be discharged with HEN. Children with neurological impairment often require HEN secondary to swallowing disorders, esophageal disorders (e.g., gastroesophageal reflux, esophageal dysmotility), and behavioral disorders (aversive feeding behaviors, sensory-based feeding disorders) (Schwartz 2003, 318). Prolonged feeding time (4–6 hours a day) may also necessitate the usage of enteral nutrition in children with neurological impairment (Vermilyea and Goh 2016, 59; Axelrod et al. 2006, S21–S22).

18.2.3 Gastrointestinal Abnormality

Gastrointestinal (GI) abnormalities that can lead to dependency on HEN are those that inhibit the structure and/or function of the GI tract. For example, congenital malformations (e.g., tracheo-esophageal fistula), intestinal failure, tumors of the GI tract, gastroparesis, and caustic ingestion (Vermilyea and Goh 2016, 60). In these instances HEN may be short term or long term depending on the degree of impact of the abnormality. Also, HEN may be the primary source of nutrition or delivered as an adjunct to parenteral nutrition.

18.2.4 Primary Therapy

HEN is used as primary therapy for the management of pediatric Crohn's disease. Research indicates that a liquid-only diet for 8–12 weeks is as advantageous in inducing remission in Crohn's disease as corticosteroid therapy (Critch et al. 2012, 299; Lochs et al. 2006, 265; Canani et al. 2006, 386). Because of the difficulty of consuming only liquids to meet nutrient requirements for 2–3 months, many children opt to deliver all or part of the nutrition via a feeding tube. After remission has been achieved, HEN is commonly used as part of the maintenance regimen.

HEN is also used to manage inborn errors of metabolism and eosinophilic esophagitis when the child is not able or willing to follow the required diet via oral intake alone (Monzka 2015, 584). For example, a child with phenylketonuria may refuse the metabolic formula orally and instead choose to receive it via a feeding tube. HEN may also be used to manage the child with uncontrollable seizures who is following a ketogenic diet given the highly restrictive nature of the ketogenic protocol and its limited palatability.

18.2.4.1 Access

The type and location of the enteral access device depends on the length of need, and the gastrointestinal anatomy and function. Adult and pediatric patients with adequate gastric function would be best served with a tube terminating in the stomach, whereas those with gastric dysfunction would best tolerate small bowel feedings. Pediatric access is addressed later in this section. For adults, short-term needs (4–6 weeks) can be met with nasogastric (NG), nasoduodenal (ND), and nasojejunal (NJ) tubes (Boullata et al. 2017, 37). The position of the tube should be confirmed radiographically prior to use (Bankhead et al. 2009). When patients are transitioning from hospital to home, it is important to obtain information on the tube tip location because there are several different manufacturers of tubes, and tube length and position can vary. Use of the auscultatory method of aspirate is unreliable in determining feeding tip location (Boullata et al. 2017, 38). Visual inspection of tube aspirate and pH should be employed to detect tube location (Boullata et al. 2017). The external tube length should be measured or marked from the nose to monitor for displacement. On occasion, small bowel tubes can migrate upward into the stomach. Changes in tolerance to feedings, increased nausea, or vomiting of tube feedings should prompt radiographic testing of the tube location. Nasal tubes can be used for enteral feeding supplementation while the patient is transitioning to an enteral diet, or to determine enteral feeding tolerance prior to placement of a long-term access, or in patients for whom long-term access is contraindicated or not desired. In patients with adequate gastric function who need long-term access, a gastrostomy tube (GT) should be placed. These tubes are larger in diameter, allowing different feeding methods and medication administration. In cases of inadequate gastric function, a gastrojejunostomy (GJT) or jejunostomy (JT) tube should be placed. Enteral tubes can be placed surgically, endoscopically, and radiographically (Gramlich et al. 2018, 4). All efforts should be made to avoid tubing not typically used for enteral feedings (e.g., drain tubes or catheters) because there is no internal or external anchoring device and connections with enteral feeding sets may not be compatible. In 1.5%–4% of cases, major complications can occur with GT placement (Strollo et al. 2017, 725). It will take 7–10 days for the tract to heal fully, so if dislodged within that time, the patient should be brought back to the healthcare institution for replacement (Strollo et al. 2017, 725). Table 18.4 highlights indications for gastric or small bowel feedings (Itkin et al. 2011). In patients with gastric dysmotility, a GJT has been useful to vent or decompress the stomach via the gastric port while feeding into the small bowel via the jejunostomy port. For patients who are concerned about the external appearance of a tube, who are active, or who are prone-sleepers, a low-profile device or skin-level device may be an option. These devices have an internal bumper and an external port or ports for gastric or jejunal feedings. Manual dexterity is needed for attaching the extension tubing to the low-profile tube in order to use enteral feeding sets or syringes for tube flush.

18.2.4.2   Maintenance of the Enteral Access

Efforts should be made to avoid skin irritation at the enteral access site. It is recommended to use mild soap and water to clean the site and avoid occlusive dressings or

---

TABLE 18.4

Select Indications/Contraindications for Gastric and Small Bowel Access

Gastric Indications
Normal gastric and small bowel motility
Adequate anatomy to place access
Small Bowel Indications
Gastric outlet obstruction
Duodenal obstruction
Gastric or duodenal fistula
Severe gastroesophageal reflux disease
Contraindications
Mechanical obstruction
Active peritonitis
Bowel ischemia
Relative Contraindications
Ascites
Recent gastrointestinal bleeding

---

placement of gauze or cut drain sponges under the external bumper (Itkin et al. 2011). Topical silver nitrate or steroid can be applied if granulation tissue develops.

Tube clogs can occur due to accumulation of formula sediment and/or improper administration of medications. Flushing the tube with 30 milliliters of water every 4 hours, before and after feedings and medications, may prevent or reduce clogging (Boullata 2017, 75).

18.3 PEDIATRIC ACCESS CONSIDERATIONS

18.3.1 OROGASTRIC

Orogastric tubes are generally not used in the outpatient setting. Rarely, they may be seen in the home patient who has a facial dimorphism that prohibits the use of a nasogastric tube. Even so, these tubes are generally replaced with a permanent tube for long-term nutrition support.

18.3.2 NASOGASTRIC

Nasogastric tubes are used for children requiring short-term enteral access (i.e., less than 12 weeks) (Lyman and Shah 2015, 568); for example, infants/children with malnutrition who are expected to become independent of nutrition support or children with altered appetite due to oncologic treatment. NG tubes can be used long term for children who are placing a tube nightly for enteral access as part of their treatment method for Crohn's disease. NG tubes are appropriate for children with little/no gastroesophageal reflux, normal gastric function, and a low risk for aspiration (Baker et al. 2007, 252). Ideally, NG tube placement should be verified using abdominal X-ray (Bankhead et al. 2009; Wathen and Peyton 2014, 16). However, repeat exposure to radiation is a concern in the pediatric cohort. Plus obtaining an X-ray to consistently verify tube placement is not feasible in the home setting. Thus, the best approach in the home setting to assure proper tube placement is to monitor tube insertion length and to measure the pH of aspirated gastric secretions (Boullata et al. 2017, 41). Gastric secretions have a pH of 1–4. The literature supports using a pH of <4 to verify correct tube placement (Irving et al. 2014, 272). Other research suggests that a pH of ≤5 may be an acceptable value to verify tube placement (Wathen and Peyton 2014, 16; Gilberston et al. 2011, 543). However, one should be cognizant that pH is not a reliable indicator for children on gastric acid-suppressive medications (Bankhead et al. 2009, 143). The auscultation method should not be used. NG tubes made of polyurethane and silicone generally can remain in place for 4 weeks before being changed (Vermilyea and Goh 2016, 60). Placement of an NG tube is not a contraindication to initiating or continuing an oral diet provided that the child is medically safe to ingest oral nutrition (Lyman and Shah 2015, 568).

18.3.3 NASOJEJUNAL

Nasojejunal tubes (NJ) are indicated for short-term enteral access and are appropriate for the child with gastroesophageal reflux, gastroparesis, aspiration risk, or acute pancreatitis. The tip of the tube should be distal to the ligament of Treitz (Nijs and

Cahill 2010, 1101). Tube placement should be verified using X-ray. Because these tubes are located in the small intestine, they are not appropriate for bolus feedings. Generally, these tubes may remain in place for 4 weeks before being replaced.

18.3.4 Gastrostomy/Gastrojejunostomy

Gastrostomy tubes are indicted for children who require enteral nutrition support long term (suggested for 12 weeks or more) (Lyman and Shah 2015, 568) and have a functioning GI tract. Conversely, GJTs are indicated for children with severe gastro-esophageal reflux who are not appropriate candidates for a Nissen fundoplication, or for children who have a GT in place but are temporarily not tolerating feeds. In this case the jejunal port should be used for pump-assisted feedings and the gastric port should be used for venting to improve feeding tolerance. Gastrostomy tubes can be replaced by the primary caregiver in the home every 3–6 months after the first tube change. GJTs cannot be changed in the home, but rather are generally changed every 3 months by an interventional radiologist (Vermilyea and Goh 2016, 62).

18.3.5 Jejunostomy

Jejunostomy tubes (JT) are indicated for children with significant gastroesophageal disease and/or gastroparesis. They are also indicated for children with a high aspiration risk. Typically these tubes are considered if enteral access is going to be needed for 6 months or longer (Lyman and Shah 2015, 569). Like GJTs these tubes are only appropriate for pump-assisted feedings. They also require routine flushing to prevent clogging.

18.3.5.1 Enteral Formula Selection

Planning the HEN regimen should take into consideration the patient's medical history, gastrointestinal capabilities, enteral access, administration method, short-term and long-term nutrition goals, and the patient/caregiver wishes.

There are enteral formulas that are manufactured for specific disease states; however, a standard polymeric formula will meet the nutritional needs of most home patients. The nutrient concentration of a polymeric formula can range from 1–2 calories/mL, and meet the Recommended Daily Allowance (RDA) for vitamins and minerals within 1.5 liters per day. Note that enteral formulas are categorized as a "medical food" under federal law. They are not considered drugs, and thus are not subject to any regulatory requirements that specifically apply to drugs (US Food and Drug Administration 2016). For a pediatric patient, the volume needed to meet the RDA is dependent on the age of the child and the type of formula being used. For example, a standard 1 calorie/mL formula is designed to meet the needs of a child 1–8 years of age in 1 liter, but for a child 9–13 years of age, 1.5 liters are required. It is important to consider the medical status of the child when choosing a formula. For example, a child that is neurologically impaired and hypotonic may do best with a calorie-reduced formula that will still provide ample protein, vitamins, and minerals for age. Fiber-containing formula may help to regulate frequency or consistency of stool. Table 18.5 describes the categories and characteristics of the various enteral formulas available. Occasionally, the patient may require a higher amount of a macronutrient, such as protein or fiber. Modular products are available that can be given

TABLE 18.5

Characteristics of Enteral Formulas and Recommendations for Use

Formula Type	Characteristics	Recommendations for Use
Polymeric	• Contain macronutrients as nonhydrolyzed protein, fat, and carbohydrate • Range in concentration from 1–2 kcal/mL • 1–1.5 liters usually meets RDA for vitamins and minerals • May be disease specific and/or contain pre- and probiotics	Patients with normal or near-normal gastrointestinal absorptive capacity
Fiber-containing	• Fiber content intended to improve the health of the GI tract, regulating frequency and/or consistency of stool by maintaining healthy GI flora • Fiber content typically below total daily fiber recommendations • May contain prebiotics in the form of fructooligosaccharides, oligofructose, or inulin • May also contain probiotics	Recommended for use among patients with diarrhea and/or to promote/maintain gut microbiota
Commercial blenderized	• Contains whole food ingredients in carton or ready-to-feed packaging • Available for adults and pediatrics	Patients with normal or near-normal gastrointestinal absorptive capacity
Homemade whole food/blenderized	• Blenderized whole foods designed to allow patients to receive qualities of food not found in standard enteral formulas, such as phytochemicals	• Due to infection/food-borne illness risk, use in medically stable patients with healed enteral access site • Best suited for patients with safe food practices and tube maintenance techniques • Should be provided as bolus/gravity drip administration to maintain safe food practices (hang time <2 hours) • RDN should be involved in development of feeding composition to ensure adequate nutrient delivery
Diabetes/glucose intolerance	• Intended to reduce hyperglycemia with macronutrient composition of 34–36% carbohydrate, 40–44% fat, and 20% protein • Fat and soluble fiber content may slow gastric emptying and prevent elevated blood glucose	Use of DM-specific enteral formulas is not currently support by strong research; instead efforts should be made to prevent overfeeding.

TABLE 18.5 (*Continued*)

Characteristics of Enteral Formulas and Recommendations for Use

Formula Type	Characteristics	Recommendations for Use
Renal	• Fluid restricted • Contains lower amounts of electrolytes, specifically potassium and phosphorus to prevent excessive deliver to patients with renal insufficiency • Protein content varies	Research does not strongly support renal formulas over standard polymeric formulas with renal insufficiency. If significant electrolyte abnormalities exist or develop, a renal formula should be considered until electrolytes stabilize. Patients receiving maintenance hemodialysis (MHD) may benefit from a renal formula with regard to electrolyte balance. In some cases a standard formula may be used in MHD patients along with monitoring electrolytes.
Elemental/Semi-elemental	• Macronutrients are hydrolyzed to maximize absorption	Intended for patients with malabsorptive disorders

Source: Brown et al. 2015. Nutr Clin Pract 30(1) pp 73, copyright © 2015 American Society for Parenteral and Enteral Nutrition. Reprinted by permission of John Wiley & Sons.

in separate doses to meet the patient's requirements. Protein modulars are available in liquid and powder forms. Fiber supplements are available as soluble fiber, and when mixed with water will dissolve and reduce risk of tube clogging.

Since the patient or caregiver will be responsible for the feedings, determination of the feeding schedule should be collaborative. Several goals can be accomplished: the patient will begin feedings and advance as tolerated to the goal volume to meet nutritional requirements, the feeding schedule and advancement will minimize complications and intolerance, and the tube feeding schedule itself is adaptable to their lifestyle. For adults with gastric access, formula can be administered intermittently (bolus, gravity drip) or by pump-assisted (cycle or continuous) method. One benefit of bolus or gravity drip is that it can mimic a mealtime schedule, and may allow flexibility in daily activities. In some cases in which oral intake has been diminished for a period of time or the patient is undergoing radiation or chemotherapy, the gravity drip method may be better tolerated than bolus, since this allows for slower infusion (over 20–30 minutes). Initiation of enteral feedings for pediatric patients will be addressed later in this section.

For adults with jejunal access, feedings are best tolerated using a pump-assisted method. Consideration should be given to a cycle infusion to allow the patient freedom from feeding equipment. The hours of infusion should be discussed with the patient/caregiver, and the tube feedings advanced accordingly. For patients with some oral intake, a nighttime cycle schedule may be ideal to supplement daytime intake. A portable feeding pump will allow flexibility with activity inside and outside the home. Table 18.6 provides recommendations on initiation and advancement.

TABLE 18.6

Enteral Access, Administration Method, and Initiation of Enteral Feedings

Access	Administration Method	Initiation
Gastric	Bolus (5–10 minutes) Gravity drip/Intermittent (20–60 minutes)	3–8 times per day, starting with 60–120 mL formula and increase by 60–120 mL each feeding or each day until goal is reached
Gastric or Small Bowel	Pump-assisted cycle (<24 hours/ day, commonly 8–14 hours/day) Pump-assisted continuous (24 hours/day)	Start at 10–40 mL/hour. For cycle schedule, increase by increments of 10–20 mL/hour every 12–24 hours depending on the length of the infusion cycle. For continuous infusion, advance by 10–20 mL/hour every 8–12 hours until goal is reached.

18.3.6 ENTERAL FORMULA SAFETY

Ensuring EN formula safety is important to reduce bacterial contamination of the enteral formula and avoid GI and infectious complications. Commercially available liquid EN products are sterilized during production, and that can be disrupted with any manipulation. Following good hygiene practices and safe hang time of the formula will reduce the risk of contamination. Follow the EN formula manufacturer's recommendations for hang times. Table 18.7 provides select practice recommendations for EN formula safety that are applicable to the home care setting.

18.4 PEDIATRIC INITIATION

Initiation of enteral feedings for a younger pediatric patient is generally done in the hospital over the course of several days to test for tolerance and advance the feeding volume (Bankhead et al. 2009, 29). However, feeds may also be initiated in the homecare setting provided that proper tube placement has been verified and caregiver support is adequate. When providing HEN to a pediatric patient it is important to implement measures that ensure safe and proper delivery of the nutrition. For example, locking the settings on the enteral pump is beneficial so that the child will not change them when touching the buttons. It is also sometimes beneficial to use clamps to secure the extension tubing to prevent separation when tugged on. For infants, running the tubing out of the bottom of a sleeper outfit for nighttime feeds prevents the infant from grabbing the tubing and disconnecting it. Applying facial tape to secure nasogastric/nasojejunal tubes is essential to reduce the incidence of tube dislodgment in infants. Using access-covering equipment (i.e., tube protective belts) can be helpful with toddlers and small children as a deterrent from playing

TABLE 18.7
Select Practice Recommendations for EN Safety in the Home Setting

1. Use a closed EN delivery system when possible.
2. Follow the manufacturer's recommendations for duration of infusion through an intact delivery device (container and administration set).
3. Do not reuse the enteral delivery device.
4. If open systems are used, follow recommended hang times and avoid topping off remaining formula, which may result in a continuous culture for exponential microbial growth.
   a. Limit infusion time for open EN feeding systems to 12 hours maximum.
   b. Change the delivery device (container and administration set) according to the manufacturer's recommendations.
5. To limit the risk of microbial growth and biofilm formation, avoid unnecessary additions to the EN administration set. If additional equipment such as 3-way stopcocks are used, follow manufacturer recommendations or facility protocol for change and cleaning practices.
6. Establish and follow protocols for preparation, handling, and storage of commercial and handmade EN.
   a. Educate those who prepare and administer EN about hand hygiene (a critical point) and safe handling of EN preparation and administration; extend education to patients and family members/caregivers who will continue this practice in the home setting.
   b. Use effective hand hygiene in all aspects of EN preparation and administration. When gloves are used, they must be clean gloves, not having been involved in other nonrelated tasks. The importance of hand washing in minimizing transference of microbial growth cannot be overstressed.
   c. Give preference to selecting systems that require minimal handling.
   d. Use a clean work surface for EN preparation.
   e. Use equipment dedicated for EN use only.
   f. Store EN formula according to the manufacturer's instructions. Store prepared or opened ready-to-feed solutions in an appropriate refrigerator, discarding any unused solutions within 24 hours of preparation or opening.
7. Keep all equipment, including syringes and containers for flush and medication administration, as clean and dry as possible. Store clean equipment away from potential sources of contamination.

Source: Adapted from Boullata et al. 2017. ASPEN Safe Practices for Enteral Nutrition Therapy. JPEN J Parenter Enteral Nutr;41:15–103. © 2017 by The American Society for Parenteral and Enteral Nutrition With permission of John Wiley & Sons.

---

with or pulling the access device, such as a gastrostomy tube. One must also consider the most appropriate regimen that will nourish the child, but also support age-appropriate development; for example, assuring that the child has a small backpack to hold the pump/formula so that they can be mobile during the day while receiving feeds. In addition, providing oral stimulation in the form of nonnutritive sucking or oral feedings, if medically safe to do so, is important to foster the development of feeding skills in children (Corkins et al. 2013, 267; Szeszycki et al. 2015, 619; Edwards et al. 2016, 620). Speech therapy services may also be needed to assist with the development of oral/motor skills.

18.4.1 Bolus and Gravity Feedings

When initiating bolus/gravity feedings, it is suggested that the regimen be initiated at 25% of the feeding goal, divided by the number of desired feedings. The volume may be increased by 25% of the feeding goal each day as tolerated (Bankhead et al. 2009, 29). It is prudent to not administer the feeding over a period of time that is less than one would expect the child to consume the formula orally since this practice may lead to intolerance of the feeding. One should also be cognizant of the child with a Nissen fundoplication. If a Nissen is intact then venting of the feeding tube after feeds may be necessary to lessen discomfort by allowing gas to escape.

18.4.2 Pump-Assisted Feedings

Guidelines suggest initiating the regimen for a child at 1–2 mL/kg/hour and advancing by 0.5–1 mL/kg/hour every 6–24 hours as tolerated until goal feedings are achieved (Bankhead et al. 2009, 29). Feedings may need to be started at a slower rate for children who are malnourished to avoid refeeding syndrome. It is best to use a non-diluted isotonic formula to reduce the risk of bacterial contamination (Bankhead et al. 2009, 29). Sterile formula in an open system can hang for up to 12 hours, unless it is being provided to a neonate in which case it should only hang for 4 hours (Boullata et al. 2017, 69. Similarly, human breast milk, non-sterile powder formulas, and modular products should only hang for 4 hours (Boullata et al. 2017, 67). For some pediatric patients a combination of pump-assisted feedings and bolus/gravity feedings may be the most appropriate method for providing HEN. For instance, some children with volume tolerance issues may do well with receiving bolus/gravity feedings during the day and pumped feedings overnight. Pump accuracy is of the utmost importance because small volumes are often administered to pediatric patients.

18.4.2.1 Monitoring

The next step in nutrition care is monitoring the therapy to be sure that the goals are achieved. Monitoring enteral therapy should take place at regular intervals as determined by the healthcare providers. Table 18.8 describes recommended monitoring parameters. The EN prescription should be reviewed accordingly based on physical exam, laboratory parameters, and transition of care (Boullata 2017, 32). Depending on clinical condition and EN tolerance, reassessment could take place every 1–4 weeks; for more stable patients, reassess at least quarterly (Boullata 2017, 93).

The enteral access should be monitored for leakage or peristomal infection. Peristomal infections are the most common complication and in most cases are mild and can be treated with antibiotics and local wound care. Stoma leakage can be caused by infection, tension on the external portion of the tube, or cleansing with irritating solutions. Patients with excessive tension between the external and internal bumpers, poor wound healing, or significant weight gain are at risk for buried bumper syndrome. The external bumper should be monitored and loosened to at least 1 cm (Itkin et al. 2011).

TABLE 18.8

Home Enteral Nutrition Monitoring

- Observations for signs and symptoms of intolerance to therapy
- Evaluation of weight changes and/or growth rates as appropriate
- Evaluation of hydration status
- Review of systems and/or physical examination
- Periodic review of biochemical, vitamin, mineral, or other pertinent laboratory data
- Assessment for clinical signs of nutrient deficiencies or excesses
- Assessment of other disease states or conditions that may affect the nutrition therapy
- Review for evidence of an interaction between the nutrition therapy and medications or other disease states
- Evaluation of functional status and performance
- Psychosocial status
- Evaluation of access device and site
- Patient/caregiver compliance with techniques and procedures
- Assessment of the need for continued therapy
- Monitoring intake (fluid, nutrient, oral) and output (urine, stool, GI losses)
- Review the appropriateness of the feeding route

Source: Adapted from Durfee et al. 2014. Nutri Clin Pract 29(4) pp 553, copyright © 2014 by American Society for Parenteral and Enteral Nutrition. Reprinted by Permission John Wiley & Sons.

18.4.2.2 Patient/Caregiver Education

The goals of education are to provide the skills needed to provide safe and effective HEN, and to reduce potential complications. Ideally, hospitalized patients transitioning to home would receive some basic education prior to discharge, then follow-up education would occur in the home. Trends have been noted with increasing home nutrition support population, decreased hospital length of stay, and decreased time for patient training in the hospital (Metzger 2010). See Table 18.9 for specific education and training needs in order to provide safe and effective therapy. Training should be aimed at the home regimen versus the hospital schedule.

For example, the home schedule could be adjusted so that patients/caregivers are not waking in the middle of the night for water flushes, adding formula, or feeding set changes.

All formula and equipment should be available in the home for comprehensive training. The patient/caregiver should be educated one on one in a quiet environment. Limitations of physical pain, dexterity, vision, hearing, or immobility may be taken into account, as well as anxiety or stress in learning a new task. The healthcare provider should provide an initial demonstration, then allow the patient/caregiver to "teach back," verbalizing the task and return demonstrate (Kornburger et al. 2013). Reassurance and encouragement should be provided with each task accomplishment.

Patient education materials used for training should have several components. The content should be accurate and based on current practice standards. The literacy level should be at a fifth- to sixth-grade level, with definitions provided for

TABLE 18.9

Patient/Caregiver Education for HEN Administration

- Name and phone numbers of resources available 24 hours per day to troubleshoot and answer questions
- The name, composition, intended use, and expected outcome of the formulation
- Medication information and administration, including dosage, route, frequency, and the potential for adverse effects and drug interactions
- Timing, method of administration, and feeding schedule
- Route of administration and duration of nutrition therapy
- Care of the enteral access device and site
- Product hang time and stability at room temperature
- Inspection of enteral products for contents and expiration date
- Clean technique for preparation of HEN, administration, and reuse of supplies and equipment
- Techniques for self-monitoring of therapy and identification of potential complications
- Proper storage of ready-to-use products and HEN formulas that require mixing
- Use and storage of enteral feeding equipment, supplies, and pump
- Proper disposal of used containers, tubing, and unused or expired feeding formulations and/or medications
- Action to be taken in the event of late or missed administration of HEN
- Process to order additional feeding formulation and supplies
- Infection prevention and control
- Basic home safety (fire, electrical, environment, mobility, bathroom)
- Information on emergency preparedness to assist patients and caregivers if an emergency should interrupt service
- Patients and caregivers shall be educated based on the teach-back method
- Patients and caregivers shall display competency in the understanding and performance of techniques

Source: Adapted from Durfee et al. 2014. Nutr Clin Pract 29(4) pp 552, copyright © 2014 by American Society for Parenteral and Enteral Nutrition. Reprinted by Permission of John Wiley & Sons.

unfamiliar words or terms (Clayton 2010). Graphics or visual presentation of information will help understanding and recall of health information. The layout of the material should be uncluttered, and type of at least 12-point font should be used. The material should be individualized to the patient/caregiver, and a chart can be used as a reminder of the schedule. Involving them in the process will help to foster learning and recall (Clayton 2010). Cultural relevance is helpful in the patient/caregiver identification with the material, so the target audience needs to be considered. Lastly, feasibility of the material refers to access to the information and materials provided in the patient's/caregiver's spoken language. There are some online videos and materials that may be helpful (ASPEN 2020; Mayo Clinic 2014; Oley Foundation 2015).

18.4.2.3   New Innovations in EN

18.4.2.3.1   Home Blenderized Tube Feedings (BTF)

Enteral feeding with blended foods was common before commercial formulas rose to prominence in the mid- and late-twentieth century. Professional preference for commercial formulas is related to lower risk of microbial contamination, nutritional predictability, and convenience. However, there has been a shift back toward blended foods among long-term enteral nutrition consumers, related to continued growing popularity of organic foods and minimally processed foods. Many patients and caregivers want to avoid common ingredients in commercial formulas, sugar and maltodextrin in particular (Weeks 2019, 1). Other motivations are emotional, including connection within families and a more normalized meal experience (Weeks 2019, 2).

While clinical evidence remains limited on the safety and efficacy, basic best-practice guidelines do exist. Patients and caregivers preparing BTF should use safe food handling techniques, avoiding cross-contamination and sanitizing equipment after each use. One study reported that in home BTF, 88% of the samples met the US Food Code criteria for safe food consumption, and 1.3% exceeded the criteria when following US Food Code guidelines (USFDA 2017; Milton et al. 2020). Once prepared, BTF should be used or refrigerated immediately. It should not be at room temperature for more than 2 hours, and refrigerated BTF should be thrown out after 24 hours (Boullata et al. 2017, 54). A high-powered blender will produce the smoothest consistency, reducing the risk of occlusion (Weeks 2019, 3). Still, clogged tubes are a higher risk with BTF, so patients with larger-bore tubes (≥14 French) are better candidates (Boullata et al. 2017, 54). Ideal BTF candidates are medically and socioeconomically stable and able to tolerate bolus feedings. Consultation with a registered dietitian will ensure consistently adequate nutrient content (Weeks 2019, 3; Walia C, et al. 2017), and resources are available (Bennett et al. 2020; Escuro 2014).

Given the growing popularity of BTF, it is no surprise that the commercial market has grown in the past decade. Companies large and small have brought blended, whole food, plant-based and/or organic food sourced enteral formulas to the market in the past several years (Weeks 2019, 1). It's important to read the ingredients carefully, since some may contain herbal extracts that may cause drug–nutrient interactions (Martin and Gardner 2017, 714). Follow the manufacturer instructions on tube size and administration. Insurance coverage remains a potential obstacle for commercial BTF formulas, which may cost more than the traditional formulas. Most insurance plans do not cover components of home BTF. However, some patients and caregivers may consider the trade-off worth it. Commercially available BTFs are available under the Healthcare Common Procedure Code (HCPC) B4149 (HCPC Codes 2020). Patient support groups (such as Oley Foundation and Tube Feeding Awareness Foundation) can be very helpful for patients and caregivers as they navigate BTF and all aspects of living with a feeding tube.

18.4.3 Pediatric Considerations in Home Blenderized Feedings

Home BTFs are becoming more commonplace in the pediatric cohort for a variety of reasons. Some caregivers believe that BTFs are better tolerated than commercial formulas in that they help to regulate bowel function and reduce gagging and vomiting. Further, with a BTF, unprocessed ingredients can be used, which is appealing to some caregivers as a means of providing their child with what they perceive as optimal nutrition. A BTF also offers a nurturing aspect to the nutrition care of a child that formula feeding does not. With a BTF caregivers may feel as if they are more involved in feeding their child and directing the nutrition that the child receives.

As with adults, there are a variety of issues that should be considered when initiating BTF. For example, the size of the feeding tube, feeding schedule, overall feeding volume, food allergies and/or intolerances, and immunosuppression should all be considered. The feeding volume and feeding schedule can be particularly problematic in pediatrics. Due to the viscosity of the blend and because it is not sterile, it is preferable for blends to be provided via bolus. However, this mode of feeding can be problematic for some children from a tolerance standpoint. In regards to tolerance, the total volume of the feedings required to meet nutrient needs may also be a barrier to providing BTF for some children (Mortensen 2006, 2; Oparaji et al. 2019, 113). For some children, usage of a commercially prepared blend may be a suitable alternative. These products have a longer hang time than homemade blends, are calorically dense, can be provided through an enteral pump, and do not have the same risk as a homemade blend for contamination.

BTF can be used in infants as young as 6 months to meet <25% of their nutritional needs. Of note, if an infant were born prematurely they should be at least 6 months corrected age before starting BTF. By age 1 year, 100% of nutritional needs can potentially be met from BTF (Walia et al. 2017, 11). One should be cognizant that a BTF for a pediatric patient is not stagnant. As the child ages, nutrient needs change and the blend will require adjusting. Thus, it is imperative that a child on a BTF receive regular medical nutrition therapy from an RDN. The RDN should analyze multiple days of the blend using a nutrition software program to assess the overall nutritional appropriateness of the blend since nutrients change depending on which ingredients are used. For example, changes in fruits and vegetables will alter the nutrient profile of the blend. The RDN should also monitor the child's anthropometrics and nutrition-related laboratory values as a means of determining the appropriateness of the blend (Malone 2005, 737).

18.4.4 ENTERAL ACCESS DESIGN

In 2006, the Joint Commission issued a sentinel event alert regarding enteral tubing misconnections (Joint Commission 2006). This alert stemmed from more than 100 incidences of enteral tubing misconnections, some with fatal outcomes, whereby small-bore connectors commonly used with medical devices were connected inappropriately with enteral tubing (e.g., enteral feedings connected with venous access). The sentinel alert called for a design change in enteral feeding connectors that would make inappropriate connections impossible (Joint Commission 2014). A re-design process was implemented by the International Organization of Standardization (ISO) in 2008 to develop a new connector that would only be compatible with enteral access. These new products, called ENFit connectors, have been developed to include the connector for the enteral set, syringes, and enteral feeding access (GEDSA 2020). The roll-out of these products began in 2015, and institutions have begun to incorporate these new devices into patient care. GEDSA has resources helpful to planning and implementation of these new devices, available at: http://stayconnected.org/tools-adopting-enfit/. Home blenderized tube feedings and commercially prepared formulas using syringe bolus administration were compared between ENFit proto-types and legacy feeding tubes. This early study showed that more force was needed for the BTF compared with the commercial tube feedings (Mundi et al. 2016). Later, this same group studied commercial EN formulas with the manufactured device. The tube sizes 14F and 24F had a significantly lower flow rate compared with other tube sizes (Mundi et al. 2018).

18.4.5 TECHNOLOGY-BASED HOME ENTERAL NUTRITION CARE

Recent changes in healthcare legislation will have a direct impact on the evolution of care of patients receiving HEN. The Health Information and Technology for Economic and Clinical Health (HITECH) Act, enacted in 2009, requires the use of electronic health records (EHRs) to improve healthcare quality, safety, and efficiency. (ONC 2014). The Patient Protection and Affordable Care Act (PPACA), enacted in 2010, includes the promotion and funding for a patient-centered medical home. "The patient-centered medical home delivery model is designed to improve quality of care through team-based coordination of care, treating the many needs of the patient at once, increasing access to care, and empowering the patient to be a partner in their own care" (HHS 2014). Strategies for clinicians to use technology to monitor HEN therapy are evolving. In 2010, Boisseau et al. used an automated tele-phone call system whereby patients could answer questions by phone and the results would be available by website to the healthcare providers (Boisseau et al. 2010). Now, patient portals have been developed in order for home patients to communicate with their healthcare providers and access their medical information. There will likely be further innovations. Use of telemedicine and facilitated support groups have been adopted utilizing mobile technology in home parenteral patients to aid in infection education and depression prevention (Nelson et al. 2017). Use of the EHRs and other technologies will hopefully aid in timely care of HEN patients and provide insight into ways to avoid or improve clinical complications.

18.4.5.1 Special Considerations in Long-Term EN Patients

Management guidelines are non-specific for monitoring patients on long-term home enteral nutrition at home (DeLegge 2002). ASPEN recommends that practitioners develop protocols that allow them to ensure that the nutrition care plan is being car-ried out as intended and the patient is able to meet their nutritional goals (Durfee et al. 2014). Prior to tube feeding initiation, a case manager, RDN, or other provider should review financial considerations with the patient/caregiver. Reimbursement levels vary based on insurance plans and diagnoses. Providers should also ensure that the patient and caregivers have adequate understanding of HEN procedures and that the home environment is appropriate for infusion (Durfee et al. 2014). Transition from HEN to an oral diet should be gradual and monitored to ensure adequacy. (Durfee et al. 2014) Discontinuation of HEN should take place when oral intake is adequate or when the care plan dictates it; for example, if a patient's advance direc-tive indicates that nutrition support is no longer appropriate (Durfee et al. 2014).

For the pediatric patient, long-term HEN requires close monitoring as the macro- and micronutrient needs change as the child ages. For instance, the calorie, protein, vitamin, and mineral needs change as an infant progresses to a toddler and then to a young child. With the evolution in needs come alterations in the type of formula provided and feeding schedule. One should be mindful to provide a formula that is designed for the age of the child so as to most appropriately meet their nutrient needs. Adult formulas should not be given to children younger than 10–13 years of age. The child's growth (weight, length/height, and head circumference for children <3 years of age), hydration status, laboratory markers, clinical status, and overall physical development should be monitored to assure that the nutrition regimen is appropriate (Corkins et al. 2013, 273). It is suggested that weight be monitored weekly, monthly, or at clinic visits and length/height be measured monthly or at clinic visits (Szeszycki et al. 2015, 618). It is also recommended that nutrient intake (calories, protein, fluid, vitamins, and minerals) be evaluated monthly. The access device needs to be assessed prior to each feeding (Szeszycki et al. 2015, 618). The device may need to be replaced periodically to accommodate periods of growth. Overall, the monitoring schedule should be developed based on the child's overall nutrition status at the time of initiation of nutrition support the child's medical condition(s), the child's age, and the tolerance to nutrition support regimen (Szeszycki et al. 2015, 616).

18.4.6 COMPLICATIONS

Pulmonary aspiration is the most acutely dangerous potential complication to enteral feedings. Caregivers can significantly reduce the risk by following guidelines. Patient position is of utmost importance to prevent regurgitation of tube feeding. Risk of aspiration is higher among patients receiving their feedings in a supine position. Therefore, maintaining a head elevation of 30–45 degrees is recommended. Patients who have difficulty protecting their airway are at risk for aspiration of their oropharyngeal secretions as well. These patients should practice or receive regular oral care and suctioning (Boullata et al. 2017, 62).

Tube clogging is another complaint common among long-term tube-fed patients. Inadequate water flushing and improper medication administration are often behind clogged feeding tubes. Minimal flushes can help prevent: flush with at least 30 mL every 4 hours during continuous feeds, before and after each bolus or gravity feed, and before and after each medication. When clogs do occur, warm water with a back-and-forth pressure is the first action recommended. Some patients do use home methods, such as meat tenderizer or carbonated drinks, but clinical evidence does not support those. A solution of pancrealipase in pH 7.9 solution has shown good results (Gramlich et al. 2018, 5–6).

Other tube complaints include discharge from the tube site, tender stoma, granulation tissue, clogs, breakage of the tube, and dislodgement (Crosby and Duerksen 2007). In a single center study, 10% of children that received GT had complications within the first year, which included cellulitis, granulation tissue, and tube malpositioning or dislodging (McSweeney et al. 2013). Although supporting studies are small and have limitations, there appears to be a strong need for close, long-term follow-up of patients with feeding tubes.

TABLE 18.10
Enteral Feeding Complications and Prevention/Treatment Suggestions

Complication	Cause	Prevention/Treatment
Aspiration	Microaspiration of saliva, regurgitation of stomach contents into airway	Feed at ≥30° angle during and remain upright for 30 min after feeding. Consider promotility agent, continuous vs. bolus feedings, small bowel feedings.
Nausea and vomiting	Feeding too quickly Formula too concentrated Intolerance to formula ingredients Incorrect positioning of patient during feeds Contaminated formula Constipation	Sit up at ≥30° angle during feeding and remain upright for 30 min after feeding. Reduce infusion rate. Allow formula to reach room temperature prior to use. Verify proper storage and preparation of formula.
Dehydration	Persistent diarrhea and/or vomiting Prolonged fever Insufficient fluid intake	Determine cause, calculate free water needs, administer fluids via tube as indicated.
Diarrhea	Formula temperature Formula infusion rate Medications Bacterial contamination Fiber Infection (parasites or bacteria) Medications (containing sugar alcohols, H2 blocking agents, lactulose, mineral-containing mixtures, antibiotics, chemotherapy)	Infuse formula at or near room temperature. Reduce infusion rate and increase hours. Consult with pharmacist regarding medications that may cause diarrhea. Ensure good hand hygiene and clean preparation surfaces. Do not use out of date formula. Rinse containers prior to opening. Store partial cans, covered, in the refrigerator for no more than 24 hours. Ensure safe water source. Equipment: Discard infusion bags after 24 hrs. When using syringes for feedings, wash with soap and water after each use. Use an enteral formula with a blend of soluble and insoluble fiber. Rule out *Clostridium difficile*. If antibiotic-related, consider formula with fructooligosaccharides (FOS) if not intolerant to FODMAP.

(*Continued*)

TABLE 18.10 (*Continued*)

Enteral Feeding Complications and Prevention/Treatment Suggestions

Complication	Cause	Prevention/Treatment
Constipation	Inadequate fluid Inadequate or absent fiber Relative or total inactivity Underlying disease Medications that may reduce GI motility	Calculate free water needs, take into account water content of EN. Assess intake of free water, increase fluids PRN via water flushes. Consider fiber-containing formula. As able and tolerated, recommend increased physical activity. Multidisciplinary interaction regarding any potential medication changes. Review medication list.
Bloating	Formula infusion rate Air in tubing FODMAP content	Decrease infusion rate and increase hours. Remove air by "priming" the tubing of feeding set.
Clogged tube	Formula clinging in tube lumen Medication clinging to tube lumen	Fill syringe halfway with very warm water (that is still comfortable to the touch). Rapidly flush small amounts at a time into the tube. If unable to flush, try clearing the tube first. Use an empty syringe and draw back the plunger; repeat until fluid flows freely. If unable to clear clog, contact your healthcare provider. Use liquid medications whenever able. Ensure that any tablet can be crushed. Crush tablets to fine powder and mix in warm water. Flush with water before and after each medication. Do not mix medications.

Source: From ASPEN 2019; Johnson et al. 2019; Mayo Foundation 2011; Wanden-Berghe C. et al. 2019.

Gastrointestinal complaints (i.e., nausea, vomiting, diarrhea, constipation, abdominal bloating) are the most frequently reported in the HEN population (Wanden-Berghe C. et al. 2019). Changes in bowel habits may occur after initiating enteral feedings. One multicenter observational study reported 63% of patients experienced one or more GI complications (Blumenstein et al. 2014, 8512). Table 18.10 outlines treatment options for common complications.

18.4.7 Factors Contributing to Diarrhea

Diarrhea is a commonly reported complication of tube feedings, both in and out of hospitals and other institutions). Reported incidence of diarrhea can vary as widely as 2% to 95%, in part due to inconsistencies in definition (Zaman et al. 2015, 5373). Diarrhea can contribute to fluid and electrolyte abnormalities. Where fecal incontinence is also present, can lead to skin breakdown with concurrent or separate wound infections (Halmos 2013, 25).

Aside from the feedings themselves, medications (especially antibiotics) and infections increase risk of diarrhea (Zaman et al. 2015, 5373). Microbial contamination is another risk for diarrhea. Strict adherence to control protocols has decreased diarrhea incidence. Such protocols include hand-washing, hang time limitations, cleaning equipment, and changing the feeding per manufacturer guidelines (Boullata et al. 2017, 67).

Fiber content in general reduces diarrhea incidence in tube-fed patients. Soy polysaccharide, a soluble fiber, is the most common fiber added to formulas. Beneficial mechanisms include its ability to hold water, increase stool bulk, and preserve gut barrier function (Zaman et al. 2015, 5377).

Prebiotics are specific, mostly soluble, fermentable fibers that provide fuel for beneficial bacteria in the colon. These gut microbes ferment prebiotics to short-chain fatty acids, the preferred food source of colonocytes. Therefore, prebiotics indirectly improve water reabsorption in the large bowel, reducing diarrhea (Zaman et al. 2015, 5373).

FODMAPs (fermentable oligo-, di-, and monosaccharides, and polyols) continue to gain attention as an exacerbating factor. The FODMAP content of enteral formulas can vary considerably, and it can also be difficult to accurately measure (Halmos et al. 2016, 1268). People with irritable bowel syndrome (IBS) respond proportionally to reductions in FODMAPs, and recognized maximum levels are <0.5 g per sitting or <3 g per day (Halmos 2013, 26). Newer studies have investigated whether FODMAP content may impact stool output in a more general patient population. One multi-center randomized double-blind study (n = 84), used formulas with three different FODMAP levels in tube-fed patients experiencing diarrhea. The low group had significantly better King's stool assessments than the moderate or high groups. Furthermore, of those with improved diarrhea, 75% were in the low FODMAP group (Yoon et al. 2015, 10–11).

18.4.8 Ethical Concerns

Nutrition support at end of life remains controversial, and the discussions can be emotionally charged. People with advanced dementia present a particularly sensitive situation. Family members may feel they are watching their loved one starve if they are no longer eating enough. They may also be concerned about overt episodes of choking. It is important for families and caregivers to understand that aspiration can still happen in patients with feeding tubes (Ijaopo and Ijaopo 2019, 2–3).

There is no true expert consensus. Many professional groups have recommended careful handfeeding over feeding tube placement. Up to 34% of nursing home residents with severe cognitive impairment receive a feeding tube, and the majority of placements occur during acute hospitalizations. Unfortunately, feeding tubes can increase medical complications. Studies suggest that up to two-thirds of patients pull their tube within 2 weeks of initial insertion. Tube replacement presents additional hospitalization requirements, increasing costs and risk of iatrogenic complications. Enteral feedings also reduce or eliminate the social interaction of handfeeding (Ijaopo and Ijaopo 2019, 3–4).

18.4.9 QUALITY OF LIFE

Quality of life (QOL) is a multifactorial concept that takes into account physical as well as psychological well-being. Social and cognitive functions play a part. Patients receiving long-term feeding face many challenges to quality of life. Gastrointestinal complaints are high among these. Other concerns include disrupted body image, restricted mobility, and interrupted sleep. A meta-analysis found that 9 of 14 included surveys reported improved quality of life after feeding tube, while 5 showed little change or decrease. Variations in results likely relate to tube type, feeding method, and underlying medical conditions. Clinicians should work with patients to address common complaints and provide early introduction to support groups (Ojo et al. 2019, 13; Chopy et al. 2015, 432). Some of the most common complaints regarding long-term HEN relate more to psychosocial aspects rather than physical issues. In a series of semi-structured interviews with 15 adult patients and 19 caregivers, they reported sleep disturbance, restricted activity, limited clothing options, finding places to do feeding while out, missing the act of eating, awkwardness in social situations, negative attitudes of others toward tube feedings, and being a burden to the family (Brotherton et al. 2006).

Considerations of quality of life (QOL) are important, particularly in light of the high mortality rates for many patients getting G-tubes (Loeser et al. 2003). Loeser's study of 211 patients confirmed a role for HEN in improving QOL as well as nutrition status (Loeser et al. 2003). In fact, their results even questioned the previous research indicating that mentally incompetent patients cannot benefit from tube feeding, since half their patients improved their competency during follow-up (Loeser et al. 2003). However, several studies do suggest worse outcomes and decreased QOL with HEN (Klek et al. 2014).

Use of HEN in pediatrics is often viewed by caregivers as a means to help their children and also improve the family dynamics (Martinez-Costa et al. 2013, 1125). For example, HEN reduces the amount of time spent feeding, which allows for more time to dedicate to other family activities. Caregivers also report feeling that their children are more appropriately nourished with HEN. However, it is important to monitor the overall well-being of the primary caregiver, who frequently is the mother, because there have been reports in the literature of increased risk for psychological distress in this population, which can affect the family dynamics (Toly et al. 2012, 8; Calderon et al. 2011, 192). Satisfaction with HEN appears to be directly related to length of time on HEN and the age at which it was started. Caregivers are more satisfied as the time on tube feedings increases and at an earlier age of initiation. With tube feedings, parents had more time to spend on interests to improve quality of life (Martinez-Costa et al. 2013, 1126–1127).

Food has tremendous emotional importance in all societies. Patients and their families tend to understand nutrition therapy better than other aspects of medical care (McMahon et al. 2005). Families and patients may choose HEN out of fear of starvation (McMahon et al. 2005). However, physiologic adaptations at end of life mean that patients do not suffer feelings of hunger. Families also need reassurance that typically the underlying disease causes death, very rarely starvation (McMahon et al. 2005).

It is important for healthcare providers to present benefits and risks openly. HEN practitioners can take the lead in helping patients best cope with their nutritional changes. Thompson presents a small qualitative study of HEN patients who identified themselves as "coping well." The patients reported adjustment on their HEN prescriptions to best fit their needs; they reported adequate initial education and good continuum of care after starting HEN (Thompson 2006). HEN practitioners should also share all available resources with patients. It is advantageous to introduce patients early on to support groups (Ojo et al. 2019, 13; Chopy et al. 2015, 432). Another qualitative study reported increased QOL with membership in the Oley Foundation, which is a national support group for home enteral and parenteral nutrition support patients (Chopy et al. 2015). Only 46% of those surveyed found out about this organization through their healthcare provider and all reported a wish that they had known about the group sooner (Chopy et al. 2015).

18.4.10 NATURAL DISASTERS

Safe HEN therapy relies on functioning water and electricity to reduce the risk of bacterial contamination, as well as home delivery of products and supplies. When a natural disaster occurs, any of these services can be interrupted, possibly for an extended period of time. Even a prolonged non-weather emergency, such as power or water outage, can impact safe HEN preparation. Therefore, pre-planning for these situations is essential (Ireton-Jones et al. 2019, 217). A checklist could be developed and provided to the HEN patient to aid in preparation for these situations (Table 18.11).

18.4.10.1 Reimbursement

Once the patient has been assessed for HEN and therapy is planned, insurance reimbursement should be explored for home therapy. Patients are typically insured by Medicare, Medicaid, or commercial/private insurance. However, the criteria under which formula and supplies are covered can vary, and clinicians can aid the process by obtaining necessary documentation of medical necessity.

18.4.11 MEDICARE

The Centers for Medicare and Medicaid Services (CMS) oversee the Medicare program. HEN (formula and supplies) are covered under Medicare Part B as a Durable

TABLE 18.11
Emergency and Disaster Planning for HEN Consumers

Items to have on hand in case of an emergency or disaster:
- Maintain a health information card or summary that is easily accessed and carried.
- Stock 1 week of bottled water for hand washing, flushes.
- Keep a stock of hand sanitizer; keep some separate for HEN use.
- Have battery-operated flashlights on hand.
- Maintain a list of emergency contacts including the HEN physician. Assure the home enteral provider has all information needed to keep in contact with the patient.
- Keep a list of local hospitals.
- Keep several extra enteral feeding bags and HEN supplies prepared (HEN emergency kit: syringes, tubing, batteries, etc.).

Have an emergency/disaster plan in place; leave early rather than staying in a potential disaster zone.

Maintain a 2–3-day supply of commercial enteral products during natural disasters (hurricanes, earthquakes, extreme weather conditions).

Maintain an adequate inventory of more specialized feeding formulas (adult and pediatric).

Especially important for pediatric patients with specialized enteral formulas (i.e., metabolic).

Source: Adapted from Ireton-Jones et al. 2019 Nutr Clin Pract 23(4); 217 © 2019 by American Society for Parenteral and Enteral Nutrition. Reprinted by Permission of John Wiley & Sons.

Medical Equipment (DME) prosthetic device. HEN is covered at 80% of the allowed amount set by Medicare. To qualify for re-imbursement the beneficiary should meet the following criteria: (a) permanent non-function or disease of the structures that normally permit food to reach the small bowel or (b) disease of the small bowel which impairs digestion and absorption of an oral diet, either of which requires tube feedings to provide sufficient nutrients to maintain weight and strength commensurate with the beneficiary's overall health status. "Permanence" under Medicare criteria is defined as greater than 3 months (CMS 1984). Coverage is not provided for psychological disorders or end-stage disease with anorexia or nausea, or home blended formula. Additional documentation may be required for pump feedings, specialized formulas, malabsorption, or feedings providing <750 or >2000 calories per day (CMS 1984).

Patients may also have Medicare secondary or supplemental insurance which may or may not cover any co-pays or the remaining 20% not covered by Medicare Part B. Medicare Advantage (also known as Medicare Part C) provides coverage by private insurers approved by Medicare and will typically follow Medicare criteria.

Private or commercial insurance coverage will vary depending on the policy contract. The insurance company will need to be contacted directly to determine the individual patient's coverage. In some cases, enteral feeding supplies will be covered, but not the formula.

Medicaid is a state-run program; therefore, coverage will vary from state to state. In 2005 the Government Accountability Office (GAO) surveyed state Medicaid reimbursement, compared to criteria of Medicare coverage. The survey questioned whether each state's Medicaid matched Medicare in five categories. The results show a patchwork of coverage with little discernable pattern (Parver and Mutinsky 2009). Clinicians should contact the Medicaid office to determine coverage (www.medicaid.gov).

18.4.12 COMMERCIAL/PRIVATE INSURANCE

Commercial insurance coverage for HEN will vary depending on the patient's individual policy. The coverage can encompass full coverage for formula and supplies, partial coverage, or no coverage at all.

18.4.13 FINANCIAL ASSISTANCE

Enteral formula companies and other medical supply providers may have programs to provide financial assistance to those uninsured or underinsured needing HEN formula and supplies. The Oley Foundation (www.oley.org) is a national support organization for HEN and parenteral nutrition patients that may have donated formula and supplies.

18.4.13.1 Home Enteral Nutrition Providers

Depending on insurance coverage, the patient may have options of who will be providing skilled nursing and home enteral formula equipment. In keeping with the ASPEN home care standards, home care equipment providers should encompass a multidisciplinary approach to the patient receiving HEN therapy. In addition, the home care provider should be able to meet the needs of those requiring more intensive nursing and nutrition monitoring. HEN providers should be knowledgeable about enteral formula equipment, enteral access, and care, and provide 24-hour on-call services.

18.5 CONCLUSION

The HEN population continues to increase yearly. The needs of these patients require a multidisciplinary approach to meet treatment goals and to keep the patient at home. Clinician expertise in the areas of assessment, intervention, and monitoring will aid in the success of HEN therapy.

18.5.1 RESOURCES

- Tube Feeding Awareness Foundation: www.feedingtubeawareness.com
- Oley Foundation: www.oley.org
- ASPEN Nutrition Support Patient Education Manual: Contains pertinent patient education material in English and Spanish
- University of Virginia GI Nutrition Support Team—Clinician Resources: https://med.virginia.edu/ginutrition/resources-for-the-nutrition-support-clinician/

REFERENCES

American Society of Parenteral and Enteral Nutrition (ASPEN). 2002. Board of directors and the clinical guidelines task force. Guidelines for the use of enteral and parenteral nutrition in adult and pediatric patients. *JPEN J Parenter Enteral Nutr.* 1SA–138SA.

American Society of Parenteral and Enteral Nutrition (ASPEN). 2019. Home Enteral Nutrition. In: Malone A. et al. (eds.), *ASPEN Enteral Nutrition Handbook*, 2nd ed., 437–443. Silver Spring, MD: American Society for Parenteral and Enteral Nutrition.

American Society of Parenteral and Enteral Nutrition (ASPEN). EN Video Inventory. 2020; www.nutritioncare.org/Guidelines_and_Clinical_Resources/EN_Video_Inventory/. Accessed 7.22.20

Axelrod D, Kazmerski K, Iyer K. 2006. Pediatric enteral nutrition. *J Parenter Enteral Nutr* 30:S21–S26.

Baker SS, Baker RD, Davis AM. 2007. *Pediatric Nutrition Support.* Sudbury, MA: Jones & Bartlett Publishers.

Bankhead R, Boullata J, Brantley S, et al. 2009. Enteral nutrition practice recommendations. *JPEN J Parenter Enteral Nutr* 33(2):122–167.

Bennett K, Hjelmgren B, Piazza J. 2020. Blenderized tube feeding: Health outcomes and review of homemade and commercially prepared products. *Nutr Clin Pract* 35(3):417–431.

Blumenstein I, Shastri YM, Stein J. 2014. Gastroenteric tube feeding: Techniques, problems and solutions. *World J Gastroenterol* 20(26):8505–8524.

Boisseau N, Burde A, Bachmann, et al. 2010 A telephone-linked computer system for home enteral nutrition. *J Telemed Telecare* 16:363–367

Boullata JI, Carrera AL, Harvey L, et al. 2017. ASPEN safe practices for enteral nutrition therapy. *JPEN J Parenter Enteral Nutr* 41:15–103.

Braegger C, Decsi T, Dias J, et al. 2010. Practical approach to paediatric enteral nutrition: A Comment by the ESPGHAN committee on nutrition. *JPGN* 51:110–122.

Brotherton A, Abbott J, Aggett P. 2006. The impact of percutaneous endoscopic gastrostomy feeding upon daily life in adults. *J Hum Nutr Diet* 19(5):355–367.

Brown B, Roehl K, Betz M. 2015. Enteral nutrition formula selection: Current evidence and implications for use. *Nutr Clin Prac* 30(1):72–85.

Calderon C, Gomez-Lopez L, Martinez-Costa, Borraz S, Moreno-Villares JM, Pedron-Giner C. 2011. Feeling of Burdon, psychological distress, and anxiety among primary caregivers of children with home enteral nutrition. *J Pediatr Psychol* 36(2):188–195.

Canani RB, Terrin G, Borrelli O, et al. 2006; Short- and long-term therapeutic efficacy of nutritional therapy and corticosteroids in pediatric Crohn's disease. *Dig Liver Dis* 38:381–387.

Centers for Medicare and Medicaid Services (CMS). 1984. National coverage determination for enteral and parenteral nutrition therapy. Medicare Coverage Database Website. www.cms.gov/medicare-coverage-database/overview-and-quick-search.aspx. Accessed 7.25.20

Chopy K, et al. 2015. A qualitative study of perceived value of membership in the Oley Foundation by home parenteral and enteral nutrition patients. *JPEN J Parenter Enteral Nutr* 39(4): 426–433.

Clayton LH. 2010. Strategies for selecting effective patient nutrition education materials. *Nutr Clin Prac* 25(5):436–442.

Corkins MR, Griggs KC, Groh-Wargo S, et al. 2013. Standards for nutrition support: Pediatric hospitalized patients. *Nutr Clin Pract* 28(2); 263–276.

Critch J, Day A, Otley A, et al. 2012; Use of enteral nutrition for the control of intestinal inflammation in pediatric Crohn disease. *JPEN J Parent Enteral Nutr* 54:298–305.

Crosby J, Duerksen DR. 2007. A prospective study of tube- and feeding-related complications in patients receiving long-term home enteral nutrition. *JPEN J Parenter Enteral Nutr* 31(4):274–277.

DeLegge M. 2002. Home enteral nutrition. *JPEN J Parenter Enteral Nutr.* 26(5):S4–S7.

Durfee SM, Adams SC, Arthur E, et al. 2014. ASPEN standards for nutrition support: Home and alternate site care. *JPEN J Parenter Enteral Nutr* 29(4):542–555.

Edwards S, Davis A, Bruce A, Mousa H, Lyman B, Cocjin J, Dean K, Ernst L, Almadhoun O, Hyman P. 2016. Caring for tube-fed children: A review of management, tube weaning, and emotional considerations. *JPEN J Parenter Enteral Nutr* 40:616–622.

Escuro A. 2014. Blenderized tube feeding: Suggested guidelines to clinicians. *Practical Gastroenterology*, December.

Gilbertson H, Rogers E, Ukoumunne O. 2011. Determination of a practical pH cutoff level for reliable confirmation of nasogastric tube placement. *J Parenter Enteral Nutr* 35:540–544.

Global Enteral Device Supply Association (GEDSA). 2020 Tools for adopting Enfit. http://stayconnected.org/tools-adopting-enfit/. Accessed July 28, 2020.

Gramlich L, Hurt RT, Jin J, and Mundi MS. 2018. Home enteral nutrition: Towards a standard of care. *Nutrients* 10(1020): 1–11.

Hall BT, Englehart MS, Blaseg K, et al. 2014. Implementation of a dietitian-led enteral nutrition support clinic results in quality improvement, reduced readmissions and cost savings. *Nutr Clin Prac* 29(5);649–655.

Halmos EP. 2013. Role of FODMAP content in enteral nutrition-associated diarrhea. *J Gastroenterol Hepatol* 29(Supp 4):25–28.

Halmos EP, Bogatyrev A, Liels KL, and Muir JG. 2016. Challenges of quantifying FODMAPs in enteral nutrition formulas: Evaluation of artifacts and solutions. *JPEN* 41(8): 1262–1271.

Hannah E, John RM. 2013. Everything the nurse practitioner should know about pediatric feeding tubes. *J Am Assoc Nurse Pract* 25:567–577.

HCPC Codes. HCPCS B-codes enteral and parenteral therapy. https://hcpcs.codes/b-codes/, Accessed August 1, 2020.

Health and Human Services (HHS). 2014. The affordable care act supports patient centered medical homes in health centers. www.hhs.gov/news/press/2014pres/08/20140826a.html. Accessed March 19, 2015.

Ijaopo EO and Ijaopo RO. 2019. Tube feeding in individuals with advanced dementia: A review of its burdens and perceived benefits. *J Aging Res*: 1–16.

Ireton-Jones C, Nishikawa K, Nishikawa R. 2019 Home parenteral and enteral nutrition during natural disasters: A guide for clinicians and consumers. *Nutr Clin Pract* 23(4): 217.

Irving S, Lyman B, Northington L, Bartlett J, Kemper C, NOVEL Project Work Group. 2014. Nasogastric tube placement and verification in children: Review of the current literature. *Nutr Clin Pract* 29:267–276.

Itkin M, DeLegge MH, Fang JC, et al. 2011. Multidisciplinary practical guidelines for gastrointestinal access for enteral nutrition and decompression from the society of interventional radiology and american gastroenterological association (AGA) Institute, with endorsement by Canadian Interventional Radiological Association (CRIA) and Cardiovascular and Interventional Radiological Society of Europe (CIRSE) *Gastroenterology* 141:742–765.

Johnson TW, Seegmiller S, Epp L, Mundi MS. 2019. Addressing frequent issues of home enteral nutrition patients. *Nutr Clin Pract* 34:186–195.

The Joint Commission Sentinel Event Alert. 2006. Tubing misconnections-a persistent and potentially deadly occurrence. www.jointcommission.org/sentinel_event_alert_issue_36_tubing_misconnections%E2%80%94a_persistent_and_potentially_deadly_occurrence/. Accessed August 1, 2020.

The Joint Commission Sentinel Event Alert. 2014. Managing risk during transition to new ISO tubing connector standards. www.jointcommission.org/resources/patient-safety-topics/sentinel-event/sentinel-event-alert-newsletters/sentinel-event-alert-53-managing-risk-during-transition-to-new-iso-tubing-connector-standards/. Accessed August 1, 2020.

Klek S, Hermanowicz A, Dziwiszek G, et al. 2014. Home enteral nutrition reduces complications, length of stay and health care costs: results from a multicenter study. *Am J Clin Nutr* 100:609–615.

Klek S, Szybinski P, Sierzega M, et al. 2011. Commercial enteral formulas and nutrition support teams improve the outcome of home enteral tube feedings. *JPEN* 35(3):380–385.

Kornburger C, Gibson C, Sadowski S, Maletta K, Klingbeil C. 2013 Using "teach-back" to promote a safe transition from hospital to home: An evidence-based approach to improving the discharge process. *J Pediatr Nurs* 28: 282–291.

Lochs H, Dejong C, Hammarqvist F, et al. 2006; ESPEN (European society for parenteral and enteral nutrition). ESPEN guidelines on enteral nutrition, gastroenterology. *Clin Nutr.* 25:260–274.

Loeser C, von Herz U, Kuchler T, Rzehak P, Muller MJ. 2003. Quality of life and nutritional state in patients on home enteral tube feeding. *Nutrition* 19:605–611.

Lyman B, Shah R. 2015. Nutrition access. In: MR Corkins (ed.), *The A.S.P.E.N. Pediatric Nutrition Support Core Curriculum*, 2nd ed., 567–582. ASPEN: Silver Spring, MD.

Malone A. 2005. Enteral formula selection: A review of selected product categories. *Practical Gastroenterol* 28:44.

Martin K, Gardner G. 2017. Home enteral nutrition: Updates, trends, and challenges. Nutr Clin Pract 32(6): 712–721.

Martinez-Costa C, Calderon C, Gomez-Lopez L, et al. 2013. Satisfaction with gastrostomy feeding in caregivers of children with home enteral nutrition, application of the SAGA-8 questionnaire and analysis of involved factors. Nutr Hosp. 28(4):1121–1128.h

Mayo Clinic. 2014. Home enteral nutrition feeding tube overview. www.youtube.com/watch?v=pqxzRyfUq6k. 2/14/14, Accessed July 24, 2020.

Mayo Foundation. 2011. *Patient Education: Tube Feeding at Home*. Rochester, MN: Barbara Woodward Lips Patient Education Center.

McMahon MM, Hurley DL, Kamath PS, Mueller PSl. 2005. Medical and ethical aspects of long-term enteral tube feeding. *Mayo Clin Proc* 80(11):1461–1476.

McSweeney ME, Jaing H, Deutsch AJ, Atmadja M, Lightdale JR. 2013. Long-term outcomes of infants and children undergoing percutaneous endoscopy gastrostomy tube placement. *J Pediatr Gastroenterol Nutr* 57(5):663–667.

Metzger LC. 2010. Education materials for home nutrition support patients. Nutr Clin Prac 25(5):451–470.

Milton DL, Johnson TW, Johnson K, et al. 2020. Accepted safe food-handling procedures minimizes microbial contamination of home-prepared blenderized tube feeding. Nutr Clin Pract 35(3):479–486.

Monzka J. 2015. Enteral nutrition support: Determining the best way to feed In: MR Corkins (ed.), *The A.S.P.E.N. Pediatric Nutrition Support Core Curriculum*, 2nd ed, 583–592. ASPEN: Silver Spring, MD.

Mortensen M. 2006. Blenderized tube feeding clinical perspectives on homemade tube feeding. *PNPG Post* 17:1–4.

Mundi MS, Duellman W, Epp L, et al. 2018. Comparison of gravity flow rates between ENFit and legacy feeding tubes. *JPEN J Parenter Enteral Nutr* 42:522–528.

Mundi MS, Epp L, Hurt RT. 2016. Increased force required with proposed standardized enteral feed connector in blenderized tube feeding. *Nutr Clin Pract* 31(6):795–798.

Mundi MS, Pattinson A, McMahon MT, et al. 2017. Prevalence of home parenteral and enteral nutrition in the United States. *Nutr Clin Pract* 32(6): 799–805.

Nelson EL, Yadrich DM, Thompson N, et al. 2017. Telemedicine support groups for home parenteral nutrition users. Nutr Clin Pract 32(6):789–798.

Nijs ELF, Cahill AM. 2010. Pediatric enteric feeding techniques: Insertion, maintenance, and management of problems. *Cardiovasc Intervent Radiol* 33:1101–1110.

Oley Foundation. 1993. *North American Home Parenteral and Enteral Nutrition Patient Registry Annual Report – 1985–1991*. Albany, NY: Oley Foundation.

Oley Foundation. Video Library. 2015, https://oley.org/page/videolibrary. Updated 2019, Accessed July 24, 2020.

Office of the National Coordinator for Health Information Technology (ONC). 2014. Health IT legislation and regulations. www.healthit.gov/topic/laws-regulation-and-policy/health-it-legislation Accessed August 1, 2020.

Ojo O, Keaveney E, Wang X, Feng P. 2019. The effect of enteral tube feeding on patients' health-related quality of life: A systematic review. *Nutrients* 11(1046): 1–16.

Oparaji J, Sferra T, Sankararaman S. 2019. Basics of blenderized tube feeds: A primer for pediatric primary care clinicians. *Gastroenterol Res* 12(3): 111–114.

Parver AK, Mutinsky SE. 2009. Enteral nutrition reimbursement-the rationale for the policy: the US perspective. *Nestlé Nutr Inst Workshop Ser Clin Perform Program* 12:53–70.

Robinson D, Walker R, Abrams SC, et al. 2018 American society for parenteral and enteral nutrition (ASPEN) definition of terms, style, and conventions used in ASPEN board of directors-approved documents. May; www.nutritioncare.org/uploadedFiles/Documents/Guidelines_and_Clinical_Resources/ASPEN%20Definition%20of%20Terms,%20Style,%20and%20Conventions%20Used%20in%20ASPEN%20Board%20of%20Directors%E2%80%93Approved%20Documents.pdf. Accessed July 18, 2020, IA.

Schwartz S. 2003. Feeding disorders in children with developmental disabilities. *Infants and Young Children* 16:317–330.

Strollo BP, McClave SA, Miller KR. 2017. Complications of home enteral nutrition: Mechanical complications and access issues in the home setting. *Nutr Clin Pract* 32(6): 732.

Szeszycki E, Cruse W, Beitzel M. 2015. Evaluation and monitoring of pediatric patients receiving specialized nutrition support In: MR Corkins (ed.), *The A.S.P.E.N. Pediatric Nutrition Support Core Curriculum*, 2nd ed., 615–639. ASPEN: Silver Spring, MD.

Thompson C. 2006. Fostering coping skills and resilience in home enteral nutrition (HEN) patients. *Nutr Clin Pract* 21:557–565.

Toly V, Musil C, Carl J. 2012. Families with children who are technology-dependent: Normalization and family functioning. *West J Nurs Res* 34(1):52–71.

US Food and Drug Administration (USFDA). 2016. Frequently asked questions about medical foods; Second edition guidance for industry. www.fda.gov/media/97726/download. Published May 2016, Accessed July 26, 2020.

US Food and Drug Administration (USFDA) 2017. Food Code 2017. Updated December 23, 2019. Accessed August 1, 2020.

Verdrell A, Rollins CJ. 2017. Drug-nutrient interactions. In: C Mueller (ed.), *The ASPEN Adult Nutrition Support Core Curriculum*, 3rd ed., 362–375. Silver Spring, MD: The American Society for Parenteral and Enteral Nutrition.

Vermilyea S, Goh V. 2016. Enteral feedings in children: Sorting out tubes, buttons, and formulas. *Nutr Clin Pract* 31:59–67.

Walia C, Van Hoorn M, Edlbeck A, Feuling MB. 2017. The registered dietitian nutritionist's guide to homemade tube feeding. *J Acad Nutr Diet* 117(1):11–16.

Wanden-Berghe C, Patino-Alonso MC, Galindo-Villardon P, Sanz-Valero J. 2019. Complications Associated with Enteral Nutrition: CAFANE Study. *Nutrients* 11:2041.

Wathen B, Peyton C. 2014. Pediatric nasogastric tube placement. *Nurs Crit Care* 9(3): 15–18.

Weeks C. 2019. Home blenderized tube feeding: A practical guide for clinical practice. *Clin Transl Gastroenterol*: 1–4.

Yoon SR et al. 2015. Low-FODMAP formula improves diarrhea and nutritional status in hospitalized patients receiving enteral nutrition: A randomized, multicenter, double-blind clinical trial. *Nutrition Journal* 14(116): 1–12.

Zaman MK, Chin K, Rai V, Majid HA. 2015. Fiber and prebiotic supplementation in enteral nutrition: A systematic review and meta-analysis. *World J Gastroenterol* 21(17): 5372–5381.

19 Home Parenteral Nutrition

Kristen Roberts

19.1 INTRODUCTION

When the GI tract is non-functional or absorption is poor due to structural and functional changes which result in malabsorption of macro and micronutrients, parenteral nutrition support can be lifesaving. When PN is required for several weeks, long-term or lifetime, it can be delivered at home and is called home parenteral nutrition (HPN). Successful delivery, maintenance, and management of HPN require a ready patient and a dedicated clinical team in the hospital and in the home. This chapter will cover initiating, monitoring, and complications and reimbursement of HPN, primarily in adults as pediatric HPN is a specialized practice. Pediatric HPN management has its own complexities – including metabolic, growth facilitation, compatibilities of formula components and psychosocial that are beyond the scope of this chapter.

19.2 HOME PARENTERAL NUTRITION

Intestinal failure (IF) is defined as a condition resulting in an inability to maintain hydration and electrolyte and nutritional status without intravenous support. For many patients with IF, home parenteral nutrition (HPN) is a life-saving modality when IF extends beyond the hospital stay (1). In the 1970s, HPN became more readily available to patients with the development of infusion pharmacy and homecare services. Over the last several decades, HPN providers have reported the main causes of IF requiring or associated with HPN as the following (2, 3):

- Surgical complications
- Bowel ischemia
- Short bowel syndrome (SBS)
- Radiation enteritis
- Inflammatory bowel disease (IBD)
- Motility disorder
- Gastrointestinal (GI) fistulae
- Bowel obstruction

Not all patients with IF are appropriate for HPN due to the complexity of the therapy. Determining appropriateness requires a team of nutrition professionals, preferably a nutrition support team (NST) or an intestinal rehabilitation center (IRC), to evaluate nutritional status, GI function, surgical anatomy, and disease severity. Specifically,

 DOI: 10.1201/9780429322570-19

these nutrition professionals include a physician, registered dietitian (RDN), registered nurse (RN), pharmacist, social worker, and case manager (2–4).

Prior to considering HPN, the home environment, social support, and reimbursement should be considered. When the patient is deemed appropriate for HPN, the nutrition care plan, selection of vascular access device (VAD), and selection of home infusion provider is initiated (3–5). The physician should oversee the full HPN evaluation process with extensive emphasis on conducting a thorough evaluation of the GI tract. The RDN plays a key role in determining the nutrition prescription with the physician and pharmacists. The nutrition prescription should achieve one or several nutrition-related goals, including recovery or maintenance of nutrition status including weight and functional status, and/or correct or prevent micronutrient deficiencies and dehydration. The RDN along with the RN contributes to educating the patient on documenting daily weights, temperatures, and intake and output records.

An essential component of the HPN process for the RN is to assist the patient in selecting a VAD. The RN ensures that the patient understands the risks and benefits to each VAD prior to making a selection (see Chapter 20). Once the VAD is selected, education on care ensues to allow the patient to be autonomous with the VAD at discharge. The pharmacist inspects the PN solution for stability and compatibility and provides recommendations for medication management in the HPN solution. Cognitive and psychosocial concerns are evaluated with the goal of assessing patient safety with a VAD and intravenous therapies in the home environment (i.e., electricity, running water, and telephone access) (6, 7). Lastly, owing to the extraneous costs of HPN, the case manager will confirm the indication for HPN with the insurance company and verify insurance benefits.

19.2.1 REIMBURSEMENT

Clinical decisions regarding patient need for HPN therapy must be made with consideration of reimbursement availability for the therapy. If a patient does not have coverage for HPN, other considerations must be made including placement in a long-term care facility or skilled nursing facility. A proficient case manager is critical to preparing the patient for discharge on HPN to ameliorate costs associated with the therapy. Knowledge of required documentation is critical for determining insurance benefits. Many patients utilize Medicare or Medicaid for HPN coverage, but the majority rely on private insurance to supplement their primary insurance coverage (8, 9). Determining insurance coverage early on in the discharge process and appropriately document the indications for HPN in the medical record is key. Medicare updated HPN coverage criteria in 2020 after 36 years. The new coverage criteria emphasize documentation strategies to clearly indicate the need for HPN. Documentation of IF and concurrent insurance approval permits the NST to complete the education sessions and stabilize the PN formula for discharge. Clinicians working in HPN (hospital and home) should ensure that they are up to date on all aspects of reimbursement for therapy (8).

19.3 HOME PARENTERAL NUTRITION: INITIATING PN

Initiation of HPN can occur in the hospital or home; however, hospital initiation is favored to minimize risk in complex cases. The American Society of Parenteral and Enteral Nutrition (ASPEN) recommends hospital initiation for patients with severe medical conditions and/or electrolyte disorders (10). This chapter will primarily address initiation of PN in the hospital. Initiation of PN in the hospital (or home) should only be started once all significant electrolyte abnormalities are corrected and the patient is metabolically stable. Once electrolyte status is stable, initiating a low-dextrose PN solution on the first day of therapy is warranted to prevent adverse events (i.e., severe hyperglycemia, cardiac dysfunction). In cases of extreme malnutrition or organ dysfunction, reaching the caloric goal may take several days to achieve and daily monitoring of laboratory parameters and weights is necessary to safely advance the PN solution. When the low-dextrose PN is tolerated (i.e., no significant electrolyte or blood sugar abnormalities), the caloric content of the solution can slowly be increased to goal calories. Once a patient is identified as appropriate for HPN, a nutrition-related goal for the PN prescription should be established, as well as other steps in the discharge process (see Figure 19.1). Patients who have an appropriate indication for PN in the home, are clinically stable, have proper access for HPN, and are capable of being educated in the safe administration of HPN, may be initiated in the home setting (10).

19.3.1 THE PN PRESCRIPTION

Macronutrient, fluid, and micronutrient components of the PN prescription are established based on the nutrition assessment completed by the RDN and the nutrition-related goals of each patient. These nutrient components are established prior to initiation and can then be adjusted in response to therapy as needed (6, 11). Total energy needs are established based on the patients' long-term goal to gain, maintain, or reduce total body weight. Calculating energy needs can be determined by multiple predictive equations or by indirect calorimetry. For most patients, 20–30 kcal/kg of body weight is sufficient for weight maintenance (6, 10, 12). Close clinical monitoring is essential since higher HPN caloric intake may be required for patients who do not meet weight gain goals outside "normal recommendations." Of these calories, lipids should be provided to prevent essential fatty acid deficiency (EFAD). Prevention of EFAD using intravenous lipid emulsion (ILE) requires a minimum of 2%–0.5% total calories delivered from linoleic (LA) and α-linolenic acid (ALA), respectively. Although ASPEN recommends that most ILE dosing not exceed 2.5 g/kg/day, most clinicians utilize a maximum of 1.0 g/kg/day for long-term HPN therapy (13). For many years, a soybean oil-based ILE (SO-ILE) was the only available ILE in the United States; if 4–8% of total HPN calories were provided as SO-ILE, LA and ALA requirements were met. SO-ILE was limited for many patients to try to prevent the deleterious effects that may be seen in patients who receive long-term high levels of omega-6 fatty acids. In 2016, a new ILE was approved for use in the United States which contained 30% soy oil, 30% MCT oil, 25% olive oil, and 15% fish oil (4-oil ILE). Another ILE contains 20% soy oil and 80% olive oil (2-oil ILE). Therefore,

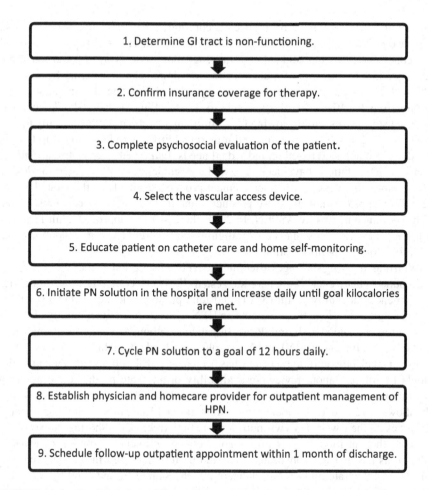

1. Determine GI tract is non-functioning.

2. Confirm insurance coverage for therapy.

3. Complete psychosocial evaluation of the patient.

4. Select the vascular access device.

5. Educate patient on catheter care and home self-monitoring.

6. Initiate PN solution in the hospital and increase daily until goal kilocalories are met.

7. Cycle PN solution to a goal of 12 hours daily.

8. Establish physician and homecare provider for outpatient management of HPN.

9. Schedule follow-up outpatient appointment within 1 month of discharge.

FIGURE 19.1 Steps for discharging a patient on home parenteral nutrition.

a greater proportion of the PN formulation must be provided as 4-oil ILE and 2-oil ILE to meet ALA and LA needs. With these new ILEs, new standards for preventing EFAD and determining the ILE requirement must be implemented. The "rule-of-thumb" of 4–8% of total calories from ILE related only to SO-ILE. When determining the amounts of 2-oil ILE or 4-oil ILE required to prevent EFAD, a greater percentage of calories from ILE must be provided to assure adequacy. In addition, the fatty acid panels for patients receiving 4-oil ILE will be different from those of patients receiving SO-ILE. Because 4-oil ILE has fish oil, Docosahexaenoic acid (DHA) and Eicosapentaenoic acid (EPA) are provided directly which may obviate the need for the former requirements for LA and ALA (13, 14). New ILEs have allowed for greater flexibility in HPN formulations in with the provision ILE which limit SO, especially for long-term HPN patients (15).

Protein (i.e., amino acids) and carbohydrate (i.e., dextrose monohydrate) requirements fluctuate based on patient tolerance, medical condition, and the response to therapy and therefore, must be adjusted accordingly (16). Typically, protein should provide 0.8–2.5 g/kg/day depending on body mass and disease severity and delivered as a concentrated amino acid solution ranging from 3% to 20% (16). Carbohydrate needs are met by infusion of a dextrose monohydrate solution ranging from 5% to 70% with each gram supplying approximately 3.4 kcal. Fluid needs can be estimated by providing 30–40 mL/kg of dry weight (6, 12, 16). Fluid delivery should cover GI and insensible losses while allowing for a minimum of 1000 mL of urine daily for the adult patient. Electrolyte, vitamin, and mineral additives should be added to the PN bag daily and adjusted based on individual needs. Estimated micronutrient requirements for PN solutions have been reviewed and guidelines are available for dosing (16). Historically, none of the trace element products available in the United States were FDA approved nor did these products contain doses of trace elements in line with recommendations by ASPEN. In 2021, the first FDA-approved adult formulation (i.e., trace elements injection 4) aligning with ASPEN recommendations (see Table 19.1 for dosing information).

With ongoing drug shortages affecting the HPN prescription, tactics for preventing micronutrient deficiencies have been suggested (12, 17). Specifically, these guidelines recommend that multivitamin (MVI) and multiple trace element (MTE) solutions should be given orally in those patients on HPN with adequate functionality of the GI tract to tolerate and absorb oral doses. In patients without adequate functionality of the GI tract, intravenous MVI and MTE solutions should be reduced from daily to 3 times per week only until the shortage has been resolved. The home infusion provider should be diligent about reviewing availability of alternate products and assuring that the patient receives the usual and recommended daily dosages as soon as supply allows. The American Society for Parenteral and Enteral Nutrition has updated resources on their website (www.nutritioncare.org/ArchivedPNShortageNews/).

Once the nutritional goals are established, the clinician formulates the HPN solution as a 3-in-1 (carbohydrate, lipid, and protein delivered in the same bag) or 2-in-1 (carbohydrate and protein delivered in the same bag and lipids given separately). Several factors determine how the PN solution is formulated, such as fluid requirements, stability parameters, presence of organ failure (i.e., hepatic, renal, and/

TABLE 19.1

Micronutrient Content of Available Products

Trace Element	Standard Daily Requirement	Trace Elements Injection 4*; American Regent™ (per mL)
Chromium	≤ 10 mcg	–
Copper	0.3–0.5 mg	0.3 mg
Manganese	55 mcg	55 mcg
Selenium	60–100 mcg	60 mcg
Zinc	3–5 mg	3 mg

* Data on Tralement® product label American Regent™.

or pulmonary diseases), and energy needs. It is not uncommon to utilize a 2-in-1 solution and a 3-in-1 solution to provide an average daily caloric and lipid intake for the week, especially as a patient is being weaned from full HPN support (12). Guidelines for maintaining stability and compatibility in 3-in-1 admixtures are listed in Table 19.2.

19.3.2 INFUSION PARAMETERS

Infusion parameters such as the infusion time, infusion rate, and tapering of the solution are established based tolerance of fluid and macronutrient infusion. Typically, HPN solutions are infused over 8–12 hours when feasible due to the psychological and hepatic benefits (18). The process of cycling a PN prescription over a shorter infusion time (<24 hours) can take several days during hospitalization. Although cycling in a long-term care facility or in the home can be done, data on the frequency and adverse events associated with this is unknown. Each adjustment to the infusion cycle requires calculation of a new infusion rate. The infusion rate is determined by calculating the total fluid volume needed in the HPN bag divided by the number of infusion hours at home (hours in the cycle). Most patients will require the HPN solution to be tapered up and down one hour to prevent blood sugar abnormalities (12). A metabolically stable patient will likely be able to tolerate a 12-hour PN cycle that tapers off over the last hour (see the following example for a patient requiring 2 L of fluid daily over 12 hours).

Main rate: 2000 mL ÷ (12 hours − ½ hour) = ~174 mL/hr × 11 hrs

Taper down rate: 174 mL/hr ÷ 2 = ~87 mL/hr × 1 hr

Infusion instructions: Start HPN solution at 174 mL/hr × 11 hrs and then decrease the infusion rate to 87 mL/hr for the last hour.

TABLE 19.2
Stability Guidelines for 3-in-1 Admixtures[1]

Nutrient	Parameters
Macronutrient	≥4% Amino acid
	≥10% Dextrose
	≥2% Lipid
Divalent Cations	Between 16–20 mEq/L
Iron	Omit iron dextran from PN solution

Boullata JI, Gilbert K, Sacks G, Labossiere RJ, Crill C, Goday P, Kumpf VJ, Mattox TW, Plogsted S, Holcombe B; American Society for Parenteral and Enteral Nutrition. ASPEN clinical guidelines: parenteral nutrition ordering, order review, compounding, labeling, and dispensing. JPEN J Parenter Enteral Nutr. 2014 Mar-Apr;38(3):334–77. doi: 10.1177/0148607114521833. Epub 2014 Feb 14. PMID: 24531708.

On the other hand, a metabolically unstable patient may require longer infusion times to gain stability (see the following example for a patient requiring 4 L of fluid daily over 18 hours).

Main rate: 4000 mL ÷ (18 hours − 1 hour) = ~235 mL/hr × 16 hrs

Taper up rate: 235 mL/hr ÷ 2 = ~118 mL/hr × 1 hr

Taper down rate: 235 mL/hr ÷ 2 = ~118 mL/hr × 1 hr

Infusion instructions: Start HPN solution at 118 mL/hr × 1 hr, then increase the infusion rate to 235 mL/hr × 16 and then decrease the infusion rate to 118 mL/hr for the last hour.

19.4 MONITORING

HPN must be monitored for complications due to the complexity of the therapy and the reported complications associated with this therapy. Monitoring should include tactics for preventing short- and long-term complications. Short-term complications include metabolic abnormalities such as fluid and electrolyte imbalances, blood glucose abnormalities, and VAD problems (i.e., occlusions, breakage, infection) (19). Long-term complications include metabolic bone disease (MBD) and liver disease. Fortunately, guidelines have been proposed for monitoring HPN patients to prevent both short- and long-term complications (see Table 19.3) (3, 12). A monitoring plan should be established with the patient prior to discharge and should include laboratory parameters, intake and output record keeping, body weight, and temperature logs (1, 12).

19.4.1 Laboratory Measurements

Laboratory parameters are assessed at baseline prior to discharge home and are tailored to each individual from that point forward. Most patients on HPN will have laboratory parameters monitored weekly after discharge with the frequency being decreased over time to monthly or fewer blood draws (see Table 19.4). This allows clinicians to identify laboratory trends that may require adjustment within the PN prescription. It is important to remember that HPN solutions are delivered a few times each month depending on the homecare pharmacy. Therefore, adjustments to the PN prescription should be subtle to avoid metabolic abnormalities between PN deliveries and blood draws.

19.4.1.1 Anthropometric and Other Measurements

Self-monitoring includes daily recording of dietary and intravenous intake, gastrointestinal losses, and body weight and temperature measurements. Prior to discharge home, patients should be educated on the importance of self-monitoring to prevent metabolic imbalances from occurring. Each component of home self-monitoring can alert the PN prescriber that adjustments in the PN prescription may be warranted (see Table 19.4). Significant fluctuations in dietary intake and GI output can quickly alter fluid and electrolyte balance requiring an adjustment of the PN prescription and/or

TABLE 19.3
Guidelines for Monitoring HPN[1]

Parameter	Baseline	Daily	Weekly	Monthly	Yearly
Laboratory Parameters					
Blood Glucose Assessment	Yes	Yes, until stable	-	-	-
Electrolytes, Blood Urea Nitrogen (BUN), and Creatinine	Yes	Yes, until stable	Yes	Yes	-
Liver enzymes and Bilirubin	Yes	Yes, until stable	Yes	Yes	-
Albumin or Prealbumin	Yes	Yes, until stable	Yes, until stable	Yes	-
Trace Elements	Yes	-	-	Every 6 months as needed	-
Vitamins	Yes, depending on disease state	-	-	Every 6 months as needed	-
Anthropometric and Other Measurements					
Intake and Output Records	Yes	Yes	-	-	-
Body Weight	Yes	Yes	-	-	-
Body Temperature	Yes	Yes	-	-	-
Dual-Energy X-ray Absorptiometry	Yes	-	-	-	Yes, as needed

[1] Davila J, Konrad D. Metabolic Complications of Home Parenteral Nutrition. Nutr Clin Pract. 2017 Dec;32(6):753–768. doi: 10.1177/0884533617735089. Epub 2017 Oct 10. PMID: 29016233.

TABLE 19.4

Acute Changes during HPN Therapy and Prescriber Considerations[1]

Reported Change	Common Differential Diagnoses	Considerations for PN Prescription
Vomiting	Exogenous toxins Mechanical obstruction Infection (viral or bacterial)	Additional IVFs and/or oral rehydration solution Adjust electrolyte and/or energy components of PN prescription
Diarrhea	Increased oral intake Medication change (type, dose) Infection (viral or bacterial) Obstruction SIBO	Additional IVFs and/or oral rehydration solution Adjust electrolyte and/or energy components of PN prescription Initiate antidiarrheal therapy as needed
Reduced stool output	Decreased oral intake Inadequate fiber or fluid intake Improved GI absorption Medication change (type, dose) Obstruction	Adjust electrolyte and/or energy components of PN prescription Adjust antidiarrheal therapy as needed
Decrease urine output	Decreased fluid intake (oral and/or IV) Dehydration	Additional IVFs and/or oral rehydration solution
Increased urine output	Increased fluid intake (oral and/or IV) Overhydration	Reduce PN fluid volume and/or infusion days per week Hold PN infusion
Decreased oral/EN intake	Worsening GI function	Adjust electrolyte and/or energy components of PN prescription Assess need for initiating IVFE
Increased oral/EN intake	Improved GI absorption	Reduce IVFE needs Adjust electrolyte and/or energy components of PN prescription Consider reducing PN infusion days
Increase in body weight	Improved GI absorption Fluid overload	Adjust electrolyte and/or energy components of PN prescription Consider reducing PN infusion days Reduce PN fluid volume and/or hold PN infusion if weight gain ≥1 lb for 2 consecutive days
Decrease in body weight	Malnutrition Decreased oral/IV intake Dehydration	Adjust electrolyte and/or energy components of PN prescription Consider increasing PN infusion days Additional IVFs and/or oral rehydration solution
Elevated body temperature	Infection (viral and/or bacterial)	Hold PN infusion until source of infection is determined

IVF: Intravenous fluids; SIBO: small intestine bacterial overgrowth; EN: enteral nutrition; IVFE: intravenous fat emulsion; IV: intravenous; CRBSI: catheter-related bloodstream infection; GI: gastrointestinal; PN: parenteral nutrition.

[1] Bering J, DiBaise JK. Home Parenteral and Enteral Nutrition. Nutrients. 2022 Jun 21;14(13):2558. doi: 10.3390/nu14132558. PMID: 35807740; PMCID: PMC9268549(; Kumpf VJ. Challenges and Obstacles of Long-Term Home Parenteral Nutrition. Nutr Clin Pract. 2019 Apr;34(2):196–203. doi: 10.1002/ncp.10258. Epub 2019 Feb 4. PMID: 30714635; Pironi L, Arends J, Bozzetti F, Cuerda C, Gillanders L, Jeppesen PB, Joly F, Kelly D, Lal S, Staun M, Szczepanek K, Van Gossum A, Wanten G, Schneider SM; Home Artificial Nutrition & Chronic Intestinal Failure Special Interest Group of ESPEN. ESPEN guidelines on chronic intestinal failure in adults. Clin Nutr. 2016 Apr;35(2):247–307. doi: 10.1016/j.clnu.2016.01.020. Epub 2016 Feb 8. Erratum in: Clin Nutr. 2017 Apr;36(2):619. PMID: 26944585.

GI-related medications (i.e., antidiarrheals, motility medications). Acute changes in fluid balance especially can easily be ascertained from daily body weights especially when blood draws are infrequent. Weight fluctuations of ≥1 pound for two consecutive days can identify significant fluid shifts associated with dehydration or over hydration (12, 19, 20). Elevated body temperature with or without tremors and chills during the PN infusion can quickly identify any infectious complications associated with the VAD (5, 20). Contacting the prescriber and/or clinical home infusion provider is warranted. These tactics for home self-monitoring can prevent significant adverse events from occurring (see Chapter 20 on PN access).

19.4.1.2 Metabolic Bone Disease

PN monitoring schedules include a baseline assessment of bone mineral status to determine the presence of metabolic bone disease (MBD). MBD is a condition of reduced bone mass such as osteomalacia and osteoporosis, which is prevalent in as many as 67% of patients on HPN (19). Nutrient deficiencies and toxicities may play a role in the pathogenesis of MBD, but a definitive cause is yet unknown (21). Historically, PN ingredients, particularly amino acid solutions, were highly contaminated with aluminum which was associated with MBD. Since this time, aluminum contamination has been minimized in HPN solutions in accordance with the FDA mandate that all manufactures list the aluminum concentration on drug packaging. This allows NSTs to accurately calculate the contribution of aluminum in the PN bag and ensure that patients are receiving less than 5 mcg/kg/d (25). Management of MBD should start with a baseline dual-energy X-ray absorptiometry (DEXA) measurement. PN prescriptions should maximize the intravenous delivery of calcium and phosphorus, supplementation of vitamin D should be given as needed and patients should be encouraged to participate in routine exercise (21). DEXA scans should be assessed at baseline and then every 6–12 months until discontinuation of HPN with abnormal readings being monitored by endocrinology (26).

19.4.1.3 Hepatobiliary Disease

PN monitoring schedules include an assessment of the liver to prevent and/or identify hepatobiliary diseases such as cholestasis, steatosis, steatonecrosis, and cirrhosis associated with HPN. Etiology of liver disease during HPN is multifactorial and has been associated with short bowel syndrome, over feeding or intolerance of enteral nutrition (19, 22, 23). Prevalence rates are largely unknown, yet monitoring schedules of HPN patients must include assessment of liver enzymes. Liver associated enzymes (LAEs), such as bilirubin, alkaline phosphatase, and aspartate transaminase (AST), as well as routine radiographic imaging of the liver and spleen can be used to assess for liver injury while on HPN (12, 19, 23). Liver biopsy, although invasive, may be the most effective tool for determining the presence of liver damage since laboratory parameters may not indicate disease until the final stages when liver transplantation is necessary. Early identification of hepatobiliary diseases during HPN is more common when followed by an NST or IRC for HPN management. Gupte and colleagues reported in a retrospective analysis of children referred for intestinal transplantation that 58% of children managed by an NST had less incidence of liver disease compared to management by a physician alone (24). The multidisciplinary approach used by an NST includes the prevention of hepatobiliary disease by preventing infectious complications associated with the VAD, providing EN when feasible, preventing overfeeding, modifying the type of ILE, and ensuring adequate micronutrient supplementation (12, 19, 23).

19.5 CONCLUSION

Selecting patients appropriate for HPN is imperative to successful outcomes. Once patients are identified as appropriate for receiving HPN, careful initiation and monitoring for potential complications reduces adverse events from occurring. Management of HPN is best by an NST or IRC and by including the patient in the establishment of the long-term goals of therapy.

REFERENCES

1. Pironi L, Arends J, Bozzetti F, Cuerda C, Gillanders L, Jeppesen PB, Joly F, Kelly D, Lal S, Staun M, Szczepanek K, Van Gossum A, Wanten G, Schneider SM; Home Artificial Nutrition & Chronic Intestinal Failure Special Interest Group of ESPEN. ESPEN guidelines on chronic intestinal failure in adults. Clin Nutr. 2016 Apr;35(2):247–307. doi: 10.1016/j.clnu.2016.01.020. Epub 2016 Feb 8. Erratum in: Clin Nutr. 2017 Apr;36(2):619. PMID: 26944585.
2. Pironi L, Goulet O, Buchman A, Messing B, Gabe S, Candusso M, Bond G, Gupte G, Pertkiewicz M, Steiger E, Forbes A, Van Gossum A, Pinna AD, Nutrition Home Artificial, and ESPEN Chronic Intestinal Failure Working Group of outcome on home parenteral nutrition for benign intestinal failure: a review of the literature and benchmarking with the European prospective survey of ESPEN. Clin Nutr. 2012;31(6):831–45. doi: 10.1016/j.clnu.2012.05.004.
3. Pironi L, Boeykens K, Bozzetti F, Joly F, Klek S, Lal S, Lichota M, Mühlebach S, Van Gossum A, Wanten G, Wheatley C, Bischoff SC. ESPEN guideline on home parenteral nutrition. Clin Nutr. 2020 Jun;39(6):1645–1666. doi: 10.1016/j.clnu.2020.03.005. Epub 2020 Apr 18. PMID: 32359933.
4. Winkler MF, Smith, CE. Clinical, social, and economic impacts of home parenteral nutrition dependence in short bowel syndrome. JPEN J Parenter Enteral Nutr. 2014;38(1 Suppl):32S–37S. doi: 10.1177/0148607113517717.
5. Kovacevich DS, Corrigan M, Ross VM, McKeever L, Hall AM, Braunschweig C. American society for parenteral and enteral nutrition guidelines for the selection and care of central venous access devices for adult home parenteral nutrition administration. JPEN J Parenter Enteral Nutr. 2019 Jan;43(1):15–31. doi: 10.1002/jpen.1455. Epub 2018 Oct 19. PMID: 30339287.
6. Bering J, DiBaise JK. Home parenteral and enteral nutrition. Nutrients. 2022 Jun 21;14(13):2558. doi: 10.3390/nu14132558. PMID: 35807740; PMCID: PMC9268549.
7. Smith CE, Yadrich D, Wright S, Ridder L, Werkowitch M, Bruce A, Bonar JRM. Themes of stressors, emotional fatigue, and communication challenges found in mobile care discussion sessions with patients requiring lifelong home parenteral nutrition infusions. JPEN J Parenter Enteral Nutr. 2021 Mar;45(3):499–506. doi: 10.1002/jpen.1854. Epub 2020 Jun 4. PMID: 32495954.
8. Allen P. Medicare Coverage for Home Parenteral Nutrition: Policy Change After Almost Four Decades; Nutrition Issues in Gastroenterology, Series #215. Practical Gastroenterology, October 2021.

9. Bonnes SL, Salonen BR, Hurt RT, McMahon MT, Mundi MS. Parenteral and enteral nutrition-from hospital to home: Will it be covered? Nutr Clin Pract. 2017 Dec;32(6):730–738. doi: 10.1177/0884533617734491. Epub 2017 Oct 10. PMID: 29016231.

10. Worthington P, Balint J, Bechtold M, Bingham A, Chan LN, Durfee S, Jevenn AK, Malone A, Mascarenhas M, Robinson DT, Holcombe B. When is parenteral nutrition appropriate? JPEN J Parenter Enteral Nutr. 2017 Mar;41(3):324–377. doi: 10.1177/0148607117695251. Epub 2017 Feb 1. PMID: 28333597.

11. Boullata JI, Gilbert K, Sacks G, Labossiere RJ, Crill C, Goday P, Kumpf VJ, Mattox TW, Plogsted S, Holcombe B; American Society for Parenteral and Enteral Nutrition. A.S.P.E.N. clinical guidelines: Parenteral nutrition ordering, order review, compounding, labeling, and dispensing. JPEN J Parenter Enteral Nutr. 2014 Mar–Apr;38(3):334–377. doi: 10.1177/0148607114521833. Epub 2014 Feb 14. PMID: 24531708.

12. Kumpf VJ. Challenges and obstacles of long-term home parenteral nutrition. Nutr Clin Pract. 2019 Apr;34(2):196–203. doi: 10.1002/ncp.10258. Epub 2019 Feb 4. PMID: 30714635.

13. Mirtallo JM, Ayers P, Boullata J, Gura KM, Plogsted S, Anderson CR, Worthington P, Seres DS, Nicolai E, Alsharhan M, Gutsul L, Mason AE. ASPEN Lipid injectable emulsion safety recommendations, part 1: Background and adult considerations. Nutr Clin Pract. 2020 Oct;35(5):769–782. doi: 10.1002/ncp.10496. Epub 2020 May 27. Erratum in: Nutr Clin Pract. 2022 Apr;37(2):482. PMID: 32460429.

14. Gramlich L, Ireton-Jones C, Miles JM, Morrison M, Pontes-Arruda A. Essential fatty acid requirements and intravenous lipid emulsions. JPEN J Parenter Enteral Nutr. 2019 Aug;43(6):697–707. doi: 10.1002/jpen.1537. Epub 2019 Mar 25. PMID: 30908685.

15. Martindale RG, Berlana D, Boullata JI, Cai W, Calder PC, Deshpande GH, Evans D, Garcia-de-Lorenzo A, Goulet OJ, Li A, Mayer K, Mundi MS, Muscaritoli M, Pradelli L, Rosenthal M, Seo JM, Waitzberg DL, Klek S. Summary of proceedings and expert consensus statements from the international summit "lipids in parenteral nutrition". JPEN J Parenter Enteral Nutr. 2020 Feb;44 Suppl 1:S7–S20. doi: 10.1002/jpen.1746. PMID: 32049392.

16. Compher C, Bingham AL, McCall M, Patel J, Rice TW, Braunschweig C, McKeever L. Guidelines for the provision of nutrition support therapy in the adult critically ill patient: The American society for parenteral and enteral nutrition. JPEN J Parenter Enteral Nutr. 2022 Jan;46(1):12–41. doi: 10.1002/jpen.2267. Epub 2022 Jan 3. Erratum in: JPEN J Parenter Enteral Nutr. 2022 Aug;46(6):1458–1459. PMID: 34784064.

17. Hassig TB, McKinzie BP, Fortier CR, Taber D. Clinical management strategies and implications for parenteral nutrition drug shortages in adult patients. Pharmacotherapy. 2014;34(1):72–84. doi: 10.1002/phar.1350.

18. Fousekis FS, Mitselos IV, Christodoulou DK. New insights into intestinal failure-associated liver disease in adults: A comprehensive review of the literature. Saudi J Gastroenterol. 2021 Jan–Feb;27(1):3–12. doi: 10.4103/sjg.sjg_551_20. PMID: 33642350; PMCID: PMC8083246.

19. Davila J, Konrad D. Metabolic complications of home parenteral nutrition. Nutr Clin Pract. 2017 Dec;32(6):753–768. doi: 10.1177/0884533617735089. Epub 2017 Oct 10. PMID: 29016233.

20. Kumpf VJ, Tillman, EM. Home parenteral nutrition: Safe transition from hospital to home. Nutr Clin Pract. 2022;27(6):749–757. doi: 10.1177/0884533612464888.

21. Buchman AL, Moukarzel A. Metabolic bone disease associated with total parenteral nutrition. Clin Nutr. 2000;19(4):217–231. doi: 10.1054/clnu.1999.0083.

22. Massironi S, Cavalcoli F, Rausa E, Invernizzi P, Braga M, Vecchi M. Understanding short bowel syndrome: Current status and future perspectives. Dig Liver Dis. 2020 Mar;52(3):253–261. doi: 10.1016/j.dld.2019.11.013. Epub 2019 Dec 28. PMID: 31892505.

23. Klek S, Szczepanek K, Scislo L, Walewska E, Pietka M, Pisarska M, Pedziwiatr M. Intravenous lipid emulsions and liver function in adult chronic intestinal failure patients: Results after 5 y of home parenteral nutrition. Nutrition. 2021 Feb;82:111029. doi: 10.1016/j.nut.2020.111029. Epub 2020 Oct 18. PMID: 33221116.

24. Gupte GL, Beath SV, Protheroe S, Murphy MS, Davies P, Sharif K, McKiernan PJ, de Ville de Goyet J, Booth IW, Kelly DA. Improved outcome of referrals for intestinal transplantation in the UK. Arch Dis Child. 2007;92 (2):147–152. doi: 10.1136/adc.2005.090068.

25. Department of Health and Human Services. Aluminum in Large and Small Volume Parenterals Used in Total Parenteral Nutrition. 1998;63(2):176–185.

26. Rhoda KM, Suryadevara S, Steiger E. Home parenteral nutrition support for intestinal failure. Surgical Clinics. 2011;91(4):913–932.

20 Parenteral Nutrition Access

Beth Lyman, Reid Nishikawa, and Marianne Opilla

20.1 INTRODUCTION

Vascular access for parenteral nutrition support at home is a challenging and complex facet of the overall therapy. Diligent maintenance and care of the access site and device by the patient or home caregiver is vital in reducing catheter related complications, extending device life, reducing hospitalizations, and improving quality of life (1).

20.2 VASCULAR ACCESS

Home parenteral nutrition (HPN) formulations are usually hyperosmolar in order to provide the nutrients and electrolytes the patient requires. The large vessels of the central venous system have the high blood flow necessary to dilute the HPN solution and prevent venous damage (2). Central venous access refers to a device whose distal tip terminates at the junction of the superior vena cava and the right atrium or the inferior vena cava above the level of the diaphragm (3).

Figure 20.1 shows the sites used for central venous catheter (CVC) placement. The most common insertion sites are the internal jugular and subclavian with the tip location in the distal superior vena cava (SVC). Other sites that may be cannulated in patients with limited venous access are the femoral vein or translumbar vessels leading into the inferior vena cava. Central venous access can also be achieved by venipuncture of the basilic and cephalic veins in the arm and the CVC is advanced to the junction of the superior vena cava and the right atrium.

CVCs appropriate for HPN infusion include the peripherally inserted central catheter (PICC), tunneled catheter, and implanted port. Each device has specific characteristics and benefits tailored to meet the patient's individual needs. Pediatric patients use the same types of devices as adults. It is recommended that placement be re-confirmed for pediatric CVCs on a yearly basis due to growth that could change the position of the catheter tip (4).

Prior to CVC insertion, careful patient assessment by the clinical insertion team helps to ensure successful placement. In addition, discussion with the patient and caregiver should include age, ability to care for self, body image, length of therapy, lifestyle characteristics, and caregiver availability. Dialogue between the patient, caregivers, and clinicians will ensure the patient receives the device most suited to their lifestyle.

DOI: 10.1201/9780429322570-20

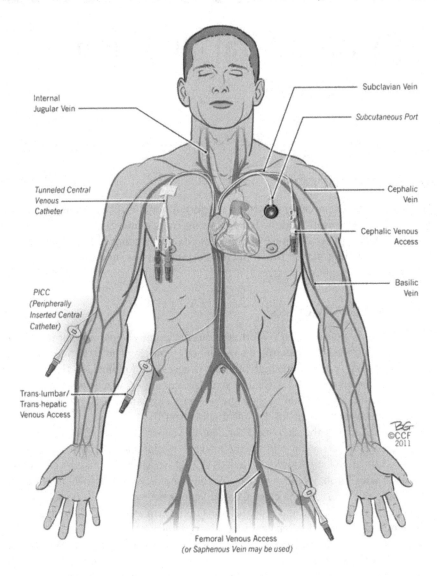

FIGURE 20.1   Venous access placement options for parenteral nutrition.

Source: Reproduced with permission from Cleveland Clinic. Parenteral nutrition: What it is, uses & types (April 19, 2022). https://my.clevelandclinic.org/health/treatments/22802-parenteral-nutrition. Accessed July 30, 2023.

CVC insertion may be performed at the bedside, in the radiology department, or in the operating room. Local anesthetic with intravenous sedation or general anesthesia may be given depending upon the individual patient's needs. CVCs are inserted by a variety of clinicians with expertise in the field. These include specially trained registered nurses, nurse practitioners, physician's assistants, and physicians.

20.3 DEVICE FEATURES

20.3.1 DESIGNS

Tunneled catheters and PICCs are available as single, double, or triple lumen. Implanted ports are single or double lumen. Multiple lumens provide access for more than one infusion but may have a higher incidence of infection due to increased manipulations at the hub. A single lumen catheter is the preferred option for patients infusing only HPN (5). Catheter lumens are either open-ended or valved at the distal tip or more proximally. An open-ended catheter requires clamping to prevent air embolism and adequate flushing to prevent clotting at the tip. Valved catheters have a pressure slit at the distal tip which opens with flush, infusion, or aspiration, but remains closed when not in use.

20.3.2 MATERIALS

The implanted port reservoir is either magnetic resonance imaging (MRI)-compatible plastic or titanium with a silicone septum. Silicone or polyurethane polymers are used for port catheters, PICCs, and tunneled catheters. Both products have superior compatibility with body tissue and fluids. The polyurethane is stiffer upon insertion but softens after placement into the body. Silicone is a very soft flexible material that is comfortable for long-term wear and compatible with most infusates and antiseptics. Polyurethane may crack with exposure to antiseptics and certain medications. Valved catheters are silicone. Although appropriate for use with HPN, polyurethane was primarily developed to administer high flow rate power injection therapies and is therefore a highly durable catheter material compared to silicone, which may tear or develop pinholes over time (6). Silicone catheters may be repaired but polyurethane CVCs cannot.

20.3.3 MEASUREMENTS

A catheter's French (Fr) size describes the circumference of the outer diameter in millimeters. The internal lumen will vary depending upon catheter design and material. Polyurethane catheters have narrower walls, so a 5 Fr polyurethane catheter has a larger internal volume than a 5 Fr silicone catheter. All types of catheters come in various lengths to accommodate different heights and weights. Silicone catheters may be trimmed to fit the anatomy of the patient, but valved and polyurethane length cannot be adjusted. French size and lumen volume may be imprinted on the hub of PICCs and tunneled catheters. The patient should receive a wallet-sized ID card which contains important catheter information and is helpful in determining measurements.

Pressure per square inch (PSI) is important to understand in the care of CVCs. Excessive PSI can cause catheter rupture. Silicone catheters are very soft and can only withstand about 40–60 PSI compared to polyurethane at 300 PSI.

20.4   CENTRAL VASCULAR ACCESS DEVICES

20.4.1   PERIPHERALLY INSERTED CENTRAL CATHETERS (PICCs)

A PICC is inserted into the cephalic or basilic vein near the antecubital fossa and advanced into the central venous system to the distal SVC. Traditionally PICCs were indicated for therapies lasting 6 months or less but have been reported to remain in place for months to years without complications (7). Figure 20.1 shows placement of a PICC. It is usually anchored in place on the skin at the insertion site using a stabilization device rather than tape or sutures. These devices reduce catheter movement at the site and within the vessel and help to prevent dislodgement (3). PICC site care is generally provided by weekly home health nursing visits to closely observe the site and maintain the stabilization device.

20.4.2   TUNNELED CATHETERS

The tunneled catheter is inserted into the vessel through a small incision or cut down and threaded into desired distal SVC tip position. Figure 20.1 shows tunneled catheter placement. A subcutaneous tunnel is created with an exit site on the chest, abdomen, or – rarely – the thigh. A Dacron cuff is placed above the exit site within the subcutaneous tissue of the tunnel. This cuff provides catheter stability, as well as a barrier against bacteria migrating from the exit site into the central venous system. Additional anchoring is provided with external sutures at the exit site. The subcutaneous tissue adheres to the Dacron cuff in 10–14 days and then sutures at the exit site can be removed. Many HPN patients and caregivers are taught to perform their own site care and in some cases a dressing is not required at the exit site once it is well healed (5). The tunnel-and-cuff feature of these catheters increases patient independence with self-care and reduces catheter malposition and dislodgement.

20.4.3   IMPLANTED PORT

The implanted port reservoir is placed in a subcutaneous pocket on the chest, abdomen, or thigh and the tubing is threaded into the central venous system. Figure 20.1 demonstrates implanted port placement in the chest area. It is completely under the skin and must be accessed for infusion with a non-coring 90-degree needle with extension to connect the HPN infusion. Once the infusion is completed, the needle can be removed or left in place for up to 7 days covered with a sterile dressing. Implanted ports are an appropriate choice for HPN patients desiring a concealed device, when infusion days are less than 5 days per week, or for patients who have intermittent HPN needs. The port site requires no dressing or routine flushing when HPN is not infusing. Careful consideration should be given before implanted ports are placed, since the needle insertion requires home health nursing, a skilled caregiver, or an individual willing to learn self-accessing.

20.5   COMPLICATIONS

20.5.1   CATHETER-RELATED BLOODSTREAM INFECTION

Catheter-related bloodstream infection (CRBSI) also called central line-associated bloodstream infection (CLABSI) is a serious complication associated with HPN therapy. Reported CRBSI rates in HPN patients range from 0.74–3.0 per 1000 catheter days (8). *Staphylococcus* species, gram-negative and fungal organisms and polymicrobial pathogens are seen in HPN-associated CRBSI (9). Catheter-related bloodstream infection may progress to bacteremia and sepsis, a leading cause of morbidity and mortality in HPN patients (10). The main portal of entry for pathogens into the bloodstream is the catheter hub and skin flora from the entry site of PICCs and implanted ports. The Dacron cuff on the tunneled catheter provides a protective barrier against migration of skin bacteria into the bloodstream.

Suspected CRBSI requires immediate medical intervention. Symptoms include fever and chills, especially at the beginning of the infusion, headache, nausea, vomiting, body aches, and malaise. Peripheral and catheter paired blood cultures should be obtained prior to initiation of antibiotics. The CDC defines CRBSI as a primary bloodstream infection with no apparent infection at another site when a CVC is in place for 48 hours or more. There must be one or more positive blood cultures and symptoms which may include fever and chills. The same pathogen must be cultured from two or more specimens drawn on separate occasions (11). When blood cannot be obtained from the CVC and/or the peripheral site, available cultures and assessment of the patient's medical condition will indicate diagnosis of CRBSI. The preferred route of treatment for HPN patients should be intravenous antibiotics since altered intestinal anatomy and gastrointestinal function may prevent absorption of oral antibiotics. Often, lock therapy is administered in conjunction with the appropriate systemic antibiotic. Locking solutions available in the United States include concentrated antibiotics and medical grade ethanol (12).

The decision to remove the CVC as part of the treatment plan is dependent upon the patient's condition. In cases of septic shock, persistent positive blood cultures, endocarditis, osteomyelitis, and fungal infections, catheter removal is indicated (1, 13). In uncomplicated gram-negative and gram-positive infections, the CVC may be salvaged (14). This is important for the HPN patient who needs to maintain a CVC for a lifetime.

Often, the therapy can be completed in the home setting after the HPN patient is symptom-free and negative blood cultures are obtained. Teaching of antibiotic administration can be completed by home health nursing or the infusion pharmacy.

Numerous risk factors have been identified as contributing to the incidence of CRBSI. Some of these include multiple therapies increasing manipulations at the hub, frequent blood draws from the catheter, use of narcotics, daily lipid infusions, pediatric age, ostomies, and multiple lumens (15). Awareness and identification of risk factors can be helpful in reducing an HPN patient's CRBSI rate.

20.5.2 Infection Prevention

Hand hygiene is the main strategy for prevention of CRBSI and should be practiced often. Antibacterial soaps or alcohol-based hand rubs are acceptable for CVC procedures (1, 5).

Disinfection is necessary with each access into the CVC port or end adapter. An antiseptic agent such as 70% alcohol, chlorhexidine and alcohol combination solution, and povidone-iodine are all acceptable when applied with a scrubbing friction technique and allowed to dry prior to access (16). Passive disinfection caps containing an alcohol foam insert are also effective when used to cover the end adapter and they offer a protective barrier against skin bacteria and ostomy or enteric tube contamination at the hub (17).

Locking solutions may be used as a preventative strategy in patients who have frequent incidents of CRBSI (5). A lock solution is instilled into the catheter and allowed to dwell for a specific time with the goal of reducing microbial biofilm within the catheter lumen. Concentrated antibiotic solutions with or without heparin, and medical grade ethanol are available as lock solutions in the United States (12). They are generally used daily or once a week.

Reduction of lab draw frequency from the CVC has been shown to reduce infection rates in HPN patients (15). Fibrin that collects within the catheter lumen and hub when blood is withdrawn provides an environment for bacteria to thrive and grow, eventually causing CRBSI. Peripheral lab draws should be encouraged whenever possible.

Catheter care should be performed with minimal conversation and in a private setting with clean work surface. Sterile gloves and masks are recommended for CVC site care with newly inserted catheters or when immune function is depressed. Well healed older catheters may not require sterile dressing and site care depending upon the individual patient and physician recommendation (5). Involvement in HPN support and networking groups has been shown to reduce the incidence of CRBSI (18).

20.5.3 OCCLUSION

CVC occlusion occurs when there is partial or complete obstruction of the CVC lumen. It presents as resistant or sluggish flushing and infusing, inability to aspirate, also known as withdrawal occlusion, and persistent increasing pump occlusion alarms. Occlusion is a significant complication that delays or interrupts therapy. The cause of occlusion is either non-thrombotic or thrombotic.

Firstly, non-thrombotic occlusion should be ruled out. All components of the CVC and infusion system should be checked for kinks, clogged filters, malfunctioning clamps, and misconnections. The entrance or exit skin sites should be examined closely for constricting sutures, tight securing devices, or crimped tubing.

Implanted ports may be more challenging to troubleshoot due to inability to visualize since they are placed under the skin. Changing or repositioning the non-coring needle may relieve an occlusion, but in most cases radiological evaluation is indicated to assess for a flipped port and kinked or separated tubing (19).

Internal mechanical causes in tunneled CVCs and PICCs may also result in occlusion and will require radiological assessment and intervention. These include kinks within the tunnel or vessel, migration of the CVC out of position, and pinch-off syndrome. Although rare, pinch-off syndrome occurs when the CVC tubing is compressed by the clavicle and the first rib. Symptoms may be intermittent during position change of the arm and shoulder, or there may be actual tearing or fracture of the CVC resulting in migration into the venous system (20). Other non-thrombotic occlusions may be caused by drug and mineral precipitate and lipid deposits within the catheter lumen. Precipitates are formed when incompatible drugs are administered without adequate flushing between each drug. Calcium, phosphorous, and magnesium may precipitate in HPN solutions when concentrations are too high. Lipid emulsion residue may also build up in the CVC lumen over time.

Incompatible drug precipitates can be avoided by not mixing drugs together in a syringe or infusion solution. Drugs should be administered individually with a 10 mL sodium chloride flush between each medication.

Pharmacy compounding protocols are established to prevent mineral precipitate in HPN solutions. Review of medications and solutions with the home care pharmacist is indicated if precipitate occlusion is suspected.

Drug and mineral precipitate may be cleared depending upon the pH of the offender. Sodium bicarbonate, sodium hydroxide, hydrochloric acid, and L-cysteine have all been shown to clear various precipitates (21). Lipid deposit occlusions are usually suspected if sluggishness or clogging occurs following a lipid infusion. Ethanol lock 70% with a 2-hour dwell time may remove lipid residue from the CVC lumen (21).

Thrombotic occlusions occur when fibrin builds up within or around the tip of the CVC lumen or non-coring needle. Thrombotic occlusions can be prevented by maintaining good catheter patency. Proper CVC flushing and use of positive or neutral end adapters prevent blood reflux into the CVC lumen (22).

A fibrinolytic drug called tissue plasminogen activator (tPA) can be used to dissolve fibrin clots within the catheter lumen. A 2 mg dose is instilled into the CVC lumen or port and allowed to dwell 30 minutes to 2 hours. Smaller doses are indicated for infants and children due to shorter catheter length. It may be repeated if patency is not restored. Alteplase is safe for use in outpatient and home settings for adult and pediatric patients without bleeding disorders and often helps to reduce emergency room and hospital visits (23). When thrombotic occlusion is not resolved by flushing or Alteplase injection, radiological studies or venogram may be indicated to determine the extent of the thrombus and further treatment plan for CVC salvage.

20.5.4 Thrombosis

Venous thrombosis is the formation of a localized clot within a vein causing narrowing or obstruction. Virchow's triad describes three factors contributing to formation of venous thrombus: vessel wall trauma, blood flow stasis, and hypercoagulability (24). Other contributing risk factors include age, cancer, diabetes, pregnancy, estrogen therapy, dehydration, immobility, multiple CVC insertions, catheter diameter, and multiple lumens (3). Symptoms of CVC-related thrombosis are extremity, face, and neck swelling and vein engorgement, pain during infusion, extremity numbness and discoloration, development of collateral vessels most often visible in the chest and neck area, pump alarms, and incomplete HPN infusions. Often thrombosis is asymptomatic and only noted when radiological studies are performed.

Prevention of thrombosis includes correct tip location at the junction of the SVC and the right atrium. Tip location proximal to the SVC junction has been shown to increase thrombosis for each type of CVC (25). Use of the smallest diameter CVC with the least number of lumens (26), maintaining good hydration, and regular exercise have been shown to help reduce thrombosis formation.

Prophylactic anticoagulation has not been shown to reduce CVC-associated thrombosis (18).

Treatment for CVC-related thrombosis includes leaving the CVC in place if tolerated and long-term anticoagulation. Increased risk for CRBSI, recurrent thrombosis, and persistent vascular occlusion are associated complications with chronic CVC thrombosis (27).

20.5.5 DISLODGEMENT

Despite sutures, securing cuffs and devices, or being totally implanted, all CVCs have the risk of becoming dislodged. This can occur with inadvertent pulling of the CVC or strenuous activity. Signs of dislodgement are leaking, cuff exposure on tunneled CVCs, longer tubing, or a moveable implanted port. Other less obvious signs are infusion problems, partial or complete occlusion, inability to aspirate, and burning or pain sensation with flush and infusion.

When dislodgement is suspected the physician should be notified immediately, infusions held, and usually radiology assessment will be required.

Dislodgement can be prevented by anchoring the CVC with a securing loop or device. Patients should be educated on ways to secure the CVC to reduce pulling, such as a securing loop. PICCs should be measured upon insertion and periodically to ensure they are not advancing out of position.

Tip migration out of the junction of the SVC and the right atrium may occur with increased intrathoracic pressure associated such as vomiting, vigorous coughing or sneezing, reduced blood flow from a disease process, tumor, or large thrombosis (24). There may be difficulty with infusion, flushing, or aspiration. The patient may complain of swishing sounds when flushing the CVC, headache, or pain or swelling in the neck, face, or shoulder (24).

20.5.6 BREAKAGE

Pulling, use of scissors, and excessive force when flushing may cause CVC rupture and damage. Small pinholes may develop over time from clamps or pinched tubing. The patient may notice a wet dressing or leakage while infusing or flushing. Internal rupture may occur with pinch-off syndrome or forced flushing and is exhibited by swelling or burning within the tunnel during flushing or infusing. A damaged and leaking implanted port catheter causes swelling into the soft tissue of the port pocket and surrounding area.

Silicone is the softest CVC material. A silicone tunneled catheter can be safely repaired with a specified kit. Repairs include a spliced section that is glued into place and can last for many years (28, 29). HPN patients should keep an individualized repair kit in their home supply stock. Polyurethane catheters are very durable and rarely develop breaks. They cannot be repaired and must be replaced if damage occurs. Implanted ports cannot be repaired and must be replaced before resuming HPN.

20.6   PATIENT EDUCATION

The HPN patient is the keeper of their lifeline and the best person to monitor and care for the CVC. In a cohort of 61 long-term HPN patients with CVCs of various kinds (PICC, tunneled, port) in place for more than 5 years, several preventative strategies related to line care as well as focused and continued patient education were effective in helping to prevent central line-associated bloodstream infections (30). In-home nursing may be initiated at the onset of HPN, but eventually the patient or family member will become the primary caregiver. Education should include the patient's ability to provide self-care for dressing changes, administration of medication and solutions, and troubleshooting the CVC device for all possible complications. It is important to identify a backup caregiver in case the patient becomes incapacitated. HPN patients should not be discharged from home health until they are able to independently return demonstrate all HPN and CVC care procedures correctly.

ACKNOWLEDGMENTS

The authors would like to acknowledge and thank Marianne Opilla, RN, BSN, CNSC, for her work on this project and dedicate this chapter to her memory.

REFERENCES

1. Kovacevich, D.S., Corrigan, M., Ross, V.M., McKeever, L., Hall, A.M., Braunschweig, C. "American Society for Parenteral and Enteral Nutrition Guidelines for the Selection and Care of Central Venous Access Devices for Adult Home Parenteral Nutrition Administration." JPEN J Parenter Enteral Nutr. Jan 2019;43(1):15–31. doi:10.1002/jpen.1455.
2. Bullock-Corkhill, Melody. "Central Venous Access Devices: Access and Insertion." In *Infusion Nursing: An Evidence-Based Approach*, 480–494. Missouri: Saunders Elsevier, 2010
3. Alexander, Mary, Gorski, Lisa A., Corrigan, Ann, et al. "Technical and Clinical Application." In *Core Curriculum for Infusion Nursing*, 1–85. Philadelphia: Lippincott Williams & Wilkins, 2014.
4. Gibbons, Sara, Richardson, Denise S. "Central Venous Catheter Care." In *Clinical Management of Intestinal Failure*, 331–358. London: CRC Press, 2011.
5. O'Grady, Naomi P., Alexander, Mary, Burns, Lillian A., et al. "Guidelines for the Prevention of Intravascular Catheter-Related Infections." *Clin Infect Dis* 52 no. 9 (2011): e162–e193.
6. Cohen, A.B., Dagli, M., Stravropoulos, S.W., et al. "Silicone and Polyurethane Tunneled Infusion Catheters: A Comparison of Durability and Breakage Rates." *J Vasc Interv Radiol* 22 no. 5 (2011): 638–641
7. Cohen, A.B., Dagli, M., Stravropoulos, S.W., et al. "Silicone and Polyurethane Tunneled Infusion Catheters: A Comparison of Durability and Breakage Rates." *J Vasc Interv Radiol* 22 no. 5 (2011): 638–641.
8. Cotogni, P., Barbero, C., Garrino, C., et al. "Peripherally Inserted Central Catheters in Non-Hospitalized Cancer Patients: 5-Year Results of a Prospective Study." *Support Care Cancer* 23 no. 2 (2015): 403–409.
9. Elfassy, Sam, Kassam, Zain, Amin, Faizan, et al. "Epidemiology and Risk Factors for Bloodstream Infections in a Home Parenteral Nutrition Program." *JPEN* 39 no. 2 (2015): 147–153.

10. Marra, A.R., Opilla, M.T., Edmond, M.B. "Epidemiology of Bloodstream Infections in Patients Receiving Long-Term Total Parenteral Nutrition." *J Clin Gastroenterol* 41 no. 1 (2007): 19–28.

11. Eriksen, M.K., Jorgensen, S.M.D., Lemming, L.E., Lal, S., Dahlerup, J.F., Hvas, C.L. "Patient Characteristics and Clinical Outcomes in a Specialised Intestinal Failure Unit: An Observational Cohort Study." Clin Nutr ESPEN. Aug 2020;38:253–262. doi:10.1016/j.clnesp.2020.04.002

12. Miller, D.L., O'Grady, N. "Guidelines for the Prevention of Intravascular Catheter-Related Infections: Recommendations Relevant to the Interventional Radiology for Venous Catheter Placement and Maintenance." *J Vasc Interv Radiol* 23 no. 8 (2012): 997–1007.

13. Bijo, J. K., Khan, Maqsood A., Speerhas, Rex, et al. "Ethanol Lock Therapy in Reducing Catheter-Related Bloodstream Infections in Adult Home Parenteral Nutrition Patients: Results of a Retrospective Study." *JPEN* 36 no. 5 (2012): 603–610.

14. Mermel, Leonard A., Allon, Michael, Bouza, Emilio, et al. "Clinical Management for the Diagnosis and Management of Intravascular Catheter-Related Infection: 2009 Update by the Infectious Diseases Society of America." *Clin Infect Dis* 49 no. 1 (2009): 1–45.

15. Dibb, Martyn J., Abraham, Arun, Chadwick, Paul R., et al. "Central Venous Catheter Salvage in Home Parenteral Nutrition Catheter-Related Bloodstream Infections: Long Term Safety and Efficacy Data." *JPEN* 40 no. 5 (2016): 699–704.

16. Buchman, Alan L., Opilla, Marianne, Kwasny, Mary, et. al. "Risk Factors for the Development of Catheter-Related Bloodstream Infections in Patients Receiving Home Parenteral Nutrition." *JPEN* 38 no. 6 (2014): 744–749.

17. The Joint Commission. "CLABSI Prevention Strategies, Techniques, and Technologies." In *Preventing Central Line-Associated Bloodstream Infections: A Global Challenge, A Global Perspective*. Oak Brook IL: Joint Commission Resources, 2012: 39–70.

18. Merrill, K. C., Sumner, S., Linford, L., et al. "Impact of Universal Disinfectant Cap Implementation on Central Line-Associated Bloodstream Infections." *Am J Infect Control* 42 no. 12 (2014): 1274–1277.

19. Smith, Carol E., Curtas, Susan, Werkowitch, Marilyn, et al. "Home Parenteral Nutrition: Does Affiliation with a National Support and Educational Organization Improve Patient Outcomes?"*JPEN* 26 no. 3 (2002): 159–163.

20. Kansagra, Akash P., Yu, John-Paul J., Naeger, David M., et al. "Risk Stratification and Radiologic Evaluation of Central Venous Port Malfunction." *JAVA* 19 no. 2 (2014): 77–83.

21. Baskin, Jacquelyn L., Pui, Ching-Hon, Reiss, Ulrike, et al. "Management of Occlusion and Thrombosis Associated with Long-Term Indwelling Central Venous Catheters." *Lancet* 11 no. 374 (2009): 159–169.

22. Ast, Daniel, and Ast, Travis. "Nonthrombotic Complications Related to Central Vascular Access Devices." *J of Infus Nurs* 37 no. 5 (2014): 349–358.

23. Hadaway, L., Richardson, D. "Needleless connectors: A Primer on Terminology." *J Inf Nurse* 33 no. 1 (2010): 22–31.

24. Baskin, J.L., Reiss, U., Wilimas, J.A., Metzger, M.L., Ribeiro, R.C., Pui, C., et al., "Thrombolytic Therapy for Central Venous Catheter Occlusion." *Haematologica* 97 no. 5 (2012): 641–650.

25. Gorski, Lisa, Perucca, Roxanne, Hunter, Mark R. "Central Venous Access Devices: Care, Maintenance, and Potential Complications." In *Infusion Nursing: An Evidence-Based Approach*, 495–515. Missouri: Saunders Elsevier, 2010.

26. DeChicco, Robert, Seidner, Douglas L., Brun, Carlos, et al. "Tip Position of Long-Term Central Venous Access Devices Used for Parenteral Nutrition." *JPEN* 31 no. 5 (2007): 382–387.

27. Ratz, D., Hofer, T., Flanders, S.A., Chopra, V. "Limiting the Number of Lumens in Peripherally Inserted Central Catheters to Improve Outcomes and Reduce Cost: A Simulation Study." *Infec Control Hosp Eipdemiol* 37 no. 7 (2016): 811–817.
28. Dibb, M., Lal, S. "Home Parenteral Nutrition: Vascular Access and Related Complications." *NCP* 32 no. 6 (2017): 769–776.
29. McNiven, C., Switzer, N., Wood, M., Persad, R., Hancock, M., Forgie, S., et al. "Central Venous Catheter Repair Is Not Associated with an Increased Risk of Central Line Infection or Colonization in Intestinal Failure Pediatric Patients." *J Pediatr Surg* 51 no. 3 (2016): 395–397.
30. Opilla, M, Nishikawa, R. "Central Venous Catheters for Home Parenteral Nutrition: Characteristics and Outcomes of Devices in Place for Five or More Years." Presented at the ASPEN Nutrition Science and Practice Conference, January 23, 2018, Las Vegas NV. *JPEN* 42, no. 2 (February 2018). jpen.1150wileyonlinelibrary.com

21 Nutritional Management of Diabetes Mellitus

Martha McHenry

21.1 OVERVIEW OF DIABETES MELLITUS

Diabetes mellitus is a chronic disease characterized by a defect in insulin secretion, ineffective insulin action, or both, that results in high blood glucose. Defects in insulin secretion can result in a substantial or absolute absence of insulin. This is often referred to as insulin deficiency and results when pancreatic beta-cells do not secrete enough insulin to keep up with the demand placed by glucose in the bloodstream. Defects in insulin action result when cells involved in glucose uptake, such as muscle cells, are unable to use insulin effectively. This results in a condition referred to as insulin resistance (American Diabetes Association 2009). One or both of these mechanisms are involved in the development and characterization of diabetes.

The number of individuals that are living with diabetes has been on a sharp rise since 2009. The International Diabetes Federation's (IDF) Diabetes Atlas reports that globally, in 2019, 463 million people were living with diabetes. That number is projected to rise, according to the IDF, by 100 million, to 578 million in just 10 years. Further, the IDF reports that in addition to cases of overt diabetes, an estimated 352 million people worldwide are living with prediabetes. While cultural foods and practices underlying diabetes differ around the world, the characteristics of diabetes do not.

Diabetes is a broad designation for a group of all metabolic disorders that have a common characteristic of marked high blood glucose. In a clinical setting, this may be referred to as hyperglycemia or high blood glucose but in an outpatient or home care setting, the colloquial term "high blood sugar" is often used. Hyperglycemia can develop through several mechanisms that range from the auto-destruction of pancreatic beta-cells resulting in little to no production of insulin, to diminished production of insulin resulting in insulin deficiency or abnormalities in how cells use insulin as in insulin resistance.

The common symptoms of hyperglycemia include but are not limited to:

- Increased thirst and urination as the body attempts to rid itself of glucose
- Blurred vision as the shape of the eyeball changes in response to hyperglycemia
- Sleepiness and fatigue after a meal as insufficient or ineffective insulin prevents glucose from entering the cells, where it can be used to produce energy
- Susceptibility to infection since a glucose-rich environment serves as the perfect medium for everyday bacteria
- Numbness and tingling in the hands and feet as blood vessels damaged by hyperglycemia fail to support the nerve tissue

 DOI: 10.1201/9780429322570-21

Chronic hyperglycemia can result in neuropathy, cardiovascular disease, kidney and vision failure, and sexual dysfunction. Acute hyperglycemia can be accompanied by ketoacidosis or nonketotic hyperosmolar syndrome. This is also known as hyperglycemic hyperosmolar syndrome/state. Patients in either one of these acute phases are often hospitalized and inpatient protocols are followed (American Diabetes Association 2015). Complications that arise from both chronic hyperglycemia and acute hyperglycemia, as well as the role played by glucose variability, will be addressed in more detail later in this chapter.

There are three common classifications of diabetes mellitus that make up the preponderance of all cases of diabetes. A fourth class consists of several uncommon types of diabetes that vary in etiology (see Table 21.1).

The classification of diabetes is typically assigned at the time of diagnosis and largely depends on the circumstances on hand at the time, such as severity of hyperglycemia, age, and other factors. An individual who exhibits signs and symptoms from more than one classification may be misdiagnosed or may be put into the fourth classification of varied etiologies (American Diabetes Association 2009).

Regardless of the classification, the end result of hyperglycemia is the same and an effective care plan for all classifications must include glycemic control as one of the primary goals.

TABLE 21.1

Classification of Diabetes Mellitus Diseases and Its Principal Distinguishing Characteristics

Classification	Type 1 Diabetes Mellitus	Type 2 Diabetes Mellitus	Gestational Diabetes Mellitus	Diabetes Due to Other Causes
Characteristics	Pancreatic beta-cell destruction resulting in complete insulin deficiency; possibly autoimmune	Progressive beta-cell dysfunction resulting in gradual insulin deficiency and/or insulin resistance	Hyperglycemia detected during the second or third trimester of pregnancy	Caused by drugs, such as steroids, monogenic syndromes such as MODY (mature onset diabetes of the young), or pancreatic diseases
Status Dependent	Insulin-dependent	Noninsulin-dependent	Noninsulin-dependent	May or may not be insulin-dependent
Onset	Predominantly in youth but can be diagnosed at any age	Usually after the age of 40 but can be diagnosed at any age and usually associated with obesity	After the first trimester of pregnancy; can be diagnosed at any age and may be associated with rapid pregnancy weight gain	Can be diagnosed at any age

21.2   DIABETES IN AMERICA

- According to the Center for Disease Control's 2019 National Diabetes Statistics Report we know the following about our target population:
  - The number of Americans with diabetes continues to climb.
  - 37.3 million, or 11.3% of the population meet the criteria are diagnosed with diabetes. In the adult only population percentage of individuals with diabetes is 14.7%.
  - 8.5 million meet the diagnostic criteria for diabetes but are undiagnosed.
  - 90%–95% of all cases of diabetes are type 2. About 5%–8% are type 1 and 2%–5% account for all other types put together.
  - The largest age group of adults with diabetes is the 65 years and older group.
- The prevalence of diabetes varies widely by race ethnicity, gender and even education level. In the CDC report, National Diabetes Statistics Report, 2019, the data indicate the following rates of prevalence among US adults with diabetes:
  - Non-Hispanic-Whites experience diabetes at a rate of 7.4% while American Indians and Alaska natives experience diabetes at the highest rate of 14.9%. In the Non-Hispanic Black community the rate is 12.1%. In the Hispanic community the rate is 11.8% and in the Asian community the rate is 9.5%.
- Further stratifications of the 2014 data showed that among Hispanic and Asian adults with diabetes, the composition or subgroups were as follows:
  - 14.4% are Mexican
  - 12.4% Puerto Rican
  - 8.3% are Central and South American
  - 6.5% are Cuban
- Among Asian American adults, the composition of subgroups is as follows:
  - 12.6% are Asian Indians
  - 10.4% are Filipinos
  - 5.6% are Chinese
  - 9.9% are "other" Asians
  - Prevalence varied also when stratified by educational level. Adults with less than a high school level eduation experienced diabetes at a rate of 13.4% while those with more than high school level education experienced diabetes at a rate of 7.1%.
- The number of individuals with prediabetes has also grown year after year.
- 96 million Americans or 38% of the American population meet the criteria for prediabetes and 80% of those individuals are unaware they have prediabetes. (CDC, National Diabetes Report, 2019).

This stratification gives an insight to the complexities of effectively treating diabetes in the United States. It's important to understand the magnitude of the diversity of persons with diabetes because it has direct implications for the dietitian. Cultural stratification can be used to drive the development of culturally relevant treatment plans that are customized to an individual's or group's

- Beliefs about diabetes and self-efficacy
- Cultural preferences for lifestyle
- Cultural preferences for food

In turn, these culturally relevant plans may be easier to adopt by the patient with diabetes, making them more sustainable over time, thereby matching the long-term nature of the disease.

21.3 THE FINANCIAL BURDEN OF DIABETES

The American Diabetes Association commissioned a study in 2012 of the costs associated with diabetes. In 2012 the cumulative cost was $245 billion. In a follow up study of the same costs in 2017, (ADA, 2018) the research shows an increase of 26% for a total of $327 billion. Of this, $237 billion was direct medical costs and $90 billion was associated with reduced productivity. Direct costs included hospital inpatient care, office visits, medications for high blood sugar and medications that treat the complications of diabetes. Indirect costs included absenteeism, reduced productivity, disability and early mortality.

- The 2017 study also showed the following:
  - The increased costs of 2017 over 2014 came primarily from the 65 and older age group putting increased pressure on Medicare.
  - Government plans covered 67% of diabetes care and commercial plans covered 31% while 2% went uninsured
  - People without insurance had 168% more emergency visits than people with insurance.
  - Men had higher diabetes-associated costs than women.
  - Non-Hispanic blacks had the highest overall health care expenditures, and 65% more emergency department visits than the population with diabetes as a whole.
  - California, Texas, Florida and New York lead the nation in diabetes-related health care costs.

As this research shows, the cost of diabetes to individuals, communities and the country as a whole is significant. Notably absent from the study were the intangible costs of diabetes. These costs can be more difficult to quantify but include intangibles such as pain and suffering, family or non-paid caregivers. Also not included is the financial cost associated with undiagnosed diabetes. In this light, confronting diabetes on all fronts, with evidence based intervention, including the home setting, is imperative (Franze, MJ 2010).

TABLE 21.2
Diagnosing Diabetes

Test	Diagnostic Threshold	Comments
HbA1c	>6.5	Added to the list of diagnostic tests in 2008 after review by an expert committee. Must be standardized to the DCCT assay to assure accuracy.
Fasting plasma glucose	>126	Must fast for at least 8 hr.
2-hour plasma glucose in OGTT	≥200	A standard protocol using 75 g of anhydrous glucose dissolved in water.
Random plasma glucose	≥200 mg/dL + symptoms of hyperglycemia	Can be done at any time.

21.4   DIAGNOSING DIABETES

Diabetes can be diagnosed through several different tests. Usual tests used in the diagnosing of diabetes are listed as fasting plasma glucose (FPG), the 2-hour plasma glucose, and the oral glucose tolerance test (OGTT), and more recently, the glycated hemoglobin test (HbA1c) has been approved as a diagnostic method in addition to its historic role of just a management tool. These tests can be used for screening, diagnosing, and management. Meeting one of the criteria listed in Table 21.2 qualifies as a diagnosis of diabetes.

Until recently, using HbA1c as a diagnostic tool was quite controversial. Since tightening the standards for this test in regard to accuracy and standardization, today, HbA1c is a popular way to diagnose and monitor diabetes care. The following are some of the reasons why HbA1c is quickly becoming a routine diagnostic tool:

- Only the HbA1c test gives a picture of the patient's chronic glycemic status.
- HbA1c is more tightly associated with the complications of diabetes such as retinopathy and cardiovascular disease than FPG.
- No fasting needed for HbA1c.
- Stress, eating, and exercising do not affect HbA1c.
- Using the same biomarker for diagnosing and managing could be useful (Enzo Bonora and Jaakko Tuomilehto 2011).

21.5   MONITORING HEMOGLOBIN A1c IN THE OUTPATIENT OR HOME SETTING

HbA1c can also be monitored in the home or outpatient setting. Care must be taken, however, to select an HbA1c monitor that meets National Glycohemoglobin

Standardization Program (NGSP) standards for accuracy. Outpatient and consulting dietitians can easily administer this test, thereby improving their value and role in the patient's care. Today, while there is no code for reimbursement for this test when administered by dietitians, a low fee with a CLIA-waived device that involves just a finger stick for the outpatient and home-bound patient until reimbursement for dietitians is recognized, could be a low-barrier out-of-pocket and billable service. In a study by Anna Chang, the following were demonstrated:

- Lay users found the A1CNow Self Check easy to use, and both lay users and HCPs were able to measure HbA1c accurately.
- An HbA1c reading was considered accurate if it was within ±13.5% of a corresponding NGSP-certified laboratory reference value.
- The A1CNow Self Check has received 2010 NGSP certification (Chang et al. 2010).

21.6 PREDIABETES

In 2003, the Expert Committee on Diagnosis and Classification of Diabetes Mellitus recognized a group of individuals who don't meet the diagnostic criteria on any of the tests discussed but have varying degrees of hyperglycemia. These individuals have prediabetes. They score too high on the IFG and IGT tests to be normal but not high enough to earn a diagnosis of diabetes. The diagnostic criteria for prediabetes are described in Table 21.3.

Individuals with IFG or IGT have a higher risk for future development of diabetes. Because HbA1c is used more commonly to diagnose diabetes in individuals with risk factors, it will also identify those at a higher risk for developing diabetes in the future. In 2009, the International Expert Committee reported that those with HbA1c levels above the laboratory "normal" range but below the diagnostic cut point for diabetes (6 to <6.5%) are at a very high risk of developing diabetes.

TABLE 21.3
Diagnostic Criteria for Prediabetes

Test	Diagnostic Threshold	Comments
Impaired fasting glucose (IFG)	100–125 mg/dL	WHO and other international organizations do not recognize this diagnostic threshold for prediabetes and use 110–125 mg/dL instead.
Impaired glucose tolerance (IGT)	140–199 mg/dL	
HbA1c	>6.0 and <6.5	Not a formal criterion. Not typically used to diagnose prediabetes.

Source: Reprinted with permission from American Diabetes Association – A position statement, *Diabetes Care*, 2015:38: S8–S16; World Health Organization, 312, 2015.

Studies show that the incidence of diabetes in people with HbA1c levels in this range is more than 10 times that of people with lower levels and may be up to 8 times higher than the incidence of diabetes found in the US population (Edelman et al. 2004) (Diabetes Care-Supplement 1, 2011).

21.7 TREATING DIABETES AND PREDIABETES

The four cornerstones of a comprehensive care plan for a person with diabetes, without regard to the type, include the following:

- Nutritional intervention
- Medication, when appropriate
- Self-monitoring of blood glucose (SMBG), when appropriate
- Physical activity

For purposes of this book, medical nutrition therapy (MNT) is the mode of nutritional intervention and is the focus of this chapter. MNT for prediabetes is very similar to MNT for diabetes. There is more focus on weight management in the care plan for prediabetes. Not all insurance plans provide MNT benefits for prediabetes.

Developing an intervention plan for diabetes and prediabetes heavily relies on the data collected for and during the assessment. Of particular importance is the data collected from the referral source, usually a primary care physician. This information may be best divided into two categories that can be helpful in organizing the intervention. One is lab values that can provide a snapshot of the patient at the time of diagnosis or referral and the second is treatment goals. An example follows:

- Lab-based data
- HbA1c at the time of referral
- FPG at the time of referral
- Kidney function values
- Glycemic treatment goals
- HbA1c target
- Fasting SMBG target, when appropriate
- Postprandial target

Treatment goals may vary from referral source to referral source and while these targets do need to be individualized, there exists marked differences in targets promoted by major diabetes institutions. Table 21.4 compares the treatment goals set forth by the American Diabetes Association (ADA), the International Diabetes Federation (IDF), and the American College of Endocrinologists (ACE). All three of these targets are used and can cause quite a bit of confusion among persons with diabetes.

TABLE 21.4

Comparison of Glycemic Targets for Persons with Diabetes

Test	ADA	IDF	ACE
HbA1c – satisfactory control	7%	6.5%	6.5%
Fasting glucose – SMBG	70–130 mg/dL	<100 mg/dL	<110 mg/dL
2-hour postprandial – SMBG	<180 mg/dL	<140 mg/dL	<140 mg/dL

Source: Reprinted with permission from American Diabetes Association – A position statement, *Diabetes Care*, 2015:38: S8–S16; aace.com and idf.org accessed March 2015.
IDF: International Diabetes Federation, 2019.

It's important for clinicians to appreciate the differences in these targets. The <180 mg/dL target held by the ADA for postprandial blood glucose corresponds to the upper limit that was chosen in patients who were allocated to the intensively treated group of the Diabetes Control and Complications Trial (DCCT). The lower value held by the International Diabetes Federation (IDF) and the American College of Endocrinology (ACE) was mainly based on the fact that 140 mg/dL is the highest value for defining the impaired glucose tolerance as a part of the oral glucose tolerance test (Monnier 2009).

A patient's treatment targets are most often set by the patient in conjunction with their primary care provider. The RD's role in target achievement is twofold.

1. To deliver medical nutrition therapy that helps the patient to meet those goals within the framework of medication and/or lifestyle changes set forth by the primary care provider
2. To communicate to the primary care provider information related to nutritional changes that directly impact a patient's success or failure to reach targets

21.8 NUTRITION ASSESSMENT FOR DIABETES MELLITUS

Nutrition assessment is a crucial first step in diabetes MNT. The assessment forms the basis for developing the intervention plan and identifying potential areas of change to a client's lifestyle and habits that will help the patient to meet their goals. The main purpose of an assessment is to gather information needed to assist in the development of individual nutrition goals and establish an appropriate nutrition intervention.

21.8.1 Preliminary Data

Before a comprehensive nutrition assessment can be performed on a patient, preliminary data must be collected. Some of these data can be obtained from the referral source but it is likely that not all of the data will be available. At a minimum, the dietitian will need the following from the referral source:

- Documented diagnosis of diabetes or prediabetes, the type and date of diagnosis, or reported duration
- The type of medication and dose if applicable
- Labs that support the diagnosis(es), HbA1c and FBG
- Labs/data that support related conditions such as kidney function or hypertension

Collecting the rest of the data then becomes a part of the assessment process with this patient. Further data needed for a complete assessment include but are not limited to the points detailed in Table 21.5 (Monk et al., 1995).

The information in each of these components is used by the dietitian to formulate an appropriate care plan that includes achievable goals and interventions that are appropriate to the outpatient or home-setting patient. After an initial consultation, regular assessment is ongoing, and is continuously modified and updated throughout the diabetes MNT process. Follow-ups are needed for several reasons.

- Collecting the necessary data before the initial consultation or even during the initial consultation with a patient, which can be difficult, making appropriate follow-ups needed to formulate a comprehensive care plan
- Monitoring of the care plan so that a patient is on track to meet the goals developed with the primary care provider
- Making modifications to the care plan as needed based on goal achievement metrics and input from the patient

The chart in Figure 21.1 is one guide for delivering MNT to persons with diabetes. Many variations are possible and should be guided by the needs of the patients, the dietitian's time, the goals of the physician, and resources at hand. While these steps originally addressed the assessment, intervention, and monitoring patients with type 2 diabetes, it is also valid and can be used with patients who have other types of diabetes and even prediabetes. Intervention and monitoring are further discussed in Figure 21.1.

21.9 NUTRITIONAL INTERVENTION FOR DIABETES

While pharmacotherapy, physical activity, and blood glucose monitoring are all components of a comprehensive care plan for diabetes, the nutritional component occupies a large portion of its overall education and nutritional management. Many patients struggle mightily with the nutritional aspect of treating diabetes (Evert et al. 2014). The ADA published a position paper that states that persons with diabetes should be referred to a registered dietitian (RD) for medical nutrition therapy or a

TABLE 21.5
Initial Nutrition Assessment

Data Needed	Metric
Clinical	Anthropometrics
	Energy needs (estimated or measured)
	Weight and weight history
	Lab values
	Treatment goals
Nutritional history	Usual intake, 24-hour recall
	Feeding habits
	Use of vitamins, minerals, and supplements
	Assessment of a disordered eating
	Previous nutrition intervention
Physical activity history	Type, frequency, physical limitations, and willingness to become more active
	Monitoring SMBG knowledge and skills
	Glucose levels and ranges
	Food intake journals and physical activity journals
	Benefits of monitoring
Psychosocial	Living situation
	Ethnic or religious beliefs
	Family and social support
	Level of stress
	Readiness for change
	Patient expectations for treatment
Economic	Education level
	Ability to purchase food and medicine
Knowledge	Understanding of the current disease state
	Survival skills
	Patient's self-management needs

Source: Adapted from *Practice Guidelines for Medical Nutrition Therapy Provided by Dietitians for Persons with Non- Insulin-Dependent Diabetes Mellitus*; Monk A. et al., *J Am Diet Assoc.*, 1995:95:999–1006.

diabetes self-management education program for nutrition counseling. The position puts forth the following goals of nutrition therapy for adults with diabetes who are non-gestational:

- To individualize nutrition needs based on personal and cultural preferences, literacy level, available resources, and willingness to make changes
- To provide practical tools for daily meal planning

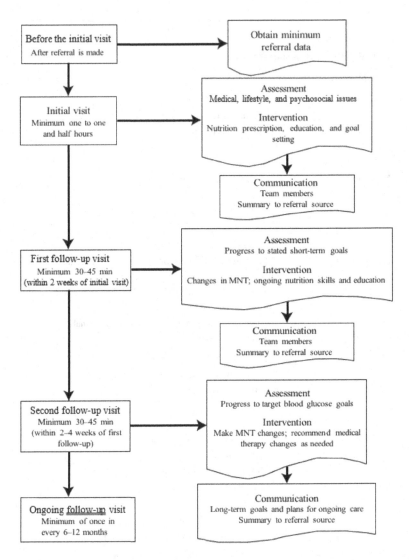

FIGURE 21.1   Flow of events in the assessment and care plan development for persons with diabetes mellitus.

Source: Adapted from Monk A et al., *J Am Diet Assoc*, 1995:95:999–1006.

- To provide positive, evidence-based information about food and the effects of foods on glycemic control (Kubota et al., 2020)
- To promote healthful eating habits that emphasize the appropriate portion size and variety so as to support
- The prescribed HbA1c target
- Blood pressure goal of 120/80

- LDL cholesterol <100 mg/dL
- Triglycerides <150 mg/dL
- HDL cholesterol >50 mg/dL for women and 40 mg/dL for men
- Body weight goal
- The prevention or delay of the complications of diabetes (Evert et al. 2014)

The Academy of Nutrition and Dietetics recommends that these goals be met in the following way:

- A series of three to four encounters with an RD lasting 45–90 min.
- The series of encounters should begin at diagnosis of diabetes or at first referral to an RD for MNT for diabetes and should be completed within 3–6 months.
- The RD should determine whether additional MNT encounters are needed.
- At least one follow-up encounter is recommended annually to reinforce life-style changes and to evaluate and monitor outcomes that indicate the need for changes in MNT or medication(s); the RD should determine whether additional MNT encounters are needed (Evert et al. 2014).

The RD needs to keep in mind that additional units of MNT can be requested and prescribed when an element of the care plan changes. For this reason, it is paramount for the patient that the RD has regular communication with the patient's primary care provider. For example, if the patient moves from an 1800-calorie meal plan to a 1500-calorie meal plan, the RD can request that the primary care provider authorizes more units of MNT so that the change can be implemented and monitored by the RD.

The following are specific, evidence-based recommendations set forth in the position statement published by the American Diabetes Association that address strategies regarding key nutrients, micronutrients, and medication and food interactions that support the goals of nutrition therapy for diabetes. These recommendations can be used as a basis for nutritional counseling during the suggested structure for MNT encounters:

- Portion control should be recommended for weight loss and maintenance.
- Carbohydrate-containing foods and beverages and endogenous insulin production are the greatest determinants of the post-meal blood glucose level; therefore, it is important to know which foods contain carbohydrates: starchy vegetables, whole grains, fruit, milk and milk products, vegetables, and sugar.
- When choosing carbohydrate-containing foods, choose nutrient-dense, high-fiber foods whenever possible instead of processed foods with added sodium, fat, and sugars.

Nutrient-dense foods and beverages provide vitamins, minerals, and other healthful substances with relatively few calories. Calories have not been added to them from solid fats, sugars, or refined starches.

- For most people, it is not necessary to subtract the amount of dietary fiber or sugar alcohols from total carbohydrates when counting the carbohydrates.
- Substitute foods higher in unsaturated fat (liquid oils) for foods higher in trans- or saturated fat.
- Select leaner protein sources and meat alternatives.
- Vitamin and mineral supplements, herbal products, or cinnamon to manage diabetes are not recommended due to lack of evidence.
- Moderate alcohol consumption (one drink/day or less for adult women and two drinks or less for adult men) has minimal acute or long-term effects on blood glucose in people with diabetes. To reduce the risk of hypoglycemia for individuals using insulin or insulin secretagogues, alcohol should be consumed with food.
- Limit sodium intake to 2300 mg/day or 1500 mg/day, depending on the patient's risks for stroke.
- Priority should be given to coordinating food with the type of diabetes medications.
- For individuals who take insulin secretagogues, a moderate amount of carbohydrate at each meal and snack is recommended.
- To reduce the risk of hypoglycemia:
  - Eat a source of carbohydrates at meals.
  - Moderate amounts of carbohydrates at each meal and snack.
  - Do not skip meals.
  - Physical activity may result in low blood glucose depending on when it is performed. Always carry a source of carbohydrates to reduce the risk of hypoglycemia.
- For individuals who take biguanides (metformin):
  - Gradually titrate to minimize gastrointestinal side effects when initiating the use.
  - Take medication with food 15 min after a meal if symptoms persist.
  - If side effects do not resolve over time (a few weeks), follow-up with a healthcare provider.
  - If taking along with an insulin secretagogue or insulin, may experience hypoglycemia.
- For individuals who take a-glucosidase inhibitors:
  - Gradually titrate to minimize gastrointestinal side effects when initiating use.
  - Take at the beginning of a meal to have maximal effect.
  - If taking along with an insulin secretagogue or insulin, may experience hypoglycemia.
  - If hypoglycemia occurs, eat something containing monosaccharides such as glucose tablets and drugs that will prevent the digestion of polysaccharides.
- For individuals who take incretin mimetics (GLP-1):
  - Gradually titrate to minimize gastrointestinal side effects when initiating use.
  - Injection of daily or twice-daily GLP-1s should be taken pre-meal.
  - If side effects do not resolve over time (a few weeks), follow up with a healthcare provider.

- If taking along with an insulin secretagogue or insulin, may experience hypoglycemia.
- Once-weekly GLP-1s can be taken at any time during the day regardless of meal times.

21.9.1 NUTRITION AND INSULIN

For individuals with type 1 diabetes and insulin-requiring type 2 diabetes:
- Learn how to count carbohydrates or use another meal-planning approach to quantify carbohydrate intake.
- The objective of using such a meal-planning approach is to "match" mealtime insulin to the carbohydrates consumed.

If on a multiple-daily injection plan or on an insulin pump:
- Take mealtime insulin before eating as directed. Some insulins act faster and last longer than others.
- Meals can be consumed at different times.
- If physical activity is performed within 1–2 hours of mealtime insulin injection, this dose may need to be lowered to reduce the risk of hypoglycemia.

If on a premixed insulin plan:
- Insulin doses need to be taken at consistent times every day.
- Meals need to be consumed at similar times every day.
- To reduce the risk of hypoglycemia, do not skip meals.
- Physical activity may result in low blood glucose depending on when it is performed. Always carry a source of quick-acting carbohydrates to reduce the risk of hypoglycemia. See how to treat hypoglycemia in Section 21.10 "Complications of Diabetes."

If on a fixed insulin plan, eat similar amounts of carbohydrates each day to match the set doses of insulin (Evert et al. 2014).

21.10 COMPLICATIONS OF DIABETES

The complications of diabetes can be categorized into two broad categories. The first category includes those that result from long-term or chronic hyperglycemia and the second category includes those that present themselves from sudden or extreme shifts in blood sugar, resulting in acute hypo- or hyperglycemia that can require medical attention.

Chronic complications that result from longer-term high blood sugar can be divided into two major categories. The first category includes complications due to damage to the major arterial vessels and the second category includes complications due to damage to the small blood vessels.

- Large-vessel damage
- Diabetic neuropathies
- Heart disease
- Small-vessel damage
- Kidney disease and kidney failure

- Retinopathy resulting in blindness
- Reproductive system dysfunction

Acute complications can include both hypoglycemia and hyperglycemia. While technically both of these can occur with any type of diabetes, acute hypoglycemia more often occurs in patients with type 1 diabetes. Care plans should include education for treatment of this condition. The typical treatment plan that is easy for the outpatient or home care dietitian to use is the rule of 15. This strategy can be found in several books about diabetes, including Dr. Alan Rubin's book, *Diabetes for Dummies*.

Diabetes ketoacidosis (DKA) and hyperglycemic hyperosmolar syndrome (HHS) are two acute, hyperglycemic conditions that can occur when blood glucose is extremely high. The most common factors that can lead to DKA or HHS are infection, inadequate insulin therapy, discontinuation of insulin therapy and other medications, pancreatitis, heart attack, stroke, and some medications. Assessing the risk of these conditions by assessing medication compliance can be included as a part of the dietitian's initial or follow-up consultation that may help in avoiding these hyperglycemic states.

- Diabetic ketoacidosis (DKA) results from a shortage of insulin and more commonly occurs in individuals with type 1 diabetes. Blood glucose of 250 or greater is a cause for concern because the production of ketones can accelerate quickly. The outpatient and home-setting dietitian should refer the type 1 patient to their primary care because DKA can have a quick onset and can be dangerous.
- The hyperosmolar hyperglycemic syndrome or state predominantly occurs in individuals with type 2 diabetes. Very high blood sugars cause severe dehydration. It is similar to DKA but without the presence of ketones. According to Ketabchi et al., a patient with a blood sugar of 600 mg/dL or greater requires medical attention; however, practically speaking, a type 2 patient with blood sugars of over 250 can also be at risk and should be monitored.

In addition to hyperglycemia causing damage to blood vessels and thereby complications, glucose variability also plays a role in the development of complications from diabetes (Smith-Palmer et al., 2014). In a systematic review of the literature that looked at glucose variability as an independent contributor to the development of diabetes complications, the following were found:

- In persons with type 2 diabetes, a positive association was consistent between increased variability and microvascular, or small-vessel complications, but not with large-vessel complications.
- In persons with type 1 diabetes, it appears that increased glucose variability plays a minimal role in both the large- and small-vessel complications (Smith-Palmer et al. 2014).

These associations found in 28 studies may be the basis for a case for using continuous glucose monitoring (CGM) in patients with type 2 diabetes. Historically, it is a practice largely confined to the monitoring of type 1 diabetes. Today, outpatient and home-setting dietitians can avail themselves of training, use, and in many cases, reimbursement for placing these monitors, even if just for short-term data gathering, on patients with type 2 diabetes. Medtronic is one provider of 3-day disposable monitors.

The life-impairing chronic complications due to diabetes are the reason that control of blood glucose is so important and why MNT care plans that treat to goal are critical. These complications can be minimized, delayed, and in some cases averted in persons with diabetes and prediabetes when nutrition therapy is integrated into the overall care plan of medication with appropriate physical activity and blood glucose monitoring.

21.11 CONCLUSION

Medical nutrition therapy in the outpatient and home care setting can offer a structured, regular intervention that can improve the outcomes and quality of life in patients with diabetes, regardless of the type. From gathering preliminary data, through the nutritional assessment and follow-up consultations, MNT must be in the context of a comprehensive plan of care that includes the goals of the primary care provider and the cultural and social aspects of the patient. MNT must be deliberate, must follow the guidelines of the best practices, and must measure and monitor the markers of progress.

21.12 HELPFUL RESOURCES FOR PROFESSIONALS

- National Diabetes Information Clearinghouse (NDIC): www.diabetes. niddk.nih.gov
- American Diabetes Association (ADA): www.diabetes.org
- Academy of Nutrition and Dietetics (AND): www.eatright.org
- International Diabetes Federation (IDF): www.idf.org/guidelines
- Weight-Control Information Network (WIN): www.win.niddk.nih.gov
- Centers for Disease Control National Diabetes Education Program (CdC-NDEP): www.cdc.gov/diabetes/ndep/index.htm www.diabetesatlas.org/upload/resources/material/20200302_133351_IDFATLAS9e-final-web.pdf

REFERENCES

American Diabetes Association. Diagnosis and classification of diabetes mellitus. Diabetes Care, 2009:32 (Suppl 1):S62–S67.
American Diabetes Association. Diagnosis and Classification of Diabetes Mellitus. Diabetes Care 1 January 2014; 37 (Suppl 1):S81–S90. https://doi.org/10.2337/dc14-S081.

American Diabetes Association. The Economic Costs of Diabetes in the US in 2017. Diabetes Care 1 May 2018; 41 (5): 917–928. https://doi.org/10.2337/dci18-0007.

American Diabetes Association. Classification and diagnosis of diabetes – A position statement. Diabetes Care, 2015:38 (Suppl 1):S8–S16.

Bonora E, Tuomilehto J. Pros and cons of diagnosing diabetes with A1c. Diabetes Care, 2011:34 (Suppl 2):S184–90.

Centers for Disease Control and Prevention. National Diabetes Statistics Report website. https://www.cdc.gov/diabetes/data/statistics-report/index.html. Accessed April 2022.

Chang A, Frank J, Knaebel J. et al. Evaluation of an over-the-counter glycated hemoglobin (A1c) test kit. Journal of Diabetes Science and Technology. 2010:4(6):1495–1503.

Edelman D, Olsen MK, Dudley TK, Harris AC, Oddone EZ. Utility of hemoglobin A1c in predicting diabetes risk. Journal of General Internal Medicine, 2004:19:1175–1180.

Evert AB, Boucher JL, Cypress M. et al. Nutrition therapy recommendations for the management of adults with diabetes. Diabetes Care, 2014:37(Suppl 1):S120–S143.

Franz MJ, Powers MA, Leontos C, Holzmeister LA, Kulkami K, Monk A, Wedel N, Gradwell E. The evidence for medical nutrition therapy for type 1 and type 2 diabetes in adults. Journal of the American Dietetic Association, 2010:110(12):1852–89.

International Diabetes Federation. IDF ᴰiabetes Atlas, 9th edn. Brussels, Belgium: International Diabetes Federation, 2019.

Kubota, Sodai et al. A review of recent findings on meal sequence: An attractive dietary approach to prevention and management of type 2 diabetes. Nutrients, 2020, Aug 19:12(9):2502. doi:10.3390/nu12092502

Monk A, Barry B, McClain K, Weaver T, Cooper N, Franz MJ. Practice guidelines for medical nutrition therapy provided by dietitians for persons with noninsulin-dependent diabetes mellitus. Journal of the American Dietetic Association, 1995:95:999–1006.

Monnier L, Claude C. Target for glycemic control: Concentrating on glucose. Diabetes Care, 2009:32 (Suppl 2):S199–S204. doi:10.2337/dc09-S310

Smith-Palmer J, Brandle M, Trevisan R. et al. Assessment of the association between glycemic variability and diabetes-related complications in type 1 and type 2 diabetes. Diabetes Research and Clinical Practice 2014:105(3):274–284.

World Health Organization. Diabetes fact sheet. 312:2015. Accessed November 21, 2015.

22 Weight Management

Lauren Lemieux and Zhaoping Li

22.1 INTRODUCTION

Clinicians play an important role in helping patients achieve clinically significant weight loss through nutrition and lifestyle counseling, and studies suggest that many patients do, in fact, want to talk to their doctor about making these changes (1). For a patient who is ready to discuss weight loss, it is helpful to learn about a prior history of weight loss or gain, dietary habits, physical activity level, family history of obesity, use of medications associated with weight gain, and barriers to losing weight (2). Furthermore, based on history and physical examination, one can screen for endocrinological disorders that can lead to weight gain such as Cushing's syndrome, polycystic ovarian syndrome, and hypothyroidism.

22.2 PERSONALIZED LIFESTYLE INTERVENTIONS FOR WEIGHT LOSS

Dietary, physical activity, and behavioral changes should be personalized to each patient, and motivational interviewing can provide a framework for eliciting patient input to develop a collaborative plan for weight loss (Table 22.1, Figure 22.1) (3). It is important to set goals based on behaviors/lifestyle that will lead to weight loss. For example, rather than just setting a goal of losing 15 lb., the patient might also plan to stop eating fast food for lunch at work and bring leftovers from dinner instead. A meta-analysis of 11 randomized controlled trials also demonstrated that motivational interviewing led to an additional mean weight loss of 1.5 kg (3). Table 22.1 shows the Ask-Tell-Ask, a motivational interviewing technique that allows the provider to provide information in a way that protects patient autonomy.

TABLE 22.1

Ask-Tell-Ask Motivational Interviewing Technique

Ask	• "What do you already know about . . ."
	• "Would it be all right if I shared some suggestions for . . ."
Tell	• Make 1–2 points that are simple and brief.
Ask	• "What do you think of what I said?"

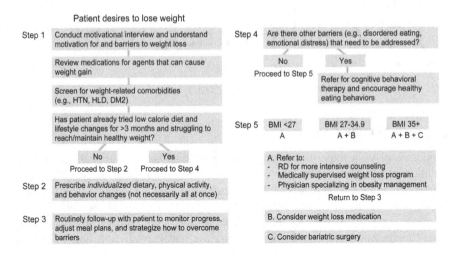

FIGURE 22.1   An approach to the patient who desires weight loss.

22.3   DIETARY APPROACHES TO WEIGHT LOSS

Studies have consistently shown that there is no perfect diet for weight loss (2, 4–6). Ultimately, successful weight loss through dietary changes involves those that a patient is able to follow long term and create a reduction in caloric intake. It is estimated that 1 lb. of fat contains 3,500 calories, so reduction in daily caloric intake by 500 calories less than what is needed to maintain weight can achieve a weight loss of 1 lb/week. Low-calorie diets typically range from 1,200–1,500 calories/day for women and 1,500–1,800 calories/day for men with adjustment based on weight and activity levels (2). Depending on the patient's current diet, it may be possible to promote weight loss by simply excluding or restricting certain food groups (e.g., fast food, processed foods, refined carbohydrates), which ultimately reduces caloric intake (2).

22.4   MACRONUTRIENT DISTRIBUTION

When it comes to *what* one should eat, there are many available diets (see Chapter 24). Some vary based on macronutrient composition, such as the ketogenic diet with ~75% of calories from fat on one end of the spectrum to a very low-fat vegan diet with 10% of calories from fat on the other. Others recommend avoiding specific foods like legumes or gluten-containing products. Another area of interest is the use of higher-protein diets for weight loss. In our practice, one strategy we may implement is recommending daily protein goals based on lean body mass (7). Ultimately, studies have not shown one distribution of macronutrients to be more effective than another for weight loss long term (4, 8, 9), and there is no consensus on the best diet for weight loss (2). Furthermore, patients often struggle to sustain overly restrictive dietary patterns. A first step might be to understand the individual's usual dietary habits and identify particular macronutrients that may be over-consumed.

22.5   QUALITY IMPROVEMENT

One approach to weight loss is to start by improving the quality of the patient's diet by reducing processed and packaged foods. A small study compared individuals fed an ultra-processed diet (e.g., processed meats, foods made with white flour and white sugar) with those fed an unprocessed diet (e.g., fish, poultry, meat, vegetables, fruits, whole grains). Although both groups received meals equivalent in calories, energy density, macronutrients, sugar, and fiber, when fed an ultra-processed diet, people consumed 500 calories more per day and gained 1 lb. over the two-week period, while those on the unprocessed diet lost 1 lb. (10).

In place of processed foods, patients should be encouraged to focus more on non-starchy vegetables and lean protein sources (e.g., white meat chicken/turkey, fish, tofu/soy, egg whites, nonfat dairy), replacing processed and refined carbohydrates with controlled portions of starchy vegetables (e.g., peas, corn, potatoes, squash), beans, whole grains, and fruits (Figure 22.2).

Dietary fats from mono- and polyunsaturated fatty acids (e.g., nuts, seeds, avocado, olives, olive oil, avocado oil, canola oil, salmon) should be encouraged in place of saturated fats (e.g., red meat, whole-fat dairy, coconut oil, palm kernel oil) and trans fats (e.g., partially hydrogenated oils), keeping in mind that fats are calorically dense (9 calories/g compared with 4 calories/g for carbohydrates or protein). Protein is also the most satiating macronutrient and nonstarchy vegetables are low in calories and high in fiber (11).

22.6   USE OF MEAL REPLACEMENTS

Meal replacements are typically high-protein, low-calorie foods (e.g., shakes) that can be used to provide adequate nutrients while controlling calories. They have been shown to be an effective tool for weight loss and weight loss maintenance by various studies including the Look AHEAD study (12–15).

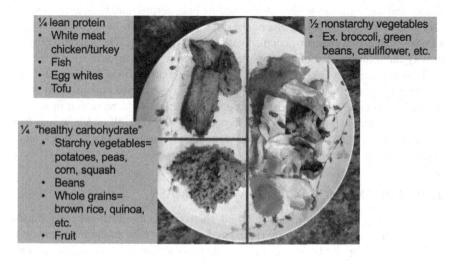

FIGURE 22.2   Healthy meal example.

Medically supervised very low-calorie diets (VLCDs), typically <800 calories/day, are a more intensive dietary regimen for weight loss compared with low-calorie diets and also utilize meal replacements. After 11–14 weeks, total weight loss has been reported to range between 14.2–21 kg (14). However, without sustained lifestyle changes after cessation of the VLCD, weight regain will occur (2, 14). Compared with low-calorie diets, long-term VLCDs were found to have greater overall and long-term weight loss (16).

22.7   SETTING REALISTIC GOALS

It is also important to discuss realistic and achievable goals with patients. With even as little as 3–5% sustained weight loss, patients may experience clinically significant reductions in blood glucose, hemoglobin A1c, triglycerides, and risk of developing type 2 diabetes. Weight loss of 5–10% can further improve the aforementioned parameters as well as blood pressure and low-density lipoprotein (LDL) and high-density lipoprotein (HDL) cholesterol levels (2, 17, 18). For nonalcoholic fatty liver disease, a target of 7–10% weight loss is recommended, since it is associated with a reduction in liver fat and fibrosis as well as remission of steatohepatitis (19). Often patients have much higher expectations for what they consider acceptable weight loss. A survey of patients prior to starting a weight loss program found that for them an acceptable weight corresponded to losing 25% of their starting body weight loss, while a disappointing weight loss was 17% (20). Another survey found that physician expectations were similarly inflated, such that an acceptable weight loss would be approximately 22%, while a disappointing weight loss was 11% (21).

22.8   EXERCISE AND HYPOCALORIC DIET

A sedentary lifestyle is one of the major contributing factors to weight gain and the obesity epidemic. Regular physical activity has been shown to improve insulin sensitivity and some studies suggest that including both aerobic and resistance exercises may be better than just doing one or the other (22). However, for significant weight loss, physical activity must be coupled with caloric restriction. The standard physical activity recommendation of 150 minutes of moderate intensity activity per week is likely to result in only 2 kg of weight loss over a 4-month period (23). A meta-analysis comparing the effect of hypocaloric diet and exercise on visceral adiposity found that in the absence of weight loss, exercise resulted in a 6.1% reduction in visceral adiposity compared with 1.1% with a hypocaloric diet (24). With 5% weight loss, hypocaloric diet plus exercise was found to reduce visceral adiposity by 21.3% versus 13.4% in the absence of exercise (24).

22.9   IMPORTANCE OF LEAN MUSCLE MASS

Depending on how weight loss is achieved, there can be a reduction in lean muscle mass. Resting energy expenditure (REE) makes up over 60% of the total amount of calories burned by the body and lean muscle mass accounts for the majority of the REE (25). Both increased protein intake and resistance exercise are recommended to prevent the loss of lean muscle mass that would otherwise accompany weight loss (11). A systematic review found that high-protein diets were more effective than lower-protein diets in preserving REE during weight loss (26). Aging is also associated with a loss of lean muscle mass, which may account for why some patients struggle to lose weight as they get older despite using methods that were previously effective. A study of 100 overweight and obese older adults (ages 55–80 years) found that a combination of a high-protein diet (1.3 g/kg) and resistance exercises (3 times/week) resulted in an increase in fat-free mass, while resistance training combined with a standard protein diet (0.8 g/kg) or a high-protein diet alone without resistance training resulted in only maintenance of lean muscle mass (27).

22.10 TYPES OF EXERCISE

High-intensity interval training (HIIT) involves brief (e.g., 30 seconds) periods of intense activity followed by a longer rest period and is typically performed over a shorter period of time compared with traditional continuous exercise. A systematic review found that HIIT can promote similar changes in terms of reduction in body fat (–2 kg) and waist circumference (–3 cm) compared with moderate-intensity continuous exercise with the added benefit that it requires 40% less time (28). When it comes to long-term weight loss maintenance, there is evidence to support regular physical activity, ideally 1 hour/day or more (29).

22.11 BEHAVIORAL STRATEGIES

Behavior changes can take various forms, including self-monitoring, stimulus control, problem solving, and contingency planning (30). Self-monitoring may involve tracking food intake, physical activity, weights, and/or behavior changes, and studies show that more frequent and more complete monitoring leads to more weight loss (31, 32). Stimulus control involves strategizing with the patient for how to anticipate and prevent overeating or eating something that is not consistent with their goals for weight loss. For example, keeping "junk" food out of the house or making the healthier options (fruits and vegetables) more visible by placing them on the kitchen counter or eye level in the refrigerator. It is also important to discuss with the patient potential obstacles they anticipate which allows for individualization of recommendations.

22.12 PHARMACOTHERAPY

Medications may be considered for patients who have participated in a high-intensity comprehensive lifestyle intervention but have been unable to achieve or sustain clinically significant weight loss. These are approved for weight loss in patients with a body mass index (BMI) ≥ 30 kg/m^2 or BMI ≥ 27 kg/m^2 with at least one obesity-related comorbidity (e.g., hypertension, diabetes, obstructive sleep apnea) in conjunction with a comprehensive lifestyle intervention (2, 33). At the time of this publication, some of the FDA-approved medications for weight loss include phentermine, phentermine/topiramate, naltrexone/bupropion, liraglutide, semaglutide, orlistat, and Gelesis100 (18, 33–35).

Weight loss medications are recommended for long-term use due to the physiologic propensity to regain weight (33). It is important when starting these medications that the patient understands that weight is typically regained if the medication is stopped. Often patients have much higher expectations for the amount of weight they will lose with a medication than what is actually seen. Based on the available published literature, in combination with a low-calorie diet and physical activity, most weight loss medications lead to approximately 5–10% total body weight loss (TBWL) on average (18–34, 36). However, semaglutide 2.4 mg demonstrated on average closer to 15% TBWL on average after 1 year making it the most effective FDA-approved medication for weight loss at the time of this publication (35). There are other medications currently being studied such as tirzepatide which are showing to be even more effective (~20% TBWL) but at this time are not FDA approved for weight loss (37). It is also recommended that if a patient has not lost at least 5% of their starting weight after 12 weeks on the medication to consider discontinuation of the medication (2, 33).

22.13   DIETARY SUPPLEMENTS

There are various over-the-counter weight loss supplements, such as *Ma huang* (*Ephedra sinica*), white bean extract, bitter orange, guar gum, raspberry ketones, chitosan, *Garcinia cambogia*, and green coffee. However, several have been associated with serious and life-threatening adverse events including arrhythmias, myocardial infarction, stroke, seizures, and liver failure (38–40). Supplements are not required to have proof of their safety or efficacy before they are on the market, since they are categorized as foods (41). Additionally, cost can be quite high, and there is the potential for drug-drug interactions. Therefore, at this time there are no over-the-counter weight loss supplements recommended for weight loss (38–40).

Caffeine has been studied in terms of its effect on thermogenesis and potential for inducing weight loss (42). A meta-analysis found that in small studies coffee intake prior to a meal reduced ad libitum intake and appetite. For appetite reduction, this was primarily seen in studies with larger volume of coffee ingestion and higher caffeine doses (43). Another meta-analysis found that subjects drinking green tea lost 1.3 kg more weight on average (44). While coffee and other caffeinated beverages may have potential benefits for weight loss, it is important to also consider what is being consumed in addition to these beverages, such as creamers, added sugars, or pastries not to mention potential adverse side effects such as increased anxiety, palpitations, and insomnia.

22.14   BARIATRIC SURGERY

Patients who have been unable to achieve or sustain clinically significant weight loss through a high-intensity comprehensive lifestyle intervention (with or without pharmacotherapy) may be considered for bariatric surgery if their BMI is ≥40 or ≥35 with at least one obesity-related comorbidity (2). Note that in 2022 the American Society for Metabolic and Bariatric Surgery (ASMBS) and International Federation for the Surgery of Obesity and Metabolic Disorders (IFSO) updated their recommendations to lower the BMI cutoffs to 35 and 30, respectively (45). Surgical options include vertical sleeve gastrectomy (VSG), adjustable gastric band (AGB), Roux-en-Y gastric bypass (RYGB), and biliopancreatic diversion with duodenal switch (BPD-DS) (46–48). VSG and AGB promote weight loss through volume restriction, while the RYGB and BPD-DS also involve malabsorption. A systematic review evaluating weight loss 10 or more years after bariatric surgery reported a mean excess body weight loss of 55.4% for RYGB and 45.9% for AGB (49). Over the years, AGB has become less commonly performed, since long-term data show that it is less effective for weight loss or obesity-related conditions (e.g., hypertension, hyperlipidemia) compared with RYGB (50). While bariatric surgery is currently considered the most effective treatment for weight loss, it involves risk (51). Furthermore, there are patients who, despite undergoing surgery, fail to lose weight; this is partly attributable to failure to maintain recommended lifestyle changes (52).

22.15 NOVEL APPROACHES

22.15.1 ENDOLUMINAL PROCEDURES

Endoscopic endoluminal procedures are an emerging area of obesity treatment that are a less-invasive alternative to bariatric surgery (53), but many of these procedures are still under investigation. These involve gastric aspiration, space-occupying procedures, and gastric reduction procedures (54–56). Gastric aspiration involves aspirating recently ingested food via a gastrostomy tube (54, 56). Intragastric ballooning, a space occupying procedure, involves endoscopic placement of a balloon filled with methylene blue or saline (53). The intragastric balloon is temporary and must be removed after 6 months; therefore, it is typically seen as a bridge to bariatric surgery (53). Finally, gastric reduction procedures, such as endoluminal suturing or plication of the stomach, are another area of active investigation, but results thus far have been mixed (54–56). For patients who have regained weight after RYGB, the purse-string transoral outlet reduction (TORe) has been shown to help promote additional weight loss and improve blood pressure and hemoglobin A1c (57).

22.15.2 MICROBIOME

Microbial dysbiosis has been implicated in the pathogenesis of obesity (58). Prenatal exposure to antibiotics and cesarean section delivery have been associated with an increased risk for childhood obesity (59). Much of our knowledge of the gut microbiome's role in obesity is based on studies involving germ-free mice. Transplantation of gut microbiota from obese mice or humans into germ-free mice leads to increased weight gain and adiposity compared with lean donors despite consuming the same diet (60–61). However, at this time there are no large, randomized control trials of probiotic or prebiotic supplements for weight loss.

22.16 INCORRECT/OUTDATED PRACTICES

A commonly held but outdated belief is that there is one specific diet that will help everyone lose weight. There is substantial variability in weight loss with different dietary patterns, from low fat to low carbohydrate to intermittent fasting, and different patterns may work better at one point in an individual's life but not later on. Studies have instead shown that the overall dietary adherence rates are the most important dietary factor leading to weight loss (2) and greater cardiovascular disease risk reduction (62, 63). Personalized nutrition, which focuses on the individual rather than groups of people, is emerging as an important tool to help our patients succeed because it aims to evaluate and incorporate one's DNA, microbiome, and metabolic response to specific foods or dietary patterns together with psychosocial environment to determine the most effective eating plan for weight management and disease prevention. Research has shown that an individual's microbiome, mood, sleep pattern, and time of meals can play a role in variations in metabolic response (64).

Many patients and providers alike believe that inability to lose weight reflects lack of motivation or willpower, which also contributes to weight stigma. The concept of calories in and calories out has been the focus of weight loss interventions and, for many healthcare providers, continues to be the primary treatment recommendation (65). Factors out of one's control, such as hormones that lead to changes in food intake and energy expenditure, can play a significant role in difficulty losing weight and weight regain. After weight loss, hormonal changes that work to restore weight can persist even up to a year after the initial weight loss (66). It is important for healthcare providers to be aware of the various barriers to weight loss. Simply assuming that failure to adhere to lifestyle recommendations is the only cause will negatively impact patient care (67).

PRACTICE PEARLS

- Successful weight loss involves a combination of dietary, physical activity, and behavioral interventions that are *personalized* to the individual patient.
- There is no one specific dietary pattern recommended for weight loss. Rather, the emphasis should be on one that promotes a caloric deficit during weight loss and a healthy pattern of eating that can be maintained long term.
- Physical activity is an important component of lifestyle changes but alone is very unlikely to result in significant weight loss.
- For patients unable to lose weight with lifestyle changes alone, additional options such as pharmacotherapy or bariatric surgery should be considered, understanding that there are various factors that contribute to weight gain outside lifestyle choices.

REFERENCES

1. Gans KM, Ross E, Barner CW, Wylie-Rosett J, McMurray J, Eaton C. REAP and WAVE: New tools to rapidly assess/discuss nutrition with patients. *J Nutr*. Feb 2003;133(2):556s–562s. doi:10.1093/jn/133.2.556S
2. Jensen MD, Ryan DH, Apovian CM, et al. 2013 AHA/ACC/TOS Guideline for the management of overweight and obesity in adults. *A Report of the American College*

of *Cardiology/American Heart Association Task Force on Practice Guidelines and The Obesity Society*. 2014;63(25 Part B):2985–3023. doi:10.1016/j.jacc.2013.11.004

3. Armstrong MJ, Mottershead TA, Ronksley PE, Sigal RJ, Campbell TS, Hemmelgarn BR. Motivational interviewing to improve weight loss in overweight and/or obese patients: A systematic review and meta-analysis of randomized controlled trials. *Obes Rev*. Sep 2011;12(9):709–723. doi:10.1111/j.1467-789X.2011.00892.x

4. Johnston BC, Kanters S, Bandayrel K, et al. Comparison of weight loss among named diet programs in overweight and obese adults: A meta-analysis. *JAMA*. 2014;312(9):923–933. doi:10.1001/jama.2014.10397

5. Shai I, Schwarzfuchs D, Henkin Y, et al. Weight loss with a low-carbohydrate, Mediterranean, or low-fat diet. *N Engl J Med*. 2008;359(3):229–241. doi:10.1056/NEJMoa0708681

6. Tobias DK, Chen M, Manson JE, Ludwig DS, Willett W, Hu FB. Effect of low-fat diet interventions versus other diet interventions on long-term weight change in adults: A systematic review and meta-analysis. *Lancet Diabetes Endocrinol*. Dec 2015;3(12):968–979. doi:10.1016/s2213-8587(15)00367-8

7. Li Z, Tseng CH, Li Q, Deng ML, Wang M, Heber D. Clinical efficacy of a medically supervised outpatient high-protein, low-calorie diet program is equivalent in prediabetic, diabetic and normoglycemic obese patients. *Nutr Diabetes*. Feb 10, 2014;4(2):e105. doi:10.1038/nutd.2014.1

8. Tobias DK, Chen M, Manson JE, Ludwig DS, Willett W, Hu FB. Effect of low-fat diet interventions versus other diet interventions on long-term weight change in adults: a systematic review and meta-analysis. *The Lancet Diabetes & Endocrinol*. 2015;3(12):968–979. doi:10.1016/S2213-8587(15)00367-8

9. Shai I, Schwarzfuchs D, Henkin Y, et al. Weight loss with a low-carbohydrate, Mediterranean, or low-fat diet. *N Engl J Med*. 2008;359(3):229–241. doi:10.1056/NEJMoa0708681

10. Hall KD, Ayuketah A, Brychta R, et al. Ultra-processed diets cause excess calorie intake and weight gain: An inpatient randomized controlled trial of ad libitum food intake. *Cell Metab*. Jul 2, 2019;30(1):226. doi:10.1016/j.cmet.2019.05.020

11. Leidy HJ, Clifton PM, Astrup A, et al. The role of protein in weight loss and maintenance. *Am. J. Clin. Nutr*. 2015;101(6):1320S–1329S. doi:10.3945/ajcn.114.084038

12. Heber D, Ashley JM, Wang HJ, Elashoff RM. Clinical evaluation of a minimal intervention meal replacement regimen for weight reduction. *J Am Coll Nutr*. Dec 1994;13(6):608–614. doi:10.1080/07315724.1994.10718456

13. Ashley JM, St Jeor ST, Perumean-Chaney S, Schrage J, Bovee V. Meal replacements in weight intervention. *Obes Res*. Nov 2001;9 Suppl 4:312s–320s. doi:10.1038/oby.2001.136

14. Johansson K, Neovius M, Hemmingsson E. Effects of anti-obesity drugs, diet, and exercise on weight-loss maintenance after a very-low-calorie diet or low-calorie diet: A systematic review and meta-analysis of randomized controlled trials. *Am J Clin Nutr*. Jan 2014;99(1):14–23. doi:10.3945/ajcn.113.070052

15. Look ARG. Eight-year weight losses with an intensive lifestyle intervention: The look AHEAD study. *Obesity (Silver Spring, Md)*. 2014;22(1):5–13. doi:10.1002/oby.20662

16. Anderson JW, Konz EC, Frederich RC, Wood CL. Long-term weight-loss maintenance: a meta-analysis of US studies. *Am. J. Clin. Nutr*. 2001;74(5):579–584. doi:10.1093/ajcn/74.5.579

17. Kushner RF, Ryan DH. Assessment and lifestyle management of patients with obesity: Clinical recommendations from systematic reviews. *JAMA*. Sep 3, 2014;312(9):943–952. doi:10.1001/jama.2014.10432

18. Ammori BJ, Skarulis MC, Soran H, Syed AA, Eledrisi M, Malik RA. Medical and surgical management of obesity and diabetes: what's new? *Diabet Med*. Dec 18, 2019. doi:10.1111/dme.14215

19. Marchesini G, Petta S, Dalle Grave R. Diet, weight loss, and liver health in nonalcoholic fatty liver disease: Pathophysiology, evidence, and practice. *Hepatology.* Jun 2016;63(6):2032–2043. doi:10.1002/hep.28392

20. Foster GD, Wadden TA, Vogt RA, Brewer G. What is a reasonable weight loss? Patients' expectations and evaluations of obesity treatment outcomes. *J Consult Clin Psychol.* 1997;65(1):79–85. doi:10.1037//0022-006x.65.1.79

21. Phelan S, Nallari M, Darroch FE, Wing RR. What do physicians recommend to their overweight and obese patients? *J Am Board Fam Med.* Mar–Apr 2009;22(2):115–122. doi:10.3122/jabfm.2009.02.080081

22. Bird SR, Hawley JA. Update on the effects of physical activity on insulin sensitivity in humans. *BMJ Open Sport Exerc Med.* 2016;2(1):e000143. doi:10.1136/bmjsem-2016-000143

23. Swift DL, Johannsen NM, Lavie CJ, Earnest CP, Church TS. The role of exercise and physical activity in weight loss and maintenance. *Prog Cardiovasc Dis.* Jan–Feb 2014;56(4):441–447. doi:10.1016/j.pcad.2013.09.012

24. Verheggen RJ, Maessen MF, Green DJ, Hermus AR, Hopman MT, Thijssen DH. A systematic review and meta-analysis on the effects of exercise training versus hypocaloric diet: Distinct effects on body weight and visceral adipose tissue. *Obes Rev.* Aug 2016;17(8):664–690. doi:10.1111/obr.12406

25. Ard JD. 17 – Obesity. In: Heimburger DC, Ard JD, eds. *Handbook of Clinical Nutrition* (4th Edition). Mosby; 2006:371–400.

26. Wycherley TP, Moran LJ, Clifton PM, Noakes M, Brinkworth GD. Effects of energy-restricted high-protein, low-fat compared with standard-protein, low-fat diets: A meta-analysis of randomized controlled trials. *Am. J. Clin. Nutr.* 2012;96(6):1281–1298. doi:10.3945/ajcn.112.044321

27. Verreijen AM, Engberink MF, Memelink RG, van der Plas SE, Visser M, Weijs PJ. Effect of a high protein diet and/or resistance exercise on the preservation of fat free mass during weight loss in overweight and obese older adults: a randomized controlled trial. *Nutr J.* Feb 6, 2017;16(1):10. doi:10.1186/s12937-017-0229-6

28. Wewege M, van den Berg R, Ward RE, Keech A. The effects of high-intensity interval training vs. moderate-intensity continuous training on body composition in overweight and obese adults: A systematic review and meta-analysis. *Obes Rev.* Jun 2017;18(6):635–646. doi:10.1111/obr.12532

29. Wing RR, Phelan S. Long-term weight loss maintenance. *Am. J. Clin. Nutr.* 2005;82(1 Suppl):222S–225S. doi:10.1093/ajcn/82.1.222S

30. Lv N, Azar KMJ, Rosas LG, Wulfovich S, Xiao L, Ma J. Behavioral lifestyle interventions for moderate and severe obesity: A systematic review. *Prev Med.* Jul 2017;100:180–193. doi:10.1016/j.ypmed.2017.04.022

31. Burke LE, Wang J, Sevick MA. Self-monitoring in weight loss: A systematic review of the literature. *J Am Diet Assoc.* Jan 2011;111(1):92–102. doi:10.1016/j.jada.2010.10.008

32. Carels RA, Darby LA, Rydin S, Douglass OM, Cacciapaglia HM, O'Brien WH. The relationship between self-monitoring, outcome expectancies, difficulties with eating and exercise, and physical activity and weight loss treatment outcomes. *Ann Behav Med.* Dec 2005;30(3):182–90. doi:10.1207/s15324796abm3003_2

33. Apovian CM, Aronne LJ, Bessesen DH, et al. Pharmacological management of obesity: an endocrine society clinical practice guideline. *J Clin Endocrinol Metab.* 2015;100(2):342–362. doi:10.1210/jc.2014-3415

34. Greenway FL, Aronne LJ, Raben A, et al. A randomized, double-blind, placebo-controlled study of gelesis100: A novel Nonsystemic oral hydrogel for weight loss. *Obesity (Silver Spring).* Feb 2019;27(2):205–216. doi:10.1002/oby.22347

35. Wilding JPH, Batterham RL, Calanna S, Davies M, Van Gaal LF, Lingvay I, McGowan BM, Rosenstock J, Tran MTD, Wadden TA, Wharton S, Yokote K, Zeuthen N, Kushner RF; STEP 1 Study group. Once-weekly semaglutide in adults with overweight or obesity. N Engl J Med. 2021 Mar 18;384(11):989–1002. doi: 10.1056/NEJMoa2032183. Epub 2021 Feb 10. PMID: 33567185.

36. Calderon G, Gonzalez-Izundegui D, Shan KL, Garcia-Valencia OA, Cifuentes L, Campos A, Collazo-Clavell ML, Shah M, Hurley DL, Abu Lebdeh HS, Sharma M, Schmitz K, Clark MM, Grothe K, Mundi MS, Camilleri M, Abu Dayyeh BK, Hurtado Andrade MD, Mokadem MA, Acosta A. Effectiveness of anti-obesity medications approved for long-term use in a multidisciplinary weight management program: A multi-center clinical experience. Int J Obes (Lond). 2022 Mar;46(3):555–563. doi: 10.1038/s41366-021-01019-6. Epub 2021 Nov 22. PMID: 34811486; PMCID: PMC8881310.

37. Jastreboff AM, Aronne LJ, Ahmad NN, Wharton S, Connery L, Alves B, Kiyosue A, Zhang S, Liu B, Bunck MC, Stefanski A; SURMOUNT-1 Investigators. Tirzepatide Once Weekly for the Treatment of Obesity. N Engl J Med. 2022 Jul 21;387(3):205–216. doi:10.1056/NEJMoa2206038. Epub 2022 Jun 4. PMID: 35658024.

38. Saper RB, Eisenberg DM, Phillips RS. Common dietary supplements for weight loss. Am Fam Physician. 2004;70(9):1731–1738.

39. Ríos-Hoyo A, Gutiérrez-Salmeán G. New dietary supplements for obesity: What we currently know. Curr Obes Rep. 2016;5(2):262–270. doi:10.1007/s13679-016-0214-y

40. Barrea L, Altieri B, Polese B, et al. Nutritionist and obesity: brief overview on efficacy, safety, and drug interactions of the main weight-loss dietary supplements. Int J Obes Suppl. 2019;9(1):32–49. doi:10.1038/s41367-019-0007-3

41. Information for Consumer on Using Dietary Supplements. FDA. Updated Aug 16, 2019. www.fda.gov/food/dietary-supplements/information-consumers-using-dietary-supplements

42. Jeukendrup AE, Randell R. Fat burners: nutrition supplements that increase fat metabolism. Obes Rev: An Official J Int Assoc Study of Obesity. 2011;12(10):841–851. doi:10.1111/j.1467-789X.2011.00908.x

43. Schubert MM, Irwin C, Seay RF, Clarke HE, Allegro D, Desbrow B. Caffeine, coffee, and appetite control: A review. Int J Food Sci Nutr. 2017;68(8):901–912. doi:10.1080/09637486.2017.1320537

44. Hursel R, Viechtbauer W, Westerterp-Plantenga MS. The effects of green tea on weight loss and weight maintenance: A meta-analysis. Int J Obes (Lond). 2009;33(9):956–961. doi:10.1038/ijo.2009.135

45. Eisenberg D, Shikora SA, Aarts E, Aminian A, Angrisani L, Cohen RV, De Luca M, Faria SL, Goodpaster KPS, Haddad A, Himpens JM, Kow L, Kurian M, Loi K, Mahawar K, Nimeri A, O'Kane M, Papasavas PK, Ponce J, Pratt JSA, Rogers AM, Steele KE, Suter M, Kothari SN. American Society for Metabolic and Bariatric Surgery (ASMBS) and International Federation for the Surgery of Obesity and Metabolic Disorders (IFSO): Indications for metabolic and bariatric surgery. Surg Obes Relat Dis. Dec 2022;18(12):1345–1356. doi: 10.1016/j.soard.2022.08.013. Epub 2022 Oct 21. PMID: 36280539.

46. Wolfe BM, Kvach E, Eckel RH. Treatment of obesity: Weight loss and bariatric surgery. Circ Res. May 27 2016;118(11):1844–1855. doi:10.1161/circresaha.116.307591

47. Welbourn R, Hollyman M, Kinsman R, et al. Bariatric surgery worldwide: Baseline demographic description and one-year outcomes from the fourth IFSO global registry report 2018. Obes Surg. Mar 2019;29(3):782–795. doi:10.1007/s11695-018-3593-1

48. Angrisani L, Santonicola A, Iovino P, et al. IFSO Worldwide Survey 2016: Primary, endoluminal, and revisional procedures. Obes Surg. 2018;28(12):3783–3794. doi:10.1007/s11695-018-3450-2

49. O'Brien PE, Hindle A, Brennan L, et al. Long-term outcomes after bariatric surgery: A systematic review and meta-analysis of weight loss at 10 or more years for all bariatric procedures and a single-centre review of 20-year outcomes after adjustable gastric banding. *Obes Surg.* 2019;29(1):3–14. doi:10.1007/s11695-018-3525-0

50. Puzziferri N, Roshek TB, 3rd, Mayo HG, Gallagher R, Belle SH, Livingston EH. Long-term follow-up after bariatric surgery: A systematic review. *JAMA.* 2014;312(9): 934–942. doi:10.1001/jama.2014.10706

51. Greenway FL. Physiological adaptations to weight loss and factors favouring weight regain. *Int J Obes (Lond).* 2015;39(8):1188–1196. doi:10.1038/ijo.2015.59

52. Odom J, Zalesin KC, Washington TL, et al. Behavioral predictors of weight regain after bariatric surgery. *Obes Surg.* 2010;20(3):349–356. doi:10.1007/s11695-009-9895-6

53. Lee HL. Role of restrictive endoscopic procedures in obesity treatment. *Clin Endosc.* 2017;50(1):17–20. doi:10.5946/ce.2017.022

54. Brunaldi VO, Galvao Neto M. Endoscopic techniques for weight loss and treating metabolic syndrome. *Curr Opin Gastroenterol.* 2019;35(5):424–431. doi:10.1097/MOG.0000000000000561

55. Carrano FM, Peev MP, Saunders JK, Melis M, Tognoni V, Di Lorenzo N. The role of minimally invasive and endoscopic technologies in morbid obesity treatment: Review and critical appraisal of the current clinical practice. *Obes Surg.* 2020;30(2):736–752. doi:10.1007/s11695-019-04302-8

56. Turkeltaub JA, Edmundowicz SA. Endoscopic bariatric therapies: Intragastric balloons, tissue apposition, and aspiration therapy. *Curr Treat Options Gastroenterol.* 2019;17(2):187–201. doi:10.1007/s11938-019-00232-7

57. Jirapinyo P, Kröner PT, Thompson CC. Purse-string transoral outlet reduction (TORe) is effective at inducing weight loss and improvement in metabolic comorbidities after Roux-en-Y gastric bypass. *Endoscopy.* 2018;50(4):371–377. doi:10.1055/s-0043-122380

58. Tabasi M, Ashrafian F, Khezerloo JK, et al. Changes in gut microbiota and hormones after bariatric surgery: A bench-to-bedside review. *Obes Surg.* 2019;29(5):1663–1674. doi:10.1007/s11695-019-03779-7

59. Mueller NT, Whyatt R, Hoepner L, et al. Prenatal exposure to antibiotics, cesarean section and risk of childhood obesity. *Int J Obes (Lond).* 2015;39(4):665–670. doi:10.1038/ijo.2014.180

60. Turnbaugh PJ, Ley RE, Mahowald MA, Magrini V, Mardis ER, Gordon JI. An obesity-associated gut microbiome with increased capacity for energy harvest. *Nature.* 2006;444(7122):1027–1031. doi:10.1038/nature05414

61. Ridaura VK, Faith JJ, Rey FE, et al. Gut microbiota from twins discordant for obesity modulate metabolism in mice. *Science.* 2013;341(6150):1241214–1241214. doi:10.1126/science.1241214

62. Dansinger ML, Gleason JA, Griffith JL, Selker HP, Schaefer EJ. Comparison of the Atkins, Ornish, Weight Watchers, and Zone diets for weight loss and heart disease risk reduction: A randomized trial. *JAMA.* Jan 5, 2005;293(1):43–53. doi:10.1001/jama.293.1.43

63. Gardner CD, Trepanowski JF, Del Gobbo LC, et al. Effect of low-fat vs low-carbohydrate diet on 12-month weight loss in overweight adults and the association with genotype pattern or insulin secretion: The DIETFITS randomized clinical trial. *JAMA.* Feb 20, 2018;319(7):667–679. doi:10.1001/jama.2018.0245

64. Berry SE, Valdes AM, Drew DA, Asnicar F, Mazidi M, Wolf J, Capdevila J, Hadjigeorgiou G, Davies R, Al Khatib H, Bonnett C. Human postprandial responses to food and potential for precision nutrition. *Nature Medicine.* Jun 11, 2020:1–0. Disclosure: TDS, SEB, AMV, FA, PWF, LMD and NS are consultants to Zoe Global Ltd ('Zoe'). JW, GH, RD, HA., JC, CB, SG, EB, PW and IL are or have been employees of Zoe.

65. Grannell A, Fallon F, Pournaras D, le Roux CW. Exploring patient beliefs and perceptions regarding obesity as a disease, obesity causation and treatment. *Ir J Med Sci*. Jul 21, 2020. doi:10.1007/s11845-020-02319-y

66. Sumithran P, Prendergast LA, Delbridge E, et al. Long-term persistence of hormonal adaptations to weight loss. *N Engl J Med*. Oct 27, 2011;365(17):1597–1604. doi:10.1056/NEJMoa1105816

67. Pearl RL, Wadden TA, Chao AM, et al. Associations between causal attributions for obesity and long-term weight loss. *Behav Med*. Apr–Jun 2020;46(2):87–91. doi:10.1080/08964289.2018.1556202

23 Obesity and Metabolic Syndrome

Michael Garcia and Zhaoping Li

23.1 INTRODUCTION

The growing prevalence of overweight and obesity and their role in the development of the most common chronic diseases remains an important public health crisis both in the United States and worldwide. As of 2016, obesity affected over one-third of adults in the United States.[1] Worldwide, nearly 2 billion adults are overweight, and nearly 110 million children and 650 million adults have obesity. The World Health Organization estimates that by 2025, 2.7 billion adults will be overweight and 1 billion adults will have obesity.[2]

The develIpment of obesity involves a complex interaction of genetics, epigenetics, environmental factors, and signals that regulate energy homeostasis. Because of its close association with obesity, metabolic syndrome is also recognized in increasing numbers. Characterized by metabolic risk factors of abdominal adiposity, dyslipidemia, elevated blood pressure, and glucose dysregulation, metabolic syndrome is associated with an increased risk of developing cardiovascular disease and type 2 diabetes.[3] The optimal approach to obesity and the risk factors of metabolic syndrome is prevention; however, early recognition and management of these related conditions is paramount to ensure individual and societal health.

23.2 DEFINITION OF OBESITY

Obesity is defined as excess fat mass that adversely affects health and life expectancy.[4] Body mass index (BMI) is often the most practical way to estimate obesity in the clinical setting with BMI $\geq$30 kg/m^2 indicating obesity; however, this index has several limitations. BMI categories were developed using the risk for morbidity and mortality in populations of European ancestry; it does not incorporate ethnic differences between BMI ranges and associated disease risk, morbidity, and mortality.[4] For example, metabolic abnormalities are seen in certain Asian populations with BMI values of 20–25 kg/m^2.[5] Furthermore, there are obese individuals that have normal metabolic profiles and a different mortality risk compared with obese individuals defined by a BMI category.[6] BMI also does not accurately measure the fat mass or lean mass of an individual. A more complete definition of obesity includes body composition analysis to measure these factors, combined with medical history and metabolic profile of an individual.[7]

DOI: 10.1201/9780429322570-23

23.3 GENETIC AND ENVIRONMENTAL INFLUENCES IN OBESITY

Obesity develops from the complex interaction between genetics, epigenetics, and environment. The "obesogenic" environment is one of positive energy balance, excess weight, and reduced physical activity, but this alone is not sufficient to cause obesity, due to the variation in weight and body fat of individuals within this environment.[4, 8] Parental BMI and overweight/obesity status is associated with risk of being overweight/obese in children.[4] This may be due in part to lifestyle variability and environment, but genetic variation also plays a role in obesity development.[4, 8]

More than 30 monogenic obesity syndromes have been reported in the literature and are characterized by obesity, cognitive impairment, dysmorphic features, and specific organ abnormalities (e.g., Prader-Willi syndrome).[4] Non-syndromic obesity is a single gene disorder with a highly penetrant form of disease, characterized by significant hyperphagia.[4] Examples include mutations leading to a deficiency of leptin, leptin receptors, and melanocortin-4 receptors (MC4R), which are involved in the regulation of energy homeostasis.[8] There are also heterozygous deleterious mutations that cause non-fully penetrant obesity.[4]

The most common form is polygenic obesity, shown in Figure 23.1,[9] in which multiple gene defects that confer susceptibility to obesity interact with epigenetic influences and the environment.[4, 8] Numerous single-nucleotide polymorphisms associated with BMI and obesity have been identified, though they collectively account for <5% of BMI and adiposity trait variation.[4, 8] Epigenetic influences, including nutrition, environment, and other prenatal and postnatal exposures alter biological functions and change gene transcription/expression without altering the DNA sequence, which both influence long-term metabolic health.[4, 8]

The environmental impact on obesity development is substantial and includes lifestyle factors, such as dietary pattern and quality, sleep, and activity levels. We frequently view obesity as the result of excess calorie consumption and reduced activity over time. This viewpoint is narrow and assumes calories are equivalent. Food and beverages uniquely affect hunger, hormones, and genetic expression in a way distinct from their caloric density.[10] Calorie type can affect calorie expenditure; for example, sugary foods, refined grains, and high-glycemic load carbohydrates have been associated with weight gain and risk for diabetes, while calorie-dense high-fat foods have the reverse association.[10]

Data from the Nurses' Health Study, Nurses' Health Study II, and the Health Professionals Follow-Up Study looked at the effects of lifestyle factors on weight gain.[11] These data showed that duration of sleep <6 hours or >8 hours showed a close association with weight gain.[11] Individual dietary factors should be evaluated in the context of their satiety effects, displacement of other foods/beverages, portion sizes, and overall dietary pattern.[11] Starches, refined grains, and processed foods were positively associated with weight gain.[11] This may be due to a lower satiety effect from these foods, which leads to increased caloric intake.[11] Increased consumption of vegetables, nuts, fruits, and whole grains was associated with less weight gain,

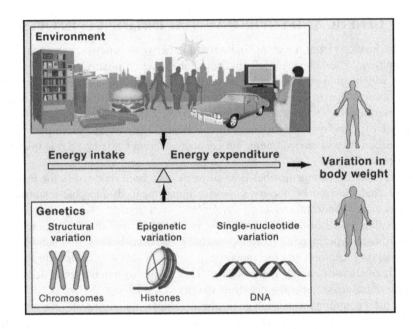

FIGURE 23.1 Contribution of genes and environmental factors to weight gain. Human adiposity is influenced by complex interactions between genetic and environmental influences. The current environment potently facilitates the development of obesity. Abundance of highly processed food has a major impact on energy intake, whereas numerous other environmental factors, such as television watching, leisure activities, and transport, negatively affect energy expenditure. In any environment, there is a variation in body fat and BMI in large part influenced by genetic variation disrupting energy homeostasis by either decreasing energy expenditure or increasing energy intake.

Source: Reprinted from van der Klaauw AA, Farooqi IS. "The hunger genes: pathways to obesity." Cell. 2015;161(1):119–132. With permission from Elsevier.

likely because higher-fiber foods slow digestion, increase satiety, and replace the consumption of more processed foods.[11] Intake of sugar-sweetened beverages was more positively associated with weight gain versus 100% fruit juice.[11] Collectively, these findings suggest that dietary quality can affect total caloric intake and thus energy balance over the long term.[11]

Emulsifiers are the most common food additive in processed foods, and are used to increase shelf life, enhance flavor, and improve texture.[12] Mayonnaise, salad dressing, fruit snacks, and frozen dinners all contain emulsifiers.[12] Studies in mice have shown that emulsifiers have several adverse effects: increased inflammation, increased adiposity, insulin resistance, and changes to the microbiome.[12] Hall and colleagues conducted an inpatient controlled trial comparing matched calorie ultra-processed foods to minimally processed foods and showed that ultra-processed foods resulted in increased energy intake, weight gain, and worsened biomarkers.[13]

23.4   THE REGULATION OF ENERGY HOMEOSTASIS

The regulation of energy balance and body weight involves a dynamic interaction between the central nervous system (CNS) and peripheral organs through neuro-hormonal mechanisms that act via afferent and efferent pathways between the two.[14] Peripheral organ systems communicate to the brain regarding energy status, including stored energy and recently ingested energy.[14] This information is integrated by the CNS to moderate food intake so that nutrients are available in the short term and stored energy is available during periods of limited energy intake (i.e., starvation).[8, 14]

Within the CNS, energy homeostasis is regulated by the arcuate nucleus in the hypothalamus, the nucleus tractus solitaris, area postrema, and dorsal vagal nucleus in the brainstem, and the amygdala in the limbic system.[14] The arcuate nucleus contains melanocortin system neurons that express pro-opiomelanocortin (POMC), a precursor for α-melanocyte stimulating hormone (α-MSH) among other peptides.[14] The arcuate nucleus contains melanocortin-4 receptor (MC4R), which is the primary receptor for α-MSH; agonist binding results in hypophagia, thermogenesis, and weight loss.[14] The arcuate nucleus also contains neurons that produce neuropeptide Y (NPY) and agouti-related peptide (AgRP), which bind their rIceptors and cause increases in food intake and weight gain.[14]

Peripheral signals that influence energy balance originate from adipose tissue, liver, pancreas, gut, and muscle.[14] Leptin and insulin reflect levels of stored energy, whereas gastrointestinal (GI) signals reflect the properties of recently ingested foods.[14, 15] Leptin is predominantly produced by white adipose tissue; it reflects energy status and total body fat and correlates more with subcutaneous fat.[14] Leptin exerts its effect in the hypothalamus, activating POMC neurons and inhibiting NPY and AgRP neurons, causing reduced feeding.[14] In the majority of obesity, leptin levels are increased; however, individuals with obesity are resistant to leptin.[14] Insulin also has an important role in energy balance.[14] Insulin levels reflect total body fat, act to decrease food intake, and correlate more with visceral fat.[14] Similar to leptin, insulin has receptors in the hypothalamus and stimulates POMC neurons while inhibiting NPY neurons.[14] However, with the chronic excess energy stores in obesity, insulin resistance diminishes the effect of elevated levels of insulin.[14]

Endocrine cells of the GI tract convey information about the nutrient content of food and contain mechanoreceptors that respond to changes in luminal volume and pressure.[15] The cells release signals that act on the liver, gallbladder, and pancreas to ensure proper digestive enzyme release.[15] These signals also activate vagal afferent neurons that innervate the GI tract to communicate to the brain to stop an ongoing meal, and thus are referred to as satiety signals.[15] Among the important satiety signals are:[14, 15]

- Cholecystokinin (CCK) from I cells (duodenal/jejunal mucosa)
- Amylin from pancreatic B cells
- Glucagon-like peptide 1 (GLP-1) from intestinal L cells
- Pancreatic tyrosine tyrosine (PYY) from intestinal L cells
- Oxyntomodulin from intestinal L cells
- Gastric leptin from P cells and chief cells

In conjunction with these signals is the phenomenon of the ileal brake, an inhibitory feedback mechanism in which ingested food activates distal intestinal signals to cause inhibition of proximal GI motility and gastric emptying.[15, 16] Ghrelin, which is produced in the stomach and proximal small intestine, acts to stimulate appetite and increase food intake.[14, 15] Peripherally, ghrelin increases gastric emptying and intestinal motility.[14] Ghrelin levels peak just prior to a meal, which suggests its role in meal initiation rather than meal size.[14, 15]

Energy homeostasis is a dynamic process in which short-acting satiety signals interact with long-acting adiposity signals to regulate body weight. Importantly, adiposity signals may affect vagal and CNS sensitivity to satiety signals from the GI tract to regulate food intake in the short term in order to achieve long-term energy balance.[17, 18]

23.5   PATHOPHYSIOLOGIC MECHANISMS IN OBESITY AND EFFECTS OF EXCESS BODY FAT

Obesity involves the accumulation of excess adiposity over time through lipids (mostly triglycerides) and increase in volume of various organs.[8] Lipids deposit mostly in subcutaneous adipose tissue in different body sites.[8] They are also stored in liposomes, organelles in different cell types that can cause adverse pathology.[8] Visceral adipose tissue (VAT) contains fewer stored lipids but is associated with the metabolic changes and chronic diseases of obesity.[8]

Adipocytes come in three types; white adipocytes are the main type in human adipose tissue.[8] They store triglycerides and cholesterol ester and release signaling molecules.[8] Brown and beige adipocytes are thermogenic and present in smaller amounts in adults.[8] Adipocytes produce and release signaling peptides, called adipokines, that regulate biological processes in different tissues.[8] Many adipokines are proinflammatory, causing chronic low-grade systemic inflammation.[8] Excess adipose tissue leads to higher levels of plasma free fatty acids, due to hydrolysis of triglycerides to free fatty acids within adipocytes.[8] Excess VAT, inflammatory cytokines, and free fatty acids lead to insulin resistance, increased sympathetic activity, and the development and progression of many obesity-associated diseases.

The role of the human gut microbiome in obesity is becoming increasingly recognized. The genetic information in the microbiome numbers more than 10 million genes, far exceeding the human genome.[19] Microbiome composition is determined by several factors: host genetic makeup, intestinal motility, pH, antibacterial proteins and mucus, medications, weight, metabolic state of an individual, and diet.[4, 19] Diet also affects microbiota gene expression.[19] Alterations in the diversity and structure of the microbiome, called dysbiosis, affects metabolic status and has an important association with obesity.[19] Animal studies have shown that transfer of gut microbiome from mice with genetic- or diet-induced obesity to germ-free mice caused an increase in fat mass and body weight.[19] Mice with obesity also exhibit an increased ratio of *Firmicutes* to *Bacteroidetes*.[19] Human studies have shown that low microbial diversity is associated with an elevated relative risk of obesity. While a precise microbial composition associated with obesity is yet to be elucidated, it is suggested that low microbial gene count, an increased ratio of *Firmicutes:Bacteroidetes*, and increased levels of fecal short-chain fatty acids (SCFAs), plasma branched-chain amino acids (BCAAs), trimethylamine *N*-oxide (TMAO), total bile acids, and lipopolysaccharide (LPS) are seen in obesity. A decrease in *Bifidobacterium* and *Akkermansia* species of gut microbes has also been implicated in obesity.[19]

The microbiome also produces metabolites important in different metabolic pathways.[19] In the cecum and colon, gut microbes ferment non-digestible dietary proteins, glycoproteins, and fibers to produce SCFAs, including butyrate, acetate, and propionate.[19] SCFAs from microbes affect colonic function, integrity, motility, and metabolism in other organs.[19] Butyrate induces intestinal cells to increase GLP-1 production, stimulates thermogenesis, fat oxidation, and mitochondrial function, and supports pancreatic β-cell function.[19] Propionate affects intestinal gluconeogenesis.[19] Microbial SCFAs may also induce secretion of PYY and leptin.[19]

In animal models and humans, elevated BCAAs and aromatic amino acids have been seen in obesity, insulin resistance, and type 2 diabetes.[19] Decreased BCAA levels are associated with improved insulin sensitivity; *Bacteroides* species in the gut may improve BCAA degradation.[19] There is ongoing research on the role of bile acids in obesity, whose metabolism is affected by the gut microbiome.[19] Another metabolite is trimethylamine *N*-oxide (TMAO).[19] Dietary components in cheese, eggs, liver, red meat, and peanuts are converted to trimethylamine and then oxidized to TMAO in the liver.[19] Research has shown the relationship of increased TMAO with hemoglobin A1c, fasting plasma glucose, plasma cholesterol levels, inflammation biomarkers, cardiovascular risk, and metabolic syndrome.[19] The association of TMAO with obesity and BMI requires further research.[19] The role of the gut microbiome and its metabolites in obesity is summarized in Figure 23.2.[19] A healthy and diverse gut microbial makeup can occur through a healthy diet and optimal weight management. Food remains an important instrument in the prevention of gut microbial dysbiosis and obesity.

Excess VAT, inflammatory cytokines, and free fatty acids characteristic of excess adiposity contribute to the pathogenesis of obesity-related disease, including liver disease, dyslipidemia, and coronary artery disease.[8] Type 2 diabetes is closely linked with visceral adiposity and inflammation. Elevated BMI and weight gain during adulthood are strong predictors of risk for developing diabetes.[20] Increased VAT also contributes to the development of hypertension, through compression of kidneys and activation of the renin-angiotensin-aldosterone system (RAAS) through adipocyte secretion of angiotensinogen.[8] Sympathetic nervous system activity increases and contributes to the development of hypertension and downstream chronic kidney disease, coronary artery disease, congestive heart failure, and stroke.[8] The physical and mechanical stress of excess adipose tissue causes joint stress of osteoarthritis, increased risk of gastroesophageal reflux disease, and excess pharyngeal soft tissue that contributes to obstructive sleep apnea.[8] Obesity is also associated with certain cancer development and an increased prevalence of mental health disorders.[8] Obesity affects many aspects of our health and contributes to the development of debilitating conditions. Early recognition and prevention can significantly improve individual and public health.

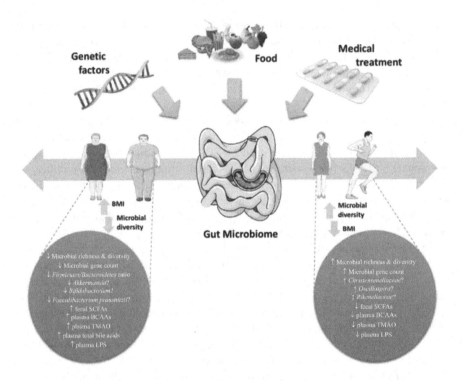

FIGURE 23.2 Overall, in obesity, there is lower microbial richness and diversity as well as lower microbial gene count than in normal-weight subjects. Most studies have demonstrated a decrease in *Akkermansia muciniphila*, *Faecalibacterium prausnitzii*, and *Bacteroidetes* and an increase in *Firmicutes*. Also, increased levels of fecal short-chain fatty acids (SCFAs) as well as elevated levels of plasma branched-chain amino acids (BCAAs), trimethylamine *N*-oxide (TMAO), total bile acids, and lipopolysaccharide (LPS) have been documented. In individuals with metabolic complications, there is a decreased abundance of *Bifidobacterium* and *Akkermansia*. In normal-weight subjects, an abundance of microbial species and microbial gene counts has been documented. Some studies have reported an increase in *Christensenellaceae*, *Oscillospira*, and *Rikenellaceae*, while there are usually lower levels of fecal SCFAs as well as plasma BCAAs, TMAO, and LPS.

Source: Images of 4 people (unchanged) and the gut (converted to grayscale) are derived from the free medical site: http://smart.servier.com/ by Servier licensed under a Creative Commons Attribution 3.0 Unported License. Reprinted from Vallianou N, Stratigou T, Christodoulatos GS, Dalamaga M. "Understanding the role of the gut microbiome and microbial metabolites in obesity and obesity-associated metabolic disorders: current evidence and perspectives." Curr Obes Rep. 2019;8(3):317–332. With permission from Springer Nature.

23.6   DEFINING THE METABOLIC SYNDROME AND ASSOCIATED RISK

Metabolic syndrome is closely associated with obesity and is characterized by interrelated risk factors that create a progressive pathophysiological state with increased risk for cardiovascular disease (CVD) and diabetes.[1, 21] The definition of metabolic syndrome has evolved over time, with important contributions from the National Cholesterol Education Program Adult Treatment Panel III, International Diabetes Federation, and the American Heart Association/National Heart, Lung, and Blood Institute.[1] The most recent unifying criteria are:

- Abdominal obesity/elevated waist circumference (population- and country-specific thresholds)
- Elevated triglycerides ≥150 mg/dL (1.7 mmol/L) or drug treatment for elevated triglycerides
- Reduced high-density lipoprotein cholesterol (HDL-C) <40 mg/dL (1.0 mmol/L) in males; <50 mg/dL (1.3 mmol/L) in females; or drug treatment for reduced HDL-C
- Elevated blood pressure: Systolic ≥130 and/or diastolic ≥85 mmHg, or antihypertensive drug treatment
- Elevated fasting glucose ≥100 mg/dL or drug treatment for elevated glucose

A clinical diagnosis of metabolic syndrome requires meeting 3 of the 5 criteria.[1] Abdominal obesity/waist circumference has been challenging to define because of its variation with other metabolic risk factors.[1] There are also differences based on sex and race/ethnicity, which cannot be captured using one set of waist circumference criteria.[1] Nevertheless, common waist circumference thresholds to define abdominal obesity are ≥80 cm or ≥88 cm in women and ≥94 cm or ≥102 cm in men, which should be adjusted based on the population in question.[1] Other variables of metabolic syndrome not specifically recognized as diagnostic criteria include high apolipoprotein B, small low-density lipoprotein particle size, endothelial dysfunction, and prothrombotic/proinflammatory states.[21]

Differences exist based on race/ethnicity, sex, and socioeconomic status, which creates phenotypic variability in metabolic syndrome.[21, 22] Analysis of the National Health and Nutrition Examination Survey (NHANES) from 1999–2010 showed that Mexican Americans of both sexes had higher prevalence of low HDL-C, high triglycerides, and high blood glucose compared with Caucasians and African Americans; African American males and females had higher prevalence of elevated blood pressure and the lowest prevalence of dyslipidemia; Caucasian males had higher prevalence of abdominal obesity but Caucasian females had lower prevalence.[22] South Asians have higher body fat content, waist-to-hip ratio, visceral fat-to-subcutaneous fat ratio, and adipocyte area than age-, sex-, and BMI-matched Caucasians.[21]

The prevalence of metabolic syndrome correlates highly with the prevalence of obesity. NHANES data from 2003–2006 showed a higher incidence of metabolic syndrome with increased weight: in men, 6.8% of normal-weight individuals had metabolic syndrome, 29.8% of overweight, and 65% of those with obesity; in women, 9.3% of normal-weight individuals had metabolic syndrome, 33.1% of overweight, and 56.1% of those with obesity.[21] This also shows that obesity alone does not confer metabolic syndrome, since there are non-obese individuals with metabolic syndrome and obese individuals without it.[21]

Metabolic syndrome confers a five-fold increased risk for type 2 diabetes and greater than two-fold risk for atherosclerotic cardiovascular disease (ASCVD) and cardiovascular mortality.[1, 21] Risk of adverse outcomes rises with a greater number of metabolic syndrome components. Examination of NHANES III data showed that individuals with metabolic syndrome had higher ASCVD risk compared with individuals with type 2 diabetes alone.[23] Metabolic syndrome also promotes a number of conditions that increase risk for multi-end-organ damage, including endocrine disorders, sleep-disordered breathing and other respiratory diseases, certain malignancies, chronic kidney disease, joint disease, nonalcoholic fatty liver disease (NAFLD), and mental health conditions.[21]

23.7 PATHOPHYSIOLOGY OF METABOLIC SYNDROME

The pathogenesis of metabolic syndrome is complex, given its multiple interrelated components. Excess VAT is a primary driver for the mechanisms that lead to metabolic syndrome.[21, 24] Prolonged excess energy intake saturates the storage and clearance capacity of subcutaneous adipose tissue. What ensues is adipocyte dysfunction, excess triglycerides, and ectopic fat deposition in liver, heart, skeletal muscle, and viscera. Insulin resistance is closely related; it is characteristically seen with VAT and leads to reduced insulin-mediated inhibition of lipolysis, with multiple subsequent effects: higher circulating free fatty acids, further lipolysis inhibition, hepatic gluconeogenesis and lipogenesis, and reduced glucose uptake in muscle.[24] Free fatty acids are lipotoxic to pancreatic beta cells, increase synthesis of triglycerides and very low-density lipoprotein, and cause vasoconstriction. VAT is metabolically active and also produces prothrombotic and proinflammatory signals. As seen in Figure 23.3,[25] excess VAT and insulin resistance cause changes that result in an increased risk of CVD.[21, 24]

VAT releases a number of adipokines, including leptin and adiponectin.[24] Adiponectin has anti-inflammatory and anti-atherogenic properties, but is present in reduced levels with excess adipose tissue. RAAS activation is also enhanced with excess adipose tissue. Adipose tissue secretes angiotensinogen, which causes increased angiotensin II that activates nicotinamide adenine dinucleotide phosphate oxidase leading to reactive oxygen species (ROS) generation. ROS trigger LDL oxidation, endothelial injury, platelet aggregation, and a cycle of inflammation, endothelial damage, and fibroblast proliferation. There is also increased production of tumor necrosis factor alpha (TNF-α) by macrophages that occurs with increased adipose tissue mass. TNF-α causes further insulin resistance, lipolysis, and inhibition of adiponectin release.[24] Figure 23.3 provides a visual summary of the pathogenic findings in metabolic syndrome.

Similar to obesity, dietary quality is important in metabolic syndrome. Independent of BMI, individuals aged 18–35 with metabolic syndrome were more likely to adhere to a Western dietary pattern compared with metabolically normal individuals, showing the importance of dietary composition.[26] Because of its close association with obesity, metabolic syndrome is also significantly tied to the gut microbiome. Gut microbial dysbiosis is associated with type 2 diabetes and the pathogenesis of NAFLD, along with other metabolic abnormalities that make up metabolic syndrome.[19]

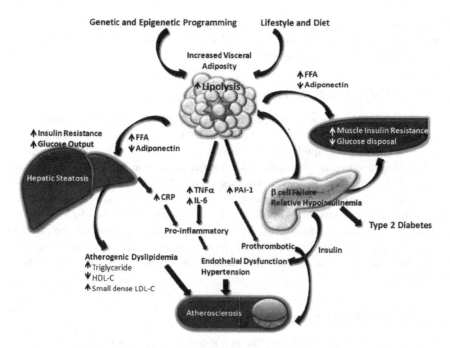

FIGURE 23.3 Proposed mechanisms for the clustering of metabolic syndrome traits and the increased risk of type 2 diabetes mellitus and cardiovascular disease. CRP: C-reactive protein; IL-6: interleukin 6; PAI-1: plasminogen activator inhibitor 1; TNFα: tumor necrosis factor α.

Source: Reprinted from Samson SL, Garber AJ. "Metabolic syndrome." Endocrinol Metab Clin North Am. 2014;43(1):1–23. With permission from Elsevier.

23.8   PREVENTION, SCREENING, AND MANAGEMENT

Primary prevention is the best treatment for metabolic syndrome. We must identify individuals at risk for metabolic syndrome through indicators such as overweight, increased susceptibility, evidence of ectopic fat deposition, and detrimental nutrition and physical activity patterns.[21] Factors such as blood pressure, lipids, BMI, and waist circumference can be measured and serially tracked to initiate aggressive management should risk factors progress. We must also recognize metabolic abnormalities not specific to the diagnostic criteria, such as NAFLD. Different metabolic abnormalities affect individuals differently and thus intervention must be individualized.

Weight loss will help improve the components of metabolic syndrome and reduce downstream risk, but treatment should also involve management of component parts with pharmacotherapy as indicated. Evaluation of data from the National Health Insurance Database of Korea showed that risk for major adverse cardiovascular events (MACE) was significantly modified based on metabolic syndrome status.[27] Individuals who recovered from metabolic syndrome based on the diagnostic criteria had reduced risk for MACE compared to those with metabolic syndrome throughout the evaluation period. Individuals who developed metabolic syndrome had increased risk compared to those who never met diagnostic criteria during the evaluation period. This shows that the risk associated with the abnormalities of metabolic syndrome may be reduced with appropriate treatment.

23.9   NOVEL APPROACHES

The dynamic development and maintenance of obesity involves a number of genetic, epigenetic, and environmental factors. Chief among environmental factors are dietary pattern and quality as well as other lifestyle variables, such as sleep and activity. Dietary quality can affect the normal regulation of energy homeostasis due to the characteristics of available foods. Dietary quality may further influence the microbiota and microbiota gene expression of an individual. Such alterations in the microbiome have been implicated in obesity and the metabolic status of an individual. Current and future research will help to further delineate the effect of dietary pattern and quality on the makeup of the microbiome and its metabolites in order to aid in the prevention and treatment of obesity and its associated metabolic conditions.

23.10   INCORRECT/OUTDATED PRACTICES

While using BMI is practical and efficient, it does not incorporate ethnic differences between BMI ranges and associated disease risk nor does it accurately measure the fat or lean mass of an individual. Body composition analysis together with medical history and metabolic profile provides a more complete definition of obesity and associated conditions. Furthermore, we must not view obesity and metabolic syndrome through a narrow lens, but rather appreciate that heritable components interact with epigenetic influences and the environment to create a risk profile for these conditions. With each degree of weight change comes a shift in how the body regulates energy balance, changes in adipokine release from adipocytes, changes in the microbiome, and effects on metabolic parameters. This creates new and different challenges in the prevention and treatment of obesity and metabolic syndrome.

23.11   CONCLUSION

Obesity and metabolic syndrome are closely associated and increasing in prevalence worldwide. Excess adipose tissue is best measured with body composition analysis rather than BMI, because of variability in metabolic measures at different BMI values. Obesity develops through the interaction of genetics, epigenetics, environment, microbiome, and signals from peripheral organs and the CNS. Excess VAT is intimately linked with insulin resistance and chronic inflammation, which together cause the increased risk and presence of multiple diseases, including type 2 diabetes and cardiovascular disease. The most effective treatment for obesity and metabolic syndrome is prevention, with early identification of individuals at risk, early aggressive management targeting weight loss, and guideline-driven treatment of metabolic abnormalities.

PRACTICE PEARLS

- The growing prevalence of worldwide overweight and obesity has led to a similar increase in the progression of metabolic syndrome.
- The most comprehensive definition of obesity includes body composition analysis to evaluate fat mass and lean mass, in conjunction with the metabolic profile of an individual.
- Dietary pattern and quality can affect energy homeostasis that is altered in obesity, as well as the gut microbiome, which is increasingly recognized for its important influence on obesity and metabolic syndrome.
- Metabolic risk factors can improve with weight loss of 5–10% of baseline weight.
- The optimal approach to obesity and metabolic syndrome is prevention; however, early recognition and management of individual risk factors and metabolic abnormalities is equally important.

REFERENCES

1. Alberti KG, Eckel RH, Grundy SM, et al. Harmonizing the metabolic syndrome: a joint statement of the International Diabetes Federation Task Force on Epidemiology and Prevention; National Heart, Lung, and Blood Institute; American Heart Association; World Heart Federation; International Atherosclerosis Society; and International Association for the Study of Obesity. *Circulation.* 2009;120(16):1640–5. doi:10.1161/CIRCULATIONAHA.109.192644.
2. Hales CM, Carroll MD, Fryar CD, Ogden CL. Prevalence of obesity among adults and youth: United States, 2015–2016. NCHS data brief, no 288. Hyattsville, MD: National Center for Health Statistics. 2017.
3. World Obesity Foundation. Prevalence of obesity. https://www.worldobesity.org/about/about-obesity/prevalence-of-obesity. 2019. Accessed January 26, 2020.
4. Pigeyre M, Yazdi FT, Kaur Y, Meyre D. Recent progress in genetics, epigenetics and metagenomics unveils the pathophysiology of human obesity. *Clin Sci.* 2016;130(12):943–86. doi:10.1042/CS20160136.
5. Yang W, Lu J, Weng J, et al. Prevalence of diabetes among men and women in China. *N Engl J Med.* 2010;362(12):1090–101. doi:10.1056/NEJMoa0908292.
6. Kramer CK, Zinman B, Retnakaran R. Are metabolically healthy overweight and obesity benign conditions? A systematic review and meta-analysis. *Ann Intern Med.* 2013;159(11):758–69. doi:10.7326/0003-4819-159-11-201312030-00008.
7. Muller MJ, Geisler C. Defining obesity as a disease. *Eur J Clin Nutr.* 2017;71(11):1256–8. doi:10.1038/ejcn.2017.155.
8. Heymsfield SB, Wadden TA. Mechanisms, pathophysiology, and management of obesity. *N Engl J Med.* 2017;376(3):254–66. doi:10.1056/NEJMra1514009.
9. Van der Klaauw AA, Farooqi IS. The hunger genes: pathways to obesity. *Cell.* 2015;161(1):119–32. doi:10.1016/j.cell.2015.03.008.
10. Ludwig DS. Lifespan weighed down by diet. *JAMA.* 2016;315(21):2269–70. doi:10.1001/jama.2016.3829.
11. Mozaffarian D, Hao T, Rimm EB, Willett WC, Hu FB. Changes in diet and lifestyle and long-term weight gain in women and men. *N Engl J Med.* 2011;364:2392–404.

12. Laster J, Bonees SL, Rocha J. Increased use of emulsifiers in processed foods and the links to obesity. *Curr Gastroenterol Rep.* 2019;21(11):61. doi:10.1007/s11894-019-0723-4.

13. Hall KD, Ayuketah A, Brychta R, et al. Ultra-processed diets cause excess calorie intake and weight gain: an inpatient randomized controlled trial of ad libitum food intake. *Cell Metab.* 2019;30(1):226. doi:10.1016/j.cmet.2019.05.020.

14. Miller GD. Appetite regulation: hormones, peptides, and neurotransmitters and their role in obesity. *Am J Lifestyle Med.* 2017;13(6):586–601. doi:10.1177/1559827617716376.

15. Strader AD, Woods SC. Gastrointestinal hormones and food take. *Gastroenterology.* 2005;128(1):175–91.

16. Pironi L, Stanghellini V, Miglioli M, et al. Fat-induced ileal brake in humans: a dose-dependent phenomenon correlated to the plasma levels of peptide YY. *Gastroenterology.* 1993;105(3):733–9.

17. Schwartz MW, Woods, SC, Porte D Jr, Seeley RJ, Baskin DG. Central nervous system control of food intake. *Nature.* 2000;404(6778):661–71.

18. Morton GJ, Cummings DE, Baskin DG, Barsh GS, Schwartz MW. Central nervous system control of food intake and body weight. *Nature.* 2006;443(7109):289–95.

19. Vallianou N, Stratigou T, Christodoulatos GS, Dalamaga M. Understanding the role of the gut microbiome and microbial metabolites in obesity and obesity-associated metabolic disorders: current evidence and perspectives. *Curr Obes Rep.* 2019;8(3):317–32. doi:10.1007/s13679-019-00352-2.

20. Colditz GA, Willett WC, Rotnitzky A, Manson JE. Weight gain as a risk factor for clinical diabetes mellitus in women. *Ann Intern Med.* 1995;122(7):481–6.

21. Sperling LS, Mechanick JI, Neeland IJ, et al. The CardioMetabolic Health Alliance: working toward a new care model for the metabolic syndrome. *J Am Coll Cardiol.* 2015;66(9):1050–67. doi:10.1016/j.jacc.2015.06.1328.

22. Beltran-Sanchez H, Harhay MO, Harhay MM, McElligott S. Prevalence and trends of metabolic syndrome in the adult U.S. population, 1999–2010. *J Am Coll Cardiol.* 2013;62(8):697–703. doi:10.1016/j.jacc.2013.05.064.

23. Alexander CM, Landsman PB, Teutsch SM, Haffner SM. NCEP-defined metabolic syndrome, diabetes, and prevalence of coronary heart disease among NHANES III participants age 50 years and older. *Diabetes.* 2003;52(5):1210–14.

24. Rochlani Y, Pothineni NV, Kovelamudi S, Mehta JL. Metabolic syndrome: pathophysiology, management, and modulation by natural compounds. *Ther Adv Cardiovasc Dis.* 2017;11(8):215–25. doi:10.1177/1753944717711379.

25. Samson SL, Garber AJ. Metabolic syndrome. *Endocrinol Metab Clin North Am.* 2014;43(1):1–23. doi:10.1016/j.ecl.2013.09.009.

26. Osadnik K, Osadnik T, Lonnie M, et al. Metabolically healthy obese and metabolic syndrome of the lean: the importance of diet quality. Analysis of MAGNETIC cohort. *Nutr J.* 2020;19(1):19. doi:10/1186/s12937-020-00532-0.

27. Park S, Lee S, Kim Y, et al. Altered risk for cardiovascular events with changes in the metabolic syndrome status: a nationwide population-based study of approximately 10 million persons. *Ann Intern Med.* 2019;171:875–84. doi:10.7326/M19-0563.

24 Nutrition/Diet Counseling and Education

Anne Roland Lee

24.1 INTRODUCTION

Historically, diet counseling had involved a rushed 2-minute diet instruction as the patient was being discharged from the hospital. We have since come to realize that the "drive-through" diet instruction does not allow for any assessment of the patient's needs or the ability to tailor the education and counseling to maximize adherence. In today's social media-influenced world, patients will seek information from many different sources. Unfortunately, not all of them are science- or evidence-based information. Often patients, especially those with undiagnosed gastrointestinal disorders, seek answers online when they fail to find them from their medical practitioner. With the increase in popularity of many restrictive diets, such as the gluten-free diet (GFD), it is imperative that patients with gastrointestinal disorders be managed by a team approach including a registered dietitian (RD) (1). It is strongly recommended that nutrition counseling shifts from the strict "one-size-fits-all" paradigm to a holistic and personalized medicine approach. Indeed, the process has shifted from one that just acquires knowledge to one that evaluates multiple factors in the client's life (social, environmental, biological) that affect the individual's food choices and dietary behavior (2).

The practice of nutrition and diet counseling, or as it is now defined as medical nutrition therapy (MNT), involves four basic steps: assessment, nutrition diagnosis, intervention, and monitoring and evaluation. While counseling is often thought of as the main focus of the nutrition intervention, each step is vital to the efficacy of optimal nutrition care. As we go through the basic steps of the counseling process, we must be mindful that the goal of nutrition education is the adoption and maintenance of behaviors that facilitate health and well-being (2). A framework for nutrition education has been developed that incorporates behavioral theories into nutrition education practices (Figure 24.1). The framework also incorporates the stages of change, the determinants of one's behavior, and the social and environmental factors affecting food choices and beliefs. These factors inform the process in order to achieve the nutrition education goals. This process is effective for individual-, group-, and community-based nutrition education programs.

DOI: 10.1201/9780429322570-24

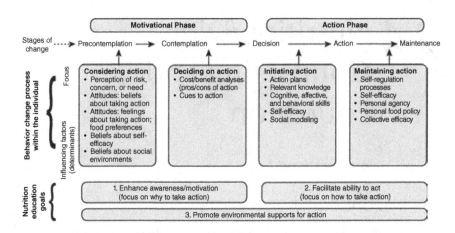

FIGURE 24.1   Conceptual framework for nutrition education.

Source: **Used with permission from I. Contento.**

24.2   PROCESS OF MEDICAL NUTRITION THERAPY (MNT)

MNT is a multidimensional process incorporating behavior theories, stages of change, and nutrition education fundamentals.

24.2.1   ASSESSMENT

The initial step in MNT is the assessment of the patient. This step is crucial whether it is the initial encounter with the patient or a follow-up. In both types of encounters, it is vital to obtain or update information pertaining to the patient's medical, psychosocial, and nutritional status. In the assessment there are six subcategories: food and nutrition history; anthropometric measures; biochemical data, medical tests, and procedures; nutrition-focused physical findings; patient history; and comparative standards.

24.2.2.1   Food and Nutrition-Related History

The food and nutrition-related history should include more than just the diet record. The food environment encompasses more than just what the individual eats. One should inquire about religious and cultural impacts on diet and intake, physical environment (college dorm/kitchen access), access to transportation to obtain food, and financial ability to obtain food. A diet recall is used to obtain good insight into the typical or usual meal pattern. To obtain detailed information on portion sizes, brands of food, snack behaviors, and other facets of the intake, a multiple pass diet recall is encouraged. The multiple pass method allows for further questions and probing on things, such as condiments added, any supplements used, cultural and religious beliefs and their impact on usual intake, who prepares the meals, and how foods are prepared. In addition to the intake record, it is important to question all aspects of daily life that affect meals and health, including physical activity frequency and duration, medication use and corresponding medical condition, food allergies or intolerances, previous dietary restrictions and/or self-selected diets, food availability, and meal preparation facilities. Beyond the direct food-related queries, one should also investigate food security, the dietary impact on one's quality of life (QoL), family life, and the ability to socialize and travel.

24.2.2.2 Anthropometric Measures

Basic anthropometric measures provide physical data to assess the individual's current nutritional status as well as the data for future comparisons and assessment. Basic measurements should include height, weight, body mass index, and growth patterns/percentile ranks. A detailed weight history should include recent weight history as well as other factors that may affect weight, such as pregnancy, menopause, and major life changes (e.g., retirement). If available, the use of a scale with body composition detail would provide additional insight into changes in body composition and distribution over time.

24.2.2.3 Biochemical Data, Medical Tests, and Procedures

The assessment should include a detailed review of serology for macro- and micronutrient levels along with procedures including endoscopy and imaging.

24.2.2.4 Nutrition-Focused Physical Findings

This section would include results from the physical examination (e.g., edema, fat, or muscle wasting) and functional tests (e.g., hand grip strength, get up and go test). If the gastrointestinal tract is involved, consider if there is increased inflammation and explore the impact on the physical acts of chewing, swallowing, or drinking.

24.2.2.5 Patient History

In this section, we assess the patient's past medical, social, and family history noting the interrelationship between these areas of one's life and the influence on health perceptions, beliefs, and healthcare. The family and medical history should include a detailed account of the extended family and their medical history as well as their functional role in the family (Is the grandparent the primary caretaker for the children while the parents work? Who is included in the family unit sharing meals? Is there more than one medical condition that must be accommodated?). In reviewing a family history, details of relevant medical conditions, follow-up testing, and ongoing care should be queried.

In addition to family history, the medical history, social history, as well as the financial and educational background of the patient should be assessed. Financial queries would include the use of Supplemental Nutrition Assistance Program (SNAP), Women, Infants, and Children (WIC) nutrition program, free school lunch, and access to food markets in the community.

Assessing the various aspects of our patients' lives will guide the recommendations for dietary intervention. The education level of the patient will also inform the RD to align the education process, resources, and materials to match the patient's needs and abilities.

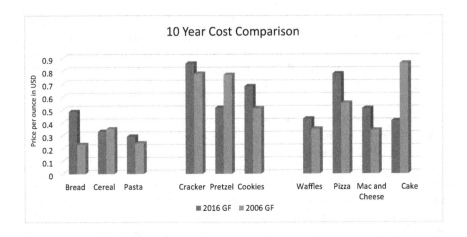

24.2.2.6   Comparative Standards

Upon completion of the full assessment, it is important to establish the patient's nutrient needs, including estimated energy, fiber, vitamin, and mineral needs. Additionally, recommendations based on body mass index (BMI), weight, and growth pattern goals should be determined.

24.2.2   NUTRITION DIAGNOSIS

According to the Academy of Nutrition and Dietetics (AND), the nutrition diagnosis describes the patient's nutrition status. A nutrition diagnosis is different from a medical diagnosis. The nutrition diagnosis is not necessarily a fixed diagnosis and should change as the patient responds to MNT. MNT should identify realistic outcomes, specific individualized interventions, with ongoing evaluation and monitoring. There are three components to a nutrition diagnosis: impact of intake, clinical or functional factors, and behavioral/environmental factors. Examples of an intake-driven diagnosis would include inadequate intake of micro- or macronutrients. A clinical-driven diagnosis would include altered metabolic status, impaired nutrient utilization, and weight status. A behavior- or environment-driven diagnosis would include resistance to dietary interventions or environmental or financial inability to adapt dietary interventions.

24.2.3   INTERVENTION

Nutrition intervention includes the nutrition prescription, which encompasses more than just the specific dietary modifications needed. There are four domains of nutrition prescription and intervention: food or nutrient delivery, nutrition education, nutrition counseling, and coordination of care. While the food and nutrient delivery section is usually a defined diet based on clinical diagnosis (e.g., low fermentable, oligo-, di-, monosaccharides, and polyols [FODMAP] diet for irritable bowel syndrome [IBS]), the nutrition education and counseling sections should be individualized to the patient's as well as the RD's abilities. If the RD does not feel comfortable with using motivational interviewing or incorporating behavioral theories, such as cognitive behavior therapy or stages of change, then use of collaborative care or referral to a skilled RD or a community agency is vital. The use of different theoretical models and counseling approaches allows the RD to provide a supportive, collaborative patient–counselor partnership to identify goals, formulate a directed strategy, and set realistic and measurable outcomes. This collaborative approach allows for a more global nutrition intervention, encompassing the domains of QoL and the individual's readiness and stage of change. It also provides supportive and knowledgeable nutrition guidance. The process allows open communication with the patient to discuss barriers of implementing a dietary change, such as anxiety, difficulty in dietary adherence in social situations, impact of symptoms on intimacy, potential negative effects of a rigid dietary regime (food avoidance behavior, disordered eating patterns), and emotional issues affecting QoL. Is the patient experiencing isolation, shame, or embarrassment? Are they experiencing frustration with navigating dietary restrictions within the work place or school? Do they have family and social support? The counselor–patient partnership also allows for time for processing and adjusting to the varied emotional and psychosocial aspects of a diet prescription. Patients' feelings can range from mourning, loss of control, anger, and anxiety to relief. Utilizing the different counseling approaches, the RD will help the patient navigate through these difficult situations.

The RD needs to counsel beyond diet and nutrients. There is the need to guide the patient on how to take ownership of the diagnosis and the treatment plan. The counseling should guide the patient to identify their barriers and support systems. The RD needs to help the patient identify the feelings associated when they encounter these barriers and identify strategies to navigate nutritionally as well as emotionally. For children in particular, counseling should include all family members that participate in the child's care. Guidance should be provided to ensure safety at school as well as avoiding situations of bullying associated with being different due to diet or diagnosis.

As many gastrointestinal disorders (e.g., IBS, celiac disease [CeD], small intestinal bacterial overgrowth [SIBO], eosinophilic esophagitis [EOE]) strongly rely on modified diets as part of their ongoing therapy, a holistic approach to nutrition counseling is important. In a study by Lee and colleagues (3), QoL was significantly impacted in individuals on a GFD. The negative impact was found to be most strongly associated with the social domain of QoL, such as dining out, social events, work-related meals, and travel. In a study by Cranney and colleagues (4), 81% of individuals reported that they no longer dine out, 91% brought their own food when traveling, and 38% avoided travel due to the difficulty of maintaining a GFD. This negative impact may have further-reaching psychological impact, including anxiety, depression, and eating disorders (5, 6).

24.2.4 MONITORING AND EVALUATION

The final step of MNT is not a finite final step, but rather a long-term ongoing process of evaluating progress and measuring outcomes. This phase of MNT should be an ongoing active phase enabling the patient to reach their desired outcome goals and providing ongoing support to maintain the prescribed outcomes. Additionally, because we are often implementing lifelong diet therapies, which restrict certain food groups in gastrointestinal disorders, there is the need to evaluate long-term effects of diet on health. Table 24.1 lists dietary considerations for various gastrointestinal disorders (7).

TABLE 24.1
Nutritional Considerations in Gastrointestinal Disorders (7)

Gastrointestinal Condition	Counseling & Education

Celiac Disease
Non-Celiac Gluten
  Sensitivity
	• Gluten-free diet
	• Avoid wheat, barley, rye, and malt
	• Avoid oats (unless labeled gluten-free)
	• Nutrients of concern:
	  • B vitamins, iron, and fiber
	  • Calcium, vitamin D

Constipation	• Increase fiber gradually and consume consistently • Use whole grains over refined grains • Add fruits, vegetables, and legumes; especially prunes and kiwifruit • Consider addition of wheat bran, wheat germ, rice bran, or flax meal • Adequate hydration
Diarrhea	• Limit foods and beverages that are high in sugar, sugar alcohols, lactose, and fructose • Avoid caffeine • Avoid spicy foods if they make symptoms worse • Small, frequent meals • Nutrients of concern: • Zinc, selenium

Eosinophilic Esophagitis	• Elimination diet process:
	  • Elimination phase
	  • Reintroduction phase
	• Top six allergen groups:
	  • Milk
	  • Soy
	  • Eggs
	  • Wheat
	  • Peanuts/tree nuts
	  • Seafood
	• Nutrients of concern depend on allergen group eliminated

Fructose Intolerance	• Low-fructose diet • Limit fructose, high fructose corn syrup, honey, molasses, agave, sorbitol, and other sugar alcohols • Limit high-fructose fruits and vegetables

TABLE 24.1 (*Continued*)
Nutritional Considerations in Gastrointestinal Disorders (7)

Gastrointestinal Condition	Counseling & Education

Gastroesophageal Reflux Disease	• Small, frequent meals
	• Sit down while eating
	• Wear loose-fitting clothes
	• Do not smoke
	• Avoid alcohol and non-steroidal anti-inflammatory drugs (NSAIDs)
	• Raise the head of your bed
	• Wait 3 hours after eating before lying down
	• Consider limiting/eliminating:
	  • Spicy foods
	  • Citrus fruits and juices
	  • Fatty, greasy, or fried foods
	  • Peppermint/spearmint
	  • Chocolate
	  • Caffeine
	  • Raw onions, garlic, or black pepper
	  • Carbonated beverages

Gastroparesis	• Small, frequent meals • Spread out intake of fat and fiber • Reduce acid reflux triggers • Limit carbonated beverages • Chew foods well • Liquids may be better tolerated • Drink fluids between meals

Inflammatory Bowel Disease	• Fiber intake depends on symptoms and severity of inflammation
	• Small, frequent meals
	• Adequate protein intake
	• Adequate hydration
	• Consider nutrient supplementation if inflammation or medications interfere with nutrient absorption:
	  • Multivitamin with minerals, including Iron
	  • Folic acid
	  • Calcium, vitamin D
	  • Vitamin B12, vitamin B6, zinc

Irritable Bowel Syndrome	• Eat meals on a regular schedule
	• Adequate fiber and fluid intake
	• Consider limiting high-fat foods
	• Low-FODMAP diet
	  • Elimination phase
	  • Challenge phase
	  • Personalization phase

Lactose Intolerance	• Low-lactose diet • Consider limiting or avoiding dairy products • Consider taking lactase supplements prior to dairy intake • Nutrients of concern: • Calcium, vitamin D

(*Continued*)

TABLE 24.1 (*Continued*)

Nutritional Considerations in Gastrointestinal Disorders (7)

Gastrointestinal Condition	Counseling & Education
Nausea/Vomiting	• Avoid foods with strong odors; cold or room temperature foods tend to have fewer odors • Try dry, starchy, or salty foods • Small, frequent meals • Limit high-fat and high-fiber foods • Adequate hydration

Ostomy	• After surgery, avoid high-fiber foods
	• Chew food slowly and well
	• Eat the largest meal in the middle of the day to decrease stool output overnight
	• Avoid acidic, spicy, greasy, and high-sugar foods that can cause diarrhea
	• Bananas, applesauce, rice, and pasta can help thicken stools
	• Limit foods that may cause gas or odor
	• To reduce gas, avoid chewing gum, drinking with straws, carbonated beverages, eating too fast, and skipping meals
	• Adequate hydration
	• Reintroduce fiber gradually as tolerated
	• Nutrients of concern:
	• Use a chewable (non-gummy) multivitamin with minerals
	  • Use a liquid calcium supplement
	  • Sodium, potassium

Pancreatitis	• Limit fat intake to 25–30% of calories • Consider choosing softer foods • Avoid alcohol • Consider pancreatic enzymes before each meal or as prescribed by your doctor • Nutrients of concern: • Fat-soluble vitamins (A, D, E, K)

Short Bowel Syndrome	• Small, frequent meals
	• Chew foods well
	• Drink fluids in between meals
	• Eat salty foods and use table salt frequently, especially if colon removed
	• Avoid foods and drinks high in sugar
	• Avoid stimulants such as caffeine and alcohol
	• Limit sugar alcohols
	• If colon intact:
	  • Choose a diet that is high in complex carbohydrates, low to moderate in fat, and adequate in protein
	  • Eat foods with soluble fiber or take a soluble fiber supplement
	  • Limit foods high in oxalate to reduce risk of kidney stones

TABLE 24.1 (*Continued*)
Nutritional Considerations in Gastrointestinal Disorders (7)

Gastrointestinal Condition	Counseling & Education
	If colon removed:
	• Choose a diet that is moderate in complex carbohydrate, moderate to high in fat, and adequate in protein
	• Adequate hydration: consider oral rehydration solution (ORS)
	• Nutrients of concern:
	• Calcium, vitamin D
	• Vitamin B12
	• Fat-soluble vitamins (A, D, E, K)
	• Magnesium, iron, copper
	• Zinc, selenium
Small Intestinal Bacterial Overgrowth (SIBO)	• Consider dietary treatments as indicated:
	• Low-FODMAP diet
	• Nutrients of concern:
	• Vitamin B12, niacin, thiamine
	• Iron
	• Fat-soluble vitamins (A, D, E)

Because diet recommendations for many gastrointestinal disorders (e.g., IBS, EOE, SIBO) restrict wheat, grains, fruits, and beans, we can use the literature on the nutritional concerns of the GFD as a model to demonstrate the need for ongoing monitoring of patients' nutritional status. One study found that many of the gluten-free products were not enriched, fortified, or naturally rich sources of folate, iron, and fiber (8). A study by Thompson and colleagues found that 37% of males and 79% of females did not meet the recommended amount of grain servings per day (9). Additionally, only 44% of female participants met their recommended intake of iron, only 46% met their recommended intake of fiber, and only 31% met their recommended intake of calcium.

Many of the nutrients lacking in the GFD are found in ancient or alternative grains. One study reviewed the impact of substituting only the grain choices of the standard GFD pattern (10). The consumption patterns of study participants were similar to Thompson's findings (9), which showed that the intake of individuals following a GFD pattern did not meet the criteria for the United States Department of Agriculture (USDA) meal or snack pattern.

The "alternate dietary pattern" substituted a higher nutrient profile grain or grain product at each meal. The change in dietary grains significantly improved the nutrient profile including increases in protein, iron, calcium, and fiber. However, in a follow-up study of grain consumption patterns, Lee and colleagues found that while the overall intake of gluten-free whole grains increased, the grains added were in an ultra-processed form (11). The most frequent processed and ultra-processed products included GF breads, bagels, cold cereals, and granola-type bars. These findings highlight the importance of nutrition monitoring and ongoing evaluation.

24.2.5 Tip Box

Encourage your patients to add the ancient grains for added nutrition!

Grain	Nutrients
Amaranth	Protein, fiber, iron, magnesium, zinc, calcium, B vitamins
Buckwheat	Protein, magnesium, B6, fiber, iron, niacin, thiamin, zinc
Millet	Protein, fiber
Oats	Protein, fiber, folate, vitamin E, zinc
Quinoa	Iron, magnesium, B vitamins, calcium, fiber
Sorghum	Fiber, iron
Teff	Protein, calcium, iron, B vitamins
Wild Rice	Fiber, protein, potassium, zinc

24.2.6 Novel Approaches

The use of telehealth may be considered a novel approach to nutrition counseling. Video visits allow the RD to instruct and guide the patient within the comfort of their home. It further allows for an interactive approach to reading labels, nutrition facts, and checking ingredients of the products on their own kitchen shelves. Nevertheless, underserved patients remain underserved due to the limited availability of technology; videoconferencing requires a smartphone, a home Internet connection, and a private room to have a conversation about personal matters. Another relatively modern approach is the use of group classes (online or in person) that allow patients to gain knowledge as well as support from the RD and each other (12).

24.2.7 Incorrect/Outdated Practices

Cookie-cutter diet sheets, diet instructions as the patient is being discharged, or the "drive-through" diet instructions are considered suboptimal and outdated practices. These practices are now recognized as neither informative nor effective; they do not allow for adequate assessment of the patient's needs or the ability to tailor the education and counseling to maximize adherence.

PRACTICE PEARLS

- Carefully consider the medical nutrition therapy process: assessment, nutrition diagnosis, intervention, and monitoring and evaluation. Important facts can be uncovered by paying attention to details of the process.
- Assess patient's medical, nutritional, and emotional needs in depth, which could include key factors of daily life (e.g., who cooks, issues of food security, education level).
- Multiple sessions are important, using telehealth if necessary for some of the follow-up visits.
- Allow time for human connection and dialog.

REFERENCES

1. National Institutes of Health Consensus Development Conference Statement. June 2004. https://consensus.nih.gov/2004/2004CeliacDisease118html.htm. Accessed April 25, 2018.

2. Contento IR. Nutrition Education; Linking Research, Theory, and Practice. 2nd edition. Burlington, MA: Jones & Bartlett Publishers Sudbury; 2011.

3. Lee AR, Diamond B, Ng D. Ciaccio E, Green PHR. Quality of life of individuals with celiac disease; Survey results from the United States. Journal of Hum Nutr Diet. 2012;25:233–238.

4. Cranney A, Zarkadas M, Graham ID, Butzner JD., Rashid M, Warren R, Molly M, Case S, Burrows V, Switzer C. The Canadian celiac health survey. Dig Dis Sci. 2007;52: 1087–1095.

5. Hauser W, Janke K-H, Klump B, Gregor M, Hinz A. Anxiety and depression in adult patients with celiac disease on a gluten free diet. World J Gastroenterol. 2012;16(22):2780–2787.

6. Wagner G, Zeiler M, Berger G, Huber WD, Favaro A, Santonastaso P, Karwautz A. Eating disorders in adolescents with celiac disease: Influence of personality characteristics and coping. Eur Eat Disor Review. 2015;23(5): 361–370.

7. Nutrition Care Manual. www.nutritioncaremanual.org/category.cfm?ncm_category_id=1&ncm_heading=Meal Plans&client_ed=1. Accessed March 23, 2020.

8. Thompson T. Folate, iron, and dietary fiber content of the gluten free diet. J Am Diet Assoc. 2000;100:1389–1393.

9. Thompson T, Dennis M, Higgins LA, Lee AR, Sharrett MK. Gluten-free diet survey: Are Americans with coeliac disease consuming recommended amounts of fibre, iron, calcium and grain foods? J Hum Nutr Diet. 2005;18:163–169.

10. Lee AR, Ng DL, Dave EJ, Ciaccio E, Green PHR. The effect of substituting alternative grains in the diet on the nutritional profile of the gluten-free diet. J Hum Nutr Diet. 2009;22:359–363.

11. Lee AR, Wolf RL, Lebwohl B, Zybert P, Green PHR. Alternative grain intake among adults with celiac disease: A prospective cross sectional study. Presented at DDW 2018.

12. Rej A, Trott N, Kurien M, Branchi F, Richman E, Subramanian S, Sanders DS. Is peer support in group clinics as effective as traditional individual appointments? The first study in patients with celiac disease. Clin Transl Gastroenterol. 2020 Jan;11(1):e00121.

25 Popular Diets for Gastroenterology

Neha D. Shah and Therezia AlChoufete

25.1 INTRODUCTION

Patients diagnosed with a gastrointestinal (GI) disorder may engage in restrictive food patterns as an effort to alleviate symptoms. The presence of GI symptoms may also lead to food aversions and thus to an impaired relationship with the diet. Nutritional impairments of unintentional weight loss, macro/micronutrient deficiencies, and sarcopenia may result as consequences. Patients attempting to follow a diet without supervision and guidance or deemed at risk for nutritional impairments should be referred to a registered dietitian (RD) specializing in GI disorders for a formal evaluation of nutrition status and for nutrition education and counseling. The evaluation assists to identify problematic weight trends, GI symptoms, nutrition patterns, and knowledge deficits to help determine interventions.

The dietitian will evaluate the indications of the diet for appropriateness as well as for nutritional adequacy for optimization. Nutrition education involves reducing knowledge deficits where present. Nutrition counseling utilizes personalized strategies for motivational interviewing and behavioral modification based on readiness to change to help the patient follow and build trust with the diet while aiming to accommodate tolerance, preferences, access, culture, and lifestyle (see Chapter 24). Engaging the patient's input throughout the process for collaboration is important to reduce barriers and optimize outcomes. Resources (e.g., food lists, meal ideas, recipes) should be provided as appropriate. Ongoing evaluation of progress with diet and nutrition status may involve an evaluation for changes in weight status, symptoms, tolerance, and in overall macro/micronutrient intake to learn of improvements and to address concerns. All food groups with personalized portions, frequency, and consistency are encouraged for consumption to promote nutritional adequacy.

This chapter will review popular diets used in gastroenterology, the evidence of claims made by these diets, and practical applications for their use in GI disorders.

25.2 LOW-FIBER DIET

Dietary fiber is a non-digestible carbohydrate found in plant-based foods such as fruits, vegetables, grains, legumes, and nuts. There are varying definitions of fiber in the literature. To standardize the definition of fiber, the Institute of Medicine (IOM) proposed the following definitions for fiber:[1]

DOI: 10.1201/9780429322570-25

- *Dietary fiber*: Defined as "non-digestible carbohydrates and lignin that are intrinsic and intact in plants"
- *Added fiber*: Defined as "isolated, non-digestible carbohydrates that have beneficial physiological effects in humans"
- *Total fiber*: Defined as "a combination of dietary and added fiber"

The physiological benefits that fiber may contribute to GI health are determined by the type and physical properties of fiber (Table 25.1).[2]

Physical properties for fiber include solubility, fermentability, and viscosity, which all determine how fiber may function within the GI tract. The physical properties of fiber are considered when developing interventions for the therapeutic use of fiber to address GI symptoms, particularly altered stool consistency, frequency, and urgency. The use of fiber has also garnered interest due to its favorable effects on the composition and diversity of the gut microbiome for overall health. The IOM has set Dietary Reference Intakes (DRIs) for daily fiber intake for children, adolescents, and adults (Table 25.2).[3] The recommendations are meant for healthy individuals; it does not set guidelines for fiber intake in chronic disease.

TABLE 25.1
Properties of Fiber

	Properties	Types of Fiber
Solubility	Refers to what extent the fiber is able to be dissolved in fluids. Fiber is further characterized as soluble and insoluble fibers.	Soluble fibers: guar gum, pectin, glucans (e.g., cantaloupe, sweet potato, oatmeal) Insoluble fibers: cellulose (e.g., skins of fruits/vegetables, celery, brown rice, nuts)
Fermentability	Refers to what extent bacteria residing in the colon can digest fiber. Fermentation of fiber by colonic bacteria results in production of short-chain fatty acids. Fiber is further characterized as fermentable and non-fermentable fibers. Many fermentable fibers are also soluble. Many non-fermentable fibers are insoluble.	Fermentable fibers: acacia gum, guar gum, pectin, glucans, inulin, fructans, galactans (e.g., beans, cauliflower, stone fruits, wheat) Non-fermentable fibers: cellulose (e.g., celery, flax, spinach, wheat bran)
Viscosity	Refers to what extent the fiber can thicken fluids. Fiber is further characterized as viscous and non-viscous fibers. Many viscous fibers are soluble and fermentable. Many non-viscous fibers can also be insoluble and may or may not be fermentable.	Viscous fibers: guar gum, pectin, glucans (e.g., banana, oat bran) Non-viscous fibers: acacia gum, cellulose, partially hydrolyzed guar gum, inulin, fructans, galactans (e.g., lentils, asparagus, rye)

TABLE 25.2
Dietary Reference Intakes for Daily Fiber Intake

Years of Age	Males	Females
Children		
1–3	19 grams of fiber	19 grams of fiber
4–8	25 grams of fiber	25 grams of fiber
9–13	31 grams of fiber	26 grams of fiber
Adolescents		
14–18	38 grams of fiber	26 grams of fiber
Adults		
19–50	38 grams of fiber	25 grams of fiber
>50	30 grams of fiber	21 grams of fiber

Although definitions and recommendations for intake exist for fiber, the definition of a low-fiber diet remains unclear regarding what type and quantity of fiber to consume. A few studies set a daily intake of 10 grams of fiber for the low-fiber diets used in the study.[4, 5] However, the studies did not indicate the type of fiber restricted. It is also unclear whether specific GI disorders may benefit from restrictions of a particular type of fiber. Foods commonly restricted in the diet are skins of fruits and vegetables, prunes, raw vegetables, whole grains, legumes, and nuts. Nutritional adequacy can be a concern for folic acid, vitamin C, and potassium with the restrictions. Animal-based foods such as meats, poultry, fish, eggs, and dairy are allowed for consumption, since there is minimal fiber in these foods.

The low-fiber diet has been traditionally used in management of gastroparesis, inflammatory bowel disease (IBD), intestinal strictures, and small bowel obstruction (SBO). In gastroparesis, fiber is thought to further delay gastric emptying and is therefore restricted.[6] The research is limited though with what type of fiber to restrict in gastroparesis. Restricting fiber in gastroparesis has also been recommended to reduce risk of phytobezoars, which is an accumulation of skins, seeds, and leaves of fruits and vegetables.[7] Fruits and vegetables that may contribute to a formation of a phytobezoar are apples, berries, persimmons, brussels sprouts, and potato skins. In IBD, the diet has been used to reduce stool output and frequency of bowel movements during active disease.[8] The studies are very limited and the diet overall has not demonstrated efficacy in IBD.[9] In intestinal strictures and SBO, the diet has been used to reduce risk of blockage that may potentially arise with excess bulk passing through a narrowed segment of small bowel. However, there are minimal studies for the use of the diet in SBO.

25.2.1 PRACTICAL APPLICATIONS

A reduction in fiber intake can be considered in the treatment and management of gastroparesis to reduce potential aggravation of delayed gastric emptying. Although there are minimal studies to support the use of the diet in intestinal strictures and

SBO, it makes practical sense to use the diet for less insoluble fiber that may contribute to bulk to reduce risk of blockage.

The rationale and evidence for the low-fiber diet should be discussed with the patient. Educational key points may also include a review of definitions, function, types, and/or food sources of fiber. The consistency of foods with fiber can be modified into a blended, mashed, or chopped consistency as needed to improve tolerance. Inclusion of small portions versus large portions of fiber at meals may also assist with tolerance.

25.3 LOW-RESIDUE DIET

The low-residue diet also restricts fiber. In contrast to the low-fiber diet, the low-residue diet may also restrict other non-fiber foods that are considered to be residue (Table 25.3).

There are varying definitions of residue used in the literature:

- Residue has been referred to as the appearance of stool after consumption of foods.[10]
- Any food that contributed to an increase in stool was also deemed to be residue.[10]
- Residue has also been referred to as crude fiber. Crude fiber in the form of cellulose, hemicellulose, and lignin are restricted in the low-residue diet.[11]

TABLE 25.3
Comparisons of the Low-Fiber Diet to the Low-Residue Diet

	Foods Allowed	Foods Restricted
Low-Fiber Diet (Restricts only fiber)	Meats	Whole grains
	Poultry	ran
	Fish	Prunes
	Shellfish	Fruit and vegetable skins
	Eggs	Raw vegetables
	Dairy	Legumes
	Refined grains	Nuts
	Oatmeal	
	Peeled or blended fruits	
	Cooked or blended vegetables	
	Creamy nut butters	
Low-Residue Diet (Restricts fiber and other non-plant-based foods)	Meat	Soft-boiled egg
	Hard-boiled egg	Whole grains
	Cottage cheese	Bran
	Rice	Milk
	Banana	Most fruits and vegetables
	Melon	Potato
	Refined grains	Legumes
		Nuts
		Butter

Early animal studies determined that fruits, potatoes, bread, lard, butter, Swiss cheese, soft boiled eggs, and milk produced the highest residue. The foods that produced the least amount of residue was gelatin, sugar, broth, hard boiled eggs, meat, liver, rice, and cottage cheese.[10]

The studies are very limited in GI disorders. The low-residue diet has been used to decrease stool output during active flares in IBD.[12] The diet has also been used as a method for bowel preparation for a colon cleanse prior to a colonoscopy. The most common bowel preparations used are magnesium citrate and polyethylene glycol. Adherence, however, is challenging to patients who find the bowel preparation difficult to complete. The diet has been shown in some studies to be comparable or superior to a clear liquid diet in its efficacy (Table 25.4).[13–15] Many of the foods restricted in the low-residue diet used for bowel preparation are also low in fiber.

TABLE 25.4
Snapshot of Studies Evaluating the Low-Residue Diet

Inflammatory Bowel Disease

- A study of 70 Italian adult patients with non-stricturing Crohn's disease randomized patients to either follow the low-residue diet or a normal Italian diet for 29 months. The low-residue diet used in the study removed whole grains and most fruits and vegetables from the diet with the exception of bananas and peeled potatoes. Patients were allowed to consume dairy in both groups. The results showed no differences in outcomes between the two groups, including any symptoms, indications for hospitalizations or surgery, complications, and nutritional status. Reintroduction of fiber was also tolerated well.[12]

Bowel Preparation prior to Colonoscopy

- A single-blind, prospective study randomized 230 adult patients to follow a clear liquid diet or a low-residue diet along with split dose oral sulfate solution a day before the colonoscopy. Patients assigned to follow the diet were allowed to choose one of three packaged meal plans. The low-residue diet primarily included eggs, yogurt, cottage cheese, chicken or turkey sandwiches using refined grains, and macaroni and cheese. The diet did not include any fruits or vegetables (with the exception of potato). The results overall showed that the patients had significantly higher satisfaction scores with the low-residue diet and there were no significant differences between the two groups of its efficacy for bowel preparation.[13]
- A single-blind study of 173 adult patients randomized the patients into two groups with one group receiving a bowel preparation of two liters of polyethylene glycol and the other group receiving one liter of polyethylene glycol with a meal kit of low-residue foods. Foods included for the diet were mussel porridge, bean paste soup, vegetable porridge, miso soup, corn soup, and orange/apple juice. The results showed that the group that received one liter of the polyethylene glycol along with low-residue foods (93%) showed similar efficacy with bowel preparation as the other group (88%) and also had higher satisfaction scores overall.[14]
- In a single-blind study of 215 patients, patients were randomized to receive a clear liquid diet or receive the low-residue diet along with a split-dose magnesium citrate preparation. The low-residue diet included meal plans from the study by Sipes et al. The results showed no significant differences in efficacy. When compared with the clear liquid diet, there were also significantly higher satisfaction scores with the low-residue diet.[15]

25.3.1 PRACTICAL APPLICATIONS

The low-residue diet is a restrictive diet due to near elimination of fiber and other non-plant based foods. Upon comparison of both the low-residue and low-fiber diets, the low-fiber diet has a greater variety of foods permitted for consumption. Any reintroduction of fiber and other foods that have been initially excluded should be commenced initially with small portions, starting with one meal in the week and eventually progressing towards multiple meals in the day.

25.4 LOW-FODMAP DIET

FODMAPs (fermentable oligosaccharides, disaccharides, monosaccharides, and polyols) are short-chain fermentable carbohydrates found in plant-based foods. The FODMAPs in the diet consist of fructans, galactans, lactose, fructose, and polyols.[16]

- *Fructans and galactans*: Oligosaccharides that are non-digestible by humans and are found in wheat, barley, rye, garlic, onion, beans, and lentils
- *Lactose*: A disaccharide with glucose and galactose and found in dairy
- *Fructose*: Monosaccharide found in fruits and honey
- *Polyols*: Sugar alcohols found in stone fruits and artificial sweeteners

Excess consumption of FODMAPs may contribute to symptoms of abdominal pain, altered bowel habits, gas, and bloating due to its osmotic effects in the small bowel. Once FODMAPs enter the colon, they may undergo bacterial fermentation resulting in excess gas production. The low-FODMAP diet is not meant to be followed long term. There are three phases of the diet: elimination, reintroduction, and personalization.[17]

- The elimination phase eliminates high FODMAPs from the diet over 2–4 weeks. During this phase, all foods high in FODMAPs are removed from the diet. Consumption of low FODMAPs and moderate FODMAPs in appropriate portions are allowed.
- The reintroduction phase adds high-FODMAP foods back into the diet over 6–8 weeks to help identify intolerance to specific FODMAPs. The reintroduction phase consists of doing trials of a high-FODMAP food in increasing portions over three days. What FODMAPs to start with is individualized. The low-FODMAP diet continues along with the trials of high-FODMAP foods.
- The personalization phase involves individualizing the diet for tolerance and variety for the long term. FODMAPs that are not tolerated well should be consumed in small portions and not daily.

The studies on the low-FODMAP diet have been primarily done in irritable bowel syndrome (IBS) and have shown significant reduction in functional symptoms of abdominal pain and bloating with implementation of the diet.[18, 19] Symptom resolution has been seen in 4 weeks of following the elimination phase of the diet. There are very limited studies on the nutritional adequacy of the diet with the few studies reporting a lower fiber, iron, and calcium intake.[20] There are also studies, although very limited, in IBD indicating that the diet may help to reduce functional symptoms in patients with IBD that have concurrent IBS (Table 25.5).[21–23] Further studies are warranted to assess long-term impact on symptoms and nutrition status.

TABLE 25.5
Snapshot of Studies Evaluating the Low-FODMAP Diet

Irritable Bowel Syndrome

- A randomized-controlled study of 92 patients with IBS-predominant diarrhea compared the effect of the low-FODMAP diet with the modified National Institute for Health and Care Excellence (mNICE) guidelines. To assist with randomization, the patients were initially screened for two weeks for an abdominal pain score of 4 or more using an 11-point rating scale and for stool consistency of Type 5 or more on the Bristol Stool Scale. They were then randomized to follow either the low-FODMAP diet (n = 45) or the mNICE diet (n = 39) for 4 weeks. The results showed patients reported a significant reduction in abdominal pain (51%) with the low-FODMAP diet when compared to the mNICE diet (23%). Improvement in bloating, consistency, frequency, and urgency of bowel movements was also seen.[18]
- A meta-analysis of 6 randomized controlled trials and 6 cohort studies found that the low-FODMAP diet significantly reduced abdominal pain and bloating. No significant differences were found in stool consistency.[19]

Inflammatory Bowel Disease

- An early pilot study of 72 adult patients with active IBD (n = 52 for Crohn's disease, n = 20 for ulcerative colitis) that followed the diet for 3 months showed that the low-FODMAP diet helped reduce abdominal pain, bloating, and diarrhea, but not for constipation. The gastrointestinal tract was not assessed for changes in inflammation.[21]
- A randomized-controlled open label study of 89 adult patients in clinical remission or have mild-moderate disease activity with IBD (n = 28 for Crohn's disease, n = 61 for ulcerative colitis) had the patients that met the Rome III criteria for IBS-like symptoms follow a low-FODMAP diet or a normal diet for 6 weeks. Patients completed the IBS Symptom Severity System and Short IBD Quality of Life questionnaire in the first week and in week 6 of the diets. Patients that were on the low-FODMAP diet experienced a significant reduction in symptoms (81%) than the patients that did not (46%), especially for those in clinical remission. A significant improvement in quality of life was also seen.[22]
- A double-blind, randomized, placebo-controlled study evaluated symptoms with re-introduction of FODMAPs in 29 adult IBD patients in remission (n = 12 for Crohn's disease, n = 17 for ulcerative colitis). The patients were randomized to a 3-day challenge with fructans, galactans, sorbitol, and glucose placebo-containing beverages; with each challenge separated by a washout period. The Global Symptom Question survey was utilized to assess adequate relief from symptoms. The results showed 62% of the patients on the fructan challenge had a significant reduction in adequate relief and had more pain, gas, bloating, and urgency. There were no significant differences found between challenges for galactans, sorbitol, and the glucose placebo, with all patients reporting adequate relief.[23]

25.4.1 Practical Applications

It is reasonable for patients diagnosed with IBS to attempt the low-FODMAP diet to alleviate symptoms. Patients with eating disorders are not appropriate for the diet due to potential psychological implications of following a restrictive diet.

Nutrition education for the diet may include its rationale, what FODMAPs exist in the diet, how FODMAPs interact with GI tract, and food sources for FODMAPs (Table 25.6).

TABLE 25.6

Food Sources for Low, Moderate, and High FODMAPs (Sample)

The diet is not meant to be followed long term and there are three Phases of the diet.
- Elimination phase: 2–6 weeks to eliminate all high-FODMAP foods
- Reintroduction phase: 6–8 weeks for reintroduction of high FODMAPs while continuing the low-FODMAP diet
- Personalization phase: Ongoing liberalization of diet based on tolerance

Low FODMAPs

Protein	Dairy	Grains	Fruits	Vegetables
Meat	Lactose-free dairy	Buckwheat	Blueberries	Bell peppers
Poultry	Cheddar cheese	Corn tortillas	Cantaloupe	Bok choy
Fish	Colby cheese	Millet	Grapes	Carrots
Shellfish	Feta cheese	Oatmeal	Kiwi	Cucumbers
Eggs	Parmesan cheese	Polenta	Mandarin	Lettuce
Tofu	Swiss cheese	Quinoa	Orange	Potatoes
Nuts (e.g., chestnuts,	Almond milk	Rice	Passion fruit	Pumpkin
peanuts, pecan,	ice milk		Papaya	Radish
walnut)			Pineapple	Spinach
Nut butters			Raspberries	Tomato
			Rhubarb	Yam
			Strawberries	Zucchini

Moderate FODMAPs

½ cup canned chickpeas			½ grapefruit	½ beetroot
≤ ½ cup canned lentils			10 boysenberries	2 brussels sprouts
< 10 almonds			< three cherries	½ celery stalk
				1 cup canned artichoke hearts

High FODMAPs

Beans	Condensed milk	Wheat	Apple	Artichokes
Chickpeas	Evaporated milk	Barley	Apricot	Cauliflower
Lentils	Cottage cheese	Rye	Dates	Mushroom
Cashews	Ricotta cheese		Dried fruit	Sugar snap peas
Pistachios	Custard		Figs	Garlic
	Ice cream		Mango	Onion
	Yogurt		Nectarine	Inulin
			Pear	Chicory root
			Peach	
			Persimmon	
			Plum	
			Watermelon	

A discussion of the three phases of the diet should take place as well with the patient. A low-FODMAP food list should be reviewed with the patient. Although the diet restricts wheat, barley, and rye, which are all sources of gluten, the diet is not meant to be strictly gluten-free. Resources for low-FODMAP cookbooks, ready-made meals, and commercial food products are all available to help the patient implement the elimination phase successfully. The patient should have a start date for the diet to allow time for the patient to become familiar with the list of low-FOD-MAP foods and obtain suitable foods and resources. It is important to emphasize that the diet is not meant to be followed long term.

If the patient continues to have symptoms despite claiming adherence to the low-FODMAP diet, the diet should then undergo an evaluation to learn consumption of portions. Barriers are important to address as well, including challenges to access and finding alternatives. If symptoms continue despite adherence to the diet, then the diet should cease. If the patient has resolution of symptoms with the diet, the reintroduction phase may commence. It would be beneficial to have the patient record a food log to track foods reintroduced and symptoms occurring after consumption of foods to learn of patterns with problematic FODMAPs.

25.5   SPECIFIC CARBOHYDRATE DIET

The specific carbohydrate diet (SCD) aims to eliminate foods composed of disaccharides, oligosaccharides, and polysaccharides from the diet. Dr. Sidney Hass in the 1920s initially utilized the SCD to treat celiac disease. Elaine Gottschall, a Canadian biochemist, later outlined the diet in her book *Breaking the Vicious Cycle* in the late 1980s after her 8-year-old daughter with ulcerative colitis experienced symptom remission from implementation of the diet in the 1950s.[24] Her daughter continued to be symptom-free many years after transitioning off the diet. The premise of the diet is that carbohydrates that do not digest well undergo bacterial fermentation, which can contribute to inflammation and injury to the GI tract. Elimination of poorly digested carbohydrates will reduce bacterial fermentation and allow the GI tract to heal. Monosaccharides are the only source of carbohydrates permitted for consumption in the diet because monosaccharides do not require digestion. Foods referred to as "illegal foods" are not allowed on the SCD and consist of all grains, dairy with high lactose content, and foods sweetened with sucrose. The diet allows for legal foods of lactose-free dairy, fresh fruits, non-starchy vegetables, and honey as its main source of carbohydrates. The inclusion of fresh meats, poultry, fish, and eggs is also permitted (Table 25.7). The diet is followed for one year while symptoms resolve and then for another year to maintain symptom resolution. Reintroduction of illegal foods to liberalize the diet can commence afterwards. If there is a recurrence of symptoms, then the diet should be followed again until symptoms resolve.

Studies have primarily evaluated the SCD in children with Crohn's disease, showing resolution of symptoms and reduction in inflammatory markers.[25–27] With the exception of vitamin D and calcium, nutritional adequacy was present for riboflavin, niacin, pantothenic acid, vitamin B6, vitamin B12, biotin, vitamin A, vitamin C, and vitamin E in diets of pediatric patients following the diet.[28] The studies are less robust in adults (Table 25.8).[29, 30]

TABLE 25.7

Foods Allowed and Foods Not Allowed on the Specific Carbohydrate Diet

Protein	Dairy	Grains	Fruits	Vegetables
Foods Allowed				
Fresh meat	Cheddar cheese		Fresh or frozen	Fresh or frozen
Fresh poultry	Colby cheese		fruits	non-starchy
Fresh fish	Gruyere cheese		Canned fruit	vegetables
Fresh shellfish	Havarti cheese		packed in its own	
Eggs	Swiss cheese		juice	
Nuts (plain)	Lactose-free yogurt		Dried fruits without	
	(homemade)		added sugar	
Foods Not Allowed				
Canned meats	Buttermilk	All grains and	Fruits with a glaze	Canned
Bacon	Cottage cheese	their associated	Canned fruits with	vegetables
Hot dogs	Ricotta cheese	flours	added sugar	Corn
Pepperoni	Sour cream			Okra
Sausage				Potatoes
Salami				Seaweed
Soy				Tomato paste
Chickpeas				Yam
Fava beans				
Mung beans				
Nuts with added				
salt or added sugar				

25.5.1 PRACTICAL APPLICATIONS

It would be acceptable for the patient diagnosed with IBD to use the SCD as a component of medical management of IBD. It is not recommended that the patient completely forgo medical therapy in lieu of diet, since we have very limited evidence to support that diet alone can promote and sustain remission. The diet should be discontinued if the patient is experiencing nutritional impairments such as unintentional weight loss or macro/micronutrient deficiencies in the setting of the diet. Because the diet includes meat, poultry, fish, eggs, and lactose-free dairy as primary protein choices, the diet is not recommended for any patient that is a practicing vegan, since the diet will significantly limit options for protein.

A discussion should take place with the patient to review the premise of the diet, the current evidence, and what types of carbohydrates are allowed and not allowed in the diet. An SCD food list should be reviewed with the patient. SCD cookbooks are available for the patient to review recipes that are easy to prepare. The diet can be initiated once the patient has learned the list of foods appropriate for consumption and the resources for implementation.

TABLE 25.8

Snapshot of Studies Evaluating the Specific Carbohydrate Diet

Pediatrics

- In a small retrospective study of 7 pediatric patients with active Crohn's disease, the SCD was administered to patients for an average of 15 months without using immunosuppressant medications. The results showed that all symptoms resolved within 3 months of following the diet. Laboratory results also showed levels for serum albumin, C-reactive protein, hematocrit, and fecal calprotectin significantly improved or reached within normal limits for all patients.[25]
- In a small uncontrolled study of 9 pediatric patients with active Crohn's disease who followed the SCD for 12 weeks, there was a reduction in disease activity indices and improvement in mucosal healing based on readings of capsule endoscopy. Seven patients continued to follow the diet for another 52 weeks. Out of the 7 patients, 2 patients showed persistent mucosal healing. The results suggest that the diet could be used as treatment, although further studies are needed to assess efficacy for mucosal healing.[26]
- A small pediatric retrospective study of 11 patients with Crohn's disease in remission followed the SCD for a year. The patients showed a significant reduction in erythrocyte sedimentation rate and improvements in hematocrit and albumin levels with the diet. The improvements were maintained after liberalization of the diet.[27]

Adults

- From a survey in a case series, 66% of 50 adult patients with IBD in remission (n = 36 for Crohn's disease, n = 9 for ulcerative colitis, n = 5 for indeterminate colitis) that self-implemented the SCD showed clinical remission after following the diet for 10 months.[29]
- A web-based survey was sent to 417 adult patients with IBD (47% with Crohn's disease, 43% with ulcerative colitis, 10% with indeterminate colitis) following the SCD. The results showed that 33% of the patients perceived clinical remission after being on the diet for 2 months and 42% of the patients maintained clinical remission at 6 and 12 months. Patients overall see clinical benefit with utilizing the SCD.[30]

25.6 GLUTEN-FREE DIET

Gluten consists of storage proteins found in wheat (gliadin), barley (hordein), and rye (secalin). A gluten-free diet eliminates all foods, beverages, and nutrition supplements produced from these grains (e.g., breads, cereals, and pastas) from the diet. Foods permitted in the diet are gluten-free foods of fresh meats, poultry, fish, eggs, dairy, fruits, vegetables, and legumes (Table 25.9).

Grains and their associated flours are allowed as long as the grains are gluten-free, such as amaranth, bean, corn, quinoa, and rice. Some foods may appear to be gluten-free, such as marinades, salad dressings, soups, and sauces; however, hidden gluten could be used to flavor the foods and is not appropriate to eat. The Food Allergen Labeling and Consumer Protection of 2004 (FALCPA) under the Food and Drug Administration (FDA) requires disclosure of the top 8 major food allergens, including wheat, in all packaged foods, supplements (e.g., fiber, vitamins), infant formula, and medical foods.[31] The inclusion of a statement that the product is wheat-free does not indicate that it is also gluten-free. As of 2013, the term gluten-free is allowed on

TABLE 25.9

Foods Allowed and Not Allowed on the Gluten-Free Diet (Sample)

- Avoid all foods made with wheat, barley, rye, and their hidden sources.
- Eat foods that are naturally gluten-free.
- Read food labels carefully to help identify gluten-containing ingredients.

Protein	Dairy	Grains	Fruits/ Vegetables	Seasonings/ Condiments/ Additives
EAT: Gluten-Free Foods				
Fresh meat	Buttermilk	Amaranth	Fresh or frozen or canned	Butter
Fresh poultry	Cottage cheese	Bean	fruits and vegetables	Honey
Fresh fish	Cream cheese	Corn		Ketchup
Fresh shellfish	Plain cheeses	Fava		Mayonnaise
Eggs	Half and half	Flax		Oils
Plain beans	Milk	Millet		Salt
Plain lentils	Yogurt	Nut		Sugar
Edamame	Sour cream	Oatmeal		Corn starch
Plain nuts		Quinoa		Potato starch
Nut butters		Potato		Rice starch
Plain tofu		Rice		Tapioca starch
		Sago		BHA/BHT
		Soy		Caramel color
		Tapioca		Citric/lactic acid
		Teff		Maltodextrin MSG
				Xanthan gum
				Yeast
AVOID: Gluten-Containing Foods				
Any meat,	Malted milk	Wheat	Any fruit or vegetable	Barley malt
poultry, fish		Barley	that is breaded or made	Brewer's yeast
that is breaded		Rye	with a gluten-containing	Malt extract
or made with		Atta	ingredient	Malt syrup
a gluten-		Dinkel		Malt vinegar
containing		Durum		Wheat germ
ingredient		Einkorn		
		Emmer		
		Farro		
		Kamut		
		Graham		
		Matzoh		
		Seitan		
		Semolina		
		Spelt		
		Triticale		

Abbreviations: BHA: butylated hydroxyanisole; BHT: butylated hydroxytoluene.

TABLE 25.10

Snapshot of Studies Evaluating the Gluten-Free Diet

- A multi-center double-blind placebo-controlled study evaluated recurrence of GI symptoms that met Rome III criteria with a gluten challenge in 140 adult patients without celiac disease or IBD that followed a gluten-free diet for three weeks. Symptom improvement was noted with the diet by 101 patients. Patients (n = 98) with positive response to the diet were randomized to ingest gluten or a placebo for seven days, followed by a crossover. A recurrence of symptoms and impaired quality of life was reported by 28 patients who completed the gluten challenge and were suspected to have NCGS.[33]
- A double-blind, placebo-controlled crossover study of 59 adult patients with self-reported NCGS that self-initiated the gluten-free diet randomized patients to either a diet with gluten, a diet with fructans, or a placebo for seven days. After doing a seven-day washout period, the patients did a crossover into another diet until all the diets were implemented. The presence of GI symptoms was measured by the Gastrointestinal Symptom Rating Scale Irritable Bowel Syndrome. The survey showed significant higher overall scores for patients following the diet with fructans versus gluten.[35]

the food label if the gluten content is <20 parts per million. The ruling does not apply to some products of meats, poultry, eggs, fruits, and vegetables whose regulation is under the United States Department of Agriculture (USDA) and some alcoholic beverages that are under the regulation of the Alcohol and Tobacco Tax and Trade Bureau (TTB). Nutritional adequacy can be a concern for folic acid, vitamins B6 and B12, vitamin D, iron, copper, and zinc.[32]

The gluten-free diet must be used as the sole treatment for celiac disease. Recently, this diet is also used in the management of non-celiac gluten sensitivity (NCGS). In contrast to celiac disease, there are no validated diagnostic biomarkers for NCGS. The term NCGS is used when celiac disease is ruled out, symptoms continue to persist with gluten consumption, and symptoms resolve with gluten elimination.[33] Symptoms of NCGS may include abdominal pain, diarrhea, gas, and bloating. Patients may also have NCGS if, after implementing the gluten-free diet, there is a recurrence of symptoms with a gluten challenge (Table 25.10). Symptom resolution with the gluten-free diet in adult IBS patients with NCGS has also been attributed to a reduction of fructans versus elimination of gluten.[34, 35]

25.6.1 Practical Applications

Patients with celiac disease must follow the gluten-free diet strictly for lifetime. Patients who have observed that their symptoms worsen with gluten consumption should have celiac disease ruled out first before attempting a gluten-free diet and if ruled out, can consider a trial of the diet to see whether the diet might help. A reduction in gluten intake can also be considered for patients who do not have celiac disease to alleviate symptoms.

Nutrition education for the diet may include its rationale, sources of gluten including hidden sources, and gluten-free foods. Although the food label may include the term "gluten-free" to ease identification of gluten, learning how to interpret food labels is critical to identifying terminology for gluten, especially hidden sources of gluten, since FALCPA does not apply to all foods and beverages. Reduction of risk of gluten cross-contamination involves using separate kitchen counters, utensils, and cookware. If a food appears to be questionable for gluten content while dining out, the server should be asked what ingredients are used to help determine if the food is gluten-free or not. It would also be helpful to learn what practices are used in the kitchen to reduce risk of cross-contamination.

25.7 MEDITERRANEAN DIET

The Mediterranean diet reflects the diet patterns of individuals living in regions alongside the Mediterranean Sea. The diet is predominately plant-based and is considered to be anti-inflammatory due to its abundance of fiber, phytonutrients, and mono- and polyunsaturated fats.[36] The diet advocates for daily consumption of whole grains, fruits, and vegetables. Legumes are consumed frequently in the week as a source of plant-based protein. Fish is the primary source of animal protein because it is a source of polyunsaturated fat. Meat, eggs, and dairy are consumed less due to their saturated fat content. Consumption of concentrated sweets is also less. Olive oil is the primary oil used to provide a rich source of polyphenols that have antioxidant and anti-inflammatory properties.[37] The frequency for daily or weekly consumption of foods included in the Mediterranean diet is also outlined, in which a high adherence to the diet will meet nutritional adequacy (Table 25.11).[38, 39]

The Mediterranean diet has primarily been used in management of diabetes, cardiovascular disorders, metabolic syndrome, and obesity.[40] There is also evidence that the diet may assist with a reduction in inflammatory markers.[41] While studies are limited in the use of the diet with GI disorders, there is interest of its use in IBD due to its potential to reduce inflammation. Further studies are warranted; however,

TABLE 25.11

Serving Sizes and Frequency for the Mediterranean Diet

* Serving sizes can vary within regions

Food Group	Foods/Fluids to Include	* Serving Size	Frequency
Animal Protein	Fish	>2 servings	Weekly
	Shellfish		
Plant Protein	Chickpeas	>2 servings	Weekly
	Beans		
	Lentils		
	Nuts		
Dairy	Cheese	2 servings	Daily
	Yogurt		
Grains	Whole grains	1–2 servings	At each meal
Fruits	Fresh and frozen fruits	1–2 servings	At each meal
Vegetables	Fresh and frozen vegetables	>2 servings	At each meal
Oils	Olive oil	1 serving	At each meal

TABLE 25.12

Snapshot of Studies Evaluating the Mediterranean Diet

- A study of 86 adult patients with Crohn's disease (n = 41 for active disease, n = 45 for remission) showed adherence to the Mediterranean diet was higher in remission. The MedDiet scoring method was utilized to calculate the mean frequency of intake of each food group within the diet in the past 6 months. The food groups included whole grain cereals, fruits, vegetables, legumes, meat, poultry, fish, dairy, olive oil, and alcohol. High scores for adherence were given to more servings in a month for fruits, vegetables, legumes, fish, and olive oil.[42]
- In a prospective observational study of 153 adult patients with ulcerative colitis who underwent pouch surgery, food frequency questionnaires were utilized to assess adherence to the Mediterranean diet. The MED score assigned points to higher frequency of intake for vegetables, fruits, legumes, nuts, grains, fish, and to less frequency of intake for alcohol, milk, and meat. A score from 0 (low adherence) to 9 (high adherence) was calculated to determine adherence. The evaluation for normal pouch or for pouchitis was assessed using the Pouchitis Disease Activity Index. Patients with decreased fecal calprotectin levels had had significantly high adherence to the diet. Patients with normal pouch were followed up to 8 years; those that had high adherence to the diet had lower rates of pouchitis.[43]
- A randomized controlled trial of 194 adult patients with Crohn's disease evaluated the efficacy of the Mediterranean diet to the SCD to achieve symptomatic remission after 6 weeks of following either diet. The patients were randomized to follow either diet for 12 weeks. For the first 6 weeks, patients consumed ready-made meals that followed the guidelines of their respective diet. In the remaining 6 weeks, the patients followed the diet on their own. The results showed that after 6 weeks on both diets, there were no significant differences found in the percentage of patients that achieved symptomatic remission or in reduction for fecal calprotectin and C-reactive protein levels.[44]

there are a few studies that have shown potential in the use of the diet in modulating inflammation (Table 25.12).

An improved quality of life as well as higher rates of inactive disease has been seen in adult patients with Crohn's disease with high adherence to the diet.[42] In adult patients with ulcerative colitis after undergoing pouch surgery, a decrease in fecal calprotectin levels and risk reduction for pouchitis was seen following high adherence to the Mediterranean diet.[43] A randomized controlled trial recently compared the efficacy of the Mediterranean diet with the SCD to achieve symptomatic remission in adult patients with Crohn's disease and found no significant differences between both diets in the percentage of patients who achieved symptomatic remission, reduction in fecal calprotectin, or reduction in C-reactive protein levels.[44] The study concluded that, given that the Mediterranean diet has greater variety and is associated with other benefits to health, it could be preferable to the SCD.

25.7.1 PRACTICAL APPLICATIONS

Patients with GI disorders are appropriate for the Mediterranean diet. A discussion should take place with the patient about the rationale for the diet and to review what plant-based foods should be consumed in greater frequency at meals. The initiation of the diet may involve using one meal in the day to include a plant-based protein along with a fruit or a vegetable at the meal. A switch to the use of olive oil as the primary oil to cook and flavor foods is needed. Resources for Mediterranean cookbooks and meal-delivery services are available. Similar to the vegetarian diet, intake of fiber must be individualized to optimize tolerance.

25.8 NOVEL APPROACHES

Evolving diet therapies have come forward over the years with a focus on the inclusion of fiber as an effort to incorporate plant-based foods. In gastroparesis, a diet with small particle sizes by modifying consistency of foods to soft and liquid forms is now recommended to ease gastric emptying.[45] Adherence to small particle size may introduce additional sources of fiber that were once restricted in the diets of patients with gastroparesis. However, a fiber restriction could still be warranted with severe gastroparesis. The low-FODMAP diet continues to be considered short-term diet therapy for patients diagnosed with IBS. There is now growing interest in its use for IBD,[23] fecal incontinence,[46] and functional dyspepsia.[47] Further studies are warranted.

25.9 INCORRECT/OUTDATED PRACTICES

Although there are limited studies to support the low-fiber diet in management of IBD in active disease, the diet continues to be utilized today with patients nearly eliminating plant-based foods. The Academy of Nutrition and Dietetics removed the low-residue diet from the Nutrition Care Manual, since there is no clear definition of residue to help quantify recommendations for intake and there is very limited evidence of the beneficial impact of the low-residue diet on GI health.[48] The diet, however, continues to be in use today. Any patient found to be following the diet should be transitioned to a low-fiber diet initially to expand food choices and, from there, to a diet without restrictions if appropriate and as tolerated.

PRACTICE PEARLS

- Acknowledge that patients diagnosed with a gastrointestinal disorder may use restrictive diet patterns and food aversions to reduce symptoms.
- Recognize that nutritional impairments of unintentional weight loss, macro/micronutrient deficiencies, and sarcopenia may result as consequences.
- Refer the patient that is following a diet without supervision or at risk for nutritional impairments (e.g., unintentional weight loss, macro/micronutrient deficiencies, sarcopenia) to an RD specializing in gastrointestinal disorders for an evaluation of nutrition status and for nutrition education and counseling.
- Collaborate with the patient to reduce barriers to interventions.
- Provide ongoing evaluation of progress with diet to aid in adjustments in the plan of care.
  Prior to commencing the patient to the diet, explain
- The rationale for the diet.
- The potential benefits of the diet, which may include a reduction in symptoms, and optimization of weight status.

- The duration that the diet should be followed for.
- A list of food allowances and restrictions.
- How to personalize portions and consistency as applicable.
- The process of elimination and reintroduction as applicable.
- Resources (e.g., food lists, meal ideas, brands, cookbooks).
  While patient is on the diet, monitor
- Any changes in weight.
- Aggravation or reduction or resolution of symptoms.
- Exclusion or inclusion of food groups for nutritional adequacy.
- Successes as reported by the patient to learn what is working well.
- Fears and barriers as reported by the patient to address concerns.
- Utilization of resources as applicable.

REFERENCES

1. Institute of Medicine. Dietary Reference Intakes: Proposed Definition of Dietary Fiber. Washington, DC: National Academies Press; 2001.
2. Eswaran S, Muir J, Chey WD. Fiber and functional gastrointestinal disorders. Official Journal of the American College of Gastroenterology| ACG. 2013;108(5):718–727.
3. Lupton JR, Brooks J, Butte N, Caballero B, Flatt J, Fried S. Dietary reference intakes for energy, carbohydrate, fiber, fat, fatty acids, cholesterol, protein, and amino acids. Washington, DC: National Academy Press; 2002, vol. 5. pp. 589–768.
4. Woolner J, Kirby G. Clinical audit of the effects of low-fibre diet on irritable bowel syndrome. Journal of Human Nutrition and Dietetics. 2000;13(4):249–253.
5. Lijoi D, Ferrero S, Mistrangelo E, et al. Bowel preparation before laparoscopic gynaecological surgery in benign conditions using a 1-week low fibre diet: A surgeon blind, randomized and controlled trial. Archives of Gynecology and Obstetrics. 2009;280(5):713–718.
6. Benini L, Castellani G, Brighenti F, et al. Gastric emptying of a solid meal is accelerated by the removal of dietary fibre naturally present in food. Gut. 1995;36(6):825–830.
7. Emerson A. Foods high in fiber and phytobezoar formation. Journal of the American Dietetic Association. 1987;87(12):1675–1677.
8. Shah ND, Parian AM, Mullin GE, Limketkai BN. Oral diets and nutrition support for inflammatory bowel disease: What is the evidence? Nutrition in Clinical Practice. 2015;30(4):462–473.
9. Pituch-Zdanowska A, Banaszkiewicz A, Albrecht P. The role of dietary fibre in inflammatory bowel disease. Przeglad Gastroenterologiczny. 2015;10(3):135.
10. Hosoi K, Alvarez WC, Mann FC. Intestinal absorption: a search for a low residue diet. Archives of Internal Medicine. 1928;41(1):112–126.
11. Kramer P. The meaning of high and low residue diets. Gastroenterology. 1964;47:649–652.
12. Levenstein S, Prantera C, Luzi C, D'ubaldi A. Low residue or normal diet in Crohn's disease: A prospective controlled study in Italian patients. Gut. 1985;26(10):989–993.
13. Sipe BW, Fischer M, Baluyut AR, et al. A low-residue diet improved patient satisfaction with split-dose oral sulfate solution without impairing colonic preparation. Gastrointestinal Endoscopy. 2013;77(6):932–936.
14. Lee JW, Choi JY, Yoon H, et al. Favorable outcomes of prepackaged low-residue diet on bowel preparation for colonoscopy: Endoscopist-blinded randomized controlled trial. Journal of Gastroenterology and Hepatology. 2019;34(5):864–869.

15. Thukral C, Tewani SK, Lake AJ, et al. Results of a community-based, randomized study comparing a clear liquid diet with a low-residue diet using a magnesium citrate preparation for screening and surveillance colonoscopies. Journal of Clinical Gastroenterology. 2019;53(1):34–39.

16. Gibson PR, Shepherd SJ. Evidence-based dietary management of functional gastrointestinal symptoms: The FODMAP approach. Journal of Gastroenterology and Hepatology. 2010;25(2):252–258.

17. Whelan K, Martin LD, Staudacher HM, Lomer MC. The low FODMAP diet in the management of irritable bowel syndrome: An evidence-based review of FODMAP restriction, reintroduction and personalisation in clinical practice. Journal of Human Nutrition and Dietetics. 2018;31(2):239–255.

18. Eswaran SL, Chey WD, Han-Markey T, Ball S, Jackson K. A randomized controlled trial comparing the low FODMAP diet vs. modified NICE guidelines in US adults with IBS-D. Official Journal of the American College of Gastroenterology| ACG. 2016;111(12):1824–1832.

19. Altobelli E, Del Negro V, Angeletti PM, Latella G. Low-FODMAP diet improves irritable bowel syndrome symptoms: A meta-analysis. Nutrients. 2017;9(9):940.

20. Staudacher HM, Kurien M, Whelan K. Nutritional implications of dietary interventions for managing gastrointestinal disorders. Current Opinion in Gastroenterology. 2018;34(2):105–111.

21. Gearry RB, Irving PM, Barrett JS, Nathan DM, Shepherd SJ, Gibson PR. Reduction of dietary poorly absorbed short-chain carbohydrates (FODMAPs) improves abdominal symptoms in patients with inflammatory bowel disease – a pilot study. Journal of Crohn's and Colitis. 2009;3(1):8–14.

22. Pedersen N, Ankersen DV, Felding M, et al. Low-FODMAP diet reduces irritable bowel symptoms in patients with inflammatory bowel disease. World Journal of Gastroenterology. 2017;23(18):3356.

23. Cox SR, Prince AC, Myers CE, et al. Fermentable carbohydrates [FODMAPs] exacerbate functional gastrointestinal symptoms in patients with inflammatory bowel disease: A randomised, double-blind, placebo-controlled, cross-over, re-challenge trial. Journal of Crohn's and Colitis. 2017;11(12):1420–1429.

24. Gottschall E, Gottschall EG. Breaking the Vicious Cycle: Intestinal Health through Diet. Kirkton, ON: Kirkton Press; 1994.

25. Suskind DL, Wahbeh G, Gregory N, Vendettuoli H, Christie D. Nutritional therapy in pediatric Crohn disease: The specific carbohydrate diet. Journal of Pediatric Gastroenterology and Nutrition. 2014;58(1):87–91.

26. Cohen SA, Gold BD, Oliva S, et al. Clinical and mucosal improvement with specific carbohydrate diet in pediatric Crohn disease. Journal of Pediatric Gastroenterology and Nutrition. 2014;59(4):516–521.

27. Burgis JC, Nguyen K, Park K, Cox K. Response to strict and liberalized specific carbohydrate diet in pediatric Crohn's disease. World Journal of Gastroenterology. 2016;22(6):2111.

28. Braly K, Williamson N, Shaffer ML, et al. Nutritional adequacy of the specific carbohydrate diet in pediatric inflammatory bowel disease. Journal of Pediatric Gastroenterology and Nutrition. 2017;65(5):533.

29. Kakodkar S, Farooqui AJ, Mikolaitis SL, Mutlu EA. The specific carbohydrate diet for inflammatory bowel disease: A case series. Journal of the Academy of Nutrition and Dietetics. 2015;115(8):1226–1232.

30. Suskind DL, Wahbeh G, Cohen SA, et al. Patients perceive clinical benefit with the specific carbohydrate diet for inflammatory bowel disease. Digestive Diseases and Sciences. 2016;61(11):3255–3260.

31. Food and Drug Administration H. Food labeling: gluten-free labeling of foods. Final rule. Federal Register. 2013;78(150):47154–47179.

32. Rondanelli M, Faliva MA, Gasparri C, et al. Micronutrients dietary supplementation advices for celiac patients on long-term gluten-free diet with good compliance: A review. Medicina. 2019;55(7):337.

33. Elli L, Tomba C, Branchi F, et al. Evidence for the presence of non-celiac gluten sensitivity in patients with functional gastrointestinal symptoms: Results from a multicenter randomized double-blind placebo-controlled gluten challenge. Nutrients. 2016;8(2):84.

34. Biesiekierski JR, Peters SL, Newnham ED, Rosella O, Muir JG, Gibson PR. No effects of gluten in patients with self-reported non-celiac gluten sensitivity after dietary reduction of fermentable, poorly absorbed, short-chain carbohydrates. Gastroenterology. 2013;145(2):320–328.

35. Skodje GI, Sarna VK, Minelle IH, et al. Fructan, rather than gluten, induces symptoms in patients with self-reported non-celiac gluten sensitivity. Gastroenterology. 2018;154(3):529–539.

36. Davis C, Bryan J, Hodgson J, Murphy K. Definition of the Mediterranean diet; A literature review. Nutrients. 2015;7(11):9139–9153.

37. Gorzynik-Debicka M, Przychodzen P, Cappello F, et al. Potential health benefits of olive oil and plant polyphenols. International Journal of Molecular Sciences. 2018;19(3):686.

38. Bach-Faig A, Berry EM, Lairon D, et al. Mediterranean diet pyramid today. Science and cultural updates. Public Health Nutrition. 2011;14(12A):2274–2284.

39. Castro-Quezada I, Román-Viñas B, Serra-Majem L. The Mediterranean diet and nutritional adequacy: A review. Nutrients. 2014;6(1):231–248.

40. Koloverou E, Esposito K, Giugliano D, Panagiotakos D. The effect of Mediterranean diet on the development of type 2 diabetes mellitus: A meta-analysis of 10 prospective studies and 136,846 participants. Metabolism. 2014;63(7):903–911.

41. Sureda A, Bibiloni MDM, Julibert A, et al. Adherence to the mediterranean diet and inflammatory markers. Nutrients. 2018;10(1):62.

42. Papada E, Amerikanou C, Forbes A, Kaliora AC. Adherence to Mediterranean diet in Crohn's disease. European Journal of Nutrition. 2020;59(3):1115–1121.

43. Godny L, Reshef L, Pfeffer-Gik T, et al. Adherence to the Mediterranean diet is associated with decreased fecal calprotectin in patients with ulcerative colitis after pouch surgery. European Journal of Nutrition. 2020;59(7):3183–3190.

44. Lewis JD, Sandler R, Brotherton C, et al. A Randomized Trial Comparing the Specific Carbohydrate Diet to a Mediterranean Diet in Adults with Crohn's Disease. Gastroenterology. Published online 2021.

45. Olausson EA, Störsrud S, Grundin H, Isaksson M, Attvall S, Simrén M. A small particle size diet reduces upper gastrointestinal symptoms in patients with diabetic gastroparesis: a randomized controlled trial. Official Journal of the American College of Gastroenterologyl ACG. 2014;109(3):375–385.

46. Menees SB, Chandhrasekhar D, Liew EL, Chey WD. A low FODMAP diet may reduce symptoms in patients with fecal incontinence. Clinical and Translational Gastroenterology. 2019;10(7).

47. Staudacher HM, Nevin AN, Duff C, Kendall BJ, Holtmann GJ. Epigastric symptom response to low FODMAP dietary advice compared with standard dietetic advice in individuals with functional dyspepsia. Neurogastroenterology & Motility. Published online 2021:e14148.

48. Cunningham E. Are low-residue diets still applicable? Journal of the Academy of Nutrition and Dietetics. 2012;112(6):960.

26 Prebiotics, Probiotics, and Synbiotics

Carla Venegas and Michael Herman

26.1 INTRODUCTION

The microbiota or gut flora in the intestines contains billions of bacteria located throughout the large colon and small bowel [1]. The phenotypic makeup of flora is highly diverse among individuals, influenced by genetic and environmental factors and previous exposures as early as childbirth [2].

The gut microbiota in healthy adults typically remains stable and is primarily composed of *Bacteroides*, *Firmicutes*, and *Actinobaceria* [3]. There is a symbiotic relationship among these dominant lines of bacteria and the host. Flora in the small bowel can influence the host's immune function by facilitating antigen presentation to its abundant lymphoid tissue. Overgrowth of bacteria in the small bowel can lead to maldigestion causing secondary bloating, diarrhea, and protein-calorie deficits. Colonic bacteria also play an important role in gut health by aiding in fermentation, digestion, and protection of the intestinal walls. Disruptions in bacterial flora homeostasis play a role in irritable bowel syndrome (IBS), inflammatory bowel disease (IBD), and severe multi-organ failure associated with the inflammatory response [4].

A possible modality to help maintain and repopulate a healthy gut flora is supplementation with prebiotics and probiotics [5]. The supportive roles they play are widespread among various bacterial species and tend to be strain-specific [6]. Variables that can affect desired health benefits include the number of colony forming units (CFU) administered, time intervals for dosing, and single- vs. multi-strain nature of formulation [5, 7, 8].

26.2 BASIC PRINCIPLES

Since the early 1900s, it has been understood that viable nonpathogenic bacteria can be utilized to change the intestinal microbiota to treat gastrointestinal disorders. In the 1960s, the term "probiotics" was coined to describe these live microorganisms that can provide health benefits to the host [6]. The term "prebiotics" then emerged later, referring to dietary, nondigestible substances that provide a fertile substrate for "healthy" bacteria, along with the term "synbiotic" – formulas containing both pre- and probiotics [9, 10].

The most used probiotic species are *Lactobacillus* and *Bifidobacterium*, but other bacteria have been utilized, like non-pathogenic *Escherichia coli*, *Bacillus*, and yeasts such as *Saccharomyces boulardii*. Commonly used prebiotics are non-digestible

DOI: 10.1201/9780429322570-26

polysaccharides and oligosaccharides, such as fructooligosaccharides (FOS), inulin, galactooligosaccharides (GOS), and lactulose [9].

As a principal mechanism of action, prebiotics and probiotics increase the amount of beneficial anaerobic bacteria in the gut and decrease potentially pathogenic microorganisms by fermenting FOS in the colon into short-chain fatty acids (SCFA), especially butyrate, providing nutrition for colonocyte health. They also stimulate pancreatic secretions and colonic blood flow [5].

Probiotics carry a dynamic ability to reduce pathogenic bacteria by (1) competing against pathogens for food and mucosal adhesion sites; (2) inhibiting overpopulation by interfering with the signaling quorum sensing system; (3) decreasing antibiotic resistance; and (4) antagonizing production of specific antimicrobial metabolites [11]. Additionally, they stimulate a balanced local and systemic immune response. Some of these effects predominate according to the strain being studied. For example, *E. coli* support epithelial barrier function, while bifidobacteria and lactobacilli stimulate mucosal immune responses [12].

26.3   USE OF PROBIOTICS IN CHRONIC CONDITIONS

26.3.1   Liver Disease

The intestinal–hepatic axis is a complex relationship between the gut flora and liver. Intestinal flora deliver metabolic, bacterial, and immune substances to the liver via the portal hepatic venous system; likewise, hepatic products, such as bile and immune factors, have an effect on intestinal function [13]. Unhealthy gut flora can disrupt the intestinal epithelial barrier, allowing bacteria DNA and endotoxins into the systemic circulation leading to a systemic inflammatory response (SIRS) in addition to accentuating intrahepatic inflammatory pathways. Underlying nonalcoholic steatohepatitis (NASH) is associated with changes in bowel gut microflora. Unfortunately, a benefit of using probiotics in NASH has not been proven in clinical outcomes [14].

The prebiotic lactulose is used for the prevention and treatment of hepatic encephalopathy secondary to cirrhosis [15]. It is metabolized in the gut to lactic acid and other organic acids. This acidification results in lower systemic ammonia by two primary mechanisms: (1) promotion of non-ammoniagenic lactobacilli growth and (2) a cathartic effect to remove trapped intraluminal ammonia [16].

26.3.2   Colorectal Cancer

Despite advances in colorectal cancer (CRC) treatment with surgery, radiotherapy, and chemotherapy, outcomes are still hampered by a high rate of side effects and complications. The most common perioperative complications after bowel resection are surgical site infections, anastomotic leak, intra-abdominal abscess, ileus, and bleeding [17]. Studies suggest a role for probiotics in reducing the risk of surgical site infections (7.1% vs. 20%), anastomotic leakage (1.2% vs. 8.8%), and improving surgical recovery time [18–21]. Despite these promising findings, research has not consistently found a positive effect of probiotics for patients who undergo abdominal surgery in general [22, 23].

26.3.3 Cancer-Associated Cachexia and Diarrhea

Probiotics have beneficial effects in patients with cancer-associated cachexia, diarrhea, and constipation [24]. A meta-analysis has shown that the use of multi-species probiotic formulations before and during chemotherapy can prevent chemotherapy-induced diarrhea and alleviate/shorten the duration in patients who experience grade 3 (>7 bowel movements [BM] per day) and grade 4 (life-threatening) diarrhea. The beneficial effects were not supported in grade 1 (<4 BM/day) and grade 2 (4–6 BM/day) diarrhea [25].

Patients with abdominal and pelvic tumors are at risk for malabsorption and changes in intestinal flora and motility due to radiation-induced diarrhea. Because of the favorable safety profile, most healthcare providers incorporate probiotics into treatment regimens for radiation-induced diarrhea, [26] although a meta-analysis of six trials using VSL#3 (*Lactobacillus casei*, *L. plantarum*, *L. acidophilus*, *L. delbrueckii*, *Bifidobacterium longum*, *B. breve*, *B. infantis*, and *Streptococcus thermophiles*) did not suggest a beneficial effect [27].

26.3.4 *Helicobacter pylori*

Concomitant use of probiotics with *Helicobacter pylori* treatment regimens can improve patient outcomes and eradication rates. A large meta-analysis demonstrated that *B. infantis* 2036 and certain stains of *Lactobacillus* improved *H. pylori* eradication rates when used in antibiotic regimens that typically had <80% eradication rates. The beneficial effects were not seen when used in combination with more effective antibiotic regimens. *H. pylori* treatment side effects were generally improved with the addition of probiotics, but only statistically significant with *S. boulardii* [28].

26.3.5 Irritable Bowel Syndrome

Meta-analyses support the role of probiotics as adjunctive treatments for symptoms related to IBS with more benefits obtained when using multi-strain species over a longer duration of time [14, 29]. *Lactobacillus* and *Bifidobacterium* were the most commonly used species in multi-strain probiotics demonstrating a beneficial effect with use of 8 or more weeks. Abdominal pain, quality of life, and general IBS symptom severity were the most improved symptoms, particularly in patients with diarrhea-predominant IBS (IBS-D) [30]. Although visceral sensitivity improved with multi-strain probiotics in some studies, results were not statistically significant [31]. The use of mono-strain probiotics for IBS tends to be more strain specific. *Bacillus coagulans* used in patients with IBS-D for 90 days demonstrated a statistically significant improvement in bloating, vomiting, diarrhea, abdominal pain, and stool frequency and consistency [32]. Other species (e.g., *Lactobacillus acidophilus* and *Saccharomyces cerevisiae*) have also been studied and shown to cause improvement in abdominal pain and general symptoms of IBS but failed to reach statistical significance when compared with placebo [33, 34]. IBS patients supplemented with 10 g of fermentable soluble fiber (psyllium) have been shown to improve abdominal pain or discomfort within two months in addition to overall improved symptom severity after three months [35].

26.3.6 INFLAMMATORY BOWEL DISEASE

Probiotic therapy should be considered for ulcerative colitis (UC). *E. coli* Nissle 17 and VSL #3 strains, supported by meta-analyses, may be as efficacious as mesalamine for inducing and maintaining remission in mild-to-moderate UC [36–38]. Rectal enemas with *Lactobacillus reuteri* have been shown to have a moderate effect in the distal colon of pediatric patients [39]. The addition of VSL#3 (3.6×10^{12} CFU/day) to conventional therapies has been shown to induce remission in patients with active UC as compared with placebo [40]. Pouchitis is inflammation and edema in the surgically constructed pouch after an ileal pouch–anal anastomosis (IPAA) for UC. Therapies with antibiotics, steroid enemas, and probiotics are common regimens for treatment. VSL#3 can aid in the treatment of an acute episode of pouchitis and as maintenance therapy to prevent future relapses [37]. The use of probiotics for disease modulation in Crohn's disease is less encouraging with no evidence to support a beneficial effect. Probiotic therapy should not be used for induction or maintenance therapy in Crohn's disease [37].

26.4 PROBIOTICS IN THE CRITICALLY ILL PATIENT

The term "critically ill patient" includes those who present with systemic inflammatory response syndrome (SIRS), require life-sustaining support (e.g., mechanical ventilation, vasopressors), or are severely injured with trauma or burns. These patients are exposed to stress factors causing significant intestinal microbiota dysbiosis, resulting in a prolonged and/or more severe inflammatory response. Described stressors include metabolic disarrangements, ischemia–reperfusion imbalance, exposure to medications like opioids which decrease gut motility, broad-spectrum antibiotics which destroy gut commensals, and inhibitors of gastric acid [41].

In non-critically ill patients, probiotic agents have been shown to successfully maintain healthy microbiota and inhibit the growth and toxin production of pathogenic bacteria, while stabilizing the epithelial barrier and modulating the host inflammatory response. There is increased interest with probiotic use in critically ill patients to restore the intestinal microbiome and ameliorate the severe inflammatory response [7, 42]. Unfortunately, studying clinical outcomes of probiotic use in critically ill patients is complicated by multiple confounding factors: lack of regulated probiotic strains; variable amount of colonies, route, and timing of administration; heterogenous nature of intensive care unit (ICU) patients; underpowered ICU studies to demonstrate outcomes; and the inherent risk of using live microorganisms in a susceptible population. Nonetheless, the potential positive impact of probiotic therapy in critical illness warrants further investigation [43].

26.4.1 ANTIBIOTIC-ASSOCIATED DIARRHEA

Critically ill patients commonly receive broad spectrum antibiotics which quickly deplete gut commensals resulting in antibiotic-associated diarrhea (AAD). This imbalance can occur with any antibiotic, appears up to 8 weeks after antimicrobial exposure, and can cause devastating consequences [42]. Probiotics in the critically ill may repopulate their intestinal flora, control the growth of pathogens, and equilibrate the immune response. However, most studies have been performed in non-critically ill patients [11].

There is strong support in the literature for efficacy *of S. boulardii, L. rhamnosus* GG, and *L. casei* DN-114 001 in preventing AAD with efficacy influenced by the strain and dosage used [11]. In one study of 135 hospitalized patients, those who received *L. casei* DN-114 001 (1.0×10^8 CFU/mL), *S. thermophiles* (1.0×10^8 CFU/mL), and *L. bulgaricus* (1.0×10^7 CFU/mL) contained in 97 mL of probiotic yogurt given orally twice a day with meals after being exposed to antibiotics, experienced less AAD (12%) compared with the placebo group (34%); the probiotics group also had no development of *C. difficile* infection [44]. *Lactobacillus* also improved acute diarrhea, traveler's diarrhea, and overall diarrhea symptoms from various causes [44]. Randomized controlled trials performed in critically ill patients, some with septic shock, demonstrated significant reductions in AAD when a soluble fiber supplement was added to standard enteral formulations, with no impact on duration of mechanical ventilation, ICU length of stay, or multi-organ failure [41].

26.4.2   C. Difficile-Associated Diarrhea

The most severe form of AAD is *Clostridioides difficile*-associated diarrhea (CDAD), which usually occurs during or after antibiotic administration (90% of the cases) and is associated with a high recurrence (30% of cases) [42]. Probiotics have been shown to decrease intestinal colonization with *C. difficile*, enhance the innate immune response, and decrease >60% risk of developing CDAD in immunocompetent patients without increasing side effects [45]. *L. rhamnosus* monotherapy is only partially efficacious, but combinations of *L. acidophilus* and *L. casei* and other combinations were shown to be consistent in preventing CDAD. A Cochrane review did not identify a clear dose-dependent effect, which could reach statistical significance [45].

A combination of *S. boulardii* with high-dose oral vancomycin (2 g/day) or metronidazole decreases recurrence of CDAD by up to 50%; but a Cochrane review found efficacy in only 1 of 4 studies using this combination [42]. To date, there is no recommendation for probiotic monotherapy for recurrent CDAD, but they may have a role as adjunctive therapy.

26.4.3   Ventilator-Associated Pneumonia

Ventilator-associated pneumonia (VAP) is a costly complication related to ICU care with onset as early as 48 hours after intubation, occurring in up to 30% of mechanically ventilated patients [42]. Reducing VAP rates with probiotics has been replicated in multiple meta-analyses, independent of the species used or route of administration. It is important to mention that while decreasing the incidence of VAP, probiotics have not impacted mortality rate in these groups [43].

26.4.4 Vancomycin-Resistant Enterococci

Vancomycin-resistant enterococci (VRE) colonization and associated infections is an emerging complication in the ICU. This particular pathogen has the ability to develop antibiotic resistance and transfer it to other pathogens, and is associated with prolonged ICU stays, antibiotic treatment, long-term dialysis, and mortality [46]. Probiotics have been used to prevent the gut colonization of VRE but evidence is still limited to a few available randomized trials with few patients [46]. One trial showed using yogurt enriched with *L. rhamnosus* GG was effective in clearing and maintaining the gut VRE-free at 4 weeks compared the placebo group, [47] but that effect was not replicated using *L. rhamnosus* Lcr35 [46].

26.4.5 Acute Pancreatitis

The use of probiotics and synbiotics in severe acute pancreatitis (AP) was initially controversial since the PROPATRIA trial raised major safety concerns surrounding their association with increased bowel ischemia and mortality [48]. Those results were subsequently attributed to methodological bias regarding selection criteria, route of administration, and the combination of soluble and insoluble fibers, [49] and have not been duplicated in other studies. New evidence has proposed reduction in infectious complications and beneficial effects of probiotics and synbiotics related to reducing bacterial translocation, favoring reduced necrosis and need for invasive intervention [50, 51].

The new concept is eco-immunonutrition, which refers to adding live *Bacillus subtilis* and *Enterococcus faecium* to enteral formulas to decrease the associated multi-organ failure seen in severe AP [50]. More randomized controlled trials are needed to clarify the efficacy in AP since a large meta-analysis including 7 randomized studies showed reduction in length of hospital stay, but no difference in infections, SIRS, or mortality [50, 52, 53]. Based on the available information, it is reasonable to consider using them in patients tolerating EN [48, 50, 52, 53].

26.4.6 Liver Transplant and Other Abdominal Surgeries

Using Synbiotic-2000 [54, 55] or live *Lactobacillus* species with a fiber-containing enteral formula after liver transplantation has shown significant reductions in infection and duration of antimicrobial therapy with trends towards decreased hospital and ICU stays [54]. Positive effects are attributed to decreasing inflammatory cytokine release, stimulating immunoglobulin secretion, and stabilizing the intestinal permeability [54, 55].

Patients undergoing other major abdominal surgeries who received different probiotic formulations (usually at high concentrations) have received similar benefits, except when probiotic dose was lower than trial dosages [56]. Randomized controlled trials have proven probiotics to be safe and effective in preventing VAP, CDAD, and AAD in selective surgical populations [42]. Patients with a pylorus-preserving Whipple procedure, given Synbiotic-Forte 2000 one hour postoperatively (immediately below the anastomosis with the Roux limb), had significantly reduced infection rates. Preparations contained 1010 CFU of each of *P. pentosaceus*, *L. mesenteroides*, *L. paracasei* subsp. *paracasei*, and *L. plantarum*, as well as inulin, oat bran, pectin, and resistant starch [21].

26.4.7 TRAUMA

Similar beneficial effects in reducing rates of infection, sepsis, ICU stay, and mechanical ventilation days have been seen in critically ill trauma patients who received probiotic or synbiotic therapy [42]. These effects were not obtained with only standard nutritional support (fiber-enhanced or peptide enteral nutrition and immunonutrition) [57].

26.5 SAFETY OF PROBIOTIC USE

The World Health Organization and the United States Food and Drug Administration (FDA) have classified probiotics as "generally regarded as safe" (GRAS) [58] but there are still questions regarding overall safety, dosing, and administration in the critically ill. Most concerns are related to the incidence of systemic infections and potential transfer of antimicrobial-resistant genes from the probiotics to other bacteria (Table 26.1) [42].

The most commonly reported adverse events (AEs) are gastrointestinal disorders and infections, followed by other low-frequency events which are described in Table 26.2. Even though endocarditis has been associated with *Lactobacillus* bacteremia, most cases have been in context of high intake of dairy products; no incidents of endocarditis arose from *Lactobacillus* given as a probiotic product [61]. A majority of the studies have not found significant differences in incidence of AEs when

---

TABLE 26.1

Potential Adverse Events after Administration of Probiotics in the Critically Ill

Concern	Related Evidence
Related Systemic Infection	• There are no reports of systemic infections in healthy populations associated with probiotic administration. • No RCT shows a single case of bacteremia or fungemia [59]. • There are case reports of probiotic-related sepsis in patients with severe immunosuppression, transplantation, prosthetic heart valves, central venous catheter, impaired intestinal transit, and poorly controlled diabetes mellitus. No related mortalities have been reported [51]. • Case series published over 50 years of use have reported 129 cases of *Lactobacillus*-related bacteremia (73 endocarditis and 39 localized infection cases) mainly associated with *L. casei*, *L. plantarum*, and *L. rhamnosus* [60] and 72 cases of *Saccharomyces*-related bacteremia or fungemia. Common strains were *S. boulardii* and *S. cerevisiae*, which are not considered true "probiotics" [60]. • In the majority of these case reports, the bacteremia or fungemia did not occur temporally (at the same time) with the administration of the probiotic.

(Continued)

TABLE 26.1 (*Continued*)
Potential Adverse Events after Administration of Probiotics in the Critically Ill

Concern	Related Evidence
Transference of Antimicrobial Resistance	• Probiotics species have their own antibiotic susceptibility–resistance patterns which may represent a resistance to common antibiotics, but due to the lack of genes on plasmids it is difficult to transfer that resistance to other species. • There are no reports of *Lactobacillus* vancomycin or aminoglycoside resistance genes being transferred to other strains of bacteria [51]. • There are no data showing that probiotic species destroy the normal flora, increase risk of colon cancer, or induce an immunosuppressive effect in susceptible populations [51].

TABLE 26.2
Safety and Adverse Events according to Studied Population

Studied Population	Type and Dose	Adverse Events (AEs)	Conclusions
Critically ill (Patients with SIRS, sepsis, trauma, burns, or receiving enteral nutrition, mechanical ventilation, or antibiotics) [4, 59].	**Strain:** • *L. rhamnosus* GR-1 (HIV patients) • *L. rhamnosus* GG (severe critically ill) **Dose:** Less than 5.0×10^{10} CFU/day **Mean duration of therapy:** 14 days (range: 7–28)	• Most common were gastrointestinal disorders (diarrhea, abdominal pain, bloating) • Infections (VAP and sepsis) • Skin disorders (rash and pruritus) • Overall incidence of AEs appears to be lower when probiotics are administered	• Currently investigated probiotic strains are safe at their evaluated dosages • Safety is not proven in chronic administration to the critically ill (all studies less than a month) • Tested dosages appear to be insufficient for maximal therapeutic effect
Gastrointestinal perioperative subgroup [4, 21, 59]	**Strain:** • *L. plantarum* (CGMCC no.1258) • *L. acidophilus* 11 • *B. longum* 88 **Dose:** Varied according the underlying disease. High daily CFU **Mean duration of therapy:** 3 days before surgery (range: 0–8) for a total of 16 days (range: 3–28)	• Most common were infections (VAP and sepsis) • Gastrointestinal disorders (diarrhea, abdominal pain, bloating) • Overall incidence of AEs appears to be lower when probiotics are administered	• Significant reduction in incidence of sepsis, bacteremia, postoperative infections, and related complications • Safety of patients receiving perioperative probiotics and synbiotics is excellent • High dosage of 2.0×1011 CFU/day have no significant AEs, and may represent a protective effect
Autoimmune disorders (RA, MS) [4, 59]	**Strain:** *B. longum* *L. johnsonii* La1 **Mean duration of therapy:** 56 days (range: 7–365)	• "Unspecified" AEs and gastrointestinal disorders were reported	• The frequency of AEs was relatively low

TABLE 26.2 (*Continued*)

Safety and Adverse Events according to Studied Population

Studied Population	Type and Dose	Adverse Events (AEs)	Conclusions
Gastrointestinal diseases (IBD, UC, Crohn's, including liver cirrhosis) [4, 59]	**Strain:** *L. acidophilus* *L. bulgaricus* *S. thermophilus* **Dose:** Varied according to underlying disease. Low daily CFU ($<2.0 \times 10^{10}$ CFU/day) **Mean duration of therapy:** 56 days (range: 7–365)	• Most common were hepatobiliary and gastrointestinal disorders. • Overall incidence of AEs appears to be lower when probiotics are administered.	• Lower incidence of AEs in populations receiving probiotics
Other high-risk populations (including cancer) [4, 31, 59]	**Dose:** Varied according to underlying disease. Low daily CFU **Mean duration of therapy:** 57 days (range: 53–70)		
Children (healthy and immune-compromised less than 18 years old) [62]	**Strain:** *L. rhamnosus* GG *S. boulardii* *L. acidophilus* NCFM *L. acidophilus* NCFM and *B. lactis* Bi-07 *L. acidophilus* and *B. bifidum* *L. casei* Shirota **Dose:** Wide range of dosages, up to a very high dosage of 1.5×10^{11} CFU/day	• Most common were gastrointestinal disorders • Allergies • Overall incidence of AEs appears to be lower when probiotics are administered • Reported bacteremia or sepsis were not related to the probiotics strains given	• Lower incidence of upper respiratory tract infections when probiotics are received • Less duration and severity of diarrhea with probiotic use

VAP: Ventilator-associated pneumonia; AE: Adverse events.

probiotics are administered to a variety of populations, and many studies have even found fewer complications in the population receiving probiotics [20, 61].

Clinical outcomes may differ according to probiotic properties and method of administration, which makes data standardization difficult to achieve and conclusions about safety supported by limited high-grade evidence [10]. Modern analysis suggests that the administration of probiotic and synbiotic strains to children [62] and immune compromised adults [59] carry no increased adverse health risk. In general, probiotics have a safe profile, but clinical indications, risks, and benefits should be considered before administration. Institutional protocols are recommended to facilitate their use in the ICU to provide maximum benefit and minimal adverse effects (Table 26.3). These results supporting the safety of probiotics and synbiotics may lead to further investigations evaluating their potential preventive and therapeutic effect with prudent surveillance in high-risk populations.

TABLE 26.3
Evidence-Based Recommendations to Optimize Probiotic Use in the Critically Ill

Criteria	Evidence-Based Recommendation
Patient Selection [11]	• Patient-appropriate clinical indication like use of antibiotics. • Weigh severity of relative contraindications like autoimmune disorders, cardiac hardware, central access catheters (especially for Lactobacillus species).
Timing of Probiotic Therapy [11, 52]	• Controversial. • For prophylaxis, administer upon introduction of the risk factor such as at onset of antibiotic therapy or upon initiation of mechanical ventilation. • As therapy, should begin at onset of disease. • There are no data related to probiotics as rescue therapy.
Type of Preparation [51, 52]	• Probiotics have been packaged as pills, capsules, packets, yogurt, and oatmeal preparations. There is no data that favors any particular method. • For patients who are on tube feeds, lactose intolerant, or otherwise nil per os, additional consideration regarding route of administration is needed. • Commercially prepared formulations of probiotics are recommended because ingredients they contain are more easily discerned; most clinical trials have utilized these products. • There is limited data regarding the use of "homemade" probiotic preparations. • The strain of probiotic utilized should be institution-specific.
Probiotics Strains [51, 52]	• Choice of probiotic preparation is also influenced by the number of strains within the product. • *L. plantarum*, *L. acidophilus*, and/or *L. rhamnosus* are preferred due to the preponderance of data available related to use of these strains. • In the critically ill, significant benefits have been seen with no more than 8 strains of probiotics. Most trials administered a single strain of probiotic demonstrating similar efficacy to those trials using multiple strains.
Dose [51, 52, 63]	• Higher doses should be utilized to maximize the benefit without concern for increase in adverse effects since rates of infectious complications are dose CFU/day independent, but efficacy decreases at low doses.
Duration of Therapy [51, 52, 56]	• Duration of probiotic therapy varies according to clinical situation. When administered for prevention of VAP, AAD, and CDAD, continue probiotics until elimination of risk factor. • Treatment regimens for probiotics should be continued for 14–21 days (the median treatment duration in clinical trials) in majority of patients.
Route of Administration [11, 51, 52]	• Enteral route predominantly used in clinical trials as colonization of the intestines is key to obtaining benefits. • Swabbing oral cavity with probiotics may lead to similar benefits as via nasoenteric tube, and may provide added benefits in mechanically ventilated patients.

VAP: Ventilator-associated pneumonia; AAD: Antibiotic-associated diarrhea; CDAD: *C. difficile*-associated diarrhea.

26.6 GUIDELINES FOR ICU PATIENTS

Recent guidelines published by the American Society for Parenteral and Enteral Nutrition (ASPEN), in conjunction with the Society of Critical Care Medicine (SCCM), in 2016 consider the use of pre- and probiotics for select medical and surgical patients correlating with the studied populations (Table 26.4) [41]. The ASPEN–SCCM recommendations are in agreement with the Canadian Clinical Practice Guidelines published in 2015 [64], but contrast with 2019 recommendations by the European Society for Clinical Nutrition and Metabolism (ESPEN) [65] which has no recommendations.

Per the European Society for Pediatric Gastroenterology, Hepatology, and Nutrition (ESPGHAN) working group [66], there is sufficient evidence to recommend a minimal daily dose of 2×10^9 CFU of *L. rhamnosus* GG and *S. boulardii* for the prevention of AAD in children. Regarding *S. boulardii*, it is important to consider its beneficial effect in children and adults, but possible detrimental consequences in the elderly [11].

TABLE 26.4
Summary American Society for Parenteral and Enteral Nutrition (ASPEN) and Society of Critical Care Medicine (SCCM) Guidelines [50]

	Recommendation
Regarding Prebiotic Use	Consider routine use of a fermentable soluble fiber as adjunctive therapy in hemodynamically stable critically ill patients who can tolerate enteral nutrition.
	For stable critically ill patients with diarrhea, give a total daily dose of 10–20 grams of a fermentable soluble fiber divided in multiple doses during the day.
Regarding Probiotics Use	Although the use of most probiotic species and strains (primarily *Lactobacillus* GG) appears to be safe in critically ill patients and have a positive effect in reducing the incidence of VAP and overall infections, the SCCM and ASPEN refrain from recommending the routine use of probiotics across the general population of ICU patients given the low-grade nature of evidence. Probiotics should be considered only for select medical and surgical patients correlating with the studied populations.
General Considerations	Future research should use standard taxonomic classification and focus on targeted probiotic supplementation to provide more conclusive evidence and support stronger, more specific evidence-based recommendations in critically ill patients.
	Due to reported cases of fungemia and worsening pancreatitis associated with the use of *Saccharomyces boulardii* in critically ill patients, its routine use cannot be recommended.
	In patients with liver transplant and other major abdominal surgeries, studied probiotic and synbiotic combinations can be considered due to the documented safety and benefit in reducing incidence of VAP, CDAD, and AAD.

26.7   NOVEL APPROACHES

26.7.1   FECAL MICROBIOTA TRANSPLANTATION

Currently, fecal microbiota transplantation (FMT) is primarily used for treatment of recurrent CDAD not responding to standard therapies, where efficacy in treating recurrent cases exceeds 90% [63, 67]. To minimize the risk of infection or other disease transmission, potential donors undergo rigorous screening including thorough history taking, serological tests, and fecal tests for parasitic, virologic, and bacterial pathogens (Table 26.5) [31].

TABLE 26.5
General FMT Recommendations

Screening for Potential Donors [59, 63]	• Donors are healthy volunteers who undergo a screening questionnaire regarding travel history, sexual behavior, sick contacts, blood transfusions, or any intervention that might increase the risk of carrying a contagious infection.
	• Exclude donors with HIV, viral hepatitis, *Dientamoeba fragilis*, *Blastocystis hominis*, *Clostridioides difficile*, and rotavirus.
	• Recommended blood screening for *T. pallidum*, *H. pylori*, CMV, Hep A, Hep B, Hep C, HIV, HTLV, JC virus, EBV, *Entamoeba histolytica*, *Strongyloides stercoralis, and schistosomas*.
	• Recommended stool test for *C. difficile*, enteric pathogens (*Salmonella, Shigela, Escherichia, Campylobacter, Listeria*), adenovirus, rotavirus, norovirus, microsporidia, giardia, cryptosporidium, isospora, and cyclospora.
	• When the recipient is an immunocompromised host, the potential donor should be screened for potential opportunistic infections.
Side Effects [65–67]	Effects related to the chosen procedure or route of administration:
	• Small risk of perforation or bleeding.
	• Potential risk of vomiting and aspiration.
	Effects related to the infusion of another human's feces:
	• Most series report minimal rates of adverse effects.
	• Mild diarrhea and abdominal cramping the same day of infusion.
Preparation of Feces [63, 66]	• After collection, cover feces as soon as possible with saline to replicate an anaerobic environment which preserves the anaerobic bacterial population.
	• Frozen stool samples are available, and this preparation appears to have no significant difference in outcomes.
	• It is recommended to infuse freshly produced stool as quickly as possible (within 6 hours of passage).
	• Dissolve feces in sterile saline. Other media like water or yogurt have been used.
	• Liquefy feces to facilitate the infusion.
	• Strain debris as much as possible.
	• Infuse slowly between 200–300 g of feces. Better outcomes have been reported with larger volumes.
Administration [65, 66]	• FMT is usually administered via fecal enemas, or upper or lower endoscopy.
	• Upper endoscopy and colonoscopy must be performed by a trained physician.
	• There is no consensus on the preferred route of infusion due to difficulties in comparing different protocols in the available literature.

TABLE 26.5 (*Continued*)
General FMT Recommendations

Number of Treatments [65, 69]	• Most patients received only one FMT treatment, but there are reports of 2 and 3 required transplants in a minority of cases.
Associated Therapy [65]	• When used for recurrent CDAD, the majority of patients receive standard antibiotic treatment prior to the FMT.
	• Some patients receive an oral whole-bowel lavage prior to FMT in the absence of any suspicious bowel obstruction. There is no data comparing performance of FMT with or without a whole-bowel lavage.

VAP: Ventilator-associated pneumonia; FMT: Fecal microbiota transplantation; CDAD: *C. difficile*-associated diarrhea.

The largest randomized trial of FMT for CDAD was stopped prematurely due to the clearly successful effect (94%) with one or two FMT infusions versus 20–30% with standard therapy [68].

26.7.2 CURRENT EXPERIMENTAL FMT USES

Obesity: Studies in male patients with metabolic syndrome who received allogenic feces from lean donors have found a temporary reduction in peripheral insulin resistance and fasting lipid profiles, suggesting an effect on whole body metabolism likely related to enhanced production of specific SCFA and restoration of normal fecal physiology. Further trials are in progress [67].

IBD: Induction of remission in adults with mild-to-moderate UC could be achieved at 8 weeks after therapy using pooled donor FMT (32%) versus autologous FMT (9%); 42% of those responding remained in steroid-free remission at 12 months [70]. A pediatric study reported 78% clinical response within one week of FMT in children with UC, 33% clinical remission, and minimal adverse events [60]. A systematic review of randomized trials and cohort studies of FMT for patients with UC demonstrated clinical remission in 42% and a clinical response in 65% with few adverse events [71]. Regarding Crohn's disease, significant adverse effects with no significant clinical improvement have been reported [67]. The use of FMT to treat IBD remains experimental.

26.8 CONCLUSION

With increasing recognition of the role intestinal dysbiosis may play in development of various diseases, influencing and restoring the microbiota with prebiotics, probiotics, synbiotics, or even with FMT has gained interest. Enthusiasm for judicious use of these therapies must be tempered, however, by the fact that no single product is a panacea and specific therapies may only be appropriate for certain populations. Future studies, possibly involving new, non-invasive intestinal stress biomarkers, may help provide better recommendations in regard to species, doses, and routes of administration along with insights about other diseases for which normalization of the intestinal microbiota may be beneficial, such as antibiotic-induced IBS, bacterial overgrowth, autoimmune diseases, and critical illness.

PRACTICE PEARLS

- The prebiotic lactulose has been used for the prevention and treatment of hepatic encephalopathy.
- Multi-strain probiotics might have benefit for reducing symptoms of IBS.
- *E. coli* Nissle 17 and VSL #3 might be effective for inducing and maintaining remission in mild-to-moderate UC.
- The addition of soluble fiber to enteral formulae has shown benefit for reducing AAD in critically ill patients.
- Probiotics and synbiotics could be considered for reducing incidence of VAP, CDAD, and AAD.

REFERENCES

1. Lozupone CA, Stombaugh JI, Gordon JI, Jansson JK, Knight R. Diversity, stability and resilience of the human gut microbiota. Nature. 2012;489(7415):220–30. doi:10.1038/nature11550.
2. Chu DM, Ma J, Prince AL, Antony KM, Seferovic MD, Aagaard KM. Maturation of the infant microbiome community structure and function across multiple body sites and in relation to mode of delivery. Nature Medicine. 2017;23(3):314–26. doi:10.1038/nm.4272.
3. Kim S, Covington A, Pamer EG. The intestinal microbiota: Antibiotics, colonization resistance, and enteric pathogens. Immunological Reviews. 2017;279(1):90–105. doi:10.1111/imr.12563.
4. Zhang CX, Wang HY, Chen TX. Interactions between intestinal microflora/probiotics and the immune system. BioMed Research International. 2019;2019:6764919. doi:10.1155/2019/6764919.
5. Markowiak P, Slizewska K. Effects of probiotics, prebiotics, and synbiotics on human health. Nutrients. 2017;9(9). doi:10.3390/nu9091021.
6. Hill C, Guarner F, Reid G, Gibson GR, Merenstein DJ, Pot B, et al. Expert consensus document. The International Scientific Association for Probiotics and Prebiotics consensus statement on the scope and appropriate use of the term probiotic. Nature Reviews Gastroenterology & Hepatology. 2014;11(8):506–14. doi:10.1038/nrgastro.2014.66.
7. Sanders ME, Guarner F, Guerrant R, Holt PR, Quigley EM, Sartor RB, et al. An update on the use and investigation of probiotics in health and disease. Gut. 2013;62(5):787–96. doi:10.1136/gutjnl-2012-302504.
8. Ebner S, Smug LN, Kneifel W, Salminen SJ, Sanders ME. Probiotics in dietary guidelines and clinical recommendations outside the European Union. World Journal of Gastroenterology. 2014;20(43):16095–100. doi:10.3748/wjg.v20.i43.16095.
9. Guarner FSM, Eliakim R, et al. WGO guidelines: Probiotics and prebiotics. World Gastroenterology Organisation Global Guidelines. 2017:1–35.
10. Organization WH. Joint FAO/WHO expert consultation on evaluation of health and nutritional properties of probiotics in food including powder milk with live lactic acid bacteria. 2001:1–50. Accessed https://www.fao.org/3/a0512e/a0512e.pdf
11. Agamennone V, Krul CAM, Rijkers G, Kort R. A practical guide for probiotics applied to the case of antibiotic-associated diarrhea in the Netherlands. BMC Gastroenterol. 2018;18(1):103. doi:10.1186/s12876-018-0831-x.

12. Howarth GS, Butler RN, Salminen S, Gibson GR, Donovan SM. Probiotics for optimal nutrition: From efficacy to guidelines. Advances in Nutrition. 2012;3(5):720–2. doi:10.3945/an.112.002501.

13. Mancini A, Campagna F, Amodio P, Tuohy KM. Gut, liver, brain axis: The microbial challenge in the hepatic encephalopathy. Food & Function. 2018;9(3):1373–88. doi:10.1039/c7fo01528c.

14. Rondanelli M, Faliva MA, Perna S, Giacosa A, Peroni G, Castellazzi AM. Using probiotics in clinical practice: Where are we now? A review of existing meta-analyses. Gut Microbes. 2017;8(6):521–43. doi:10.1080/19490976.2017.1345414.

15. Sharma P, Agrawal A, Sharma BC, Sarin SK. Prophylaxis of hepatic encephalopathy in acute variceal bleed: a randomized controlled trial of lactulose versus no lactulose. Journal of Gastroenterology and Hepatology. 2011;26(6):996–1003. doi:10.1111/j.1440-1746.2010.06596.x.

16. Frederick RT. Current concepts in the pathophysiology and management of hepatic encephalopathy. Gastroenterology and Hepatology (N Y). 2011;7(4):222–33.

17. Darbandi A, Mirshekar M, Shariati A, Moghadam MT, Lohrasbi V, Asadolahi P, et al. The effects of probiotics on reducing the colorectal cancer surgery complications: A periodic review during 2007–2017. Clinical Nutrition (Edinburgh, Scotland). 2019. doi:10.1016/j.clnu.2019.11.008.

18. He D, Wang HY, Feng JY, Zhang MM, Zhou Y, Wu XT. Use of pro-/synbiotics as prophylaxis in patients undergoing colorectal resection for cancer: A meta-analysis of randomized controlled trials. Clin Res Hepatol Gastroenterol. 2013;37(4):406–15. doi:10.1016/j.clinre.2012.10.007.

19. Yang Y, Xia Y, Chen H, Hong L, Feng J, Yang J, et al. The effect of perioperative probiotics treatment for colorectal cancer: Short-term outcomes of a randomized controlled trial. Oncotarget. 2016;7(7):8432–40. doi:10.18632/oncotarget.7045.

20. Liu Z, Qin H, Yang Z, Xia Y, Liu W, Yang J, et al. Randomised clinical trial: The effects of perioperative probiotic treatment on barrier function and post-operative infectious complications in colorectal cancer surgery – a double-blind study. Alimentary Pharmacology and Therapeutics. 2011;33(1):50–63. doi:10.1111/j.1365-2036.2010.04492.x.

21. Kotzampassi K, Stavrou G, Damoraki G, Georgitsi M, Basdanis G, Tsaousi G, et al. A Four-probiotics regimen reduces postoperative complications after colorectal surgery: A randomized, double-blind, placebo-controlled study. World Journal of Surgery. 2015;39(11):2776–83. doi:10.1007/s00268-015-3071-z.

22. Komatsu S, Sakamoto E, Norimizu S, Shingu Y, Asahara T, Nomoto K, et al. Efficacy of perioperative synbiotics treatment for the prevention of surgical site infection after laparoscopic colorectal surgery: A randomized controlled trial. Surgery Today. 2016;46(4):479–90. doi:10.1007/s00595-015-1178-3.

23. Peitsidou K, Karantanos T, Theodoropoulos GE. Probiotics, prebiotics, synbiotics: Is there enough evidence to support their use in colorectal cancer surgery? Dig Surgery. 2012;29(5):426–38. doi:10.1159/000345580.

24. Herremans KM, Riner AN, Cameron ME, Trevino JG. The microbiota and cancer cachexia. International Journal of Molecular Sciences. 2019;20(24). doi:10.3390/ijms20246267.

25. Leventogiannis K, Gkolfakis P, Spithakis G, Tsatali A, Pistiki A, Sioulas A, et al. Effect of a preparation of four probiotics on symptoms of patients with irritable bowel syndrome: Association with intestinal bacterial overgrowth. Probiotics Antimicrob Proteins. 2019;11(2):627–34. doi:10.1007/s12602-018-9401-3.

26. Giralt J, Regadera JP, Verges R, Romero J, de la Fuente I, Biete A, et al. Effects of probiotic *Lactobacillus casei* DN-114 001 in prevention of radiation-induced diarrhea: results from multicenter, randomized, placebo-controlled nutritional trial. International Journal of Radiation Oncology — Biology — Physics. 2008;71(4):1213–9. doi:10.1016/j.ijrobp.2007.11.009.

27. Liu M-M, Li S-T, Shu Y, Zhan H-Q. Probiotics for prevention of radiation-induced diarrhea: A meta-analysis of randomized controlled trials. PLoS One. 2017;12(6):e0178870-e. doi:10.1371/journal.pone.0178870.

28. Dang Y, Reinhardt JD, Zhou X, Zhang G. The effect of probiotics supplementation on *Helicobacter pylori* eradication rates and side effects during eradication therapy: A meta-analysis. PLoS One. 2014;9(11):e111030-e. doi:10.1371/journal.pone.0111030.

29. Dale HF, Rasmussen SH, Asiller OO, Lied GA. Probiotics in irritable bowel syndrome: An up-to-date systematic review. Nutrients. 2019;11(9). doi:10.3390/nu11092048.

30. Dale HF, Rasmussen SH, Asiller Ö, Lied GA. Probiotics in irritable bowel syndrome: An up-to-date systematic review. Nutrients. 2019;11(9). doi:10.3390/nu11092048.

31. Ludidi S, Jonkers DM, Koning CJ, Kruimel JW, Mulder L, van der Vaart IB, et al. Randomized clinical trial on the effect of a multispecies probiotic on visceroperception in hypersensitive IBS patients. Neurogastroenterology & Motility. 2014;26(5):705–14. doi:10.1111/nmo.12320.

32. Majeed M, Nagabhushanam K, Natarajan S, Sivakumar A, Ali F, Pande A, et al. *Bacillus coagulans* MTCC 5856 supplementation in the management of diarrhea predominant irritable bowel syndrome: A double blind randomized placebo controlled pilot clinical study. Nutrition Journal. 2016;15:21. doi:10.1186/s12937-016-0140-6.

33. Lyra A, Hillilä M, Huttunen T, Männikkö S, Taalikka M, Tennilä J, et al. Irritable bowel syndrome symptom severity improves equally with probiotic and placebo. World Journal of Gastroenterology. 2016;22(48):10631–42. doi:10.3748/wjg.v22.i48.10631.

34. Pineton de Chambrun G, Neut C, Chau A, Cazaubiel M, Pelerin F, Justen P, et al. A randomized clinical trial of *Saccharomyces cerevisiae* versus placebo in the irritable bowel syndrome. Digestive and Liver Disease. 2015;47(2):119–24. doi:10.1016/j.dld.2014.11.007.

35. Moayyedi P, Quigley EM, Lacy BE, Lembo AJ, Saito YA, Schiller LR, et al. The effect of fiber supplementation on irritable bowel syndrome: A systematic review and meta-analysis. American Journal of Gastroenterology. 2014;109(9):1367–74. doi:10.1038/ajg.2014.195.

36. Kruis W, Fric P, Pokrotnieks J, Lukas M, Fixa B, Kascak M, et al. Maintaining remission of ulcerative colitis with the probiotic *Escherichia coli* Nissle 1917 is as effective as with standard mesalazine. Gut. 2004;53(11):1617–23. doi:10.1136/gut.2003.037747.

37. Shen J, Zuo ZX, Mao AP. Effect of probiotics on inducing remission and maintaining therapy in ulcerative colitis, Crohn's disease, and pouchitis: meta-analysis of randomized controlled trials. Inflammatory Bowel Disease. 2014;20(1):21–35. doi:10.1097/01.MIB.0000437495.30052.be.

38. Losurdo G, Iannone A, Contaldo A, Ierardi E, Di Leo A, Principi M. *Escherichia coli* Nissle 1917 in ulcerative colitis treatment: Systematic review and meta-analysis. Journal of Gastrointestinal and Liver Diseases. 2015;24(4):499–505. doi:10.15403/jgld.2014.1121.244.ecn.

39. Oliva S, Di Nardo G, Ferrari F, Mallardo S, Rossi P, Patrizi G, et al. Randomised clinical trial: the effectiveness of *Lactobacillus reuteri* ATCC 55730 rectal enema in children with active distal ulcerative colitis. Alimentary Pharmacology and Therapeutics. 2012;35(3):327–34. doi:10.1111/j.1365-2036.2011.04939.x.

40. Astó E, Méndez I, Audivert S, Farran-Codina A, Espadaler J. The efficacy of probiotics, prebiotic inulin-type fructans, and synbiotics in human ulcerative colitis: A systematic review and meta-analysis. Nutrients. 2019;11(2). doi:10.3390/nu11020293.

41. Taylor BE, McClave SA, Martindale RG, Warren MM, Johnson DR, Braunschweig C, et al. Guidelines for the provision and assessment of nutrition support therapy in the adult critically Ill patient: Society of Critical Care Medicine (SCCM) and American Society for Parenteral and Enteral Nutrition (A.S.P.E.N.). Critical Care Medicine. 2016;44(2):390–438. doi:10.1097/ccm.0000000000001525.

42. Urben LM, Wiedmar J, Boettcher E, Cavallazzi R, Martindale RG, McClave SA. Bugs or drugs: Are probiotics safe for use in the critically ill? Current Gastroenterology Reports. 2014;16(7):388. doi:10.1007/s11894-014-0388-y.

43. Petrof EO, Dhaliwal R, Manzanares W, Johnstone J, Cook D, Heyland DK. Probiotics in the critically ill: A systematic review of the randomized trial evidence. Critical Care Medicine. 2012;40(12):3290–302. doi:10.1097/CCM.0b013e318260cc33.

44. Hickson M, D'Souza AL, Muthu N, Rogers TR, Want S, Rajkumar C, et al. Use of probiotic *Lactobacillus* preparation to prevent diarrhoea associated with antibiotics: randomised double blind placebo controlled trial. BMJ. 2007;335(7610):80. doi:10.1136/bmj.39231.599815.55.

45. Goldenberg JZ, Yap C, Lytvyn L, Lo CK, Beardsley J, Mertz D, et al. Probiotics for the prevention of *Clostridium difficile*-associated diarrhea in adults and children. Cochrane Database of Systematic Reviews. 2017;12:Cd006095. doi:10.1002/14651858. CD006095.pub4.

46. Kampmeier S, Kossow A, Clausen LM, Knaack D, Ertmer C, Gottschalk A, et al. Hospital acquired vancomycin resistant enterococci in surgical intensive care patients – a prospective longitudinal study. Antimicrobial Resistance and Infection Control. 2018;7:103. doi:10.1186/s13756-018-0394-1.

47. Karki S, Land G, Aitchison S, Kennon J, Johnson PD, Ballard SA, et al. Long-term carriage of vancomycin-resistant enterococci in patients discharged from hospitals: a 12-year retrospective cohort study. Journal of Clinical Microbiology. 2013;51(10): 3374–9. doi:10.1128/jcm.01501-13.

48. Besselink MG, van Santvoort HC, Buskens E, Boermeester MA, van Goor H, Timmerman HM, et al. Probiotic prophylaxis in predicted severe acute pancreatitis: A randomised, double-blind, placebo-controlled trial. Lancet (London, England). 2008;371(9613):651–9. doi:10.1016/s0140-6736(08)60207-x.

49. Bongaerts GP, Severijnen RS. A reassessment of the PROPATRIA study and its implications for probiotic therapy. Nature Biotechnology. 2016;34(1):55–63. doi:10.1038/nbt.3436.

50. Zhang MM, Cheng JQ, Lu YR, Yi ZH, Yang P, Wu XT. Use of pre-, pro- and synbiotics in patients with acute pancreatitis: A meta-analysis. World Journal of Gastroenterology. 2010;16(31):3970–8. doi:10.3748/wjg.v16.i31.3970.

51. Manzanares W, Lemieux M, Langlois PL, Wischmeyer PE. Probiotic and synbiotic therapy in critical illness: A systematic review and meta-analysis. Critical Care (London, England). 2016;19:262. doi:10.1186/s13054-016-1434-y.

52. Warren M, McCarthy MS, Roberts PR. Practical application of the revised guidelines for the provision and assessment of nutrition support therapy in the adult critically Ill patient: A case study approach. Nutrition in Clinical Practice: Official Publication of the American Society for Parenteral and Enteral Nutrition. 2016;31(3):334–41. doi:10.1177/0884533616640451.

53. Karakan T, Ergun M, Dogan I, Cindoruk M, Unal S. Comparison of early enteral nutrition in severe acute pancreatitis with prebiotic fiber supplementation versus standard enteral solution: A prospective randomized double-blind study. World Journal of Gastroenterology. 2007;13(19):2733–7. doi:10.3748/wjg.v13.i19.2733.

54. Rayes N, Seehofer D, Theruvath T, Schiller RA, Langrehr JM, Jonas S, et al. Supply of pre- and probiotics reduces bacterial infection rates after liver transplantation – a randomized, double-blind trial. American Journal of Transplantation: Official Journal of the American Society of Transplantation and the American Society of Transplant Surgeons. 2005;5(1):125–30. doi:10.1111/j.1600-6143.2004.00649.x.

55. Sawas T, Al Halabi S, Hernaez R, Carey WD, Cho WK. Patients receiving prebiotics and probiotics before liver transplantation develop fewer infections than controls: A systematic review and meta-analysis. Clinical Gastroenterology and Hepatology: Official Clinical Practice Journal of the American Gastroenterological Association. 2015;13(9):1567–74.e3; quiz e143–4. doi:10.1016/j.cgh.2015.05.027.

56. McNaught CE, Woodcock NP, MacFie J, Mitchell CJ. A prospective randomised study of the probiotic *Lactobacillus plantarum* 299V on indices of gut barrier function in elective surgical patients. Gut. 2002;51(6):827–31. doi:10.1136/gut.51.6.827.

57. Kotzampassi K, Giamarellos-Bourboulis EJ, Voudouris A, Kazamias P, Eleftheri-adis E. Benefits of a synbiotic formula (Synbiotic 2000Forte) in critically Ill trauma patients: Early results of a randomized controlled trial. World Journal of Surgery. 2006;30(10):1848–55. doi:10.1007/s00268-005-0653-1.

58. Fijan S. Microorganisms with claimed probiotic properties: An overview of recent literature. International Journal of Environmental Research and Public Health. 2014;11(5):4745–67. doi:10.3390/ijerph110504745.

59. Van den Nieuwboer M, Brummer RJ, Guarner F, Morelli L, Cabana M, Claasen E. The administration of probiotics and synbiotics in immune compromised adults: Is it safe? Benef Microbes. 2015;6(1):3–17. doi:10.3920/bm2014.0079.

60. Kunde SPA, Bonczyk S, Kunde S, Pham A, Bonczyk S, et al. Safety, tolerability, and clinical response after fecal transplantation in children and young adults with ulcerative colitis. Journal of Pediatric Gastroenterology and Nutrition. 2013;56:597–601. \

61. Cannon JP, Lee TA, Bolanos JT, Danziger LH. Pathogenic relevance of Lactobacillus: A retrospective review of over 200 cases. European Journal of Clinical Microbiology & Infectious Diseases: Official Publication of the European Society of Clinical Microbiology. 2005;24(1):31–40. doi:10.1007/s10096-004-1253-y.

62. van den Nieuwboer M, Brummer RJ, Guarner F, Morelli L, Cabana M, Claassen E. Safety of probiotics and synbiotics in children under 18 years of age. Benef Microbes. 2015;6(5):615–30. doi:10.3920/bm2014.0157.

63. Gough E, Shaikh H, Manges AR. Systematic review of intestinal microbiota transplantation (fecal bacteriotherapy) for recurrent Clostridium difficile infection. Clinical Infectious Diseases. 2011;53(10):994–1002. doi:10.1093/cid/cir632.

64. Committee CCPG. The 2015 Clinical Practice Guidelines. 2015. https://www.critical-carenutrition.com/resources/cpgs/past-guidelines/2015.

65. ReintamBlaser A, Deane AM, Starkopf J. Translating the European Society for Clinical Nutrition and Metabolism 2019 guidelines into practice. Current Opinion in Critical Care. 2019;25(4):314–21. doi:10.1097/mcc.0000000000000619.

66. Szajewska H, Canani RB, Guarino A, Hojsak I, Indrio F, Kolacek S, et al. Probiotics for the prevention of antibiotic-associated diarrhea in children. Journal of Pediatric Gastroenterology and Nutrition. 2016;62(3):495–506. doi:10.1097/mpg.0000000000001081.

67. van Nood E, Speelman P, Nieuwdorp M, Keller J. Fecal microbiota transplantation: Facts and controversies. Current Opinion in Gastroenterology. 2014;30(1):34–9. doi:10.1097/MOG.0000000000000024.

68. You DM, Franzos MA, Holman RP. Successful treatment of fulminant *Clostridium difficile* infection with fecal bacteriotherapy. Annals of Internal Medicine. 2008;148(8):632–3. doi:10.7326/0003-4819-148-8-200804150-00024.

69. Kelly CR, Kahn S, Kashyap P, Laine L, Rubin D, Atreja A, et al. Update on fecal microbiota transplantation 2015: Indications, methodologies, mechanisms, and outlook. Gastroenterology. 2015;149(1):223–37. doi:10.1053/j.gastro.2015.05.008.

70. Costello SP, Hughes PA, Waters O, Bryant RV, Vincent AD, Blatchford P, et al. Effect of fecal microbiota transplantation on 8-week remission in patients with ulcerative colitis: A randomized clinical trial. JAMA. 2019;321(2):156–64. doi:10.1001/jama.2018.20046.

71. Shi Y, Dong Y, Huang W, Zhu D, Mao H, Su P. Fecal microbiota transplantation for ulcerative colitis: A systematic review and meta-analysis. PLoS One. 2016;11(6):e0157259. doi:10.1371/journal.pone.0157259.

27 Eating Disorders in Gastroenterology

Christina T. Gentile

27.1 INTRODUCTION

Eating disorders (EDs) are complex biopsychosocial conditions characterized by severe disturbances in eating behavior, resulting in psychosocial impairment and reduced quality of life.[1, 2] EDs are associated with serious medical complications, such as electrolyte abnormalities, malnutrition, arrythmia, and hypoglycemia.[3] Gastrointestinal (GI) symptoms frequently co-occur with EDs and complicate the identification of an ED. The chronicity of GI symptoms can also increase the risk of disordered eating behaviors (DEBs),[4] which can impact digestive functioning and treatment outcomes.

The overlap of GI problems with EDs and DEBs have been reviewed in the literature.[4–6] Patients may present with GI disturbances (Table 27.1), such as constipation and early satiety[5, 6] and DEBs can complicate medical and nutritional management.[6–10]

The relationship between Gi disorders, DEBs, and EDs has shown the following:

- High rates of postprandial fullness and epigastric pressure in bulimia nervosa[7]
- DEBs are associated with disturbed GI sensitivity and motor physiology[8]
- Food avoidance is common in patients with inflammatory bowel disease (IBD)[9]
- Long-term dietary restraint in celiac disease may increase the risk of DEBs[11]
- Crohn's disease (CD) and anorexia nervosa (AN) are frequent comorbidities[12]

Screening is necessary to identify risk factors (Table 27.2) and interactions with the GI disorder.

27.2 OVERVIEW OF EATING DISORDERS

The diagnostic categories of anorexia nervosa (AN), bulimia nervosa (BN), binge-eating disorder (BED), and avoidant/restrictive food intake disorder (ARFID) – as described in the *Diagnostic and Statistical Manual of Mental Disorders, Fifth Edition* (5th ed.; *DSM-5*) – are reviewed in the subsequent section. These disorders are mutually exclusive of one another such that the presence of one precludes the presence of another.[16]

DOI: 10.1201/9780429322570-27

TABLE 27.1

GI Disturbances in Anorexia Nervosa and Bulimia Nervosa

Anorexia Nervosa (AN)	Bulimia Nervosa (BN)
Constipation	Bloating
Abdominal pain	Flatulence
Early satiety	Constipation
Postprandial fullness	Decreased appetite
Slow gastric emptying	Borborygmi
Nausea	Nausea

TABLE 27.2

Potential Risk Factors in GI Populations

Irritable Bowel Syndrome[13–15]	Celiac Disease[10, 11, 14, 15]	Inflammatory Bowel Disease[9, 14]
• Fear of gut sensations	• Poor disease adjustment	• Fear of disease activity
• GI symptom anxiety	• Burden of GFD*	• Disease burden
• Unremitting GI episodes	• Strict dietary restraint	• Higher food avoidance with
• Skipping meals	• Food preoccupation	disease activity or history of
• Fear of trying new or	• Emotional distress with	strictures
unfamiliar foods	weight gain from GFD	• Increased anxiety and BID
• GI symptoms and BID*	• BID and weight status	during flare-ups
• Self-initiated dietary	• Limited food variety	• Weight gain, BID, and
restrictions	• Fear of gluten exposure	corticosteroid treatment
• Fear of reintroduction phase	• Deliberate ingestion of	• Surgical intervention,
of FODMAP diet	gluten for weight loss	adjustment, and BID
• Embarrassment and shame	• High levels of anxiety	• Fear of GI discomfort
about symptoms	• Poor QoL	• Fatigue and poor QoL
• Poor QoL*	• Financial resources	• Anxiety or depression
• History of ED	• History of ED	• History of ED

* BID: body image dissatisfaction; QoL: quality of life; GFD: gluten-free diet.

27.2.1 ANOREXIA NERVOSA

Anorexia nervosa (AN) is a serious condition that has the highest mortality rate of all psychiatric disorders, with death resulting from medical complications or suicide. AN is characterized by a significantly low body weight from caloric restriction (below minimally normal for adults) with severity based on body mass index (BMI) (Table 27.3); an intense fear of weight gain or engagement in behaviors that interfere with weight gain (purging and/or non-purging behaviors) (Table 27.4); and a severe disturbance in body image perception.[16] Fear of weight gain does not alleviate with weight loss.[17] Subtypes describe the behavioral presentation over the last 3 months and includes

TABLE 27.3
AN Severity Specifiers

Level of Severity	Body Mass Index (BMI)
Mild	≥ 17 kg/m^2
Moderate	16–16.99 kg/m^2
Severe	15–15.99 kg/m^2
Extreme	<15 kg/m^2

TABLE 27.4
Examples of Purging and Non-Purging Behaviors

Purging Behaviors	Non-Purging Behaviors
Self-induced vomiting	Excessive exercise
Laxatives	Fasting
Diuretics	Skipping meals
Enemas	Food restriction
Suppositories	Diet pills

recurrent binge eating and/or purging (binge-eating/purging type; AN-BP) or predominant dietary restriction, fasting, and/or exercise (restricting type; AN-R).[16]

27.2.2 BULIMIA NERVOSA

Bulimia nervosa (BN) involves repeated episodes of binge eating (the consumption of an objectively large amount of food) within a discrete period of time (two hours) that are accompanied by a perceived loss of control. Binge eating is followed by inappropriate compensatory behaviors (ICBs) that function to prevent weight gain. ICBs may also serve to temporarily alleviate distress and discomfort (e.g., guilt associated with binge episode). ICBs include purging (e.g., self-induced vomiting, laxative misuse, or enemas) and non-purging methods (e.g., skipping meals or excessive exercise). While individuals with BN usually engage in several methods to compensate for binges, self-induced vomiting is one of the most common behaviors. ICBs are also features that are observed in AN or other specified feeding and eating disorder (OSFED).[16]

Binge eating and ICBs both occur at least once a week for 3 months. Severity of BN is based on the frequency of ICBs per week (Table 27.5). Body weight and shape have an excessive influence on self-evaluation and contribute to the maintenance of BN. Low self-esteem, dysphoric mood, and feelings of shame or disgust are common features. If an individual meets the behavioral and cognitive criteria for both AN-BP and BN, a diagnosis of AN-BP is assigned, since AN takes precedence due to low body weight.[16]

TABLE 27.5
BN Severity Specifiers

Level of Severity	Inappropriate Compensatory Behaviors (ICBs)
Mild	1–3 episodes of ICBs per week
Moderate	4–7 episodes of ICBs per week
Severe	8–13 episodes of ICBs per week
Extreme	14 or more episodes of ICBs per week

TABLE 27.6
BED Severity Specifiers

Level of Severity	Frequency of Binge Episodes
Mild	1–3 binge episodes per week
Moderate	4–7 binge episodes per week
Severe	8–13 binge episodes per week
Extreme	14 or more binge episodes per week

27.2.3 BINGE-EATING DISORDER

BED includes recurrent episodes of binge eating in the absence of ICBs that occur at least weekly over 3 months, with severity based on the average frequency of binges per week (Table 27.6). The occurrence of a binge is accompanied by a loss of control and an elevated level of distress. Three or more of the following indicators must be present to meet diagnostic criteria:

- Eating more rapidly than normal
- Eating past the point of fullness
- Eating a large amount of food while not physically hungry
- Eating alone secondary to embarrassment about eating behaviors
- Feelings of disgust, depression, and/or guilt after eating[16]

27.2.4 AVOIDANT/RESTRICTIVE FOOD INTAKE DISORDER

Avoidant/restrictive food intake disorder (ARFID) involves clinically significant dietary restriction or food avoidance, resulting in a persistent inability to meet nutritional or energy needs. ARFID is associated with at least one of the following: significant weight loss or severe nutritional deficiency; dependence on enteral tube feeding or nutritional supplementation; and/or marked psychosocial impairment. Common behavioral signs of ARFID are shown in Table 27.7. ARFID is not diagnosed when the following is present:

- Feeding behaviors that are related to a cultural practice (e.g., religious fast)
- Limited availability or access to food resources

TABLE 27.7

Behavioral Signs of ARFID

Sensory-Based Avoidance	Lack of Interest	Fear-Based Avoidance
Heightened sensitivity to food (taste, temperature)	Low appetite; forget to eat; feel full more quickly	Intense fear of and avoidance to prevent an adverse outcome (choking, vomiting, pain)

- Developmentally appropriate behavior (e.g., picky eating in toddlers)
- Restriction due to body disturbance or weight concerns (e.g., as in AN)
- Eating disturbance that is explained by a medical or psychiatric disorder

Those with fear-based consequences may have had a past traumatic event related to food, eating, or illness.[16] Patients with GI disorders may have significant anxiety about GI symptom episodes and engage in restrictive diets to prevent feared consequences, such as abdominal pain, nausea, constipation, or diarrhea. Fear of GI symptoms (e.g., abdominal pain), coupled with avoidance behaviors (e.g., restriction in the variety of food and/or volume of dietary intake), perpetuate anxiety and may result in food avoidance that generalizes to other similar food items.

Careful assessment of ARFID in GI populations is necessary to differentiate it from other diagnoses (AN, obsessive–compulsive disorder, major depressive disorder, or autism spectrum disorder) or determine if the behaviors are better explained by an adjustment disorder (e.g., coping with a new diagnosis), GI symptom-specific anxiety, or patient-specific factors (e.g., poor understanding of a prescribed diet). Providers should consider the degree to which fear-based consequences are adversely impacting medical status (e.g., nutritional deficiencies or significant weight loss), psychosocial functioning (e.g., avoidance of social engagements, distress in social eating situations, and/or difficulties with interpersonal relationships), and overall quality of life. A patient can receive a diagnosis of ARFID if the eating disturbance is out of proportion to what is expected for the GI disorder and requires clinical attention.

27.3 SCREENING AND ASSESSMENT IN GI POPULATIONS

Early recognition of DEBs can mitigate the onset of an ED and concurrent medical consequences (Table 27.8). Screening is important when considering dietary interventions (e.g., elimination diet) or prescribed medical diets (e.g., gluten-free diet for celiac disease). Warning signs should also be considered in the context of the individual psychosocial implications of the GI disorder (e.g., fear of symptoms in public, embarrassment about diarrhea, body dissatisfaction due to distension, patient's explanatory model of disease).

27.3.1 EFFECTIVE INTERPERSONAL COMMUNICATION SKILLS

Central to an effective evaluation is a patient-centered approach that facilitates collaboration between the patient, provider, and multidisciplinary team. Communication

TABLE 27.8
Examples of Cognitive-Affective and Behavioral Signs of DEBs

Behavioral Signs	Cognitive-Affective Signs
Dietary restriction or avoidance	Inflexible rules about food or eating
Uncontrollable eating	Preoccupation with weight or shape
Chewing or spitting out food	Body dissatisfaction
Frequent dieting or fasting	Irritability or sadness
Self-induced vomiting	Frequent worry or rumination
Ingestion of trigger foods	Obsessive thought patterns
Social withdrawal	Perfectionistic traits
Sleep problems	Dichotomous thinking

TABLE 27.9
Interpersonal Communication Skills for Providers

Verbal Skills	Non-Verbal Skills
Validate emotional responses	Appropriate eye contact
Use reflective listening	Relaxed, open posture
Acknowledge difficulties	Head nodding
Provide summaries	Leaning slightly forward
Foster hope and team-based care	Facial expression
Elicit feedback from the patient	Tone of voice

skills (Table 27.9) that promote trust and warmth are likely to enhance the effectiveness of the encounter (e.g., patient–provider trust, patient satisfaction, openness to disclose current challenges).

Sensitivity to individual factors during the encounter is essential. This includes personality traits (e.g., neuroticism, alexithymia), mood (e.g., depressed), affect (e.g., tense), and motivation (e.g., ambivalence). Fatigue, pain, or discomfort may interfere with engagement and is further complicated by severe medical complications (e.g., malnourishment and cognitive performance).

27.3.2 CLINICAL INTERVIEW

The use of open- and closed-ended questions will depend on the clinical rationale and availability of time. Potential screening areas include the following: GI symptom severity, level of adjustment, and distress; emotional responses to GI problems; current eating behaviors, ICBs, and dietary restriction; food-related beliefs and concerns about weight, body image, and eating; and past history of an ED. Additional areas that may warrant further evaluation include distress with dietary expansion or reintroduction; progressive dietary restriction despite medical recommendations; fear-based food aversions; and the use of avoidance or control behaviors to manage

GI symptom episodes (e.g., skipping breakfast to prevent diarrhea at work or use of laxatives to "feel empty" before an event). Providers will also benefit from assessing the sociocultural context (e.g., cultural health beliefs, food security, access to health-care, and quality of social support) to identify the social interactions among DEBs and the GI disorder.

27.3.3 SCREENING MEASURES FOR EATING DISORDERS

Screening measures (Table 27.10) and interview-based methods (Table 27.11) can assist with identifying risk factors and augment data obtained from the medical record, clinical interview, and multidisciplinary team. Data should be interpreted with caution because validity with GI populations is limited at this time. Instead, providers may benefit from using these measures as a tool to guide the clinical con-versation and facilitate further evaluation. An in-depth review of these measures is documented elsewhere.[18–20]

TABLE 27.10
Screening Measures for Eating Disorders

Measure	Description
Screen for Disordered Eating (SDE)[21]	5-item screener for AN, BN, and BED
Eating Attitudes Test-26 (EAT-26)[22]	26-item measure to screen for disordered eating attitudes and behaviors
Clinical Impairment Scale (CIS)[23]	16-item measure to assess psychosocial impairment due to an eating disorder
Eating Disorder Examination-Questionnaire (EDE-Q)[24]	28-item measure to assess eating disorder pathology
Binge Eating Disorder Screener-7 (BEDS-7)[25]	7-item measure for binge eating behaviors
Nine-Item ARFID Screen (NIAS)[26]	9-item measure to screen for avoidant and restrictive eating behaviors
Food Neophobia Scale (FNS)[27]	10-item measure to screen for fear and avoidance of new or unfamiliar foods

TABLE 27.11
Interview-Based Measures for Eating Disorders

Measure	Description
Eating Disorder Assessment for DSM-5 (EDA-5)[28]	Semi-structured interview
Eating Disorder Examination 17.0D (EDE)[29]	Investigator-based interview
Eating Pathology Symptoms Inventory – Clinician Rated Version (EPSI-CRV)[30]	Semi-structured interview

TABLE 27.12

Screening Measures for Psychological Distress

Measure	Description
Patient Health Questionnaire-9 (PHQ-9)[33]	9-item measure to screen for depression
Beck Depression Inventory (BDI-II)[34]	21-item measure to assess depression
Generalized Anxiety Disorder 7 (GAD-7)[35]	7-item measure to screen for anxiety
Beck Anxiety Inventory (BAI)[36]	21-item measure to assess anxiety severity
Hospital Anxiety and Depression Scale (HADS)[37]	14-item measure to screen for anxiety and depression in medical populations
Depression, Anxiety, and Stress Scale-21 (DASS-21)[38]	21-item measure to assess the emotional states of depression, anxiety, and stress

27.3.4 PSYCHIATRIC COMORBIDITY

Mood (e.g., major depressive disorder, bipolar disorder), anxiety (e.g., generalized anxiety disorder, panic disorder, social phobia), trauma (e.g., post-traumatic stress disorder), and substance use disorders (e.g., alcohol, opioids) frequently co-occur with EDs.[16, 31, 18, 19] Suicide attempts are common in AN and BN,[16] and the risk is increased with comorbid depression, substance use, or borderline personality disorder.[17, 31] Distress measures (Table 27.12) are used to screen for possible psychiatric symptoms and the psychometrics are reviewed elsewhere.[20, 32] Interpretation should be made with caution to determine if mood is attributed to the current GI episode, somatic symptoms (e.g., fatigue), or medical complications (e.g., nutrient deficiency on cognitive processes).

27.4 RECOMMENDATIONS FOR BIOPSYCHOSOCIAL TREATMENT

Patients with risk of DEBs or an ED and/or psychiatric comorbidities are appropriately referred to a mental health specialist (e.g., psychologist) for diagnostic evaluation and will also need an evaluation by the physician to determine if there are any medical complications that warrant attention. The Academy for Eating Disorders has published guidelines for standards of care; these are available in multiple languages. The type of treatment will depend on the severity of ED pathology, medical instability, psychiatric comorbidities, and functional impairment.[39, 40]

27.5 NOVEL APPROACHES

Patients with DEBs that do not require an intensive level of treatment (medically and psychiatrically stable) are likely to benefit from a biopsychosocial approach that includes a multidisciplinary team (e.g., gastroenterologist, GI-specialized registered dietitian, and health psychologist) for integrative, evidence-based treatment that supports whole-person wellness. An example of a clinical pathway for multidisciplinary care is presented in Figure 24.1. Clinical awareness of DEBs and the implementation of effective communication skills amongst the multidisciplinary team are key for screening, management, and coordination of care.

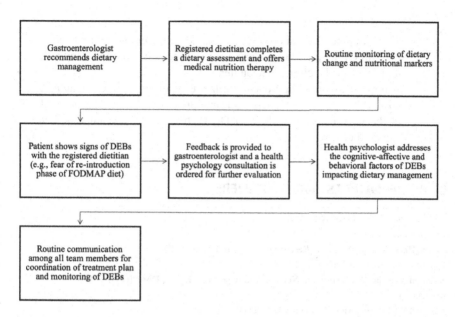

FIGURE 27.1   Referral to registered dietitian and health psychologist for patient with DEBs.

Collaboration with a GI registered dietitian and GI health psychologist (or mental health specialist) provides comprehensive support that is tailored to the unique needs of the patient (e.g., evaluate potential risk factors prior to dietary management; support adjustment to a prescribed medical diet; address GI symptom-specific anxiety or maladaptive thoughts interfering with dietary adherence; and/or provide skills-based training to enhance self-efficacy with GI symptom management.

27.6   CONCLUSION

DEBs and EDs are common in GI populations and providers should consider the psychosocial implications of the GI disorder on daily functioning (including prescribed medical diets) and the sociocultural context of the patient. Treatment will depend on medical and psychiatric severity and warrants further evaluation by a physician and psychologist. Patients that do not need intensive treatment are likely to benefit from an integrative approach that includes collaboration with a registered dietitian and psychologist for improved GI symptom management and to reduce the risk of progressively worsening DEBs.

PRACTICE PEARLS

- DEBs and/or EDs can contribute to the maintenance of GI symptoms, interfere with treatment outcome, and markedly diminish quality of life.
- Proper screening of DEBs and/or EDs in GI populations is essential for improved management and mitigating medical consequences.
- Medical standards of care are available at the Academy for Eating Disorders.

- Screening measures should be interpreted with caution because validity with GI populations is limited at this time and should be used as a tool to guide the clinical encounter.
- A multidisciplinary approach that includes a registered dietitian and GI health psychologist can provide comprehensive care that is tailored to the patient for patients with DEBs that do not warrant a higher standard of care.

27.8 RESOURCES FOR PROVIDERS

Academy for Eating Disorders (AED)
www.aedweb.org/home

Eating Disorders Coalition for Research, Policy, and Action (EDC)
www.eatingdisorderscoalition.org/

National Association of Anorexia Nervosa and Associated Eating Disorders (ANAD)
www.anad.org/

National Eating Disorders Association (NEDA)
www.nationaleatingdisorders.org/

National Institute of Mental Health (NIMH)
www.nimh.nih.gov/health/topics/eating-disorders/index.shtml

REFERENCES

1. Hudson, J. I., Hiripi, E., Pope, H. G., & Kessler, R. C. (2007). The prevalence and correlates of eating disorders in the national comorbidity survey replication. *Biological Psychiatry*, *61*(3), 348–358. https://doi.org/10.1016/j.biopsych.2006.03.040
2. Engel, S. G., Adair, C. E., Hayas, C. L., & Abraham, S. (2009). Health-related quality of life and eating disorders: A review of update. *International Journal of Eating Disorders*, *42*(2), 179–187. https://doi.org/10.1002/eat.20602
3. Birmingham, C. L., & Levine, M. P. (2015). The Wiley handbook of eating disorders (Wiley clinical psychology handbooks). In L. Smolak & M. P. Levine (Eds.), *Medical Complications and Diagnosing Eating Disorders* (1st ed., pp. 170–182). Retrieved from https://doi.org/10.1002/9781118574089.ch14
4. Satherley, R., Howard, R., & Higgs, S. (2015). Disordered eating practices in gastrointestinal disorders. *Appetite*, *84*, 240–250. https://doi.org/10.1016/j.appet.2014.10.006
5. Sato, Y., & Fukudo, S. (2015). Gastrointestinal symptoms and disorders in patients with eating disorders. *Clinical Journal of Gastroenterology*, *8*(5), 255–263. https://doi.org/10.1007/s12328-015-0611-x
6. McKinlay, A., & McKay, R. (2018). Multidisciplinary management of eating disorders. In J. Morris & A. McKinlay (Eds.), *How Do Medical Conditions Interact with Eating Disorders and How Are They Managed in This Context?* (pp. 63–90). https://doi.org/10.1007/978-3-319-64131-7
7. Santonicola, A. (2012). Prevalence of functional dyspepsia and its subgroups in patients with eating disorders. *World Journal of Gastroenterology*, *18*(32), 4379. https://doi.org/10.3748/wjg.v18.i32.4379

8. Janssen, P. (2010). Can eating disorders cause functional gastrointestinal disorders? *Neurogastroenterology & Motility*, *22*(12), 1267–1269. https://doi.org/10.1111/j.1365-2982.2010.01621.x

9. Bergeron, F., Bouin, M., D'Aoust, L., Lemoyne, M., & Presse, N. (2018). Food avoidance in patients with inflammatory bowel disease: What, when and who? *Clinical Nutrition*, *37*(3), 884–889. https://doi.org/10.1016/j.clnu.2017.03.010

10. Satherley, R., Howard, R., & Higgs, S. (2015). Disordered eating practices in gastrointestinal disorders. *Appetite*, *84*, 240–250. https://doi.org/10.1016/j.appet.2014.10.006

11. Satherley, R., Howard, R., & Higgs, S. (2016). The prevalence and predictors of disordered eating in women with coeliac disease. *Appetite*, *107*, 260–267. https://doi.org/10.1016/j.appet.2016.07.038

12. Ilzarbe, L., Fàbrega, M., Quintero, R., Bastidas, A., Pintor, L., García-Campayo, J., . . . Ilzarbe, D. (2017). Inflammatory bowel disease and eating disorders: A systematized review of comorbidity. *Journal of Psychosomatic Research*, *102*, 47–53. https://doi.org/10.1016/j.jpsychores.2017.09.006

13. Mari, A., Hosadurg, D., Martin, L., Zarate-Lopez, N., Passananti, V., & Emmanuel, A. (2019). Adherence with a low-FODMAP diet in irritable bowel syndrome. *European Journal of Gastroenterology & Hepatology*, *31*(2), 178–182. https://doi.org/10.1097/meg.0000000000001317

14. David, J., Culnan, E., & Ernst, L. (2017). Adolescents with diet-related chronic health conditions (DRCHCs) and unique risk for development of eating pathology. *Journal of Child and Adolescent Behavior*, *05*(02). https://doi.org/10.4172/2375-4494.1000340

15. Quick, V. M., Byrd-Bredbenner, C., & Neumark-Sztainer, D. (2013). Chronic illness and disordered eating: A discussion of the literature. *Advances in Nutrition*, *4*(3), 277–286. https://doi.org/10.3945/an.112.003608

16. *American Psychiatric Association: Diagnostic and Statistical Manual of Mental Disorders: Diagnostic and Statistical Manual of Mental Disorders* (5th ed.). Arlington, VA: American Psychiatric Association, 2013.

17. Gray, E., Murray, H., & Eddy, K. (2015). The Wiley handbook of eating disorders (Wiley clinical psychology handbooks). In L. Smolak & M. P. Levine (Eds.), *Diagnosing Anorexia Nervosa* (1st ed., pp. 95–104). Retrieved from https://doi.org/10.1002/9781118574089.ch14

18. Smolak, L., & Levine, M. P. (2015). *The Wiley Handbook of Eating Disorders (Wiley Clinical Psychology Handbooks)*. Retrieved from https://doi.org/10.1002/9781118574089

19. Walsh MD, B. T., Attia MD, E., Glasofer PhD, D. R., & Sysko PhD, R. (2015). *Handbook of Assessment and Treatment of Eating Disorders*. Washington, DC: American Psychiatric Association Publishing.

20. Baer, L., & Blais, M. A. (2010). *Handbook of Clinical Rating Scales and Assessment in Psychiatry and Mental Health (Current Clinical Psychiatry)* (2010 ed.). Boston: Humana.

21. Maguen, S., Hebenstreit, C., Li, Y., Dinh, J. V., Donalson, R., Dalton, S., . . . Masheb, R. (2018). Screen for disordered eating: Improving the accuracy of eating disorder screening in primary care. *General Hospital Psychiatry*, *50*, 20–25.

22. Garner, D. M., Olmsted, M. P., Bohr, Y., & Garfinkel, P. E. (1982). The Eating Attitudes Test: Psychometric features and clinical correlates. *Psychological Medicine*, *12*(4), 871–878. https://doi.org/10.1017/s0033291700049163

23. Bohn, K., Doll, H. A., Cooper, Z., O'Connor, M., Palmer, R. L., & Fairburn, C. G. (2008). The measurement of impairment due to eating disorder psychopathology. *Behaviour Research and Therapy*, *46*(10), 1105–1110. https://doi.org/10.1016/j.brat.2008.06.012

24. Fairburn, C. G., & Beglin, S. J. (2008). Eating disorder examination questionnaire (6.0). In C. G. Fairburn (Ed.), *Cognitive Behavior Therapy and Eating Disorders*. New York: Guilford Press.

25. Herman, B. K., Deal, L. S., DiBenedetti, D. B., Nelson, L., Fehnel, S. E., & Brown, T. M. (2016). Development of the 7-item binge-eating disorder screener (BEDS-7). *The Primary Care Companion for CNS Disorders.* https://doi.org/10.4088/pcc.15m01896

26. Zickgraf, H. F., & Ellis, J. M. (2018). Initial validation of the nine item avoidant/restrictive food intake disorder screen (NIAS): A measure of three restrictive eating patterns. *Appetite, 123,* 32–42. https://doi.org/10.1016/j.appet.2017.11.111

27. Pliner, P., & Hobden, K. (1992). Development of a scale to measure the trait of food neophobia in humans. *Appetite, 19*(2), 105–120. https://doi.org/10.1016/0195-6663(92)90014-w

28. Sysko, R., Glasofer, D. R., Hildebrandt, T., Klimek, P., Mitchell, J. E., Berg, K. C., Peterson, C. B., Wonderlich, S. A., & Walsh, B. T. (2015, July). The eating disorder assessment for DSM-5 (EDA-5): Development and validation of a structured interview for feeding and eating disorders. *International Journal of Eating Disorders, 48*(5), 452–63.

29. Fairburn, C., Cooper, Z., & O'Connor, M. (2014). Eating disorder examination (Edition 17.0D; April 2014). Updated from Fairburn C. G., Cooper, Z., & O'Connor M. E. (2008). Eating disorder examination (Edition 16.0D). In: C. G. Fairburn, *Cognitive Behavior Therapy and Eating Disorders* (pp. 265–308). New York: Guilford Press, 2008.

30. Forbush, K. T., Wildes, J. E., Bohrer, B. K., Chapa, D. A., & Hagan, K. E. (2018). *Eating Pathology Symptoms Inventory: Clinician Rated Version.* Kansas: Lawrence.

31. Lock, J. D. (2018). *Pocket Guide for the Assessment and Treatment of Eating Disorders* (1st ed.). Washington, DC: Amer Psychiatric Pub Inc.

32. Benyamini, Y., Johnston, M., & Karademas, E. C. (2016). *Assessment in Health Psychology, a Volume in the Series Psychological Assessment Science and Practice* (2nd ed.). Boston, MA: Hogrefe Publishing.

33. Kroenke, K., Spitzer, R. L., & Williams, J. B. W. (2001). The PHQ-9. *Journal of General Internal Medicine, 16*(9), 606–613. https://doi.org/10.1046/j.1525-1497.2001.016009606.x

34. Beck, A. T., Steer, R. A., & Brown, G. K. (1996). *Manual for the Beck Depression Inventory-II.* San Antonio, TX: Psychological Corporation.

35. Spitzer, R. L., Kroenke, K., Williams, J. B. W., & Löwe, B. (2006). A brief measure for assessing generalized anxiety disorder. *Archives of Internal Medicine, 166*(10), 1092–1097. https://doi.org/10.1001/archinte.166.10.1092

36. Beck, A. T., Epstein, N., Brown, G., & Steer, R. A. (1988). An inventory for measuring clinical anxiety: Psychometric properties. *Journal of Consulting and Clinical Psychology, 56,* 893–897.

37. Zigmond, A. S., & Snaith, R. P. (1983). The hospital anxiety and depression scale. *Acta Psychiatrica Scandinavica, 67*(6), 361–370. https://doi.org/10.1111/j.1600-0447.1983.tb09716.x

38. Lovibond, S. H., & Lovibond, P. F. (1995). *Manual for the Depression Anxiety Stress Scales* (2nd ed.). Sydney: Psychology Foundation. ISBN 7334–1423–0.

39. Yager, J., Devlin, M. J., Halmi, K. A., Herzog, D. B., Mitchell, J. E., Powers, P., & Zerbe, K. J. (2014). Guideline watch (August 2012): Practice guideline for the treatment of patients with eating disorders, 3rd edition. *Focus, 12*(4), 416–431. https://doi.org/10.1176/appi.focus.120404

40. Hilbert, A., Hoek, H. W., & Schmidt, R. (2017). Evidence-based clinical guidelines for eating disorders. *Current Opinion in Psychiatry, 30*(6), 423–437. https://doi.org/10.1097/yco.0000000000000360

28 Nutrition, Diet, and Health
Resources

Carol Ireton-Jones

Nutrition care in the outpatient setting may be the key to disease prevention and/or managing progression. It is hard to name a disease process that does not have a nutrition component. Gastrointestinal (GI) disease may significantly affect nutrition status through intake, assimilation, and metabolism. Disease states such as diabetes and cancer may affect nutrition status and involve nutrition intervention. Malnutrition continues to be a problem while the incidence of overweight and obesity rises. The gut microbiome has an ever-increasing importance in unlocking better health. What one eats makes a difference in health, performance, and quality of life.

Nutrition is complex. Every person is different and has different tastes, experiences, and customs about food. A country as large as the United States not only has differences in the areas of the country as to what people eat but also different labels for foods such as "Southern food," "soul food," "comfort food," "Creole," "hearty Midwestern," and even "funeral food." Diversity and the integration of different cultures also brings in different types of foods. In the United Kingdom, ethnic diversity and therefore food diversity has been recognized as a factor in disease prevention and treatment (1). Being culturally competent in healthcare provision recognizes social and cultural considerations in care delivery (2). Absolutely imperative is communicating nutrition principles using a person's traditional, familiar, and accessible foods. Providing nutrition care must encompass an understanding of the individual's requirements and goals as well as their ability to maintain or make changes related to nutrient intake.

28.1 HEALTHY EATING

Healthy eating is rather complex. In fact, what is healthy eating? Is there one healthy diet? Healthy eating or a healthy diet might be described as the consumption of a variety of foods that meet an individual's nutrient needs. There are resources to help define and prepare a healthy diet. The US Dietary Guidelines and MyPlate give suggestions for including nutritious foods and understanding portion sizes (3, 4). Several medically credible sources have online presences and may provide a starting point in gathering information on the components of a healthy diet (5–7). The Mediterranean diet encourages fruits, vegetables, and whole grains, and there are variations to the diet that have been offered (8). According to US News and World

DOI: 10.1201/9780429322570-28

reports, the Mediterranean diet and DASH diet (which stands for dietary approaches to stop hypertension) come in at #1 and #2 as "Best Overall Diets" and have for several years in a row based on nutritional value, ease of use, and effectiveness to help manage chronic disease (9). Healthy People 2030 focuses on helping people get the recommended amounts of healthy foods – fruits, vegetables, and whole grains – to reduce their risk for chronic diseases and improve their health (10). The goal of nutrition care is to provide the most varied, delicious, easy nutrition plan that decreases or prevents food- or diet-related symptoms and improves or maintains health.

28.2 CHALLENGES IN NUTRITION

A nutritious diet can be had for all including those individuals that have a preference for or commitment to a specific diet such as vegan, vegetarian, low-fat, low-carbohydrate, or an eating style such as multiple small meals or circadian rhythm. Any nutrition regimen that avoids extremes can "probably" provide adequate nutrition. Those that focus solely on one macronutrient (protein, for example) or leave out classes of foods (for example, dairy-free or grain-free) will lack important individual nutrients which can lead to poor nutrition.

Along with managing new and chronic diseases, a major concern in the United States is the presence of overweight and obesity. When a person's weight is higher than what is considered to be a normal weight for a given height, this is described as being overweight or having obesity (11–13). There are many diet plans and programs as well as surgical procedures for weight loss. Weight loss is a journey and requires expert guidance. Weight management, metabolic syndrome, and obesity are addressed in Chapters 22 and 23.

Along with the cultural considerations mentioned previously, sensitivity and respect for a person's body habitus is important. In addition, person-first language provides a foundation for "collaborative treatment environments that promote respect, human dignity, and hope" (14). Therefore, a person is no longer a "diabetic" or obese – they are a person with diabetes or a person with obesity (14). Condition-first language can negatively affect motivation to change and increase stigmatization (15).

Food and eating have many connotations from enjoyment of being with friends and family, to nourishment for a life change such as pregnancy or an athletic or recreational sports event, to health maintenance or repair. People may have an illness, disease process, or disorder that changes their ability to tolerate certain foods. They may have challenges with eating – whether amount, types of foods, composition of the food, or method of receiving nutrition.

An evidence-based approach to diet and nutrition management is key. In practice, a multidisciplinary team can address many elements of care – diagnosis, treatment, medications, psychosocial support, and diet. A qualified, experienced, evidence-based registered dietitian has the specialized knowledge to combine food and nutrition expertise to develop an appropriate eating plan. Nutrition intervention usually involves food changes and may include reducing or modifying certain foods while creating a nutritionally adequate diet. Take for example two evidenced based nutrition interventions: the gluten-free diet for celiac disease, a lifelong elimination of gluten-containing foods; and the low-FODMAP diet, used with IBS, which includes elimination and reintroduction of specific foods. Chapter 25 provides information on several popular diets for people with gastrointestinal disorders.

Other "diets," especially many found by searching the Internet, may be very restrictive and eliminate many foods without adequate or any supportive evidence. Two relatively new concepts in nutrition are avoidant or restrictive food intake disorder (ARFID) and orthorexia "an obsessive focus on eating healthy" (16, 17). When creating a nutrition plan, a comprehensive evaluation should consider the potential for ARFID, orthorexia or other disordered eating which could result in food avoidance and fear of eating. Implementation of any kind of nutrition "plan" may need to be modified to prevent further exacerbation of these disorders (18). Chapter 27 addresses eating disorders and challenges for people with gastrointestinal disorders.

There are challenges to following a specialized diet such as eating at home versus away from home or social or peer pressure to eat which has been described related to people who receive home parenteral or enteral nutrition (19). In a study of adults with short bowel syndrome who received home parenteral nutrition, the ability to consume food was an important aspect of a positive quality of life regardless of the nutritional content absorbed from the food (20).

28.3 MALNUTRITION

Malnutrition in the United States is present in children, adults, and the elderly at many socioeconomic levels. In US hospitals the prevalence of malnutrition in the hospital is 20–50% (pediatric and adult patients) (21, 22). Estimates are likely to be similar in long-term care and outpatient or homecare although data is lacking. Improving food accessibility as well as nutrition interventions for disease treatment and prevention are needed to improve nutrition status. This is a focus for organizations such as the American Society for Parenteral and Enteral Nutrition (www.nutritioncare.org) and the Academy of Nutrition and Dietetics (www.eatright.org) with available tools and resources for identifying and addressing malnutrition (23–25).

28.4 THE GUT MICROBIOME

"You are what you eat," is a quote from Anthelme Brillat-Savarin who wrote, in *Physiologie du Gout, ou Meditations de Gastronomie Transcendante, 1826*: "Dismoi ce que tu manges, je te dirai ce que tu es" [Tell me what you eat, and I will tell you what you are] (26). This old quote has new life especially as it relates to the human gut microbiota. This microbiota comprises trillions of microorganisms that have many functions including immune function and metabolism (27, 28). The type and amount of food consumed affects the microbiota and may have a crucial role in obesity, diabetes, and diseases such as inflammatory bowel disease (28). The microflora are also affected by medications. Antibiotics have been shown to decrease gut bacteria, although a recent study showed that while this may affect immune competence, glucose tolerance was not affected (29). Stool sample testing may be used to determine the presence of a parasite, the presence of *Clostridium difficile* in intractable diarrhea, or for increased fat content due to malabsorption but is not useful in determining how to treat the gut microbiome (30). Because there are millions of bacteria not only in the stool but also in the intestinal wall, a stool sample does not define the bacteria milieu in the GI tract (31). Although gut microbial dysbiosis certainly occurs, attempting to make a nutrition or probiotic recommendation based on the stool data is complex with many factors to consider (32).

Probiotics and prebiotics are being used to influence the gut microbiome; however, much more research is needed (see Chapter 26). The future of nutrition, prevention of disease, and disease management will incorporate managing and modifying the gut microbiota. Many components of understanding and manipulating the gut microbiome remain under investigation.

28.5 UNPROVEN NUTRITION

Registered dietitian nutritionists (RDNs) are food and nutrition experts who understand the unique interactions of foods, diet, and nutrition in the body. Registered dietitians have specialized training and education as well as the credential of RD or RDN (33). RDNs who specialize in clinical care may work in hospitals, outpatient clinics, community/public health, research, government agencies, and private practice. RDNs work hand in hand with physicians, nurses, pharmacists, and other members of the healthcare team. The role of the RDN in assessing nutrition status of the critically ill patient and collaborating with the medical and surgical team regarding route of nutritional support, nutritional access, fluid and electrolyte issues, and selecting enteral feeding products continues to be recognized as a vital part of the critical care (34). For pediatric patients with type 1 and type 2 diabetes, the RDN provides multifactorial nutrition care, including assessing growth and development, eating behaviors, food choices, and meal patterns. Improved glycemic control and delayed onset of diabetes complications have been demonstrated when pediatric patients and their families have access to a skilled RDN (35). Dietitian-led nutrition education has been shown to better manage lipid levels and aid in weight management and improve adherence and outcomes for patients with irritable bowel syndrome following the low FODMAP diet (18, 35). Each of the chapters in this book reviews GI and related disorders in which nutrition and an RDN play an essential role in care and management. Evidence-based nutrition uses the best available scientific evidence to help prevent, treat, and manage nutrition in health and disease. Evidence-based nutrition should also be combined with clinical experience (36). People, especially those with GI symptoms may seek out non-evidence-based therapies or tests often because the time to diagnosis may be protracted. The desire to have a "test" or confirmation that certain foods cause specific symptoms has led to a plethora of products that often have a placebo effect. For example, tests to assess food "sensitivities" are marketed; however, at the time of this publication there is no evidence-based test for food sensitivities since these typically test serum IgG or IG4 antibodies to foods or white blood cell reactions to food using flow cryptography which is not relatable to a food reaction (37). Other non-evidence-based tests used to evaluate food-related symptoms include hair analysis, electrodermal testing, and applied kinesiology. Testing for food allergies is determined by testing for food-mediated IgE changes and is quite different from a food "sensitivity" test (37). Chapters 12 and 13 cover this important topic.

A recent term "anti-science aggression" can also relate to nutrition since so much misinformation on food, cooking, and agriculture, as well as medicine, is distributed through social media channels (38). Some of the reliable resources on social media include Food Science Babe, Dr. Timothy Caufield, Abby Langer, Neva Cochran, and Dr. Joe Schwarcz. Even in 1952, it was noted that unfounded (now non-evidence-based) claims were being made to promote the use of "unbalanced diets" lacking in essential nutrients (39). To avoid receiving poor nutrition advice and care, consider these points: (1) if it sounds too good to be true, it probably is; (2) if the clinician – dietitian, nurse, pharmacist, physician – has a product to sell that directly relates to what the clinician found was "missing" in the blood, diet, etc. – beware; (3) if it goes against scientific and clinical evidence because "it has worked for others" (no data); and (4) if there is a list of good foods and bad foods with no evidence for elimination or reintroduction. Pseudoscience is everywhere – especially in nutrition when the experiment may be on an n of 1.

28.6 CONCLUSION

Nutrition – "eating" is a personal and individual experience. Nutrition science is ever changing and evolving, with some of the "discoveries" turning out to be fine tuning of previously known therapies through better research techniques. Today, the best advice may be to eat a variety of fresh, in-season foods, be active, and avoid stress – easier said than done – and, to seek specialists in the evidence-based practice of nutrition. Nutrition care provided by a registered dietitian that is knowledgeable about the disease process and the effects of food in the body can individualize recommendations for the best possible nutrition plan.

REFERENCES

1. Szczepura A. Nutrition in an ethnically diverse society: What are some of the key challenges? Proc Nutr Soc. 2011 May;70(2):252–262. Doi: 10.1017/S0029665111000085.
2. Kirmayer LJ. Rethinking cultural competence. Transcultural Psychiatry. 2012;49(2):149–164. Doi: 10.1177/1363461512444673
3. www.nal.usda.gov/human-nutrition-and-food-safety/dietary-guidance
4. www.myplate.gov/
5. www.eatright.org
6. www.heart.org/en/healthy-living/healthy-eating/eat-smart/nutrition-basics/what-is-a-healthy-diet-recommended-serving-infographic
7. www.hsph.harvard.edu/nutritionsource/healthy-eating-plate/
8. https://my.clevelandclinic.org/health/articles/16037-mediterranean-diet
9. https://health.usnews.com/best-diet/best-diets-overall
10. https://health.gov/healthypeople
11. Defining Adult Obesity. Centers for disease control and prevention. June 7, 2021. Accessed January 29, 2021. www.cdc.gov/obesity/adult/defining.html
12. Fryar CD, Carroll MD, Afful J. Prevalence of overweight, obesity, and severe obesity among adults aged 20 and over: United States, 1960–1962 through 2017–2018. NCHS Health E-Stats, Centers for Disease Control and Prevention. 2020. February 8, 2021. Accessed January 29, 2021. www.cdc.gov/nchs/data/hestat/obesity-adult-17-18/obesity-adult.htm External link

13. Fryar CD, Carroll MD, Afful J. Prevalence of overweight, obesity, and severe obesity among children and adolescents aged 2–19 years: United States, 1963–1965 through 2017–2018. NCHS Health E-Stats, Centers for Disease Control and Prevention. January 29, 2021. Accessed April 22, 2021. www.cdc.gov/nchs/data/hestat/obesity-child-17-18/over-weight-obesity-child-H.pdf External link (PDF, 352 KB)

14. Bialonczyk D, Dickinson J, Reece J, Kyle T, Close K, Nadglowski J, Johnson K, Garza M, Pash E, Chiquette E. Person-first language in diabetes and obesity scientific publications: Are we making progress? Presented as a poster at the American Diabetes Association 82nd scientific sessions, June 2022. Diabetes. 2022;71(Suppl 1):929-P https://doi.org/10.2337/db22-929-P

15. Crocker AF, Smith SN. Person-first language: Are we practicing what we preach? J Multidiscip Healthc. 2019 Feb 8;12:125–129. Doi: 10.2147/JMDH.S140067. PMID: 30799931; PMCID: PMC6371927.

16. www.nationaleatingdisorders.org/learn/by-eating-disorder/arfid

17. Scarff JR. Orthorexia nervosa: An obsession with healthy eating. Fed Pract. 2017; 34(6):36–39.

18. Scarlata K, Catsos P, Smith J. From a dietitian's perspective, diets for irritable bowel syndrome are not one size fits all. Clin Gastroenterol Hepatol. 2020;18:543–545.

19. Tillman EM, Ireton-Jones C. To eat or not to eat: A commentary on eating issues that affect home parenteral nutrition and home enteral nutrition consumers. Nutr Clin Pract. 2016 Apr;31(2):155–157. Doi: 10.1177/0884533616629637.

20. Winkler MF, Smith CE. Clinical, social, and economic impacts of home parenteral nutrition dependence in short bowel syndrome. JPEN J Parenter Enteral Nutr. 2014 May;38(Suppl 1):32S–37S. doi: 10.1177/0148607113517717.

21. White JV, Guenter P, Jensen G, Malone A, Schofield M. Consensus statement: Academy of Nutrition and Dietetics and American Society for Parenteral and Enteral Nutrition: Characteristics recommended for the identification and documentation of adult malnutrition (undernutrition). JPEN J Parenter Enteral Nutr. 2012;36(3):275–283.

22. Cass AR, Charlton KE. Prevalence of hospital-acquired malnutrition and modifiable determinants of nutritional deterioration during inpatient admissions: A systematic review of the evidence. J Hum Nutr Diet. 2022 Dec;35(6):1043–1058. Doi: 10.1111/jhn.13009. Epub 2022 Apr 26. PMID: 35377487; PMCID: PMC9790482.

23. White JV, Guenter P, Jensen G, Malone A, Schofield M. Consensus statement: Academy of Nutrition and Dietetics and American Society for Parenteral and Enteral Nutrition: Characteristics recommended for the identification and documentation of adult malnutrition (undernutrition). JPEN J Parenter Enteral Nutr. 2012;36(3):275–283.

24. Skipper A, Coltman A, Tomesko J, Charney P, Porcari J, Piemonte TA, Handu D, Cheng FW. Position of the Academy of Nutrition and Dietetics: Malnutrition (undernutrition) screening tools for all adults. J Acad Nutr Diet. 2020 Apr;120(4):709–713. Doi: 10.1016/j.jand.2019.09.011.

25. www.nutritioncare.org/guidelines_and_clinical_resources/Malnutrition_Solution_Center/

26. www.phrases.org.uk/meanings/you-are-what-you-eat.html. Accessed December 17, 2015.

27. Wu H, Tremaroli V, Backhed F. Linking microbiota to human disease: A systems biology perspective. Trends Endocrinol Metab. 2015;26(12):758–770.

28. Cresci GA, Bawden E. Gut microbiome: What we do and don't know. Nutr Clin Prac. 2015;30(6):734–746.

29. Mikkelsen KH, Frost M, Bahl MI, et al. Effects of antibiotics on gut microbiota, gut hormones, and glucose metabolism. PloS One. 2015;10(11): e0142352.

30. Ireton-Jones C, Weisberg MF. Management of irritable bowel syndrome: Physician-dietitian collaboration. Nutr Clin Pract. 2020 Oct;35(5):826–834. Doi: 10.1002/ncp.10567

31. Wang L, Alammar N, Singh R, et al. Gut microbial dysbiosis in the irritable bowel syndrome: As systematic review and meta-analysis of case-controlled studies. J Acad Nutr Diet. 2020;120(4):565–586.

32. Su GL, Ko, CW, Bercik P, et al. AGA clinical practice guidelines on the role of probiotics in the management of gastrointestinal disorders. Gastroenterology. 2020. https://doi.org/10.1053/j.gastro.2020.05.059

33. www.cdrnet.org/certifications/registered-dietitian-rd-certification

34. Patel JJ, Mundi MS, Taylor B, McClave SA, Mechanick JI. Casting light on the necessary, expansive, and evolving role of the critical care dietitian: An essential member of the critical care team. Crit Care Med. 2022 Sep 1;50(9):1289–1295.

35. Steinke TJ, O'Callahan EL, York JL. Role of a registered dietitian in pediatric type 1 and type 2 diabetes. Transl Pediatr. 2017 Oct;6(4):365–372.

36. Johnston BC, Seivenpiper JL, Vernooij RWM, de Souza RJ, Jenkins DJA, Zeraatkar D, Bier DM, Guyatt GH. The philosophy of evidence-based principles and practice in nutrition. Mayo Clin Proc Innov Qual Outcomes. 2019 May 27;3(2):189–199.

37. Kelso JM. Unproven diagnostic tests for adverse reactions to food. J Allergy Clin Immunol Pract. 2018; 6(2):362–365.

38. Goudarzi Sara. Viral spread: Peter Hotez on the increase of anti-science aggression on social media. January 30, 2023. https://thebulletin.org/2023/01/viral-spread-peter-hotez-on-the-increase-of-anti-science-aggression-on-social-media/#post-heading.

39. QUACKERY in the field of nutrition. Am J Public Health Nations Health. 1952 Aug;42(8):997–998. Doi: 10.2105/ajph.42.8.997. PMID: 14952609; PMCID: PMC1526178.

SUGGESTED RESOURCES

- https://conscienhealth.org/about-conscienhealth/
- *DASH Diet for Dummies* and *Hypertension Cookbook for Dummies*
- American Society for Parenteral and Enteral Nutrition (www.nutritioncare.org)
- Academy of Nutrition and Dietetics (www.eatright.org)
- www.dummies.com/how-to/content/dash-diet-for-dummies-cheat-sheet.html
- www.quackwatch.com
- https://www.fns.usda.gov/
- https://www.fda.gov/food
- https://www.eatright.org/
- https://conscienhealth.org/
- https://www.acsh.org/
- https://foodintegrity.org/
- https://foodinsight.org/

TO FIND A REGISTERED DIETITIAN

Dietitian Directory located on AGA GI Patient Center website: (https://patient.gastro.org/)

Find a Nutrition Expert (Academy of Nutrition and Dietetics): www.eatright.org/find-a-nutrition-expert

Index

Page numbers in **bold** indicate tables and *italics* indicate figures.

A

α-linolenic acid (ALA), 230, 300–301
α-melanocyte-stimulating hormone α-MSH, 355
α-MSH, *see* α-melanocyte-stimulating hormone
A/C, *see* Adriamycin/Cytoxan
AAAs, *see* aromatic amino acids
AASLD, *see* American Association for the Study
    of Liver Diseases
AAP, *see* American Academy of Pediatrics
abdominal pain
    ARFID, 417
    EGID, 165
    EoE, 129, 161
    fiber, 75, 77
    FODMAP diet, 381, **382**
    IBD, 54, 56, 61–62
    IBS, 43–45, 49–50, 397
    IgE-mediated allergies, 146
    NCGS, 388
    obstruction, 226
    SIBO, 104, 112, 118
    as side effect, **233**, **402**
absorption
    copper, 180
    decreased, **13**, 56–57, 76, 208
    fluid, 40–42
    monosaccharide, 47–48, 77
    nutritional, 35–40, 64, 93, 98–104, 112,
        176–178, 208, 268, **306**, **371**
absorptive capacity, 36, 42, 77, 98, 102–104, 226,
    276
ABW, *see* actual body weight
Academy of Nutrition and Dietetics (AND), 2, 58,
    218, 333, 337, 368, 391, 427
Acetaminophen toxicity, 195, 197
ACG, *see* American College of Gastroenterology
acquired immunodeficiency syndrome (AIDS),
    111, 116
activities of daily living, 6, **205**
actual body weight (ABW), 5–6, 236
acute disease, 2, 57
acute liver failure (ALF)
    acetaminophen-induced, 195, 197
    amino acid metabolism, 197
    complications, *188*
    hepatic function, 187–188, **195**, 199–200
    hypoglycemia, 196–194
    metabolic derangements, 197

nutritional intervention, 198–199
nutritional assessment, 196, 199
ADA, *see* American Diabetes Association
adenocarcinomas of the esophagus (AE), 234–235
adipocytes, 229, 356, 362
adiponectin, 177, 179–180, 360
AdjBW, *see* adjusted body weight
adjustable gastric band (AGB), 345
adjusted body weight (AdjBW), 6
Adriamycin/Cytoxan (A/C), 233, 237
AE, *see* adenocarcinomas of the esophagus
AGA, *see* American Gastroenterological
    Association; Antigliadin antibody
AGB, *see* adjustable gastric band
agouti-related peptide (AgRP), 355
AGREE conference, 128
AgRP, *see* agouti-related peptide
AIDS, *see* acquired immune deficiency syndrome
ALA, *see* α-linolenic acid
alanine aminotransferase (ALT), 175, 180–181
albumin, 190, 193, 199, 204, 207, **267**, **305**, **386**
alcohol consumption, 178, 208, 221, 230,
    235–236, 334
ALF, *see* acute liver failure
allergic rhinitis, 132, 144, 146, 158
ALT, *see* alanine aminotransferase
ambulatory pH testing, 19, 30
American Academy of Pediatrics (AAP), 151
American Association for the Study of Liver
    Diseases (AASLD), 178–179, 196
American College of Gastroenterology (ACG),
    45, 50, 129
American Diabetes Association (ADA), 325,
    329–330 333, 337
American Gastroenterological Association (AGA),
    62, 251
American Society for Gastrointestinal Endoscopy
    (ASGE), 21, 24–26
American Society for Metabolic and Bariatric
    Surgery (ASMBS), 344
American Society of Anesthesiologists, 24, 26
American Society of Parenteral and Enteral
    Nutrition (ASPEN), 2, 198, 268, 285,
    293, 300, 302, 405
amino acids, 36, 38–39, 52, 99, 117, 190, 197,
    240; *see also* AAAs; BCAAs
ammonia
    elevated, 198, 207–208, 396
    metabolism, 187–188, *189*, 193

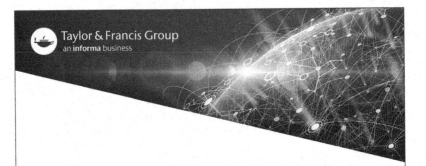

Printed in the United States
by Baker & Taylor Publisher Services